Neural and Behavioural Plasticity

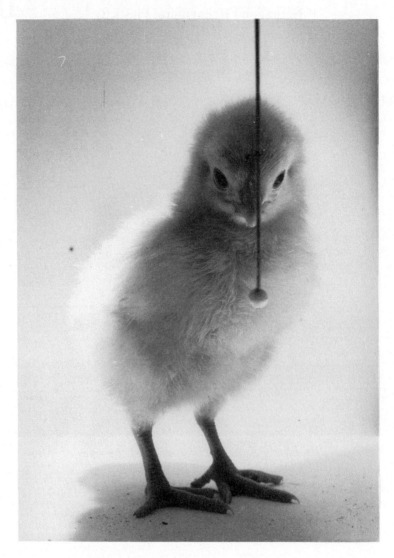

Chick and bead (photograph: Colin Atherton)

Neural and Behavioural Plasticity

THE USE OF THE DOMESTIC CHICK AS A MODEL

Edited by
R. J. ANDREW

School of Biological Sciences
University of Sussex

OXFORD UNIVERSITY PRESS
OXFORD   NEW YORK   TOKYO
1991

Oxford University Press, Walton Street, Oxford OX2 6DP

Oxford New York Toronto
Delhi Bombay Calcutta Madras Karachi
Petaling Jaya Singapore Hong Kong Tokyo
Nairobi Dar es Salaam Cape Town
Melbourne Auckland
and associated companies in
Berlin Ibadan

Oxford is a trade mark of Oxford University Press

Published in the United States
by Oxford University Press, New York

© The contributors listed on pp. xi–xii, 1991

British Library Cataloguing in Publication Data
Neural and behavioural plasticity.
1. Animals. Behaviour. Neurophysiological aspects
I. Andrew R. J.
591.188
ISBN 0-19-852184-7

Library of Congress Cataloging in Publication Data
Neural and behavioural plasticity / edited by R. J. Andrew.
Includes bibliographical references and index.
1. Learning–Research–Methodology. 2. Memory–Research–
Methodology. 3. Neuroplasticity–Research–Methodology.
4. Chicks–Behavior. I. Andrew, R. J.
QP408.N47 1991   153.1'5–dc20   90-7913
ISBN 0-19-852184-7

Typeset by CentraCet, Cambridge
Printed in Great Britain
by Bookcraft (Bath) Ltd
Midsomer Norton, Avon

To Diana

Preface

The domestic chick has been used with great success in studies of early learning of the processes of memory formation, and of the location and nature of learning-induced change. Despite its importance, much of this work is relatively less widely known than corresponding studies in mammals.

In September 1988, a conference was held at the University of Sussex which brought together for the first time representatives of almost all the laboratories, which at that time were investigating learning, learning-induced change, and memory formation in the chick. At this meeting there was general agreement that the time had come to present together a number of research programmes using the chick, in order to show the implications of each for the others, and for studies of memory formation as a whole.

This book is the result. It consists in the main of commissioned reviews by authors who have themselves been responsible for much of the recent advances in the area which they cover. In addition, since the anatomy of the bird brain has only recently come to be at all well understood, and since it differs markedly from that of the mammalian brain, two chapters are devoted to the special features of the bird brain and to a consideration of homologies with mammalian structures. Work on the chick is set in a wider context by comparison of memory formation in chick and rat, which reveals remarkable correspondences between chick and mammal.

It is our hope that many workers will be attracted to the alternative approaches to some of the central problems of learning and neural plasticity, which are possible in the chick. The book opens with an introduction to techniques of experiments on the chick, which may help such new recruits. The many advantages of the chick, and the advances in knowledge which they have made possible, are set out in the book itself. It only remains for me to thank all the authors for their enthusiasm, hard work, and (where needed) patience.

Brighton   R. J. A.
December 1990

Contents

Contributors

C. *Allweis*, Department of Physiology, Hebrew University, Hadassah Medical School, Israel

R. J. *Andrew*, School of Biological Sciences, University of Sussex, Brighton BN1 9QG, UK

P. P. G. *Bateson*, Sub-Department of Animal Behaviour, University of Cambridge, Madingley, Cambridge CB3 8AA, UK

D. *Beniston*, Department of Psychology, University of California at Berkeley, USA

E. L. *Bennett*, Department of Psychology, University of California at Berkeley, USA

J. J. *Bolhuis*, Department of Zoology, University of Cambridge, Downing Street, Cambridge CB2 3EJ, UK

P. G. *Clifton*, Laboratory of Experimental Psychology, University of Sussex, Brighton BN1 9QG, UK

P. J. *Colombo*, Department of Psychology, University of California at Berkeley, USA

J. E. *Davey*, Department of Zoology, University of Cambridge, Downing Street, Cambridge CB2 3EJ, UK

D. C. *Davies*, Department of Anatomy, St George's Hospital Medical School, Cranmer Terrace, Tooting, London SW17 0RE, UK

M. *Dharmaretnam*, Department of Zoology, Eastern University, Chenkalady, Sri Lanka

J. L. *Dubbeldam*, Department of Organismal Zoology, Leiden University, The Netherlands

M. E. *Gibbs*, School of Behavioural Sciences, La Trobe University, Bundoora, Victoria, Australia

S. *Crowe*, School of Behavioural Sciences, La Trobe University, Bundoora, Victoria, Australia

O. *Güntürkün*, Allgemeine Psychologie, Universität Konstanz, D-7750 Konstanz, FRG

G. Horn, Department of Zoology, University of Cambridge, Downing Street, Cambridge CB2 3EJ, UK

M. H. Johnson, MRC Cognitive Development Unit, 17 Gordon Street, London WC1H 0AH, UK

J. P. Kent, Ballyrichard House, Arklow, Co. Wicklow, Eire

D. W. Lee, Department of Psychology, University of California at Berkeley, USA

J. L. Martinez Jr, Department of Psychology, University of California at Berkeley, USA

B. J. McCabe, Department of Zoology, University of Cambridge, Downing Street, Cambridge CB2 3EJ, UK

K. T. Ng, School of Behavioural Sciences, La Trobe University, Bundoora, Victoria, Australia

T. A. Patterson, Department of Psychology, University of California at Berkeley, USA

L. J. Rogers, Physiology Department, University of New England, Armidale, NSW 2531, Australia

S. P. R. Rose, Brain and Behaviour Research Group, Biology Department, Open University, Milton Keynes MK 7 6AA, UK

J. A. P. Rostas, Neuroscience Group, Faculty of Medicine, University of Newcastle, NSW 2308, Australia

M. R. Rosenzweig, Department of Psychology, University of California at Berkeley, USA

G. Schulteis, Department of Psychology, University of California at Berkeley, USA

P. A. Serrano, Department of Psychology, University of California at Berkeley, USA

R. M. Stephenson, School of Biological Sciences, University of Sussex, Brighton BN1 9QG, UK

M. G. Stewart, Brain and Behaviour Research Group, Biology Department, Open University, Milton Keynes MK7 6AA, UK

L. Workman, Department of Behavioural and Communication Studies, Polytechnic of Wales, Pontypridd, Mid Glamorgan, UK

Introduction

R. J. Andrew

Domestic chicks have long been recognized as ideal material for the study of early learning. Almost one hundred years ago, Spalding (1893) was impressed by the range of behaviour which chicks would show soon after their first opportunity to see; the interaction of predispositions and learning has been studied in chicks ever since. After Lorenz (1935) described imprinting on the mother in birds as a kind of learning which he felt to be in many ways *sui generis*, interest in learning in the chick increased.

More recently, filial imprinting in the chick proved ideal in the hands of Horn, Bateson, and Rose for work on learning-induced change. Another task (involving the inhibition of pecking at an ill-tasting bead) has also been valuable, by allowing (for example) the demonstration of sharply timed phases in memory formation by Gibbs and Ng. Work based on these tasks is now in many respects as advanced as corresponding programmes in mammals.

The dependence of biochemical and structural change in neurons on specific learning has been established with unusual rigour in the chick (e.g. Chapters 8, 10). At least three cerebral structures (intermediate medial hyperstriatum ventrale, lobus parolfactorius, paleostriatum augmentatum) have shown to undergo learning-induced change. The involvement of these structures in learning has been further confirmed by the effect of lesions and of the local application of amnestic agents. Both procedures suggest the involvement of a further structure, the lateral neostriatum. Different structures have been shown to come into play at different times following learning, and the same structures may play a different part in the right and the left hemisphere.

Indeed, almost all lines of investigation now agree on the existence of profound differences between processes in the right and left hemispheres of the chick. This is true of learning-induced change, whether molecular or ultrastructural, of the functioning of cerebral structures, and of mechanisms underlying phases of memory formation.

These last are one of the most striking features of memory formation in the chick, which is divided by sharply defined transitions into a series of phases; recently, evidence for closely corresponding phases in the rat has become convincing. The nature of the processes underlying phases is discussed in several chapters. New possibilities are raised by the demonstration that the transitions between phases largely coincide with the timings of brief episodes of good retrieval which recur cyclically following learning.

The chick continues to be of great importance for the study of the development of behaviour and of the CNS. The complex interactions of maturing predispositions and abilities with the effects of learning are unusually well understood. Unexpected phenomena (such as brief and consistently timed periods of left- or right-hemisphere dominance during development) continue to be discovered, and will in due course call for new physiological and anatomical investigations.

A number of features of the young chick have facilitated research. The unossified skull roof allows intracranial injection with a minimum of disturbance. This, coupled with a learning task which takes no more than 10 seconds to administer, has made possible the construction of very detailed timecourses, both for the ability to retrieve and for changes in sensitivity to a variety of amnestic agents. The fact that the chick hatches from an egg, and does so at a very advanced stage of development, is also important. It means that experience can be readily controlled both in the late fetus and immediately after hatching; there is no awkward period (as in the mammals which are most commonly studied) in which perceptual and motor mechanisms are maturing, and it is not clear exactly what can be perceived or performed. Very early learning has therefore been readily accessible to study: it is probably partly as a result of this that it has been possible to demonstrate learning-induced change so unambiguously.

REFERENCES

Lorenz, K. Z. (1935). Der Kumpan in der Umwelt des Vogels. *Journal für Ornithologie*, **88**, 137–213, 289–413.
Spalding, D. A. (1873). Instinct: with original observations on young animals. *Macmillan's Magazine*, **27**, 282–93. Reprinted in *British Journal of Animal Behaviour*, 1954, **2**, 2–11.

PART I

Introduction to the use of the chick in experiment

1

The chick in experiment: techniques and tests

GENERAL
R. J. Andrew

The first question facing an investigator who wishes to use chicks is whether to use males or females (or both). There are marked sex differences in many tests, including some which are commonly used to study learning (Chapters 18, 20, 21); in other cases, where data are available only for males, sex differences may well occur. It is worth noting that there is a consistent tendency across strains for females to hatch earlier and for early hatching chicks to be more vigorous (Davies and Payne 1982). In very young chicks it thus may be difficult to separate effects of time since hatching and effects of sex. If large batches of chicks (say 100) are necessary for a single experiment, as is the case in work on the pharmacology of memory formation, then it is usual to use only males and to obtain them from a commercial hatchery.

If conditions during, or at hatching have to be manipulated experimentally, then eggs must be incubated in the laboratory. It may be worth doing this in some experimental programmes in order to provide more natural conditions in late fetal life. Rogers (1982) has shown that exposure of the egg to light at this time produces lateralized control of copulation and attack, together with asymmetry in visual pathways (Chapter 20). It may be advantageous to standardize light exposure (or its absence) for some purposes. Such exposure might well determine (for example) the way in which post-hatching experience of light affects responsiveness to imprinting objects (Moltz and Stettner 1961; 'priming', Section D; Chapter 5).

The other feature of normal development which is absent in the incubation is vocal interaction with the mother (Chapter 6). It is likely, therefore, that incubator-hatched chicks are to some extent affected by sensory deprivation; whether this has any important consequences for studies of learning and its central consequences, when using chicks in the first or second day of life, remains to be seen.

Once chicks are removed from the incubator or from the travelling boxes in which they are held in groups, they need special care. Chicks learn to feed and drink very quickly if they first encounter food (scattered rather thinly on the cage floor) and water in the company of several other chicks. Social facilitation is then marked (p. 101). If chicks must be isolated (below), then they should be encouraged to drink by dipping the bill in their drinking fountain. Feeding will be promoted if a few grains are dropped on the floor in front of the chick. Even on the first day of life, when yolk reserves are high, it is good practice to make sure chicks are feeding and drinking if they are not to be held in an incubator. Commercial chick foods ('starter' or 'mash') are entirely satisfactory (unless contaminated by mites, which may be visible as drifts of fine dust on the surface of undisturbed food in containers). The constituents of such foods vary with batch and season, which is a possible source of variation between experiments.

Young chicks are not capable of maintaining body temperature in air which is substantially cooler than that in an incubator (38–40°C), without an external heat source. A radiant heat source such as a 40 W tungsten bulb, suspended above the open top of the cage has the advantage that the chick can itself regulate its heat intake by moving within the cage. The cage floor should not conduct heat readily: paper towelling over a more permanent glazed paper covering to a wooden surface is satisfactory; paper over a metal floor is not.

This simple solution commits the investigator to continuous light. Chicks still show 24 hour cycles of behaviour under such regimes, and time of day may affect the outcome of tests (Reymond and Rogers 1981; Chapter 6). The effects of varying light/dark cycles have been little studied.

A convenient cage design is four-walled with open top and bottom, either as single units or in blocks of four or five (Gibbs and Ng 1977). It is sometimes important to familiarize chicks with the layout of an experimental area in order to reduce visual exploration, distraction or even attempts to escape during test. This can be done very successfully by the use of cages through the transparent fronts of which the test area can be seen (Klein and Andrew 1986).

The rapid growth of chicks means that cages of different design and larger size are needed after the first 2–3 days. Food hoppers become necessary and then a shift to mesh floors by day 5 or 6 to prevent any accumulation of droppings within the cage; previous to this, floor paper should be changed daily.

Barbiturate anaesthesia has commonly been used (40 mg/kg sodium pentobarbitone: Miles 1972; 0.1 ml/50 g Equithesin: Horn and McCabe 1974). Anaesthetic and lethal doses can be close together, and there is marked variation with age. Ether is satisfactory when only brief immobility is needed. In the first few days of life this can best be done by using a long glass vial, whose aperture is the right size to make a loose fit around the chick's beak in front of the eyes. Ether is applied to a cotton wool plug at the bottom of the vial, which is so positioned as to be out of any direct contact with the chick. The chick will rapidly become still, and then briefly struggle with a series of soft peeps; its bill should be removed from the vial just as these die away.

Chicks of any age may be humanely killed by exposure in small groups to carbon dioxide gas, preferably with some admixture of air (which may be provided by leaving the lid of the chamber open for half a minute or so). EEC guidelines recommend against carbon dioxide for birds younger than 7 days because it is unsuitable for altricial nestlings; in the UK, therefore, it must be specified as a procedure in Home Office licences.

A complete stereotactic atlas for the chick brain was prepared by Youngren and Phillips (1978); separate atlases for diencephalon and midbrain are also available (Andrew and Oades 1973; De Lanerolle and Andrew 1974).

BEHAVIOUR
R. J. Andrew

Nearly all the work described in the chapters which follow rests on two responses, pecking at small objects or approaching (or following) imprinting objects. The chick has in fact quite a rich behavioural repertoire, much more of which could be profitably used in experiment. Aggressive and sexual behaviour can be evoked in young male chicks by simple stimuli, such as are also capable of bringing about imprinting and evoking social responses (Andrew 1964b, 1966). The lateralization of the control of such behaviour is discussed in Chapter 20.

Escape responses provide a useful index of the extent to which a stimulus or situation is found aversive or frightening. They include (a) avoidance and fleeing, if there is a particular evoking stimulus; (b) attempts to get through obstacles: the head and body are swung from side to side with the bill against the obstacles (e.g. cage wall); (c) looking up, sometimes accompanied by alternate crouching and going erect, which may pass into direct jumps at the walls. The time taken to return to undisturbed behaviour (Andrew and Clayton 1979) is often revealing in tests which attempt to measure the effectiveness of novelty, or aversive training. Sustained preening is one reliable marker of such a return; note that brief preening (such as one or two brief applications of the bill to the upper chest or wing) occurs as a displacement activity (e.g. in extinction tests). Search over, and pecking at the floor are other useful markers of undisturbed behaviour.

Head shaking, eye closure, throat movements, with rejection movements of the tongue, are all usual consequencs of pecking at a bead which is coated with the aversant methylanthranilate; they are used, therefore, in aversive bead tests to pick out those chicks which have been successfully trained (p. 17 *et seq.*). However, head shaking is also evoked by novel and conspicuous visual stimuli, even when there has been no pecking. It also occurs, sometimes together with body shaking, at the point in time when the chick shifts from one behaviour to another (Clayton and Andrew 1979).

Perhaps the behaviours most neglected by experimenters are the calls of the chick. A full treatment is given by Andrew (1963, 1969*a*, 1975). Two groupings of calls deserve mention here:

1. *Short calls (twitter to short trill).* Twitters as originally defined by Collias and Joos (1953) were short, sharply ascending calls; at slightly higher intensity, they are equally brief, but descending. They have been termed 'pleasure calls' because they are evoked by the sight of the object to which the chick is imprinted and by the sight of food. After training, twitters are also given to conditioned stimuli (such as light illumination) for food (Andrew 1964*a*, 1969*a*). At highest intensity, short trills take their place: here the stimulus (such as a novel insect or bead) is on the edge of evoking avoidance, and the chick may at the same time back and raise its head feathers. Conversely, when chicks are held in completely familiar surroundings, from which alerting sounds and sights are excluded, they will feed in complete silence (Andrew and de Lanerolle 1974). Twitters are thus associated with periods of enhanced responsiveness and alertness. Small lesions in the anterior intercollicular area both mute and prevent such enhancement of response (de Lanerolle and Andrew 1974; Andrew and de Lanerolle 1974).

2. *Peeps and warbles.* Peeps (distress calls) are characteristic long loud calls, which are reliably evoked by separation from social companion or familiar surroundings, or by discomfort (e.g. cold). They commonly accompany fleeing, and are evoked by conditioned stimuli for punishment (Andrew 1969*a*, 1973). If the evoking conditions continue the chick may assume a resting attitude (leg flexure, head withdrawal, and eye closure); this can be distinguished from normal undisturbed sleep by the continuing vocalization, which now takes on a continuous warbling quality.

All of these behaviours provide potentially valuable additional measures for learning tasks: in imprinting studies a useful index of attachment to an object is its ability to abolish escape and peeps in a strange environment (e.g. in ducklings, Hoffman *et al.* 1972); use of the sharp transition from peeps to twitter makes the measure more sensitive (Bateson 1964).

In the passive avoidance test using beads, so standardly used in the chick (p. 17 *et seq.*), the first presentation of a bead often evokes a short trill or even avoidance, with peeps; this is particularly likely if the bead is relatively large and blue, for example.

When, during pre-training with clean beads, behaviour shifts to active pursuit and vigorous pecking, twitters become common. Conversely, when a bead of the type which tasted unpleasant at training is presented at first, the chick may shake its head (suggesting specific recollection of the taste), and avoid and peep (suggesting recollection of an unpleasant experience).

The most interesting possibility is that calling may give a measure of the type and effectiveness of the reinforcement associated with response to a stimulus. Intracranial self-stimulation in the chick is usually accompanied by vocalization (Andrew 1967, 1969b). Key operation is normally preceded by twitters, and stimulation itself usually results in a reduction in calling; a rebound follows which may involve short calls or peeps, according to which central structure is stimulated. It is usually assumed that intracranial self-stimulation is driven relatively directly by activation of reinforcement mechanisms; if this is so, then the rebound of calling may be associated with such activation.

LEARNING IN THE CHICK: AN INTRODUCTION
R. J. Andrew

Ever since the work of Spalding (1873), there has been recurring interest in the sort of visual learning which chicks can carry out soon after hatching, and so with minimal visual experience. Most of this book has grown out of such interest. However, it is worth noting that psychologists continue to turn to the chick to try to resolve theoretical issues: day-old chicks were used by Robinson *et al.* (1976) to show that prior experience of making errors was not necessary for errorless discrimination learning. Attempts have been made to extend investigation of conditioning to the late fetus (Sedlaçek 1962, 1964) using, for example, swallowing as the UCR, saccharin solution as the UCS and a tone as the CS.

The two tasks most usual in work on chick learning and their variants are considered in later separate sections. However, a remarkable variety of other tasks have been used and may be more suitable for particular purposes than either the aversive bead task or imprinting.

Effective positive reinforcers include radiant heat provided in a cool environment (Wasserman 1973), food (Oades and Messent 1981), water (Andrew 1969a), intracranial self-stimulation (Andrew 1967), and access to, or opportunity to view a social partner or imprinting object (below, and Chapters 5 and 8). Operant conditioning has most usually involved pecking a key. Scaled down versions of pigeon keys are suitable: the addition of a central bead helps shaping and the bead can then be removed. Visual discrimination, using two trans-illuminated keys, can be readily established (Oades and Messent *loc.cit.*) Choice between two visual patterns, one in each of a pair of adjacent goal boxes, is learned for warm air reinforcement (McCabe *et al.* 1982).

The chick has been much used for studies which explore the limits conventionally assigned to the properties of reinforcers. 'Autoshaping', in which the animal comes to direct responses at the source of a CS for reinforcement (rather than simply using it as a cue to predict the arrival of, say, food) has been much studied in chicks (Zolman *et al.* 1977; Woodruff and Starr 1978). The behaviour used in response has been shown to be initially appropriate to the CS, but then to shift in form towards behaviour appropriate to the reinforcer: thus, at first, chicks peck vigorously at a small light which signals the arrival of heat, but this progressively shifts into snuggling behaviour (Wasserman 1973).

Classic Pavlovian procedures have also been used in the chick, such as conditioning the movement of the nictitating membrane (Davies and Coates 1978).

Conditioned aversions can readily be established in the chick if lithium chloride is administered following consumption of a sweet solution with a novel colour (Gaston 1977; Genovese and Brown 1978), or a novel food (Gillette *et al.* 1980). Such aversions can be transferred to discriminatory stimuli (Gillan 1979); they can already be established on the first day of life (Hale and Green 1988). Extinction of conditioned aversions is opposed by androgens, as in the rat (Clifton and Andrew 1987).

Perhaps the aspect of learning in the chick which has most surprised psychologists is the powerful effect of the behaviour of other conspecifics on the acquisition and permanence of food preferences. Work has concentrated on the effects of seeing others peck. Models are effective: when a simple model can be seen pecking at one out of a number of types of small targets, a chick (which is prevented from approaching the model by a transparent screen) will begin itself to peck at that type of grain (Turner 1964). Such learning results in relatively stable preferences, even though the targets are not edible, in training carried out on days 1, 2, or 3 (Suboski and Bartashunas 1984). In the absence of model movement, sharp taps will facilitate pecking (Suboski 1987). If chicks see their fellows pecking at food through an aperture of a particular shape, they acquire a preference for that shape of aperture, which is relatively resistant to extinction (Meyer and Frank 1970). The effect is not restricted to feeding: a chick can acquire a preference for a particular type of drinking fountain by seeing fellows drink, whilst it itself is only able to drink from a separate and different fountain (Franchina *et al.* 1986).

Predispositions are thus of great importance in chick learning and must be carefully borne in mind in experimental design. Visual releasers not so far mentioned include:

1. Eye-like patterns. These are important in imprinting (Chapters 5, 8); however, they also maintain tonic immobility in frightened and immobilized chicks (Gallup 1977); the most effective configuration is discussed by Gagliardi and Gallup (1976).
2. Colour. The same preference for the red and blue ends of the spectrum is present (Mayer and Hailman 1976) in responses to the imprinting objects and in pecking (despite contrary claims: Schaefer and Hess 1959), and so may affect both of the standard learning tasks discussed in later sections. A complicating effect is that stressing and frightening conditions increase preference for green (David and Fischer 1978).

Other modalities remain to be studied. Response to particular features of the calls of broody hens is briefly touched on in Chapter 6. Olfaction should not be ignored: avoidance of blood by naive chicks appears to depend partly on olfactory cues (Jones and Black 1979).

Finally, a range of specific tasks deserves brief mention:

a. Learning to orient by close, and by distant cues to find food buried under sawdust (Rashid and Andrew 1989).
b. Open field test. Distress calls and attempts at escape have both been used as measures of fear in a chick placed in a strange environment (Andrew 1975c; Jones 1977; Gallup and Suarez 1980). The test has advantages for rapid screening of a variety of manipulations for behavioural effects which might otherwise be missed. However, it suffers in chicks, as in rats, from the fact that immobility may reflect either freezing or relaxed behaviour. This presents particular difficulties in chicks, which when placed in a fully enclosed open field, often pass from initial tense freezing to apparently normal sleep, without even moving (Andrew, personal observation).
c. Novel object. The evocation of fear responses in the home cage by the introduction of a novel object has the advantage that it is possible to use the return to normal maintenance activity as one measure (Andrew and Clayton 1979; Jones and Black 1980). In the open field the disappearance of disturbance of behaviour is difficult to establish.
d. Distraction and persistence in approach to food in a runway (Archer 1974a). The same test is readily adaptable to studies of extinction (Archer 1974b).
e. Zanforlin (1981; Vallortigaro and Zanforlin 1986) has used discrimination between visual stimuli presented on the lids of boxes or at the end of Y-maze arms to examine which features are used to segregate objects or stimuli as distinct perceptual units.

FILIAL IMPRINTING

Measuring preference and differential responsiveness *P. P. G. Bateson*

Tests of whether a subject responds more strongly to one stimulus rather than another may be conducted and analysed in a variety of ways. Several important issues arise when considering such tests.

a. Should the stimuli be living animals, stuffed animals, audio- or visual recordings, or models?
b. Should the stimuli be presented simultaneously or successively?
c. Should the same object be tested once or repeatedly?
d. Should the types or rates of response to the stimuli be compared in terms of absolute or relative differences?

Each method has its own advantages and drawbacks and these need to be considered carefully before proceeding with a study. What follows is largely drawn from Martin and Bateson (1986).

Stimuli

Living animals are the richest and most natural type of choice stimulus, but they have several potential drawbacks. First, the stimulus animals are liable to interact with the test subject, making it difficult to decide who chooses whom. Sometimes these interactions can be eliminated if the stimulus animals are made unaware of the subject's presence by using one-way screens. Even if one-way screens are used, though, the behaviour of the stimulus animals is likely to change with successive tests as they become habituated. If, on the other hand, different individuals are used as models in successive tests they may behave differently from one another. Finally, because a living animal does provide such a rich and complex stimulus, it can be difficult to know precisely which features of the stimulus influenced the subject's choice.

Stuffed animals and recordings have many of the advantages of living stimuli and, in addition, they are not influenced by the subject. Furthermore, the effectiveness of particular features of the stimuli can be analysed by selective removal or alteration of different parts of the choice stimuli. This type of manipulation is particularly easy with audio and video tape-recordings. However, the responses of the test animal may be greatly reduced if presented with a stuffed stimulus animal rather than a real one.

Models can be surprisingly effective as test stimuli. They are relatively simple to make and, since their characteristics can be varied systematically, the result obtained with them are easily analysed. However, responses to models are often greatly reduced compared with those to more natural stimuli.

Simultaneous or successive tests?

In principle, comparison between stimuli presented at the same time provides the more sensitive measure of preference, while presentation of each stimulus in turn provides the more rigorous test. However, drawbacks of both methods of testing need to be considered.

Simultaneous presentation may be distracting to the subject and also tends to be highly unnatural. The subject may become 'trapped' by its first choice, simply because it happens to be facing one way and approaches the stimulus it is facing. Finally, withdrawing from one stimulus may be incorrectly interpreted as approaching the other (or vice versa). This last problem can sometimes be overcome by providing a three-way choice, with a 'blank' (no-stimulus) choice in addition to the two-choice stimuli.

Successive presentation may be insensitive if the subject responds at the maximum possible level to each of several stimuli when it cannot make simultaneous comparisons between them. More seriously, successive tests may be confounded by order effects because the subject becomes generally more (or less) responsive to all stimuli during the course of testing. Such effects may be allowed for by varying the order of presentation for different subjects, or by presenting two stimuli (A and B) in the order A,B,B,A (see McCabe *et al.* 1982).

Repeated testing?

On the face of it, the more information that a given subject provides the better. Testing the subject many times is likely to enhance the reliability of the results. However, the subject may simply stop responding if it is tested too many times and, more seriously, its preferences may be influenced by repeated exposure to the stimuli. This effect is seen, for example, in imprinting experiments with domestic chicks, when the birds start to form a preference for the novel stimulus with which the familiar stimulus is being compared (e.g. Bateson 1979). Also remember that all the data provided by one subject must only be used as one member of the sample in subsequent statistical analysis since, in this context, the results of repeated tests with the same subject must not be treated as though they were statistically independent (Machlis *et al.* 1985). For this reason, increasing the time spent testing one subject has rapidly diminishing returns.

Analysing and presenting data

If each subject's reaction to a stimulus is recorded as an all-or-nothing response (for example, 'approaches the stimulus'), the simplest method of presenting the results is in terms of how many subjects responded to each stimulus. However, this measure of response is relatively crude. If quantitative measures of how much or how many times each subject responded to the stimuli were obtained (which they should have been if at all possible), forms of analysis that use this additional information are preferable.

Absolute differences in responsiveness are obtained by subtracting the responses to stimulus B from the response to stimulus A. This provides a single score for each subject. If the same subject has been tested repeatedly, the mean of the differences in response to the two stimuli should be used as that subject's score. The scores for all subjects can then be analysed statistically by means of a matched-pairs test, such as a Wilcoxon signed-ranks test or a matched-pairs t test.

Response ratios can be calculated in a variety of ways, a particularly useful form being:

$$\text{Responses to A}/(\text{Responses to A} + \text{Responses to B})$$

If the subject has always responded to A and never to B, its score will be 1.0. Conversely, if it has responded to B but not A, its score will be 0. The chance level of response is 0.5. If more than two stimuli have been used, the divisor is the total number of responses to all the stimuli and the chance score is 1.0 divided by the number of stimuli used (for example, 0.25 in the case of four stimuli).

Subjects which fail to respond to either stimulus (non-responders) can cause problems in the analysis stage (particularly if this is done on a computer), since calculating their scores involves dividing by zero. This problem can be dealt with by either (a) systematically excluding the scores of all non-responders, or (b) arbitrarily assigning a chance-level score (0.5 for a two-choice test) to all non-responders.

For the purpose of statistical analysis, each subject provides one value, which is the difference between its ratio score and the chance level. These difference scores are analysed with a matched-pairs test, as in the case of absolute differences. It is worth noting that, for various reasons, scores obtained by the ratio method tend to be unevenly distributed, with modes at either end of the distribution between 0 and 1.0. This non-normal distribution of scores may render invalid certain types of statistical analysis, but can sometimes be corrected by transformations (such as arcsine) of the data (see Martin and Bateson 1986).

Results based on absolute rather than ratio scores will be greatly affected by those individuals that have responded strongly in the tests. By contrast, the ratio method is more sensitive to variation within individuals, even when considerable variation is found between individuals. Indeed, it is logically possible for the two methods to generate contradictory results if the high-responding individuals have a preference for stimulus A and the low-responders a preference for B. For this reason, it is wise to analyse results both ways and, if the two methods generate different conclusions, consider carefully why the differences have arisen. The apparent contradiction may itself be interesting.

Procedures *J. J. Bolhuis and M. H. Johnson*

Chicks have usually been reared in visual isolation up to the commencement of imprinting. They are hatched in a dark incubator either each within a separate container or (more practically) are transferred to separate containers in another incubator after hatching. Such transfer may be done in the dark or under dim green light, on the assumption that, since green objects are relatively ineffective in eliciting approach (Schaefer and Hess 1959; Kovach 1971; Mayer and Hailman 1976), any momentary sight of objects will be relatively ineffective.

The imprinting stimulus has been presented in a variety of ways: for example, a flashing light behind a wire mesh screen (Hoffman and Segal 1983), or an arena in which the chick follows an object moving in a circle (Gottlieb 1965). We place the chicks in wire mesh running wheels in a heated training cabinet (Horn 1985). In each cabinet there are three wheels that have solid sides so that the animals cannot see each other. The wheels are so placed that the animals are facing a conspicuous object at a distance of around 50 cm. The number of revolutions of the running wheels towards and away from the conspicuous object can be recorded by means of a system of magnets and reed switches attached to the wheel and its base. The sensitivity of this measurement can be altered by varying the number of magnets on a wheel.

The stimuli used by Horn and collaborators are either flashing lights or rotating objects (e.g. stuffed jungle fowl) that are lit by means of spotlights or from within (e.g. McCabe *et al.* 1981; Horn 1985). One object commonly used is a rotating red box that is lit from within by a 24 W light (McCabe *et al.* 1981). Bolhuis and Trooster (1988) changed the intensity of this light to vary its relative attractiveness.

The length of training used varies from a few minutes to several hours. Horn and his collaborators have frequently used two periods of 1 hour, separated by 1–1.5 hours in a dark incubator. During training a 5 W white light, placed above the running wheels, is kept on continuously. Several procedures have been used to increase the effectiveness of exposure. First, exposure of the animals to white light ('priming'), before the start of training has been shown to enhance subsequent imprinting (Bateson and Wainwright 1972). Second, the animals are not exposed to the object continuously, but in bouts, separated by periods in which the stimulus is not visible to the chicks (e.g. 50 s on/10 s off in each minute). Bolhuis and Johnson (1988) contrasted a fixed interval/fixed duration schedule of exposure with a variable interval/variable duration exposure schedule.

Two hours after training the latter schedule led to a significantly greater preference for the training object than the former. An advantage of the variable interval/variable duration schedule of exposure is that 20 minutes' exposure or even less are sufficient to achieve a significant preference for the training object.

A third procedure used to increase the effectiveness of exposure to an object is to play back a tape with maternal calls or call surrogates (e.g. Gottlieb 1965; Bateson 1979).

Several studies have used an operant task to expose the animal to a conspicuous object (e.g. Bateson and Reese 1968; Gaioni *et al.* 1978; Johnson *et al.* 1985; Johnson and Horn 1986, 1987). In the study of Johnson and Horn (1986; cf. Bateson and Reese 1968), each chick was placed in an operant box (42 × 18 × 30 cm), the walls of which were painted matt black. One side of the box was made of wire mesh. The stimulus was placed approximately 35 cm from the apparatus and in front of the wire mesh wall. In the floor of the box were two pedals made conspicuous by black and white chequer patterning. Whilst the chick stood on one of the pedals, the imprinting object was illuminated and rotated; this ceased as soon as the chick left the pedal. Depression of the other pedal had no effect. For half the birds the effective pedal was on the right and for half on the left. Each training session was terminated either after 45 minutes or when a criterion of nine correct operations out of ten had been reached. Chicks were held to have learned the task if they reached criterion in either of two training sessions given within about 2 hours of each other.

One of the advantages of the operant training method is that imprinting and operant learning can be studied simultaneously, involving the same stimuli. Johnson and Horn (1986) have used this method to investigate the differential effects of lesions on these types of learning. Bolhuis and Johnson (1988) found that operant control over the presentation of the conspicuous stimulus did not enhance imprinting over what occurred in yoked controls. Several authors have used an instrumental task with the chicks' vocalization (rather than pedal pressing) as the operant, with similar results (e.g. Hoffman and Segal 1983; Ten Cate 1986).

The principles of measurement of preferences have already been considered. A convenient way of obtaining a response ratio with a running wheel, is to expose the chick for short periods (2–4 minutes) to either the training stimulus (T) or a novel object (N) on a schedule such as T-N-N-T (Bolhuis *et al.* 1986). Variation in schedule seems to have little affect on the resulting measure (McCabe *et al.* 1981). Wheel revolutions away from the stimulus are rare; they may be ignored or subtracted from revolutions towards it. The response ratio is then (in revolutions): approach to T/ approach to (T + N).

Bateson and Wainwright (1972) used a simultaneous choice test. Here a wire mesh running wheel was so mounted on a railway that attempts by the chick to approach a stimulus actually caused the chick to be carried away from it. Two measures were used: (i) position on the railway (i.e. distance from object) at which the chick reversed the direction of running; (ii) the difference between total revolutions towards the familiar, and towards the novel object. The variability of (i) and (ii) suggested the percentage of total approach which is directed to the familiar stimulus as the preferable measure of performance. This may be particularly sensitive when fine discriminations are being measured, such as recognition of an individual stuffed fowl (Johnson and Horn 1987).

Differences between sequential and simultaneous tests using the running wheel (e.g. Johnson *et al.* 1985; Bolhuis *et al.* 1985) may be due to differences in the distance which the chick has to run in order to move the trolley a given distance (see Johnson *et al.* 1985, for further discussion).

AVERSIVE BEAD; A ONE-TRIAL PASSIVE AVOIDANCE TASK

Introduction *R. J. Andrew*

This task is of great importance in that it was used to establish the detailed temporal structure, and the pharmacology of memory formation in the chick; it continues, with imprinting, to be the main basis for work on chick memory formation. It has the advantage of being relatively natural: in the field a chick will readily peck at small moving objects (which are usually arthropods), and if one tastes unpleasant, no doubt the chick learns not to peck again at objects of that sort.

Laboratory studies of such learning have been shown that the visual properties of the 'prey' are important, as well as its bad taste. The acquisition of aversion is quicker when targets contrast with the background, irrespective of target colour (Roper and Redston 1987). Intrinsic properties are of great importance: at least one common pattern of warning coloration, black and yellow striping, is spontaneously avoided, even in the absence of any experience of bad taste or other punishment (Schuler and Hesse 1985). Roper and Cook (1989) show that black alone is as effective as black and yellow; unexpectedly, red and black striping is attractive. Increasing size also increases the likelihood of avoidance. This holds even if size is increased in only one dimension: elongated prey such as mealworms are not at once eaten by naive chicks; instead they may be pecked with the closed bill or picked up and carried in a characteristic rapid run (Hogan 1966; Mench and Andrew 1986).

Colour also affects response to the small beads used in the ill-tasting bead task. The ease of elicitation of pecking shows a U-shaped dependence on wavelength in the very young chick, so that both red and blue beads are very effective (review Andrew *et al.* 1981). However, blue beads are also more likely to evoke avoidance, and this affects at least one phenomenon important in the aversive bead task: competition (Chapters 18, 19) between pre-training and training (which can be marked with red beads) cannot be obtained with blue beads (Andrew *et al.* 1981). It would be worth using blue beads in the standard task when a memory particularly resistant to disruption is desirable.

Size is also important. Even 5 mm beads can evoke avoidance responses: small beads were introduced in pre-training because they appeared to minimize such behaviour. There is no detailed study of the dependence of avoidance on size of sphere, but the testosterone-facilitated pecking (which largely represents the removal of the inhibition of pecking due to increasing size) becomes marked with spheres somewhere between 5 and 15 mm in diameter (Clifton and Andrew 1983).

The other visual property of commonly used targets which deserves comment here is reflectivity: shiny metallic beads may be effective in the evocation of pecking because of their resemblance to water drops. An auditory cue of importance in some variants of the task is the sharp tapping used to alert chicks just before pre-training (in particular); such sounds strongly promote pecking in naive chicks (above).

At the first introduction of the standard task (Cherkin and Lee-Teng 1965), it involved presentation of a 7 mm sponge, moistened with the ill-tasting substance methylanthranilate. A wide variety of stimuli, some quite large, were used subsequently: a 3 mm shiny steel ball (Lee-Teng and Sherman 1966); a 3 × 5 mm microminiature lamp (Cherkin 1972); a 'banana plug' (an electrical connector: Mark and Watts 1971). Subsequent work has standardly used either small metal spheres or glass beads; methylanthranilate softens many plastics. A second common change in procedure has been the addition of pre-training.

The next section describes current procedures in the La Trobe laboratory from which has come the largest body of work using the task; it also explores a number of more general issues. Variation in procedures for the task between laboratories is then summarized, followed by separate discussion of housing, pre-training and training.

La Trobe procedure *K. T. Ng, M. E. Gibbs, and S. Crowe*

Introduction

Day-old chicks, normally black Australorp-white Leghorn cockerels, are obtained from a local hatchery on the morning of each experiment. The chicks are delivered in cardboard boxes housing approximately 100 chicks in each box, with each box divided by cardboard dividers into four compartments. A number of holes in the lid and sides of the boxes allow

Table 1.1   Outline of behavioural procedures

Experimental stage	Activity	Stimulus	Approximate interval between steps (min)
Stage 1	Placed in boxes in *pairs*		
Stage 2	Pre-training trial 1	Chrome bead + water	30
	Pre-training trial 2	Chrome bead + water	20
Stage 3	Pre-training trial 3	Red bead + water	20
	Pre-training trial 4	Blue bead + water	2–3
Stage 4	Training trial	Red bead + MeA	30
Stage 5	Test trial 1	Dry red bead	Required TTI
	Test Trial 2	Dry blue bead	2–3

MeA = methyl anthranilate
TTI = interval between training and test

light to filter into the boxes. On arrival at the laboratory, the chicks are kept in the delivery boxes for approximately 30 minutes prior to being placed in pairs in wooden experimental boxes (20 × 25 × 20 cm) with chick mash *ad libitum*. The experimental boxes are arranged in blocks of five boxes. Typically, 20 different chicks are used for each data point, with the 20 chicks housed in two blocks of five boxes each, placed on two shelves. Each laboratory normally houses no more than 12 blocks of boxes (i.e. 120 chicks). The temperature in each laboratory is maintained at 22–26°C by red light bulbs (60 W) suspended above the experimental boxes.

The experimental protocol is outlined in Table 1.1. Briefly, 30 minutes after placement in the experimental boxes, chicks are exposed to a pre-training trial with a small chrome bead (2 mm diameter), attached to a straight wire, and coated with water. The attention of each pair of chicks is attracted by tapping lightly on the front of the box and the bead is introduced into the box for up to 20 seconds. This pre-training trial is followed by a second similar pre-training trial. Following the second chrome bead trial, a red glass bead (4 mm diameter), dipped in water, is presented to each pair of chicks for 10 seconds. The number of pecks and the latency to first peck at this bead (and that presented next) are recorded for each chick using a manually operated handset connected to a computer. All chicks in each group of 20 are given this pre-training trial before being presented with a blue glass bead (4 mm diameter), dipped in water, for 10 seconds.

The training trial is started 30 minutes after the last pre-training trial. Each pair of chicks is presented for 10 seconds with a red glass bead, identical to that used in the pre-training trial, but coated with the chemical aversant methylanthranilate. The number of pecks and the latency to first peck for each chick are recorded. Chicks which fail to peck at the training bead on this trial or which fail to show the typical disgust reactions of beak-wiping and distress calls are eliminated from data analyses at the end of the experiment. In general, no more than 10 per cent of chicks are eliminated for this reason.

Retention tests are carried out at various times after the training trial. These consist of a 10 second presentation of a dry red bead, identical to that used in the training trial, to each pair of chicks in a block of 20, followed by a 10 second presentation of a dry blue bead, also identical to that used in the pre-training trial. The number of pecks and the latency to first peck for each chick are recorded for each of the retention trials.

In all our experiments, unless we are explicitly interested in the effects of isolation, chicks are pre-trained, trained and tested in pairs. In a number of other laboratories (e.g. Patterson *et al*. 1986) chicks are typically trained and tested in isolation. It is also the case that in some of these laboratories chicks are not pre-trained. Undoubtedly, differences also exist in the general laboratory layout, in details of experimental procedure, and in the training protocol.

There appears to be no doubt that isolating day-old chicks results in increased stress (de Vaus *et al*. 1980), as evidenced by increases in distress calls. For reasons related possibly to the increased levels of stress hormones as a result of isolation, the use of isolated chicks results in a marked change in the nature of the retention function (de Vaus *et al*. 1980). Both isolation and corticosterone treatment result in an extension of the duration of intermediate memory, with the second transient retention deficit normally observed in paired chicks about 55 minutes after training occurring at a much later time (Chapter 17). This effect of isolation may account in part for the differences in results obtained in our laboratories and those obtained by Patterson *et al*. (1986).

Copying in paired chicks

A potential problem with pre-training, training and testing chicks in pairs is that the behaviour of one of the chicks may affect the behaviour of the other chick. To determine the extent of such dependencies, we conducted two experiments in which chicks were housed in pairs in wooden boxes (20 × 25 × 20 cm) with a clear Perspex divider placed diagonally in the box, in order to separate the chicks physically but not visually or auditorily. One chick of each pair was trained, the other untrained; otherwise the two chicks were subject to identical experimental procedures. For each

Table 1.2 Effect of copying behaviour on responses of day-old chicks trained on a single trial passive discriminated avoidance learning trial.

		Non-blind condition		% pairs			Blind condition		% pairs	
		% avoiding	DR	correct	n		% avoiding	DR	correct	n
		Red Blue					Red Blue			
A tested	A	82 24	0.928	71	17	A	94 17	0.975	77	18
before B	B	12 6	0.493			B	22 6	0.514		
B tested	A	82 18	0.914	71	17	A	88 12	0.951	76	17
before A	B	18 18	0.491			B	24 0	0.632		

A = trained chicks; B = untrained chicks; DR = discrimination ratio. Any chick failing to peck the blue bead at retention test is excluded. DR for any given chick then equals the number of pecks at the red bead divided by the total number of pecks at red and blue beads.

experiment, two groups of ten pairs of chicks were used. In one group, the trained chick of each pair was tested for retention first, while in the other group, the untrained chick was tested first.

For both experiments, all pre-training procedures were carried out by a research assistant, and the same experimenter both trained and tested the chicks. In the first experiment, the experimenter knew which chick in each pair had been trained. In the second experiment, however, chicks were randomly interchanged between compartments after the training trial by the research assistant, so that the experimenter was unaware of the training history of the chicks during retention tests. The discrimination ratios (legend: Table 1.2) for these experiments are reported in Table 1.2, as are the number of pairs of chicks which exhibited correct responses (i.e. trained chick avoiding the previously aversive red bead and the untrained chick pecking it). All retention tests were carried out 180 minutes after the training trial.

While there is a tendency for chicks in the 'blind' experiment to show higher levels of avoidance of the red bead, lower levels of avoidance of the blue bead, higher discrimination ratios and higher percentage pairs of chicks showing the appropriate responses, the differences are small. In any event, the results suggest that interdependencies were less obvious in the 'blind' experiment, a finding which is counter-intuitive to the expectation that experiment bias would lead to lower levels of dependencies in the 'non-blind' experiment. When the results are compared with a control group of chicks pre-trained by a research assistant, trained by one experimenter, and tested by a different experimenter, in pairs without a divider in the box, it is clear that the level of dependency arising from using paired chicks is not substantial and would not materially affect the results reported from our laboratories.

Box position effects

In almost all our experiments, a different group of 20 chicks is used for each data point on each experimental day. Chicks are housed in pairs in experimental compartments (20 × 25 × 20 cm). These compartments are arranged in blocks of five by dividing a large wooden box into five compartments. Each group of chicks is housed in two such blocks, and the blocks are placed on two wooden shelves, one above the other. Thus, half the group of chicks within each group are in close proximity to each other. The possibility arises of position effects arising both from proximity to other chicks and from the fact that one block of ten chicks is placed at a higher level than the other.

To determine whether there are such positional effects, we present the cumulated per cent of chicks in each box position that avoided the red training bead during retention tests carried out at times corresponding to the intermediate and long term stages of our postulated three stages of memory processing (Ng and Gibbs, 1988: Chapter 13), from a random selection of our published reports. Short-term memory times of test were omitted, as were retention tests carried out at 15 and 55 minutes post-learning when chicks typically do not avoid the red bead. The results (Fig. 1.1) clearly show that there are no significant box position effects.

The effects of pre-training

A major procedural difference between laboratories is in the use of pre-training trials. All the chicks in our experiments, unless otherwise stated, are given two pre-training trials with a small chrome bead, followed by one pre-training trial with a red glass bead, and one with the blue glass bead, with all beads coated with water. To examine the effects of pre-training, 15 groups of 20 chicks each were pre-trained, trained, and tested normally at 45 minutes (6 groups), 75 minutes (6 groups), and 100 minutes (3 groups) after training (Fig. 1.2). A further 15 groups of 20 chicks each were not pre-trained but left in the experimental boxes for the same time as the pre-trained chicks, then trained and tested at the above times. For the six groups tested at 100 minutes (Fig. 1.2c), different experimenters were used to train and test the chicks. A research assistant was used for all pre-training trials, and in all cases, the experimenter(s) was 'blind' as to which groups had been pre-trained. The study was conducted in three separate experiments on three different experimental days, as shown in Fig. 1.2. The results suggest a slightly lower level of retention at all training-test intervals used for the groups not pre-trained. Of greater significance is the clear observation that groups not pre-trained showed considerably greater variability in retention levels both within and across

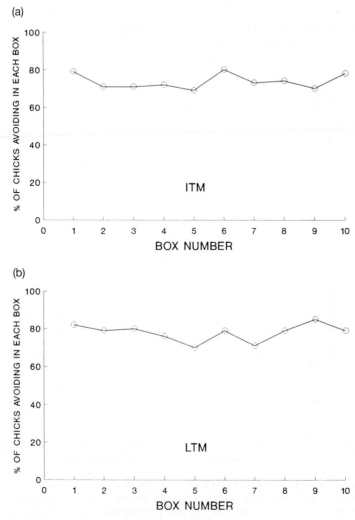

Fig. 1.1   Percentage of chicks avoiding the aversive red bead in each box from (a) a total of 63 pairs of chicks from 17 experiments tested between 20 and 50 min post-learning, under saline or non-drug conditions, and (b) a total of 75 pairs of chicks from 12 experiments, tested between 60 and 180 min post-learning, under saline or non-drug conditions. Boxes are numbered from 1 to 10: 1–5 are on the top shelf of the block and 6–10 on the bottom. 1 and 6, 2 and 7 and corresponding succeeding numbers thus occupy similar positions.

training-test intervals. This finding is particularly important in view of the issue of lack of variability in our published data raised by Roberts (1987; Ng and Gibbs 1987). It would appear that pre-training of the chicks increases retention levels and reduces variability. For the pre-trained

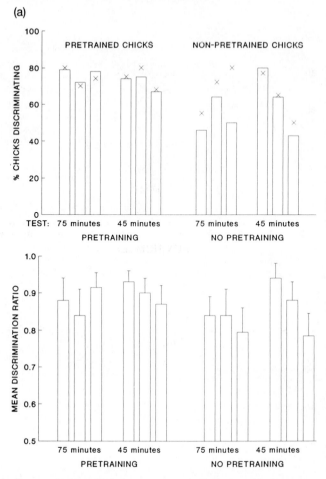

Fig. 1.2   Effect of pre-training versus not pre-training chicks on retention after training on a single trial passive discriminated avoidance learning task, as measured by per cent of chicks avoiding the red and pecking the blue bead, and by mean discrimination ratio, defined as the number of pecks at the blue bead divided by the total number of pecks at the blue and the red bead for each chick pecking the blue bead on the retention test. The percentage of birds avoiding the red bead at test, before exclusion of birds which failed to peck the blue bead, is shown by a cross; SEM are shown as bars. Intervals between training and testing were 45, 75 or 100 minutes. Panels (a) and (b) show two replications which both involved 45 and 75 minute groups; panel (c) shows an experiment with a 100 minute group only. (Parts (b) and (c) are on pp. 25 and 26, respectively.)

groups, the percentage of chicks avoiding the red bead on the retention tests remain within the relatively narrow range of 80–90 per cent found in our previously published results. With the non-pre-trained groups, these percentages range mainly between 50 and 95 per cent.

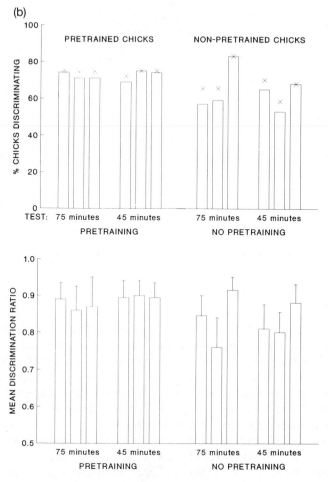

Fig. 1.2 See caption on p. 24.

'Blind' versus 'non-blind' experiments

In pharmacological experiments where the effects of different pharmacological treatments or where dose–response functions are being investigated, it is possible and desirable to carry out 'blind' experiments, where the experimenter involved in the training and/or testing of chicks is not aware of the treatment received by any given group of chicks. In experiments where interest is in the nature of the retention function, it is more difficult, but just as desirable, to maintain 'blind' procedures, especially when the training-test intervals in any given experimental day show a wide range (e.g. 5 min–180 min). The absence of 'blind' procedures in these experiments can give rise to conscious or unconscious bias in the single trial

(c)

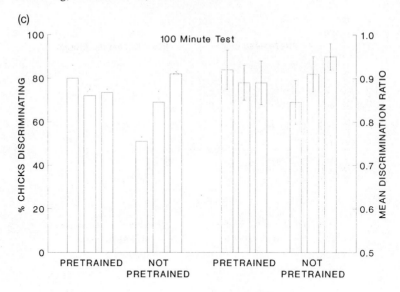

Fig. 1.2   See caption on p. 24.

passive avoidance task that we use with day-old chicks. To check on this possibility, we ran a series of several experiments in which a research assistant pre-trained the chicks, one experimenter trained the chicks and another experimenter tested the chicks. Neither experimenter was aware of the training-retention interval to be used with each independent group of 20 chicks, the schedule being prepared by a third experimenter. The experiments were grouped so that training-test intervals within any one experiment were kept in a narrow range in order to permit 'blind' testing. For training-test intervals between 5 and 30 minutes and between 40 and 70 minutes an interval of 15 minutes and 55 minutes respectively, was also included. These are times when chicks are expected to show a transient retention deficit (Ng and Gibbs 1988). The composite retention function obtained from these experiments is reported in Fig. 1.3. The results from the 'blind' experiments essentially confirm our previous findings, both with respect to the nature of the retention function and the levels of retention obtained. Again, it would appear that the lack of variability in a number of our published retention functions, pointed to by Roberts (1987), cannot be attributed to experimenter bias *per se*. This is particularly so since the 'blind' function exhibits the two points of temporary retention deficit at 15 and 55 minutes following the learning trial found in our previous experiments. Furthermore, it is interesting to note that the lack of variability observed previously, and in the 'blind' experiment, with percentage avoidance of the red bead as an index of retention, is also found with the continuous, and therefore more sensitive measure using discrimination ratios.

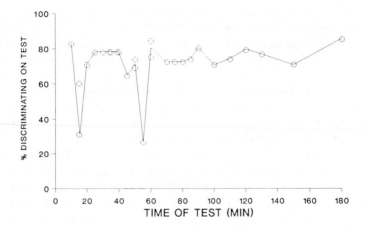

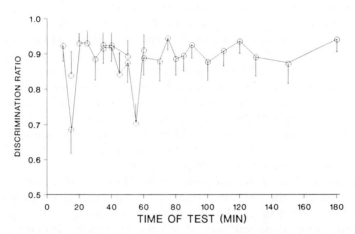

Fig. 1.3 Retention functions for 'blind' and 'non-blind' retention tests for chicks trained on a single trial passive discriminated avoidance learning task. SEM are shown as bars.

Pre-training, training, and test: variation between procedures
R. J. Andrew

The procedures commonly used at the four laboratories responsible so far for most of the work which is based on this task, are summarized in Table 1.3. This by no means exhausts variations of the task. Davies and Payne (1989), for example, used a 6 mm red bead, without pre-training, placed chicks for 5 minutes in a test area before training, and held them singly in an incubator for 3 hours before test, which again was after 5 minutes isolation; presentations were up to 60 s at training and 30 s at test, unlike the more usual 10 s. A variety of combinations of bead types have been used in pre-training at Sussex, and have been shown to affect response at test in different ways (e.g. Clifton *et al.* 1982); a single red presentation has the advantage of making precise timing easier.

There has been little attempt to examine the effects of variations in procedure, partly no doubt because in general results agree between laboratories, despite such variations (Chapters 13–19). However, it was shown in the previous section that when using the La Trobe procedure, pre-training reduces variability, and increases the proportion of birds which inhibit pecking at test. It is likely that habituation of pecking at the red bead due to pre-training contributes to the latter effect (Andrew and Brennan 1985). Habituation in the absence of training reduces pecking rates; in combination with training, it is likely slightly to increase the proportion of birds not pecking at all. A second possible effect of pre-training is more important. Presentation of the red bead in pre-training is likely to compete with the establishment of a trace based on training with an ill-tasting red bead; the effect is likely to change rapidly (Chapter 19) with slight changes in the interval between pre-training and training over the interval of 30–33 minutes, which is usual in the La Trobe procedure (Table 3). It is possible that such slight changes tend to occur systematically within blocks of ten cages in the La Trobe procedure: this would be the case if the pre-training presentations of red and blue beads each took (in total across the block) slightly less time than the corresponding period of training the block. If so, this would tend to generate within each block one or two birds in which competition was unusually effective, and which were therefore unusually likely to peck at test.

This minor effect is in itself unimportant. However, if present, it would provide exactly the sort of systematic change in the behaviour of a proportion of birds in each block which is needed to explain the significant departure from expected variability between blocks demonstrated by Roberts (1987; see previous section).

Competition between pre-training and training, particularly when enhanced by hormones such as testosterone (Chapter 18), offers many opportunities for the study of the temporal structure of memory formation, as well as insights into the processes which go on at different times. Competition usually occurs only when a bead similar to that used in training is also used in pre-training. However, this is not true when very short intervals are used: pre-training with a blue bead then opposes training with a red one (Clifton *et al.* 1982). This sort of approach is particularly suited to the dissection of the earliest stages of memory formation, since the first presentation does not involve an unpleasant tasting substance, likely to linger in the bill, or any other reinforcer whose

Table 1.3

	Pre-train	Train	Test
La Trobe	Begin-30-C-20-R-(2 to 3)-B	-30-R*-x-	-R-(2 to 3)-B
Sussex	Begin-One Day-W-5-W-10-R-5-B-	-120-R*-x-	-R-5-B
Berkeley	Begin-	-120-S*-x-	-S
Open University	Begin-120-W-5-W-5-W-C-	-10-C*-x-	-C

The summary of each procedure beings with the time at which the chicks are placed in their cages (shown by 'Begin'). The intervals between bead presentations are then given in minutes. The abbreviations which are used for types of bead are as follows:

La Trobe (Gibbs and Ng 1977):   C=chrome, 2mm; R=red glass, 4 mm; B=blue glass, 4 mm. Age: day 1

Sussex (Andrew *et al.* 1981):   W=white plastic, 2.5 mm; R=red glass, 4 mm; B=blue glass, 4 mm. Age: day 2

Berkeley (Patterson *et al.* 1986):   S=stainless steel, 3 mm. Age : day 2

Open University (Rose and Jork 1987):   W=white, 2.5 mm; C=chrome 4 mm. Age: day 1 (beginning of day 2)

In general, presentations were for about, or up to 10 s; * = bead coated with methylanthranilate (or water if a control group was included). In the La Trobe procedure beads are wet with water at pre-training; both dry and wet beads have been used at different times at Sussex, as have other combinations of types of bead (text).

Chicks were housed in pairs, except at Berkeley, where they were held in groups until the beginning of the experiment, when they were placed singly in the experimental chambers.

after-effects are likely directly to change behaviour for anything up to several minutes.

A particularly versatile bead for such experiments consists of a hollow glass sphere (6 mm), with an internal coating of paraffin wax to diffuse the light with which it is internally illuminated though a light guide, running the length of the mounting rod (Andrew and Brennan 1985). The colour can be rapidly changed without affecting other parameters.

The use of water on the surface of beads may have effects beyond that intended, which is to provide a bead which looks like the training bead with its coat of methylanthranilate, but which is tasteless. It is possible that some positive reinforcement is provided by such beads. Chicks can sometimes be seen to make drinking movements after pecking them; indeed pecks directed at water drops are probably a usual way by which chicks learn to drink. Wet beads are used at pre-training under the La Trobe procedure shown in Table 1.3; they are used at training to provide control groups under the Open University procedure. Test under all procedures shown in Table 1.2 involves dry beads, which is perhaps illogical if the only consideration is to retain the exact appearance of the training bead.

Milder aversants than pure methylanthranilate are valuable tools. Cherkin (1972) used a dispersion of methylanthranilate (1.25 per cent) in water, and found that retention of inhibition of pecking was initially good, but that it fell away by 24 hours. Crowe *et al.* (1989) found that memory loss occurred under these conditions at about 50 minutes after training. Procedures of this sort are examined further in later chapters (Chapters 15 and 17); they offer an interesting approach to the investigation of the processes involved in the estabishment of a long-term trace.

The advantages of the precise timing of events in memory formation which is allowed by this task are so important that it is worth emphasizing the features which make precise timing possible. Training and test each take at most 10 s; the beginning of each is conventionally taken as the exact time of presentation, and crucial events within a presentation, such as first peck, vary by only a few seconds in relation to this. As all procedures take place in the home cage, variation in the timing of entries of beads at the beginning of a presentation can realistically be held to less than ±5 s, so long as care is taken to alert the chick (e.g. by tapping on the cage wall), and to make sure that it is facing the entry point, just before bead entry. The administration of drugs can and should be timed as carefully as presentations. With practice and an automatic syringe, injections can be carried out at a rate of one every 15 seconds, and this matches the fastest reasonable rate of testing (a test every 30 s). The choice of duration of steps in a timecourse is important. The shortest step which has so far commonly been used is (not surprisingly) 5 minutes, but finer resolution is certainly required over crucial sections of time-courses (e.g. 1 minute, Andrew and Brennan 1985). If, as is desirable, accurate timing is to be combined with a fully balanced pseudorandom distribution of treatments (including variation in intervals between presentations or presentation and injections), then quite complex schedules are necessary. Almost invariably these generate regular breaks in the otherwise rapid sequence of presentation (and injection, if this is included); such breaks are in any case almost essential if concentration is to be sustained. Two workers are needed, even if no drug administration is involved. One presents beads, whilst the other uses the schedule to control which chick receives what treatment at what time. Especially when combined with double-blind procedures for drug administration, such schedules make it quite impossible for the worker presenting the beads to have any expectation of likely outcomes for any particular chick.

Finally, the choice of measure deserves some consideration. In general, the response of pecking has been the only one considered. When only one type of bead is used at test, the choice is between whether a bird pecks or not, and the number of pecks made (which may vary from zero to perhaps a dozen in the case of a red bead). The first is the classic measure; the second is amenable to parametric analysis, and may reveal effects which are missed by the first (e.g. Chapter 19).

When a second bead ('neutral') of a type different from that used at training is also presented at test, a variety of more complex measures become possible. In both the La Trobe procedure and the Sussex variant, the neutral bead is presented second. As a result, it is impossible to be sure how far depression of pecking at the neutral bead, which is brought about by training (or other treatments), represents failure to discriminate (or rather to make use of the ability to discriminate) the two types of bead. Response to the neutral bead under these conditions might also be affected by short-term after-effects of the presentation of the red bead (e.g. habituation), as well as by longer-term extinction of inhibition of pecking due to a non-reinforced trial. Designs in which the order of presentation is balanced across groups are possible, but have not been used, no doubt because they would halve the group sizes for the standard measure of responses to the training bead, presented first. Andrew and Brennan (1985) showed that response to the neutral bead presented alone at test varies with interval between training and test in a way which gives information inaccessible to analysis of response to the training bead.

In view of evidence that rates of pecking at training and neutral beads can vary independently, it is probably best to use rates of pecking at the neutral bead (rather than some composite measure: below) as the main measure for the neutral bead; (Pecks at neutral minus Pecks at training bead) is a simple secondary measure which picks out treatments which greatly reduce differences in response to the two types of bead.

However, response to the neutral bead can be used in other ways. It is convenient to be alerted at once to the possibility that failure to peck at the training bead may reflect not excellent retention, but some general depression of behaviour due to a particular treatment; if the neutral bead is pecked, then such depression is unlikely (Gibbs and Ng 1977). However, it may not be always safe to draw the alternative conclusion when neither type of bead is readily pecked: disturbances of memory may result in an unusual degree of transfer of inhibition of pecking at the neutral bead (Chapter 19). Ng (Chapter 13) suggests that chicks which fail to peck the neutral bead at test should be excluded from analysis. My preference would be to avoid such exclusion on the grounds that failure to peck is likely to be only the most extreme variant of the reduction in pecking, which is itself the most informative type of change in response to the neutral bead.

Other behavioural measures deserve consideration. Failure at test to peck at the training bead correlates well with responses such as trilling and backing or turning away from the bead; such behaviour can reveal marked differences along time-courses when inhibition of pecking is consistently very marked (Chapter 19). Head shaking, a response which commonly occurs on tasting the methylanthranilate (MeAn), and which has often been used as one criterion of successful training, also occurs sometimes at test; it too varies with time between training and test.

32   R. J. Andrew

Housing: variations between procedures

Introduction   R. J. Andrew

Two main types of housing are in use. At Berkeley, following the procedures introduced by Cherkin, chicks are housed singly in small cartons (white cylindrical, 8.3 × 17.8 cm: below). Other laboratories (Sussex, Open University) use variants of the cages introduced at La Trobe (Gibbs and Ng 1977) and, like La Trobe, house in pairs (or, at Sussex, with a substitute for the partner: below). Isolation stresses chicks, and the resulting hormonal changes markedly affect the timing of transitions in memory formation (above, and Chapters 13, 17 and 19). Pairing prevents such stress. If it is necessary to hold chicks singly and at the same time study undisturbed timing of events in memory formation, some substitute for the partner must be provided. A table tennis ball suspended within the cage is very effective (Chapter 21). Alternatives are considered below (see also Montevecchi and Noel 1978).

Paired, individual, and pseudo-paired housing   M. R. Rosenzweig,
E. L. Bennett, J. L. Mortimer Jr, D. Beniston, P. Columbo, D. W. Lee,
T. A. Patterson, G. Schulteis, and P. A. Serrano

A variety of methods for housing chicks have been compared recently in our laboratory to determine their relative advantages and disadvantages for training and testing. The conditions examined included paired, individual, and pseudo-paired housing. In the paired housing condition, two chicks were placed in a rectangular compartment as reported previously by Gibbs and Ng (1977). Individually housed chicks were each placed in a cardboard cylinder as described previously (Patterson *et al.* 1986, 1989*b*). Chicks in pseudo-paired conditions were individually housed in a manner that mimicked some aspects of the paired-housing condition. In one pseudo-paired condition, chicks were housed in a white rectangular box subdivided into five paired compartments. The central divider was made of clear Plexiglas, allowing chicks in adjacent compartments to view but not physically contact each other. In a second pseudo-paired condition, chicks were housed in a similar rectangular box, but the central divider was opaque and a mirror was mounted on one wall of the compartment to allow each chick to view its own image.

Comparisons were made between chicks housed individually in boxes with a transparent divider (TD), mirrored wall (MW), or in cardboard cylinders (CC). Chicks were housed 2 hours before training in separate rooms for each housing condition.

Training. During training, chicks in the MW condition exhibited the fewest distress signs, including jumping against the Plexiglas cover of the box or making distress peeps. Chicks housed in the TD condition showed slightly more distress activity, while CC-housed chicks were the most active and distressed. During one-trial peck-aversion training with no pre-training, 93 per cent of chicks in the CC condition ($n=60$) pecked at the aversive bead; this is a very satisfactory level of training. Chicks in the TD and MW conditions were more startled than CC chicks at the presentation of the training bead, and they showed 90 per cent ($n=60$) and 75 per cent ($n=40$) training, respectively. In the physically paired (PP) condition, 75 per cent of the chicks trained ($n=40$). Our standard CC condition showed significantly better training than either the MW or PP chicks ($\chi^2=6.7$, $p < 0.05$). No interactions were observed between the effects of drug or saline injection and the per cent of chicks that trained in any particular housing condition, for the agents we examined. Therefore, while pseudo-paired chicks were calmer than chicks housed in cardboard cylinders prior to training, they were more easily startled and did not train better than the isolated chicks.

Housing comparisons were also made using a pre-training protocol resembling, but not identical with that reported by Gibbs and Ng (Table 1.1: Chapter 13). Briefly, each chick was presented with a sequence of chrome pre-training beads at intervals of approximately 10 minutes, followed by presentation of a red bead, which had been dipped in methylanthranilate. Any chick that pecked at the training bead was considered to have trained successfully regardless of previous behaviour. Prior to training, chicks in the MW condition showed the fewest distress signs, followed by PP-, TD-, and CC-housed chicks, respectively. With this protocol, 55 per cent of PP chicks ($n=160$) trained successfully; this was the housing condition used by Gibbs and Ng. Only 33 per cent of the CC-housed chicks ($n=200$), 10 per cent of TD-housed chicks ($n=40$) and 25 per cent of MW-housed chicks ($n=40$) pecked at the training bead. With pre-training, the PP chicks trained significantly more frequently than chicks in the other conditions ($p < 0.01$); the CC chicks trained more frequently than the TD chicks. There was a tendency for fewer chicks in each condition to peck at successive presentations of pre-training beads. These percentages are far below the rate of training reported by Gibbs and Ng and far below the percentages for our method, which does not include pre-training. Perhaps the methods of Gibbs and Ng are very sensitive to the level of skill and experience of the experimenter, or perhaps they reflect strain differences which we discuss in our chapter. Certainly, our procedure with individual housing and no pre-training is simple to use and yields clear results that are, for comparable experiments, usually similar to those of other laboratories.

We agree that it would be desirable to show discrimination learning, that is, that chicks avoid the colour associated with the aversive substance but do not avoid a bead of another colour. For this reason we conducted several experiments in which a red bead was coated with MeAn and a blue bead was coated with water. Pre-training with chrome beads was used, as in the work of Gibbs and Ng. The results showed, first, that many chicks did not train satisfactorily after the pre-training, and second that about as many chicks avoided both the red and blue beads as avoided the red bead alone; few chicks avoided blue but pecked at red or avoided neither. Thus with the White XL chicks and in our laboratory the discrimination effect is not strong.

It appears, then, that each laboratory has worked out details of procedures that are appropriate for its subjects and local conditions and that the various laboratories are engaged in productive research with many concordant results.

Drug administration   *R. J. Andrew*

Systemic administration is best done by injection into a fold of skin pinched between the fingers along the keel of the sternum. The needle should run rostrad and parallel to the keel. Long-term action of steroid hormones has commonly been produced by the use of appropriate slow release esters but silastic implants are sometimes preferable (Clifton and Andrew 1989).

The most important special feature of drug administration in the chick is the ease of intracranial injection. The unossified character of the skull roof allows this to be done freehand with as little (or less) disturbance as results from subcutaneous injection. Although the blood-brain barrier is poorly developed in young chicks, there is usually little information about the ease with which any particular drug enters the CNS; direct administration avoids any potential problems of entry. More importantly, localization of effects predominantly to one or other hemisphere can be achieved (Bell and Gibbs 1977; Chapters 15 and 19). Two approaches have been taken to further localization. One is to use a superimposed cap which guides the needle more accurately (Davis *et al.* 1982); well localized zones of action have been confirmed with this technique (Patterson *et al.* 1986; Chapter 15). The other, which is valuable in wide exploration, is to aim freehand injections to a broad zone, and then to plot entry points after death (Chapter 16). After reflecting the scalp, entry can be seen as a red point. A transparent cap, whose undersurface is a negative cast of the upper surface of the skull, can then be superimposed, and the entry point plotted using a 2 mm graticule on the upper surface of the cast. Depth (as usual with intracranial injection in the chick) is controlled by length between stop and needle tip.

Although localization within one hemisphere has been demonstrated, caution needs to be exercised when trying to identify particular structures which might be involved. Not only are all structures along the track of entry directly exposed to the drug, but reflux is marked, so that the surface of the brain is likely to be rapidly affected. Rosenzweig (Chapter 15) discusses these issues further.

Other tasks involving pecking at small objects *R. J. Andrew*

Learning can be measured using pecking at beads as the main measure, without exposure to aversive tasks. If beads are presented for periods, and at intervals which are precisely timed, habituation of pecking occurs along standard timecourses. So far this has chiefly been used in studies of lateralization, comparing birds using right or left eyes only (Chapter 21). Here advantage is taken of the fact that change in almost any property of the bead can dishabituate pecking: the degree of habituation gives a measure of the extent to which the change is judged to be important. A related test began with 60 second presentation of the bead, which is sufficient for pecking to be replaced by repeated turning away; retention was measured by the readiness to turn away at test (Andrew and Brennan 1985).

Combination of tasks of this sort with the administration of amnestic agents, and the systematic variation of intervals between presentations, is yet to be fully explored (but see Chapter 19). The absence of aversive taste or other negative reinforcement and the possibility of quite subtle investigation of processes of stimulus analysis, would allow much to be done which is difficult or impossible with the classical aversive bead task.

Other tasks involve the presentation of food. They are suitable for chicks older than 3 days: it becomes so difficult to evoke pecking by the presentation of beads in chicks after the third day that bead tasks are of little use thereafter. Food-based tasks can also be used on day 3 (Mench and Andrew 1986) and probably day 2, but some prior period of experience of food is necessary before the task.

The most extensively used task of this sort is the pebble floor task introduced by Dawkins (1971), and modified by Andrew and Rogers (1972). In the simplest form of the task, familiar food grains are scattered amongst pebbles of roughly similar size and appearance, which are firmly attached to the substrate; in contrast, the food is loose and can be swallowed. The rate at which pecks at pebbles decline provides a measure of learning, although its detailed interpretation requires caution (Chapter 21). The task has been used in studies of the effects of amnestic agents (Gibbs and Ng 1977); it differs from the passive avoidance task in that learning is followed over a series of closely spaced experiences. Temporary storage of information is likely to be of great importance, and this may explain a striking effect of ethacrynic acid (Rogers *et al.* 1977): the agent prevents any change during training, but subsequent test shows that learning has nevertheless occurred (see also Chapter 14).

Related tasks use two familiar types of food grain (e.g. red and yellow coloured), and measure runs of choice of one or other (Andrew 1972). In the past, such tasks have been used to study stabilization of attention by steroid hormones: stabilization extends the period for which one type of food is selected, once such selection has begun (Andrew 1983). However, they may be useful in the study of amnestic agents affecting the earliest stages of memory formation.

Unpleasant tasting food has also been used (e.g. 'aversive wheat' task: Gibbs and Ng 1977): this allows the use in older chicks of a closer parallel to the bead passive avoidance task.

DRUG STUDIES: GENERAL ISSUES
R. J. Andrew

The use of a variety of drugs as amnestic agents following ill-tasting bead tasks is considered at length in later chapters. However, it should be noted here that a smaller number of studies have applied such agents following imprinting. Lecanuet *et al.* (1976) were able to disturb imprinting by halothane anaesthesia induced immediately after good following had been achieved. Benzodiazepines have also been shown to impair imprinting (Venault *et al.* 1986).

Enhancement of learning by drugs has also been studied in chicks. Low concentrations of the convulsant ether flurothyl applied immediately after learning (using the ill-tasting bead task) increase the resulting inhibition of pecking at test (Cherkin *et al.* 1975; Gerbrandt *et al.* 1977). The same has been described for arginine vasotocin (Davis *et al.* 1982). When agents have to be applied immediately after an aversive task, it is necessary also to consider whether aversive consequence of the agent itself may be involved in any effect (e.g. Chapter 15). The competition procedure (pp. 28–9) offers a complementary approach: enhancement by agents given following the first (non-aversive) experience has been shown for steroid hormones (Chapter 18) and for noradrenalin (Stephenson 1981; Andrew 1985). In the case of imprinting, ACTH analogues have been shown to facilitate approach to the imprinting object but not to affect subsequent preference (Martin and Van Wimersma Greidanus 1978). However, benzodiazepine antagonists do enhance acquisition of imprinting (Venault *et al.* 1986).

Chicks have also been used in studies of the pharmacology of 'emotional behaviour'. Panksepp *et al.* (1980, 1984) review the evidence that distress, including separation-induced peeping, depends upon neural systems which use opioid (perhaps CRF) peptides.

Manipulation of dopaminergic systems affects a variety of behaviours in chicks in a way suggesting action on attention to conspicuous or valent stimuli (De Lanerolle and Millam 1980). Some of these effects survive decerebration and are likely to be mediated at midbrain level (De Lanerolle 1978). Dopaminergic pathways appear to be important in sustaining tonic immobility in chicks (Ettinger and Thompson 1978), although not unexpectedly other systems are also involved (e.g. noradrenergic and cholinergic: Thompson and Joseph 1978; Gagliardi and Thompson 1977). Motor effects of both dopaminergic and cholinergic systems have been described (Sanberg 1983). Motor stereotypy (especially involving pecking) is obvious and has been antagonized by dopamine receptor blockers (Ayiteh-Smith and Addae-Mensah 1983).

SUBCELLULAR FRACTIONATION
J. A. P. Rostas

Techniques for the preparation of subcellular fractions enriched in synaptic structures work equally well with adult brains from chicken and rat. However, brains from newly hatched or young immature chickens behave differently during fractionation. The reasons for this are as follows.

1. The postsynaptic density is much thinner in immature synapses than in adult.
2. The adhesion of the pre- and postsynaptic membranes across the synaptic cleft is relatively weak in newly hatched chicken brain.
3. The postsynaptic density in newly hatched chicken brain is structurally fragile and easily disrupted by detergents.
4. There is a relative lack of myelin in newly hatched chicken brain.

Synaptosomes provide a convenient model system for the study of the nerve terminal *in vitro*. They are also prepared as the first stage in the purification of subsynaptic structures such as synaptic plasma membranes, synaptic vesicles and postsynaptic densities. Therefore anything that alters the properties or isolation of synaptosomes also affects the purification of other synaptic structures.

Synaptosomes

Standard homogenization condition applied to adult brain from chicken and rat produce intact synaptosomes, most of which have intact synaptic clefts with attached postsynaptic membranes and postsynaptic densities. The same conditions applied to newly hatched chicken brain produce intact synaptosomes, most of which have lost their postsynaptic element (Rostas *et al.* 1984). This change is unlikely to be due to different sizes or geometries of the contact zones, resulting in altered mechanical properties, as the average length of the contact zones does not change in the posthatch period (Rostas *et al*. 1984). Rather, they are probably due to weaker adhesion across the synaptic cleft. The lack of attached postsynaptic element and thinness of the postsynaptic densities significantly decreases both sedimentation rate and equilibrium density of the immature synaptosomes. This is because the major determinants of the sedimentation properties of synaptosomes are size, mitochondrial content and the size (mass) of the attached postsynaptic density and associated postsynaptic element (Dunkley *et al*. 1988; Jarvie, Harrison, Weinberger, Baker, Rostas and Dunkley, unpublished).

The altered sedimentation properties of the synaptosomes mean that fractionation steps replying on sedimentation rate require somewhat higher centrifugation speeds or longer times in order to sediment the majority of the synaptosomes and maintain yield. To sediment synaptosomes from newly hatched brain we routinely use 20 000 g_{av} for 20 minutes (using 0.32 M sucrose at 4°C in a fixed angle rotor) to prepare the initial P2 fraction as compared with 10 000–15 000 g_{av} for 10–20 minutes which is normally used with adult rat (or chicken) brain. This results in a slightly higher degree of contamination of the P2 and final synaptosome fractions by light membranes from the Golgi apparatus and endoplasmic reticulum. If both purity and yield were important for an experiment, the optimum centrifugation conditions would have to be derived empirically for each age. Fortunately, most experiments depend more on maximal yield than purity, so that approximate corrections to the centrifugation conditions are sufficient. In equilibrium density gradient centrifugation the synaptosomes tend to shift to lighter fractions. For most discontinuous gradient procedures this would make little difference, since they use only two or three steps in the gradient with large differences in density between the steps. However, with the more sensitive and rapid nonequilibrium Percoll gradient procedure (Dunkley *et al*. 1988) there is a significant shift in the distribution of synaptosomes to lighter fractions.

By the end of the first week posthatch, the adhesion across the synaptic cleft has strengthened sufficiently to permit the isolation of many synaptosomes with attached postsynaptic elements (we have not determined the precise time-course of this change). The thickening of the postsynaptic densities is a much slower process, which does not attain the mature state until 8–10 weeks post-hatch (Rostas and Jeffrey 1981; Weinberger and Rostas 1988; see also Chapter 7). Using the Percoll gradient procedure, synaptosomes from 1–2-week chickens are still shifted to lighter fractions and the adult distribution is attained gradually as the postsynaptic density thickens (Jarvie, Harrison, Weinberger, Baker, Rostas and Dunkley, unpublished).

There is relatively little myelin in a newly hatched chicken brain because myelination is largely a post-hatch process in chickens. This means that, despite the change in sedimentation properties of the synaptosomes, there is comparatively little contamination of synaptosome fractions with myelin in the newly hatched chick.

Synaptic junctions and postsynaptic densities

The mature postsynaptic density is a highly conserved and stable structure that resists homogenization and preserves its morphology to a remarkable extent when isolated attached to synaptosomes. Postsynaptic densities are also resistant to extraction with mild detergents, and can be isolated in good yield and purity by a number of procedures involving selective solubilization (Cotman and Taylor 1972; Cohen *et al.* 1977; Matus and Taff-Jones 1978; Gurd *et al.* 1982). When these methods are applied to adult chicken brain the yields and purities of the fractions obtained are virtually identical to those obtained from adult rat brain. If the synaptosomes used as the starting point for these methods are prepared using the greater centrifugation forces needed for newly hatched chicken brain, the yields of the final fraction are higher than expected due to the presence of contaminating lighter membranes (Rostas *et al.* 1979).

When these selective solubilization techniques are applied to newly hatched chicken brain the degree of solubilization achieved by these detergents is far greater than that in the adult (Rostas and Jeffrey 1981; Murakami *et al.* 1986). Therefore, in newly hatched chickens, it is preferable to use methods which use some crosslinking to stabilize synaptic structures before detergent extraction (Cotman and Taylor 1972; Gurd *et al.* 1982), to avoid the use of very strong detergents such as N-lauryl sarcosinate (Rostas and Jeffrey 1981) and to lower the concentration of the detergent used (Murakami *et al.* 1986) The gross fragility of the postsynaptic density observed in the newly hatched brain is no longer apparent by the end of the first post-hatch week, although the amount of postsynaptic density material which can be isolated is much less than that from the adult brain, because the amount of postsynaptic density material does not reach adult levels until 8–10 weeks post-hatch (Rostas and Jeffrey 1981; Rostas *et al.* 1983). It is not known whether the apparently coincident disappearance of the fragility of the synaptic cleft to homogenization and the fragility of the postsynaptic density to detergents is due to a functional link between the two.

HISTOLOGICAL METHODS
M. G. Stewart

General

Birds are warm blooded vertebrates whose body fluids are fairly similar in ionic and osmotic composition to those of mammals. Therefore, histological methods for chick neurohistology, whether for whole brain autoradiography, light and electron microscopy, Golgi studies, or immuno-cytochemistry, are essentially similar to those used for the mammalian CNS.

For light and electron microscopy, procedures should follow those well established for mammals (Glauert 1974) but the following details may be useful.

Fixation

Fixation of domestic chick CNS tissue post-hatch, especially from birds of a few days of age, does not always, in practice, prove to be a simple matter. One contributory reason is that despite the fact that chicks are born in a precocial state, their CNS is in a phase of continuing development. Blood vessels at this age are also very thin and susceptible to damage. In a region of the forebrain known as the intermediate and medial hyperstriatum ventrale (IMHV) and in the lobus parolfactorius (LPO), synaptogenesis is still occurring, whereas neuronal numbers are declining (Curtis *et al.* 1989; Hunter and Stewart 1989). As in pre-hatch tissue, there is a considerable amount of space present in the neuropil which does not disappear until approximately 9 days of age, when the tissue assumes an appearance more similar to that of the adult.

Obtaining good fixation of tissue in young post-hatch chicks can be a frustrating business; apparently well fixed tissue (judging from the stiffness of the chick's head and the firmness of the brain), sometimes proves to be very poorly preserved. The following protocol has been used successfully in the Open University for a number of years as detailed in Stewart *et al.* (1984), and Hunter *et al.* (1989).

Composition of fixatives for light and electron microscopy

The description given is for electron microscopy. Similar fixatives and procedures are used also for light microscope studies, except that glutar-aldehyde is normally omitted and the concentration of paraformaldehyde is increased to 4 per cent. In all cases chicks are anaesthetized intraperito-neally with pentobarbitone (Sagatal), 0.15 ml for a 2-day-old chick, followed by perfusion fixation using a peristaltic pump. Gravity feed perfusion will also suffice, but it is not so easy to control the rate of flow.

1. *Perfusion.* A cannula (0.1 ml syringe tip with the sharp end removed) is placed in the left ventricle and a cut made in the right atrium to drain out blood (and later the perfusate). Perfusion is made via a peristaltic pump at low pressure, first with 15 ml of 0.9 per cent saline (0.9 g NaC1/l

in distilled water) to flush out blood, and then approximately 100 ml of primary fixative (see below) at room temperature. There is little advantage in our experience in using fixation at body temperature. The chick should go rigid, showing tetanic contractions within a short time of the fixative passing through the blood system. If it does not the perfusion should be abandoned: the brain preservation will probably be poor. However, even if it goes rigid, the brain is not necessarily well fixed, so 50 per cent more animals than required should be perfused.

2. *Primary fixative*. This comprises a mixture containing glutaraldehyde (final concn 2 per cent) and paraformaldehyde (final concn 2 per cent) in 0.1 molar sodium cacodylate buffer (pH 7.3); phosphate buffer can also be used but is less satisfactory. After primary fixation the brains can then be dissected out into a bottle containing the primary fixative, and either left in a refrigerator overnight, or regions of interest can be removed immediately. It is crucial for good ultrastructural preservation to ensure the brain is kept moist and that physical trauma be reduced to a minimum when tissue is dissected from the brain. The size of the samples should be not more than 1 mm^3, or 2 mm^3 at absolute maximum.

3. *Secondary fixation*. Following 2 washes in 0.1 M cacodylate buffer, tissue is placed in 2 per cent osmium tetroxide in 0.1 M cacodylate buffer (pH 7.3) for 30 minutes–1 hour. This stage must be carried out in a fume cupboard as (ideally) should the primary fixation.

4. *Wash* sample in 0.1 M cacodylate buffer for 10 minutes.

5. *Dehydrate*

50% ethanol	10 min
70% ethanol	15 min
80% ethanol	10 min
95% ethanol	5 min
100% ethanol (two changes)	20 min each
100% ethanol (dried over molecular sieve)	20 min

6. *Embedding*. Spurr's resin is very convenient (because it infiltrates the tissue relatively quickly) but any embedding resin may be used (e.g. Araldite: Ciba-Geigy). If Araldite is used the dehydration and embedding schedule may be slightly different and propylene oxide must be used after the 100 per cent stage.

1:1 Spurr's resin/100% ethanol	2 hours
100% Spurr's resin	overnight
100% fresh Spurr's resin	4 hours
Embed in flat moulds at 60°C	24 hours

We normally code the samples and put a number on a very small piece of paper inserted into one end of the mould.

Immunocytochemistry

For pre-embedding immunocytochemistry the chicks are perfused as described above and the immunoreaction is carried out before the embedding procedure. However, as with any immunocytochemistry procedure in mammals, the composition of the fixative will have to be modified depending on the nature of the antigen to be localized and the manner of production of the antibody. For example, in immunocytological localization of the amino acid neurotransmitter GABA (γ-aminobutyric acid) we have used a low concentration of glutaraldehyde in the primary fixative because higher glutaraldehyde concentrations produce greater non-specific staining.

For post-embedding immunocytochemistry, tissue is prepared in the manner described for electron microscopy (using normal strength glutaraldehyde and paraformaldehyde), post-fixed in osmium tetroxide and embedded in resin blocks. Sections are cut at 0.5–1.0 μm thickness and immunostaining carried out on the sections. For the immunogold technique the immunoreaction can be carried out on ultrathin sections collected on coated grids. The protocols followed are precisely those described for use in mammals. Some recent papers providing full details of procedures used for pre- and post-embedding immunocytochemistry for localization of GABA in the young chick are: Curtis and Stewart (1986); Csillag *et al.* (1987; 1989).

Autoradiography

The most common autoradiographic procedures used in behavioural studies in young chicks are either in studies of 2-deoxyglucose metabolism, or in receptor autoradiography. Radiolabelled ligands or other isotopes can be injected intraperitoneally or intracerebrally before killing the chicks (for *in vivo* autoradiographic studies), or isotope labelling can be carried out *in vitro* on frozen brain sections.

Light fixation with 0.1 per cent paraformaldehyde improves the ease with which the brain can be handled, but even such a low level of fixation may interfere with the binding of some ligands. It also necessitates the use of anaesthetics, which may pose problems for autoradiographic studies. Therefore it is desirable to remove the brains from freshly killed chicks without any fixation and to do so as quickly as possible. Brains should be immersed in isopentane for cryoprotection to prevent shattering of the brain during freezing; separation of the forebrain from the hind brain also helps to prevent this. The brains in isopentane are then frozen rapidly by immersion in liquid nitrogen and may be stored at −70°C for a time, as required, before cryostat sectioning and labelling with isotope (if to be done *in vitro*), and preparation for film-apposition autoradiography. Some details of the protocols for 2-deoxyglucose autoradiography are given in Kossut and Rose (1984) and for *in vitro* receptor autoradiography in Stewart *et al.* (1988) and Csillag *et al.* (1988).

Golgi studies

The standard procedures used in the mammalian CNS are effective with the chick brain for Golgi impregnation using either rapid Golgi, or the longer processing time of Golgi–Kopsch (Csillag *et al.* 1987; Tombol *et al.* 1988*a,b,c*; Patel and Stewart 1988). For Golgi studies to be carried out by light microscopy using the rapid Golgi method only 4–8 per cent paraformaldehyde (without glutaraldehyde) is used in the perfusing fixative, followed by the relevant Golgi impregnation protocol (Valverde 1970). For studies to be carried out at both light and electron microscope level (which will therefore involve gold toning: Csillag *et al.* 1987), the initial perfusing fixative contains a mixture of 1 per cent glutaraldehyde and 1 per cent paraformaldehyde.

TECHNIQUE FOR CANNULATION TO ALLOW FOR SUBSEQUENT
MICROINJECTION INTO THE IMHV OF THE AWAKE CHICK
J. E. Davey, B. J. McCabe, and G. Horn

Chicks are anaesthetized and the feathers surrounding the auditory meati are clipped to facilitate the insertion of the earbars when mounting the head of the chick in a stereotaxic apparatus. A horizontal bar, positioned 8 mm below the earbars, is inserted between the upper and lower mandibles and pressed gently against the hinge of the beak.

The skin overlying the skull is incised and the fronto-parietal (f/p) suture identified. A guide cannula 6 mm in length (21 SWG) is held in a pin chuck, specially modified by attaching a rod to the collar of the chuck; only a small force on the rod is then needed to rotate the collar, permitting the guide cannula to be released from the chuck without lateral movement. The cannula, in the pin chuck, is mounted in the vertical arm of the stereotaxic apparatus and positioned 2.75 mm anterior to the f/p suture and 0.75 mm lateral to the midline. At this point, a flap of skull is incised and reflected to expose the underlying dura. With a second cut the dura is incised to expose the brain. A further single slit is made in the skull at a point approximately 3 mm anterior and 3 mm lateral to the first incision. A small stainless steel insect pin (125 μm diameter) is prepared by coiling it twice at one end. This pin (the support pin) is slipped into place by inserting the first turn of the coil under the skull, through the anterior slit; the second turn is then above the skull (Cipolla-Neto *et al.* 1979). The guide cannula is lowered to the surface of the brain and advanced to a final position 1 mm below the brain surface.

Cyanoacrylate adhesive (RS Components Ltd) is applied to the base of the guide cannula, support pin and the surrounding skull, particularly posterior to the guide cannula, and across the f/p suture. Care is taken to avoid any glue touching the surface of the brain. When the adhesive is set, dental acrylic ('Simplex Rapid', Howmedica International Ltd) is applied over the cyanoacrylate adhesive in order to secure the position of the cannula and support pin. When the acrylic has cured, the guide cannula is released from the pin chuck. The distance between the guide cannula and the support pin is measured and a second stainless steel insect pin is cut to the appropriate length. A loop is made at each end of the pin, one loop being placed over the guide cannula and the other over the support pin, forming a bridge. More acrylic is then applied to secure this bridging pin. Care is taken to ensure that no dental acrylic or glue invades the contralateral side of the skull if any further surgical intervention is to be carried out on the contralateral side. The chicks are left to recover in a warm dark incubator, after closing the incision.

To inject, chicks are held in the hand, whilst an injection cannula (27 SWG) is inserted into the guide cannula. A small collar is attached to the injection cannula 7.5 mm from its tip. Accordingly, when the injection cannula is inserted up to the collar, this cannula protrudes 1.5 mm from the end of the guide cannula (2.5 mm below the surface of the brain). The injection into IMHV may then be made.

TECHNIQUE FOR REMOVING IMHV FROM THE CHICK BRAIN
G. Horn

Removal of dorsal part of skull

Decapitate the chick with heavy scissors. The line of transection should be close to the posterior surface of the skull. In any case trim the tissue away from the posterior surface of the skull to expose the foramen magnum. Hold the head in one hand and, with fine surgical pointed scissors (e.g. iris scissors), cut the skin overlying the skull. The cut should be in the midline. Exert gentle lateral traction on the skin flaps to expose the skull. Insert one blade of the scissors into the foramen magnum, directing the point upwards in the midline. Divide the vertical plate of cartilage which forms the posterior wall of the skull (Fig. 1.4a,i,1). Continue the cut onwards in the line of the sagittal suture to the anterior boundary of the cranial cavity (Fig. 1.4a,ii,1 continued). When making this cut ensure that the tip of the lower blade of the scissors inside the skull is directed upwards, to minimize the risk of damaging the underlying cerebral tissue. The next cut is made at right-angles to the first cut (Fig. 1.4*a*,ii,2). Place the lower blade of the scissors approximately 1 mm behind the fronto-parietal suture (Fig. 1.4*a*,ii) and cut the dorsal and lateral surface of the skull (Fig. 1.4*a*,ii,iii,2). Rotate the head and repeat the procedure (Fig. 1.4*a*,ii,3), continuing the cut down the lateral surface of the skull, mirroring the corresponding cut *2* (Fig. 1.4*a*,iii). Rotate the skull so that its anterior end is nearest to you. Insert one blade of the scissors into the anterior end of the previous midline cut (Fig. 1.4*a*,ii,1). The blade should be on the floor of the skull immediately above the roof of the orbit. The blade should remain on the floor of the skull for the cut that is now to be made. Cut round the lateral (Fig. 1.4*a*,iii,4) and posterior wall (Fig. 1.4*a*,i,4) of the skull. Repeat this cut on the other side of the skull (cut *5* corresponding to cut *4* of Fig. 1.4*a*,i; see also Fig. 1.4*a*,i,5). The roof of the skull is now divided into two parts. Use toothed forceps to gently prise the roof of one half of the skull away from the base. Repeat this procedure for the remaining half. The brain is now exposed, lying attached to the base of the skull. The dura mater will probably have been removed with the skull cartilage but if not, gently pull from its attachment to the skull any dura that remains.

Exposure of ventricular surface of hyperstriatum ventrale

The description of the procedure for this exposure refers first to the left hemisphere and reference should be made to Fig. 1.4*b*. The sides of the skull base, with the brain attached, should be grasped in one hand. Using a pair of microsurgery scissors, for example 11 cm spring action microvascular (Adventitia, Weiss, Wigmore Street, London W1H 0DN), cut into the posterior wall of the ventricle (Fig. 1.4*b*,i,ii). The lower blade of the scissors is gently inserted into the ventricle and the cut continued dorsally and medially (Fig. 1.4*b*,iv). The blade of the scissors is then withdrawn. The outer surface of the lower blade of the scissors, used as a blunt spatula, is then lowered into the cerebral fissure and the two hemispheres gently separated by 1 or 2 mm. The lower blade of the scissors is reintroduced into the ventricle and the cut, along the dorso-medial part of the roof, continued forward (Fig. 1.4*b*,iii,v). The cut is continued forward for just over half the length of the hemisphere. As this cut is made, it is helpful to remove the scissors from the ventricle and, using the flat surface of the lower blade again, gently to press the lower part of the medial wall downwards into the cerebral fissure. This procedure allows a clear view of the floor of the ventricle, and also of the medial wall of the right cerebral hemisphere. When the incision has been completed, use the flat surface of the lower blade of the scissors to push laterally the roof of the ventricle. At the dorso-lateral margin of the ventricle, the floor and roof of the ventricle are united (Fig. 1.4*b*,iii upper and lateral boundary of the ventricle, v.1.).

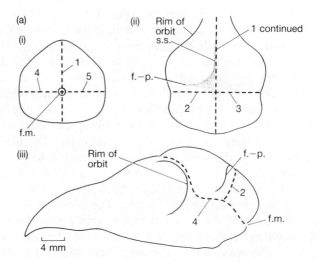

Fig. 1.4 Procedure for removing the left IMHV. Highly diagrammatic. (a) Removal of the skull. The numbered broken lines indicate the sequence of cuts into the skull. (i) Posterior view of the skull, (ii) dorsal view of the skull, (iii) lateral view of head. Scale bar, 4 mm. See also part (b) overleaf.

The roof may then be separated from the floor either by cutting the reflected roof, or by a gentle scraping movement of the blunt surface of the lower blade of the scissors. A diagram of the left hemisphere at this stage of the procedure is shown in Fig. 1.4*b*,vi.

Removal of IMHV

The shiny floor of the ventricle comprises mainly the ventricular surface of the hyperstriatum ventrale. Before cutting, again depress the medial wall of the roof downwards into the cerebral fissure. For the next procedure a sharp scalpel blade with a straight cutting edge is required. The blade should be of a standard used for human surgery, since these are sharpest. The one I use is Swann-Morton stainless steel sterile surgical blade No. 11 (Swann-Morton Ltd, Sheffield S6 2BJ, England). After several IMHVs have been removed it is worth changing the blade if it appears to become blunt. The posterior approximately 1 mm of the exposed ventricular surface comprises part of the posterior neostriatum and most caudal part of the hyperstriatum ventrale. These are removed by the first cut (Fig. 1.4*b*,vii,1). For the second cut (Fig. 1.4*b*,vii,2) the flat surface of the blade should be held in the coronal plane as for cut 1. Cut 2 is placed approximately 1 mm anterior to the midpoint between the anterior and posterior poles of the hemisphere (see Horn *et al.* 1979; Horn 1981). The point of the blade is introduced into the cerebral hemispheres. When the

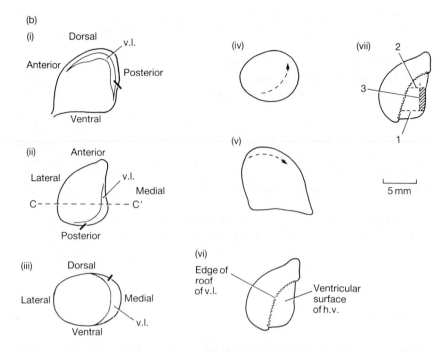

Fig. 1.4 (b) Removal of left IMHV from brain. The short black lines indicate scissor cuts. Broken lines with arrow heads indicate line and direction of cuts. (i) Lateral view of left hemisphere in a parasagittal plane. (ii) Dorsal view of brain indicating region of lateral ventricle (v.1.). (iii) Coronal section of brain along line C--C′ of drawing b,ii. (iv) Posterior view of brain to show line of cut to expose the posterior part of the lateral ventricle. (v) Medial view of left cerebral hemisphere showing line of cut. (vi) Dorsal view of left hemisphere after roof of ventricle has been removed. (vii) Sequence of incisions to remove the left IMHV, the dorsal surface of which is indicated by the hatched zone. Other abbreviations: f.m., foramen magnum; f.-p., fronto-parietal suture; h.v., hyperstriatum ventrale; s.s., sagittal suture.

point is approximately 3 mm below the surface of the hemisphere cut 2 is made; the cut should be extended laterally for approximately 2 mm (i.e. the incision is approximately 2 mm deep). The scalpel blade is then removed from the brain and aligned along the sagittal plane, approximately 0.5 mm lateral to the medial boundary of the exposed floor of the ventricle. The tip of the blade should be just anterior to cut 2. Cut 3 (Fig. 1.4*b*,vii,3) is then made downwards and slightly medially. The incision should begin anteriorly with short strokes as if cutting a slice of bread, and proceed caudally. The 'plate' of cerebral tissue removed is the bulk of IMHV. The sample should be approximately 2–2.4 mm long in the antero-posterior plane, 1.5–2.0 mm deep in the vertical plane and approximately

0.5 mm thick. If the tissue that is removed exceeds 1 mm thickness it will contain part of the neostriatum. The tissue should weigh between 2.0 and 2.5 mg.

A similar procedure is used to remove the right IMHV. If both IMHVs are to be removed, the procedure described above is varied slightly. After exposing the floor of the ventricle of the left hemisphere (i.e. after the procedure which results in a view similar to that illustrated in Fig. 4*b*), the floor of the right cerebral ventricle is exposed. After placing cut 2 (Fig. 4*b*,vii,2), the blade of the scalpel is rotated 180° and the same incision made in the right hemisphere. After completing the procedure for removing the left IMHV the right IMHV is removed. After some practice the whole procedure may be completed within 4 minutes of decapitating the chick.

The IMHV extends roughly from A 6.4 to A 9.6 in the stereotaxic atlas of the two-week chick brain constructed by Kuenzel and Masson (1988). This corrects for the larger size of the older brain and for shrinkage in fixation (Horn *et al.* 1979).

REFERENCES

Andrew, R. J. (1963). Effects of testosterone on the behaviour of the domestic chick. *Journal of Comparative and Physiological Psychology*, **56**, 933–40.
Andrew, R. J. (1964*a*). Vocalization in chicks, and the concept of 'stimulus contrast'. *Animal Behaviour*, **12**, 64–76.
Andrew, R. J. (1964*b*). The development of adult responses from responses given during imprinting by the domestic chick. *Animal Behaviour*, **12**, 542–8.
Andrew, R. J. (1966). Precocious adult behaviour in the young chick. *Animal Behaviour*, **14**, 485–500.
Andrew, R. J. (1967). Intracranial self-stimulation in the chick. *Nature*, **213**, 847–8.
Andrew, R. J. (1969*a*). The effect of testosterone on avian vocalizations. In *Bird vocalizations*, R. A. Hinde, pp. 97–130. Cambridge University Press.
Andrew, R. J. (1969*b*). Intracranial self-stimulation in the chick and the causation of emotional behaviour. *Annals of the New York Academy of Sciences*, **159**, 625–39.
Andrew, R. J. (1972). Changes in search behaviour in male and female chicks, following different doses of testosterone. *Animal Behaviour*, **20**, 741–50.
Andrew, R. J. (1975). Effects of testosterone on the calling of the domestic chick in a strange environment. *Animal Behaviour*, **23**, 169–78.
Andrew, R. J. (1983). Specific short-latency effects of oestradiol and testosterone on distractibility and memory formation in the young domestic chick. In *Hormones and behaviour in higher vertebrates*, (ed. J. Balthazart, E. Pröve, and R. Gilles), pp. 463–73. Springer-Verlag, Berlin.
Andrew, R. J. (1985). The temporal structure of memory formation. *Perspectives in Ethology*, **6**, 219–59.

Andrew, R. J. and Brennan, A. (1985). Sharply timed and lateralised events at time of establishment of long-term memory. *Physiology and Behaviour*, **34**, 547–56.

Andrew, R. J. and Clayton, D. A. (1979). Effects of testosterone on investigation of stimulus change by the domestic chick. *Behaviour*, **69**, 135–44.

Andrew, R. J., Clifton, P. G., and Gibbs, M. E. (1981). Enhancement of effectiveness of learning by testosterone in domestic chicks. *Journal of Comparative and Physiological Psychology*, **95**, 406–17.

Andrew, R. J. and de Lanerolle, N. (1974). The effects of muting lesions on emotional behaviour and behaviour normally associated with calling. *Brain, Behaviour and Evolution*, **10**, 377–99.

Andrew, R. J. and Oades, R. D. (1973). Escape, hiding and freezing behaviour elicited by electrical stimulation of the chick diencephalon. *Brain, Behaviour and Evolution*, **8**, 191–210.

Andrew, R. J. and Rogers, L. J. (1972). Testosterone, search behaviour and persistence. *Nature*, **237**, 343–6.

Archer, J. (1973). The influence of testosterone on chick behaviour in novel environments. *Behavioural Biology*, **8**, 93–108.

Archer, J. (1974*a*). The effects of testosterone on the distractibility of chicks by irrelevant and relevant stimuli. *Animal Behaviour*, **22**, 397–404.

Archer, J. (1974*b*). Testosterone and behaviour during extinction in chicks. *Animal Behaviour*, **22**, 650–5.

Ayiteh-Smith, E. and Addae-Mensah, I. (1983). Effects of wisanine and dihydrowisanine on aggressive behaviour in chicks. *European Journal of Pharmacology*, **95**, 139–41.

Bateson, P. P. G. (1964). Changes in chicks' responses to novel moving objects over the sensitive period for imprinting. *Animal Behaviour*, **12**, 479–89.

Bateson, P. (1979). Brief exposure to a novel stimulus during imprinting in chicks and its influence on subsequent preferences. *Animal Learning and Behaviour*, **7**, 259–62.

Bateson, P. P. G. and Reese, E. P. (1968). Reinforcing properties of conspicuous objects before imprinting has occurred. *Psychonomic Science*, **19**, 379–80.

Bateson, P. P. G. and Wainwright, A. A. P. (1972). The effects of prior exposure to light on the imprinting process in domestic chicks. *Behaviour*, **42**, 279–90.

Bell, G. A. and Gibbs, M. E. (1977). Interhemispheric engram transfer in chick. *Neuroscience Letters*, **13**, 163–8.

Bolhuis, J. J. and Johnson, M. H. (1988). Effects of response-contingency and stimulus presentation schedule on imprinting in the chick (*Gallus gallus domesticus*). *Journal of Comparative Psychology*, **102**, 61–5.

Bolhuis, J. J., Johnson, M. H., and Horn, G. (1985). Effects of early experience on the development of filial preferences in the domestic chick. *Developmental Psychobiology*, **18**, 299–308.

Bolhuis, J. J., McCabe B. J., and Horn, G. (1986). Androgens and imprinting: differential effects of testosterone on filial preference in the domestic chick. *Behavioral Neuroscience*, **100**, 51–6.

Bolhuis, J. J. and Trooster, W. J. (1988). Reversibility revisited: stimulus-dependent stability of filial preferences in the chick. *Animal Behaviour*, **36**, 668–74.

Cherkin, A. (1972). Retrograde amnesia in the chick: resistance to the reminder effect. *Physiology and Behavior*, **8**, 948–55.

Cherkin, A. and Lee-Teng, E. (1965). Interruption by halothane of memory consolidation in chicks. *Federal Proceedings*, **24**, 328.

Cherkin, A., Meinecke, R. O., and Garman, M. W. (1975). Retrograde enhancement of memory by mild flurothyl treatment in the chick. *Physiology and Behaviour*, **14**, 151–8.

Cipolla-Neto, J., Horn, G., and McCabe, B. J. (1979). A method for recording unit activity from the brain of the freely moving chick. *Journal of Physiology*, **295**, 8–9P.

Clayton, D. A. and Andrew, R. J. (1979). Phases of inhibition and response during investigation of stimulus change by the domestic chick. *Behaviour*, **69**, 36–56.

Clifton, P. G. and Andrew, R. J. (1983). The role of stimulus size and colour in the elicitation of testosterone facilitated aggressive and sexual responses in the domestic chick. *Animal Behaviour*, **31**, 878–86.

Clifton, P. G. and Andrew, R. J. (1987). Gonadal steroids and the extinction of conditioned taste aversions in young domestic fowl. *Physiology and Behaviour*, **39**, 27–31.

Clifton, P. G. and Andrew, R. J. (1989). Contrasting effects of pre- and post-hatch exposure to gonadal steroids on the development of vocal, sexual and aggressive behaviour of young domestic fowl. *Hormones and Behaviour*, **23**, 572–89.

Clifton, P. G., Andrew, R. J., and Gibbs, M. E. (1982). Limited period of action of testosterone on memory formation in the chick. *Journal of Comparative and Physiological Psychology*, **96**, 212–22.

Cohen, R. S., Blomberg, F., Berzins, K., and Siekevitz, P. (1977). The structure of post-synaptic densities isolated from dog cerebral cortex: I. Overall morphology and protein composition. *Journal of Cell Biology*, **74**, 181–203.

Collias, N. E. and Joos, M. (1953). The spectrographic analysis of sound signals of the domestic fowl. *Behaviour*, **5**, 175–88.

Cotman, C. W. and Taylor, D. (1972). Isolation and structural studies on synaptic complexes from rat brain. *Journal of Cell Biology*, **55**, 696–711.

Crowe, S. F., Ng, K. T., and Gibbs, M. E. (1989). Effect of retraining trials on memory consolidation in weakly reinforced learning. *Pharmacology Biochemistry and Behavior*, **33**, 889–94.

Csillag, A., Bourne, R. C., Kalman, M., Boxer, M. I., and Stewart, M. G. (1989). Opioid receptors in the brain of the domestic chick (*Gallus domesticus*): (^{3}H) Naloxone binding *in vitro* followed by quantitative autoradiography. *Brain Research*, **479**, 391–6.

Csillag, A., Bourne, R. C., Patel, S., Stewart, M. G., and Tombol, T. (1989). Localization of GABA-like immunoreactivity in the ectostriatum of domestic chicks: GABA immunocytochemistry combined with Golgi impregnation. *Journal of Neurocytology*, **18**, 369–79.

Csillag, A., Stewart, M. G., and Curtis, E. M. (1987). GABA-ergic structures in the chick forebrain: autoradiography combined with GABA immunocytochemistry. *Brain Research*, **437**, 283–97.

Curtis, E. M. and Stewart, M. G. (1986). Development of GABA-immunoreactivity in chick hyperstriatum ventrale and cerebellum: light and electron microscopical observations. *Developmental Brain Research*, **30**, 189–99.

Curtis, E. M., Stewart, M. G., and King, T. S. (1989). Quantitation of synaptic, neuronal and glial development in the intermediate and medial hyperstriatum ventrale (IMHV) of the chick *Gallus domesticus*, pre- and post- hatch. *Developmental Brain Research*, **48**, 105–18.

Davies, D. C. and Payne, J. M. (1982). Variation in chick sex ratios during hatching. *Animal Behaviour*, **30**, 931–2.

Davies, D. C. and Payne, J. M. (1989). Amnesia of a passive avoidance task due to the β_2-adrenoceptor antagonist ICI 118551. *Pharmacology, Biochemistry and Behaviour*, **32**, 187–90.

Davis, J. L. and Coates, S. R. (1978). Classical conditioning of the nictitating membrane response in the domestic chick. *Physiological Psychology*, **6**, 7–10.

Davis, J. L., Pico, R. M., and Cherkin, A. (1982). Arginine vasopressin enhances memory retroactively in chicks. *Behavioural and Neural Biology*, **35**, 242–50.

Davis, S. J. and Fischer, G. J. (1978). Chick colour approach preferences are altered by cold stress: colour pecking and approach preferences are the same. *Animal Behaviour*, **26**, 259–64.

Dawkins, M. S. (1971). Perceptual changes in chicks: another look at the 'searching image' concept. *Animal Behaviour*, **19**, 556–74.

De Lanerolle, N. C. (1978). The effect of amphetamine on the behaviour of decerebrate domestic chicks. *Comparative and Biochemical Physiology*, **50c**, 75–7.

De Lanerolle, N. C. and Andrew, R. J. (1974). Midbrain structures controlling vocalization in the domestic chick. *Brain, Behaviour and Evolution*, **10**, 354–76.

De Lanerolle, N. C. and Millam, J. R. (1980). Dopamine, chick behaviour and states of attention. *Journal of Comparative and Physiological Psychology*, **94**, 346–52.

De Vaus, J. E., Gibbs, M. E., and Ng, K. T. (1980). Effects of social isolation on memory formation. *Behavioural and Neural Biology*, **29**, 473–89.

Dunkley, P. R., Heath, J. W., Harrison, S. M., Jarvie, P. E., Glenfield, P. J., and Rostas, J. A. P. (1988). A rapid Percoll gradient procedure for isolation of synaptosomes directly from an S1 fraction: homogeneity and morphology of subcellular fractions. *Brain Research*, **441**, 59–71.

Ettinger, R. H. and Thompson, R. W. (1978). The role of dopaminergic systems in the mediation of tonic immobility (animal hypnosis) in chickens. *Bulletin of the Psychonomic Society*, **12**, 301–2.

Franchina, J. J., Dyer, A. B., Zaccaro, S. J., and Schulman, A. H. (1986). Socially facilitated drinking behaviour in chicks (*Gallus domesticus*): relative effects of drive and stimulus mechanisms. *Animal Learning and Behaviour*, **14**, 218–22.

Gagliardi, G. J. and Gallup, G. G. (1976). Effect of different pupil to size ratios on tonic immobility in chickens. *Bulletin of the Psychonomic Society*, **6**, 58–60.

Gagliardi, G. J. and Thompson, R. W. (1977). Cholinergic blockade and tonic immobility in chickens. *Bulletin of the Psychonomic Society*, **9**, 343–5.

Gaioni, S. J., Hoffman, H. S., DePaulo, P., and Stratton, V. N. (1978). Imprinting in older ducklings: some tests of a reinforcement model. *Animal Learning and Behavior*, **6**, 19–26.

Gallup, G. G. (1977). Tonic immobility: the role of fear and predation. *Psychological Record*, **1**, 41–61.

Gallup, G. G. and Suarez, S. D. (1980). An ethological analysis of open-field behaviour in chickens. *Animal Behaviour*, **28**, 368–78.

Gaston, K. E. (1977). An illness-induced conditional aversion in domestic chicks: one-trial learning with a long delay of reinforcement. *Behavioral Biology*, **20**, 441–53.

Genovese, R. F. and Browne, M. P. (1978). Sickness-induced learning in chicks. *Behavioral Biology*, **24**, 68–76.

Gerbrandt, L. K., Eckhardt, M. J., Davis, J. L., and Cherkin, A. (1977). Retrograde enhancement of memory with flurothyl: electrophysiological effects in chicks. *Physiology and Behaviour*, **19**, 729–34.

Gibbs, M. E. and Ng, K. T. (1977). Psychobiology of memory: towards a model of memory formation. *Biobehavioral Reviews*, **1**, 113–36.

Gibbs, M. E., Richdale, A. L., and Ng, K. T. (1987). Effects of excess intracranial aminoacids on memory: a behavioural survey. *Neuroscience and Biobehavioural Reviews*, **11**, 331–9.

Gillan, D. J. (1979). Learned suppression of ingestion: role of discriminative stimuli, ingestive responses and aversive tastes. *Journal of Experimental Psychology : Animal Behavioral Processes*, **5**, 258–72.

Gillette, K., Martin, G. M., and Bellingham, W. P. (1980). Differential use of food and water cues in the formation of conditioned aversions by domestic chicks (*Gallus gallus*). *Journal of Experimental Psychology : Animal Behavioral Processes*, **6**, 99–111.

Glauert, A. (1974). *Techniques in electron microscopy*, Vol. 3, Part 1. North-Holland, Amsterdam.

Gottlieb, G. (1965). Imprinting in relation to parental and species identification by avian neonates. *Journal of Comparative Physiology and Psychology*, **59**, 345–56.

Gurd, J. W., Gordon-Weeks, P. R., and Evans, W. H. (1982). Biochemical and morphological comparison of post-synaptic densities prepared from rat, hamster and monkey brains by phase partitioning. *Journal of Neurochemistry*, **39**, 1117–24.

Hale, C. and Green, L. (1988). Effect of early ingestional experiences on the acquisition of appropriate food selection by young chicks. *Animal Behaviour*, **36**, 211–24.

Hoffman, H. S. and Segal, M. (1983). Biological factors in social attachments: a new view of a basic phenomenon. In *Advances in analysis of behaviour*, Vol. 3 (ed. M. D. Zeiler and P. Harzem), pp. 41–61. John Wiley, London.

Hoffman, H. S. Ratner, A. M., and Eiserer, L. A. (1972). Role of visual imprinting in the emergence of specific visual attachments in ducklings. *Journal of Comparative and Physiological Psychology*, **81**, 399–409.

Hogan, J. A. (1966). An experimental study of conflict and fear: an analysis of behaviour of young chicks towards a mealworm. *Behaviour*, **27**, 273–89.

Horn, G. (1981). Neural mechanisms of learning: an analysis of imprinting in the domestic chick. *Proceedings of the Royal Society of London, Series B*, **213**, 101–37.

Horn, G. (1985). *Memory. Imprinting and the brain*. Clarendon Press, Oxford.

Horn, G. and McCabe, B. J. (1974). A method for recording with minimal artifact the e.e.g. of unanaesthetised, newly hatched chicks. *Journal of Physiology*, **245**, 38–9P.

Horn, G., McCabe, B. J., and Bateson, P. P. G. (1979). An autoradiographic study of the chick brain after imprinting. *Brain Research*, **168**, 361–73.

Hunter, A and Stewart, M. G. (1989). The synaptic development of the lobus parolfactorius of the chick, *Gallus domesticus*. *Experimental Brain Research*, **78**, 425–36.

Johnson, M. H., Bolhuis, J. J., and Horn, G. (1985). Interaction between acquired preferences and developing predispositions during imprinting. *Animal Behaviour*, **33**, 1000–6.

Johnson, M. H. and Horn, G. (1986). Dissociation of recognition memory and associative learning by a restricted lesion of the chick forebrain. *Neuropsychologia*, **24**, 329–40.

Johnson, M. H. and Horn, G. (1987). The role of a restricted region of the chick forebrain in the recognition of individual conspecifics. *Behavioral Brain Research*, **23**, 269–75.

Jones, R. B. (1977). Sex and strain differences in the open-field responses of the domestic chick. *Applied Animal Ethology*, **3**, 255–61.

Jones, R. B. and Black, A. J. (1979). Behavioural responses of the domestic chick to blood. *Behavioural and Neural Biology*, **27**, 319–29.

Jones, R. B. and Black, A. J. (1980). Feeding behaviour of domestic chicks in a novel environment: effects of food deprivation and sex. *Behavioral Processes*, **5**, 173–83.

Klein, R. M. and Andrew, R. J. (1986). Distraction, decisions and persistence in runway tests using the domestic chick. *Behaviour*, **99**, 139–56.

Kovach, J. K. (1971). Effectiveness of different colours in the elicitation and development of approach behaviour in chicks. *Behaviour*, **38**, 154–68.

Kuenzel, W. J. and Masson, M. (1988). *A stereotaxic atlas of the brain of the chick* (Gallus domesticus). Johns Hopkins University Press, Baltimore and London.

Lecanuet, J. P., Alexinsky, T. and Chapouthier, G. (1976). The following response in chicks: conditions for the resistance of consolidation to a disruptive agent. *Behavioural Biology*, **16**, 291–304.

Lee-Teng, E. and Sherman, S. M. (1966). Memory consolidation of one-trial learning in chicks. *Proceedings of the National Academy of Sciences*, **56**, 926–31.

McCabe, B. J., Cipolla-Neto, J., Horn, G., and Bateson, P. P. G. (1982). Amnestic effects of bilateral lesions placed in the hyperstriatum ventrale of the chick after imprinting. *Experimental Brain Research*, **48**, 13–21.

McCabe, B. J., Horn, G., and Bateson, P. P. G. (1981). Effects of restricted lesions of the chick forebrain on the acquisition of filial preferences during imprinting. *Brain Research*, **205**, 29–37.

Machlis, L., Dodd, P. W. D., and Fentress, J. C. (1985). The pooling fallacy: problems arising when individuals contribute more than an observation to the data set. *Zeitschrift fur Tierpsychologie*, **68**, 201–14.

Mark, R. F. and Watts, M. E. (1971). Drug inhibition of memory formation in chickens. Long-term memory. *Proceedings of the Royal Society of London, Series B*, **178**, 439–54.

Martin, P. and Bateson, P. P. G. (1986). *Measuring behaviour*. Cambridge University Press.

Martin, J. T. and van Wimersma Greidanus, T. B. (1978). Imprinting behavior: influence of vasopressin and ACTH analogues. *Psychoneuroendocrinology*, **3**, 261–9.

Matus, A. I. and Taff-Jones, D. H. (1978). Morphology and molecular composition of isolated post-synaptic junctional structure. *Proceedings of the Royal Society of London, Series B*, **203**, 135–51.

Mayer, S. and Hailman, J. P. (1976). Similarity of approach a ıd pecking preferences for spectral stimuli in domestic chicks: absence of a mirror-image relation. *Journal of Comparative and Physiological Psychology*, **90**, 185–9.

Mench, J. A. and Andrew, R. J. (1986). Lateralization of a food searclı task in the domestic chick. *Behavioural and Neural Biology*, **46**, 107–14.

Meyer, M. E. and Frank, L. H. (1970). Food imprinting in the domestic chick: a reconsideration. *Psychonomic Science*, **19**, 43–5.

Miles, F. A. (1972). Centrifugal control of the avian retina I: Receptive field properties of retinal ganglion cells. *Brain Research*, **48**, 65–92.

Moltz, H. and Stettner, L. J. (1961). The influence of patterned-light deprivation on the critical period for imprinting. *Journal of Comparative and Physiological Psychology*, **54**, 279–83.

Montevecchi, W. A. and Noel, P. E. (1978). Temporal effects of mirror-image stimulation on pecking and peeping in isolate, pair- and group-reared domestic chicks. *Behavioral Biology*, **23**, 531–5.

Murakami, K., Gordon-Weeks, P. R., and Rose, S. P. R. (1986). Isolation of post-synaptic densities from day old chicken brain. *Journal of Neurochemistry*, **46**, 340–8.

Ng, K. T. and Gibbs, M. E. (1987). Less-than-expected variability in evidence for three stages in memory formation: a response. *Behavioral Neuroscience*, **101**, 126–30.

Ng, K. T. and Gibbs, M. E. (1988). A biological model for memory formation. In *Information processing by the brain* (ed. H. Markowitsch). Hans Huber, Toronto.

Oades, R. D. and Messent, P. R. (1981). Testosterone administration in chicks affects responding in the presence of task irrelevant stimulus changes. *Behavioral and Neural Biology*, **33**, 93–100.

Panksepp, J., Meeker, R., and Bean, N. J. (1980). The neurochemical control of crying. *Pharmacology and Biochemistry of Behavior*, **12**, 437–43.

Panksepp, J., Normansell, L., Siviy, S., Rossi, J., and Zolovick, A. J. (1984). Casomorphins reduce separation distress in chicks. *Peptides*, **5**, 829–31.

Patel, S. and Stewart, M. G. (1988). Changes in dendritic spine structure in the medial hyperstriatum ventrale of the domestic chick, *Gallus domesticus*, following passive avoidance training. *Brain Research*, **449**, 34–46.

Patterson, T. A., Alvarado, M. C., Warner, I. T., Bennett, E. C., and Rosenzwieg, M. R. (1986). Memory stages and brain asymmetry in chick learning. *Behavioural Neuroscience*, **100**, 856–65.

Patterson, T. A., Schulteis, G., Alvarado, M. C., Martinez, J. L. Jr., Bennett, E. L., Rosenzweig, M. R., and Hruby, V. J. (1989). Influence of opioid peptides on memory formation in the chick. *Behavioral Neuroscience*, **103**, 429–37.

Rashid, N. and Andrew, R. J. (1989). Right hemisphere advantage for topographical orientation in the domestic chick. *Neuropsychologia*, **27**, 937–48.

Reymond, E. and Rogers, L. J. (1981). Diurnal variation in learning performance in chickens. *Animal Behaviour*, **29**, 241–8.

Roberts, S. (1987). Less-than-expected variability in evidence for three stages in memory formation. *Behavioral Neuroscience*, **101**, 1, 120–5.

Robinson, P. W., Foster, D. F., and Bridges, C. V. (1976). Errorless learning in newborn chicks. *Animal Learning and Behaviour*, **4**, 266–8.

Rogers, L. J. (1982). Light experience and asymmetry of brain function in chickens. *Nature*, **297**, 223–5:

Rogers, L. J. (1986). Lateralization of learning in chicks. *Advances in the Study of Behaviour*, **16**, 147–89.

Rogers, L. J. and Anson, J. M. (1979). Lateralization of function in the chicken forebrain. *Pharmacology, Biochemistry and Behaviour*, **9**, 735–40.

Rogers, L. J., Oettinger, R., Szer, J., and Mark, R. F. (1977). Separate chemical inhibition of long-term and short-term memory: contrasting effects of cyclohex- imide, ouabain and ethacrynic acid on various learning tasks in chickens. *Proceedings of the Royal Society of London*, **196**, 171–95.

Roper, T. J. and Cook, S. E. (1989). Responses of chicks to brightly coloured insect prey. *Behaviour* , **110**, 276–93.

Roper, T. J. and Redston, S. (1987). Conspicuousness of distasteful prey affects the strength and durability of one-trial avoidance learning. *Animal Behaviour*, **35**, 739–47.

Rose, S. P. R. and Jork, R. (1987). Long-term memory formation in chicks is blocked by 2-deoxygalactose, a fucose analogue. *Behavioural and Neural Biology*, **48**, 246–58.

Rostas, J. A. P., Brent, V. A., and Guldner, F. H. (1984). The maturation of post-synaptic densities in chicken forebrain. *Neuroscience Letters*, **45**, 297–304.

Rostas, J. A. P., Guldner, F. H., and Dunkley, P. R. (1983). Maturation of post- synaptic densities in chicken forebrain. In *Molecular pathology of nerve and muscle: noxious agents and genetic lesions* (ed. A. D. Kidman, J. K. Tomkins, N. A. Cooper, and C. Morris), pp. 67–79. Humana Press, New Jersey.

Rostas, J. A. P. and Jeffrey, P. L. (1981). Maturation of synapses in chicken forebrain. *Neuroscience Letters*, **25**, 299–304.

Rostas, J. A. P., Pesin, R. H., Kelly, P. T., and Cotman, C. W. (1979). Protein and glycoprotein composition of synaptic junctions prepared from discrete synaptic regions and different species. *Brain Research*, **168**, 151–67.

Sanberg, P. R. (1983). Dopaminergic and cholinergic influences on motor behavi- our in chickens. *Journal of Comparative Psychology*, **97**, 59–68.

Schaeffer, H. R. and Hess, E. H. (1959). Colour preferences in imprinting objects. *Zeitschrift fur Tierpsychologie*, **16**, 161–72.

Schuler, W. and Hesse, E. (1985). On the function of warning colouration: a black and yellow pattern inhibits prey attack by naive domestic chicks. *Behavioral Ecology and Sociobiology*, **16**, 249–55.

Sedlaçek, J. (1962). Notes on the characteristics of the temporary connection in chick embryos. *Physiologia Bohemoslovenica*, **11**, 307–18.

Sedlaçek, J. (1964). Further findings on the conditions of formation of the temporary connection in chick embryos. *Physiologia Bohemoslovenica*, **13**, 411–19.

Sluckin, W. (1972). *Imprinting and early learning*. Methuen, London.

Spalding, D. A. (1973). Instinct, with original observations on young animals. *Macmillans Magazine*, **27**, 282–93. Reprinted in 1954, *British Journal of Animal Behaviour*, **2**, 1–11.

Stephenson, R. M. (1981). Memory processing in the domestic chick (*Gallus gallus*): a psychopharmacological investigation. D. Phil thesis. University of Sussex, UK.

Stewart, M. G., Chmielowska, J., Kalman, M., Bourne, R. C., Csillag, A., and Stanford, D. (1988). Autoradiographic localization of ³H-muscimol receptors in the chick CNS. *Brain Research*, **456**, 387–91.

Stewart, M. G., Rose, S. P. R., King, T. S., Gabbott, P. L. A., and Bourne. R. (1984). Hemisphere asymmetry of synapses in chick medial hyperstriatum ventrale following passive avoidance training: a stereological study. *Developmental Brain Research*, **12**, 261–9.

Suboski, M. D. (1987). Environmental variables and releasing-valence transfer in stimulus-directed pecking of chicks. *Behavioural and Neural Biology*, **47**, 262–74.

Suboski, M. D. and Bartashunas, C. J. (1984). Mechanisms for social transmission of pecking preference to neonatal chicks. *Journal of the Experimental Analysis of Behaviour*, **10**, 182–94.

Ten Cate, C. (1986). Does behaviour contingent stimulus movement enhance filial imprinting in Japanese quail? *Developmental Psychobiology*, **19**, 607–14.

Thompson, R. W. and Joseph, S. (1978). The effect of norepinephine on tonic immobility in chickens. *Bulletin of the Psychonomic Society*, **12**, 123–4.

Tombol, T., Csillag, A., and Stewart, M. G. (1988*a*). Cell types of the hyperstriatum ventrale of the domestic chicken, *Gallus domesticus*: a Golgi study. *Journal für Hirnforschung*, **29**, 319–34.

Tombol, T., Csillag, A., and Stewart, M. G. (1988*b*). Cell types of the paleostriatal complex of the domestic chicken, *Gallus domesticus*: a Golgi study. *Journal für Hirnforschung*, **29**, 493–507.

Tombol, T., Magloczky, Z., Stewart, M. G., and Csillag, A. (1988*c*). The structure of the chicken ectostriatum: I. Golgi study. *Journal für Hirnforschung*, **29**, 525–46.

Turner, E. R. A. (1964). Social feeding in birds, *Behaviour*, **24**, 1–45.

Vallortigaro, G. and Zanforlin, M. (1986). Position learning in chicks. *Behavioural Processes*, **12**, 23–32.

Valverde, F. (1970). The Golgi Method. In *Contemporary methods in neuroanatomy*. (ed. W. J. Nauta and S. O. E. Ebbesson), pp. 12–31. Springer-Verlag, Berlin.

Venault, P., Chapouthier, G., Prado de Carvalho, L., Simiaud, J., Moore, M., Dodd, R. H., and Rossier, J. (1986). Benzodiazepine impairs and beta-carboline enhances performance in learning and memory tasks. *Nature*, **321**, 864–6.

Wasserman, E. A. (1973). Pavlovian conditioning with heat reinforcement produces stimulus-directed pecking in chicks. *Science*, **181**, 875–7.

Weinberger, R. P. and Rostas, J. A. P. (1988). Developmental changes in protein phosphorylation in chicken forebrain: II. Calmodulin stimulated phosphorylation. *Developmental Brain Research*, **43**, 259–72.

Woodruff, G. and Starr, M. D. (1978). Autoshaping of initial feeding and drinking reactions in newly hatched chicks. *Animal Learning and Behaviour*, **6**, 265–72.

Youngren, O. M. and Phillips, R. E. (1978). A stereotaxic atlas of brain of three-day-old domestic chick. *Journal of Comparative Neurology*, **181**, 567–99.

Zanforlin, M. (1981). Visual perception of complex forms (anomalous surfaces) in chicks. *Italian Journal of Psychology*, **8**, 1–16.

Zolman, J. F., Hall, J. A., and Sahley, C. L. (1977). Effects of isolation rearing on keypecking in young domestic chicks. *Bulletin of the Psychonomic Society*, **10**, 506–8.

PART II

Anatomy

Introduction

R. J. Andrew

The differences between the organization of the forebrain in birds and mammals have made it difficult in the past to extrapolate mammalian findings to the chick. This may have had its advantages, in that initial search for structures important in learning was not restricted by hypotheses currently popular in mammalian work. However, our understanding of the avian forebrain is now sufficiently advanced (Dubbeldam, Chapter 2) as not only to allow profitable comparison with mammals, but also to make clear that the different organization of the forebrain in birds and mammals makes them complementary as experimental material.

The existence in birds of two major divisions, into one or other of which most forebrain structures fall (the Wulst, and the structures derived from the dorsal ventricular ridge), appears at first sight to be quite different from anything found in mammals. However, as Dubbeldam shows, in the case of the visual projections much the same division can be recognized in mammals and birds, with the avian pathway from retina to thalamus to Wulst corresponding to the mammalian thalamo–striate system, and the avian retinal–tecto–rotundo–ectostriatal pathway (together with the associated neostriatal projection: Chapter 3) to the mammalian colliculo–thalamo–temporal pathway. It remains to be seen whether all sensory modalities are divided in this way in birds : somatosensory inputs are, but auditory projections may lack Wulst representation in the strict sense.

The striking separation of the two divisions of the visual projections in birds has provoked many attempts to study their functioning in isolation (Güntürkün, Chapter 3). The surprising conclusion seems to be that either division by itself can support standard visual discrimination tasks using frontal vision with remarkable (but not complete) success.

It may be time to take the known anatomy of the two divisions into account in framing hypotheses. In both Anuran amphibia (Ingle 1982) and mammals (Dean *et al.* 1989), there is evidence that the optic tectum (superior colliculus) is responsible both for targeting responses, such as prey catching, and for avoidance of large looming objects. Any projection from the tectum is thus likely to carry information about the presence of such stimuli and the likelihood of responses to them. The potential independence in birds of the functioning of midbrain visual systems is made clear by their ability to perform visually guided behaviour in the absence of the forebrain (Chapter 3). On the other hand, the extensive projections of the visual Wulst back on to the thalamic and visual nuclei and the tectum suggests that the Wulst plays an important part in modulating the functioning of thalamic and midbrain visual structures. Its connections would allow this to be done on the basis of information reaching it directly, and also by relay from the rotundal route.

Both of the main learning tasks used in the chick employ stimuli of a sort to which tectal mechanisms are likely to be sensitive. It will be of great interest to discover what roles the two divisions of the visual system in the forebrain play in imprinting and the bead pecking task. An extreme possibility is raised by Rogers (Chapter 20), who presents evidence which suggests that, under some conditions at least, the visual Wulst is relatively inactive in the young chick.

When we turn to the anatomical differences between birds and mammals, it becomes clear that the most important of these all reflect two different principles of segregation of categories of neurons. As Dubbeldam notes (Chapter 2), the whole of input structures such as nu. basalis must correspond (at the most) to layers 3 and 4 of mammalian cortex. This unexpected segregation holds for the Wulst as well: IHA, like the ectostriatum, may be compared to layer 4. The principle is particularly obvious for the rostral and intermediate archistriatum, which is the main output relay for sensory and motor structures derived from the dorsal and ventricular ridge. It is as though much of layers 5 and 6 of the whole mammalian sensorimotor and sensory cortex had been brought together in a single block, far removed from the site of corresponding layers 2 to 4.

Segregation is perhaps also more complete in birds for structures involved in particular levels of processing. The hyperstriatum ventrale (HV), within which lies the IMHV which plays such a central part in studies reported in this book, is a clearly demarcated slab of tissue lying between the Wulst and the main derivatives of the dorsal ventricular ridge. Dubbeldam (Chapter 2) demonstrates a pattern which is remarkably standard across modalities: within the zone of the HV which receives visual inputs (for example) the two major visual routes finally converge. Return projections allow the HV to affect the functioning of both routes and (presumably) to transfer information between them. The HV has a major output via the archistriatum, which may affect sensory or motor structures, or more probably both; the connections of IMHV are more specifically considered in Chapter 8. It will be interesting to see whether multimodal projection areas (such as are described in Chapter 3) follow the same pattern with respect to HV.

In view of the unambiguous and profound involvement of the IMHV in learning, the identification of structures in mammals corresponding to it, and to the HV as a whole, becomes important. Horn (1985, p. 252) compares IMHV with prefrontal and cingulate cortex; prefrontal connections to the basal ganglia are matched, as he notes, by projections from

IMHV to the palaeostriatum augmentatum (PA). Such connections are standard for areas of the HV (Chapter 2); this suggests a wider comparison of HV with the cortical parts of the circuits from cortex to basal ganglia which feed back to restricted sections of the cortical areas of origin via the thalamus (Alexander *et al.* 1986). On this argument HV might correspond in addition to prefrontal, to orbitofrontal areas, and in addition to cingulate, to areas of temporal cortex. This is given particular interest by the finding (Rose, Chapter 10; Stewart, Chapter 11) that both PA and lobus parolfactorius (LPO) are involved in learning and show learning-induced change. The PA and LPO correspond to the mammalian basal ganglia (corpus striatum, Chapter 2). It is perhaps unexpected to find the basal ganglia involved in such functions, but there is increasing evidence for the involvement of the basal ganglia *sensu lato* in cognitive processes (Alexander *et al.* 1986), and for their association with forebrain structures connected to amygdala and hippocampus.

It seems likely that other forebrain structures will be found to be involved in learning in the chick. Stephenson (Chapter 16) provides evidence for the involvement of a posterior structure, which could be either hippocampus or the posterior pole of the neostriatum. It seems certain that the hippocampus will play a significant part in learning. Dubbeldam notes that HV connections with the hippocampus (and with the amygdalar section of the archistriatum) need further investigation. However, perhaps the biggest gap in our knowledge is of structures corresponding to entorhinal cortex and subiculum in the bird.

Finally, a site of permanent storage, separate from IMHV (S': Horn, Chapter 8) remains to be identified. Candidates are suggested in later chapters (LPO, Rose, Chapter 10; lateral neostriatum, Davies, Chapter 12). The lateral neostriatum has the interesting property of receiving from the HV and projecting to the output structures of the archistriatum.

REFERENCES

Alexander, G. E., Delong, M. R., and Strick, P. L. (1986). Parallel organization of functionally segregated circuits linking basal ganglia and cortex. *Annual Review of Neuroscience*, **9**, 357–81.

Dean, P., Redgrave, P., and Westby, G. W. M. (1989). Event or emergency? Two response systems in the mammalian superior colliculus. *Trends in Neurosciences*, **12**, 137–46.

Horn, G. (1985). *Memory, imprinting and the brain*. Oxford University Press.

Ingle, D. J. (1981). Brain mechanisms of visual localization by frogs and toads. In *Advances in vertebrate neuroethology* (ed. J. P. Ewert, R. R. Capranica, and D. J. Ingle), pp. 177–226. Plenum, New York.

2

The avian and mammalian forebrain: correspondences and differences

J. L. Dubbeldam

Birds and mammals make up the two classes of homoiothermic verte-brates. The two groups have many features in common, but show striking differences in other aspects. Both groups possess large brains, but the forebrains have completely different appearances in cross-section. The design of the avian forebrain is basically similar to that in reptiles, whereas the organization of the mammalian neocortex is novel. This chapter provides a general outline of the avian forebrain, which may serve as a framework for the following chapters. The organization of specific regions of the avian forebrain will be discussed and comparisons with the mam-malian situation will be made.

The aim of much comparative neuroanatomical research is to look for similar traits in the organization of the brains of different vertebrates. Birds and mammals represent parallel phylogenetic lines that diverged long ago in evolution. For this reason some authors prefer the use of the term homoplasy instead of homology (i.e. the possibility of tracing structures back to a common ancestor), in comparison of structurally similar parts of the brain between the two groups. For a more elaborate discussion of this issue, see for example Campbell and Hodos (1970) and Northcutt (1981). In the present discussion we will stick to the term homology to indicate morphological correspondence between structures. Another possibility is that structural similarity is the result of a convergent development of analogous structures. The term analogy is used to indicate that elements serve the same function. Since comparable functions (com-parable functional demands) require comparable structural solutions, the term 'functional homology' has been used; however, this term is confusing and should be avoided.

Clearly homology and analogy are not mutually exclusive. In compara-tive anatomy a set of criteria is needed to recognize the homology of elements. In classic comparative anatomy these criteria were position, shape, structure and ontogeny. In comparative neuroanatomy cytoarchi-tectonics, the pattern of connections (hodology), histochemical character-istics and embryological data are commonly used as criteria. Nauta and Karten (1979) introduced the concept of homologous cell populations:

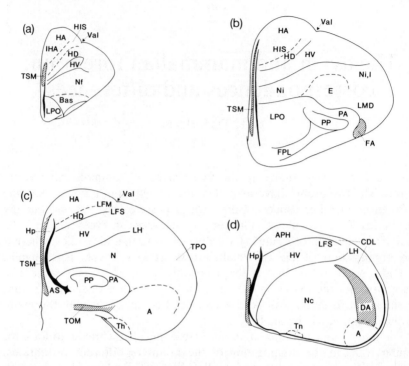

Fig. 2.1   Four cross-sections of the chicken telencephalon, at intervals of about 2.5 mm. Redrawn after the atlas of van Tienhoven and Juhasz (1962); Youngren and Phillips (1978) provide an atlas of the 3-day-old chick. See list of abbreviations, p. 89.

those neuron pools in different species can be considered homologous that are interconnected in the same way. To recognize analogy or convergence both function and structure should be studied.

A GENERAL OUTLINE OF THE AVIAN BRAIN

For a long time the avian forebrain was assumed to consist of an overdeveloped corpus striatum with only a rudimentary cortical region, *viz*. the eminentia sagittalis or Wulst (cf. Ariens Kappers *et al.* 1936). This view is still reflected in the commonly used nomenclature. In cross-sections a number of thick cell layers can be recognized that are called palaeostriatum, neostriatum, hyperstriatum, and ectostriatum (Fig. 2.1). Since the fifties the interpretation of the telencephalic organization has changed considerably. Källen (1953), using embryological evidence, was the first to

Table 2.1 Areas possibly containing homologous telencephalic cell groups. Compare Fig. 2.1 for arrangement of the layers

Mammals	Birds
Isocortex	*Eminentia sagittalis* (Wulst)
	Hyperstriatum accessorium (HA)
	Nucleus intercalatus of HA (IHA)
	Hyperstriatum intercalatum supremum (HIS)
	Hyperstriatum dorsale (HD)
	Dorsal ventricular ridge:
	Hyperstriatum ventrale (HV)
	Neostriatum (N)
	Ectostriatum (E)
	Nucleus basalis (Bas)
	Archistriatum (rostral part) (A)
Hippocampus	*Hippocampus*
Amygdala	Archistriatum (medial + caudal part)
Corpus striatum	*Palaeostriatum complex*:
Caudate-putamen	Palaeostriatum augmentatum (PA)
	+ Lobus parolfactorius (LPO)
Globus pallidus ext	Palaeostriatum primitivum (PP)
int	Nucleus intrapeduncularis (INP)
Nucleus accumbens	*Nucleus accumbens*

point out that large parts of the avian forebrain, including the dorsal ventricular ridge as well as the Wulst, should be considered pallial (i.e. potentially equivalent to cortex) rather than subpallial structures. The dorsal ventricular ridge can be defined as the part of the telencephalon developing between the dorsal and middle ventricular sulci (Ulinski 1983); it protrudes into the lateral ventricle. Large areas of the avian telencephalon can thus be considered equivalent to the mammalian neocortex (Table 2.1).

In 1970 Nauta and Karten distinguished an internal and an external striatum. In their interpretation the internal striatum in birds consists mainly of the palaeostriatal complex, including the lobus parolfactorius (LPO), and corresponds to the mammalian corpus striatum. The external striatum, comprising the dorsal ventricular ridge (DVR) and Wulst, contains cell groups homologous to those in the mammalian neocortex. It comprises endstations of ascending systems, telencephalic 'motor' output areas and large areas with predominantly intratelencephalic connections. Perhaps it is possible to compare the populations of neurons in these respective regions with cell groups in specific layers of the cortex. The arrangements of cells and their afferent and efferent connections are quite different in mammals and birds, though in some areas a strong resemblance in organization can be recognized.

Impressive differences in organization and cytoarchitectonic differentiation exist between the brains of different groups of birds (Stingelin 1958). As will be pointed out, some of these differences may be related to behavioural specializations of the respective species. For this reason the birds form a very suitable group for a comparative functional and anatomical study of brain organization. In the following discussion various species will be considered, but it is the aim to sketch a generalized picture of the organization of the avian forebrain that can be used in comparison with mammalian brain organization. Avian telencephalic organization has repeatedly been discussed before (e.g. Karten 1969; Cohen and Karten 1974; Benowitz 1980). The focus of the present overview will be on the principles of organization of the respective brain areas.

HISTOCHEMISTRY OF THE AVIAN FOREBRAIN

Before discussing connectivity, some histochemical data will be reviewed in order to see whether these can help to elucidate some aspects of the forebrain organization. Data about the distribution of some neuroactive chemicals (or neuromediators, Nieuwenhuys 1985) are compiled in Table 2.2. From this survey it is clear that the palaeostriatal complex, with its subdivisions including LPO and nucleus accumbens (Acc), can be characterized quite well. Some differences between sets of data can be ascribed to the fact that different authors do not always use the same subdivisions: thus LPO seems sometimes to be included in the palaeostriatum augmentatum (PA). For other parts of the telencephalon the picture arising from the available data is at best sketchy. Various authors suggest similarities between specific avian and mammalian brain areas. However, a cursory comparison of the data of Table 2.2 and those from the studies of Nieuwenhuys (1985) and Palkovitz (1984) does not provide a very satisfactory picture.

Correspondence between PA + LPO and the mammalian caudate–putamen is suggested by the distribution of cholinergic elements and the reactivity for dopamine, GABA, somatostatin, and substance P (also cf. Hall *et al.* 1984), but for the distribution of neurotensin, enkephalin, or endorphin (for example) the correspondence is not so evident. The histochemical similarity between palaeostriatum primitivum (PP) and the external pallidum is less convincing. The hippocampus in both birds and mammals is characterized by the presence of cholinergic elements, GABA, enkephalin and somatostatin. Again it is difficult to identify the avian amygdala using mammalian characteristics. For other pallial areas data are still too incomplete to reach a reliable conclusion.

It is questionable whether the presence of one specific mediator allows the homologization of cell groups. How tricky this can be is demonstrated by a series of observations by Divac and co-workers (Divac and Mogensen 1985; Divac *et al.* 1985, 1988). Initially, these authors suggested that the posterodorsolateral neostriatum (TPO, DA) in the pigeon could be the equivalent of the mammalian prefrontal cortex, mainly on histochemical and biochemical evidence. However, in a comparison of different breeds of pigeon significant differences in the content of catecholamine in the various brain parts were found. It may be too early to reach a final conclusion about the usefulness of histochemical data to characterize homologous pallial cell groups.

INTERNAL STRIATUM AND BASAL GANGLION

The paleostriatum augmentatum (PA) and primitivum (PP), the lobus parolfactorius (LPO) and nucleus intrapeduncularis (INP) are the main components of the internal striatum. PA, LPO, and INP contain large numbers of medium size perikarya, PP a small number of large cells. The combination of histochemical and hodological data (Parent and Olivier 1970; Karten and Dubbeldam 1973) delineates the avian palaeostriatal-lobus parolfactorius complex as the equivalent of the mammalian corpus striatum. These data and the results of more recent studies have been discussed in several reviews (Webster 1979; Reiner *et al.* 1984; Parent 1986), which sustain the original conclusion. The pattern of afferent and efferent fibres is a key feature of the mammalian corpus striatum. The afferents of the caudate–putamen complex derive from the cerebral neocortex, from the intralaminar thalamic nucleus and from the substantia nigra, pars compacta. The globus pallidus and substantia nigra, pars reticulata are the major recipients of the caudate–putamen efferents.

Figure 2.2 summarizes the pattern of connections of the palaeostriatal complex in birds. Projections from the overlying layers appear to correspond to the neocortical projections in mammals. Several intratelencephalic sources of PA afferents have been described: TPO and other lateral regions of the neostriatum in the pigeon (Brauth *et al.* 1978), the frontal part of the neostriatum (Nf) in the mallard (Dubbeldam and Visser 1987) and goose (Veenman and Gottschaldt 1985). In the anseriform birds this projection from Nf is clearly topographically organized; this is reminiscent of the topographic neocortical projection upon the caudate–putamen (e.g. Veening *et al.* 1980). LPO receives projections from Nf and the hyperstriatum ventrale (HV) (Bons and Olivier 1986: quail, Dubbeldam and Visser 1987: duck). PA and LPO both receive afferents from the dorsal thalamus (Wild 1987*a*). However, an intralaminar thalamic nucleus cannot be

Table 2.2 Neuromediators in avian forebrain

	ACh[1] rec.	AChE[2]	id.[3]	id.[4]	Cat.[5] term.	DA[6] rec.	DA[7]	MAO[2]	GABA[8] rec.	GABA[9] c	GABA[9] np
HA	++	±		–	+	+++		++		++	++
HIS	+++	–		–	++			±		++	++
HD	+++	±		–	+			+		++	++
HV	+++	±	c	–		+++		+	+/++	++	++
N	++	++	c	–	±			+		++	++
L	±			–						++	++
E	+	+		–	±	–		–	+	++	++
Bas	++			–				–		++	++
CDL	++			–						?	?
Ad*		++		–		+++		+		++	++
v*	++	±		–				+++		++	++
1*				++						?	?
Hp	+	±–+	c	–				+++		++	++
APH	+			–					+		
AS	+++	–	c	±				+++	±	++	++
LPO	+++			+++	++	++	+++			+++	+++
PA	+++	+++		+++	++	++	+++	+++	+/++	+++	++
PP	±	–		–	–	±		+	+++	+	+++
INP	++			++			+++			+++	–
Acc	+++	+++		++			+++	++		+	++
VP**	–		c							+	++

±, +, ++, +++: low–high concentration; -: explicit negative finding; ?: not mentioned.
c: cells, np: neurophil, rec.: receptors, cat.: catecholamine, term.:terminalia

[1] Wächtler (1985), Dietl et al. (1988): pigeon
[2] Kusunoki (1969): Uroloncha, mallard. MAO: monoamine oxidase
[3] Davies and Horn (1983), cells projecting upon HVcI): chicken
[4] Dubbeldam C.S. (unpublished): mallard (in lat. and caudolat. zone A: ++); Parent and Olivier (1970): pigeon, not in A
[5] Bagnoli and Casini (1985): pigeon; Lewis et al. (1981): zebra finch (catecholaminergic terminalia). Divac et al. (1988) mention differences between races of pigeons
[6] Dietl and Palacios (1988): pigeon, dopamine
[7] Parent and Olivier (1970): monoamine (dopamine?)
[8] Dietl et al. (1988b): pigeon
[9] Domenici et al. (1988): pigeon, 'GABA-like immunoreactivity'
  * Ad, v, l: dorsal, ventral and lateral zones of archistriatum
** VP: ventral paleostriatum; for further explanation: see list of abbreviations, p. 89

identified with any certainty in birds (Webster 1979). The intense cate-cholamine fluorescence that can be induced in PA and LPO can be traced back to an input from cholinergic cell bodies in the midbrain tegmentum (substantia nigra, pars reticulata; Dubé, cited by Parent 1986). PA also

Table 2.2 *Cont.*

	Endorph[10]	1.Enk[10]	mEnk[11,12]	SP[13] c.	v.	Somato[14] statin	Neuro-[15,16] tensin	LANT[16]
HA	±	–					++	–
HIS	±	–					+	–
HD	±	–	c/v					–
HV	±	–					+++	–
N	+	–		±			+++(NC)	–
L							+	–
E				±			+	–
Bas								–
CDL						±		–
Ad	++	+					++	–
v	++	+						–
1	++	+						–
Hp		+				++	±	
APH			v				±	
AS	+++	+++	++			v		
LPO	+++	+	c	+++	++	++	–	+
PA	+	+	c	++	+	++	–	+
PP	+	+	v	±	+++		–	+
INP		–		–				–
Acc			c	–				
VP					+++			+

[10] Bayon *et al.* (1980): pigeon
[11] De Lanerolle *et al.* (1981); Blähser and Dubois (1980): chicken
[12] Reiner *et al.* (1984*b*): pigeon, 'enkephalin-like activity'
[13] Reiner *et al.* (1983): pigeon, substance P; dynorphin co-occurs with SP cells in rostral PA; c: cells, v: fibres
[14] Takatsuki *et al.* (1981): budgerigar
[15] Brauth *et al.* (1986): pigeon, neurotensin binding places
[16] Reiner and Carraway (1987): pigeon, Lys[8]-Asn[9]-Neurotensin[8-13]

receives a dopaminergic projection from the n. pedunculopontinus tegmenti, pars compacta. PA sends its efferents to PP, whereas the lateral LPO projects mainly upon the midbrain tegmentum through the ansa lenticularis (AL). PP is another source of AL fibres with projections upon a series of thalamic and midbrain nuclei. This arrangement of cell groups and fibre systems shows strong parallels to that of the mammalian corpus striatum. The similarity of this pattern and the histochemical correspondences indicate homology of the avian palaeostriatal complex with mammalian caudate-putamen + globus pallidus.

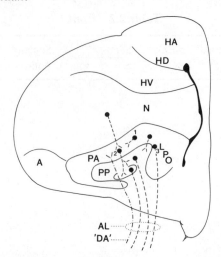

Fig. 2.2 Pattern of connections of the avian 'corpus striatum'. 'DA' indicates the dopaminergic projection from the midbrain tegmentum (substantia nigra). 1 = PA containing intrinsic neurons that are characterized by the presence of acetylcholine and somatostatin; 2 = PA projection neurons, characterized by dynorphin, substance P and/or enkephalin; 3 = lateral LPO neurons characterized by dynorphin, substance P and GABA. Histochemical data taken from Reiner *et al.* (1984*a*). See list of abbreviations, p. 89.

There is some doubt about the status of INP. Karten and Dubbeldam (1973) suggested that INP may correspond to the internal segment of the globus pallidus. Histochemical data, however, contradict this suggestion, as it is almost devoid of substance P- and enkephalin-immunoreactive fibres (Table 2.2). In the duck INP receives a direct input from Nf (Dubbeldam and Visser 1987). In general, there may be some doubt about the precise identification of this cell group in the different species of birds.

Most characteristic is the high content of AChE in the neuropil of PA and the low content in PP. Parent (1986), citing the work of Dubé, suggests that large, intensely stained AChE cells in PA and PP may correspond to the magnocellular cholinergic elements comprising the mammalian n. basalis of Meynert.

The ventral paleostriatum (only recently defined: VP) contains small to medium size cells. It is bordered by the lateral forebrain bundle and the ventral surface of the telencephalon. Fibres from this area descend with the ansa lenticularis (Kitt and Brauth 1981; Dubbeldam and Visser 1987) and may extend as far as the parvocellular reticular formation of the myelencephalon (Bout 1987). In the duck it also has connections with the lateral belt of the archistriatum and lateral intermediate neostriatum (Ni, l) (Dubbeldam and Visser 1987). It receives input from the overlying part of LPO and (perhaps) the medial neostriatum. It has been suggested that this ventral palaeostriatum is homologous with the mammalian substantia innominata (Parent 1986).

THE EXTERNAL STRIATUM OR PALLIAL REGION

As has already been pointed out, the external striatum of birds and the mammalian cerebral cortex contain the pallial cell groups. There is, however, a striking difference in organization between the two structures. In birds two large components can easily be recognized, the dorsal ventricular ridge (DVR) and the eminentia sagittalis or Wulst. These areas are assumed to contain the 'neocortical' cell populations. In addition, the Wulst contains the dorsomedial cortex, usually termed hippocampus + parahippocampal area in birds. DVR and Wulst each have a comparable and characteristic organization. Both include a component which gives rise to a large extratelencephalic fibre system: the archistriatum (A) with the occipitomesencephalic tract in the DVR, the hyperstriatum accessorium (HA) with the septomesencephalic tract in the Wulst. Quite often these two fibre systems together have been compared to the mammalian corticobulbar and -spinal (pyramidal) tract. Each of the two fibre systems in birds has its own trajectory and terminal fields.

The significance of the bipartition of the 'neocortical' part of the external striatum is not clear, but may have something to do with different roles in the organization of avian behaviour or merely reflect a different ontogenetic origin.

THE EMINENTIA SAGITTALIS

The Wulst is an area with a distinct cortical appearance. Possibly it corresponds to the reptilian dorsal cortex. Four layers can be distinguished from dorsal to ventral: (1) The hyperstriatum accessorium (HA); this is, in the pigeon, a broad, superficial layer with medium size cells; (2) The nucleus intercalatus of HA (IHA), a granular cell layer; (3) The n. intercalatus superior (HIS) with scattered, medium size cells; (4) The hyperstriatum dorsale (HD) with relatively large cells. IHA is the recipient of thalamic afferents conveying two sensory modalities, *viz.* somatosensory information in the most rostral part of the Wulst and visual information in the more caudal part (Fig. 2.3).

The somatosensory input was recorded for the first time in the pigeon by Delius and Bennetto (1972); recent studies by Wild (1987*b*) and Funke (1988) provide additional and more specific information. Both authors described projections from the nucleus dorsalis intermedius ventralis

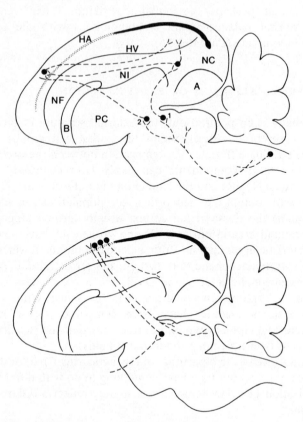

Fig. 2.3 Diagrams showing the somatosensory (*upper panel*) and visual (*lower panel*) projection areas in the eminentia sagittalis (Wulst). 1 = Nucleus dorsolateralis posterior (DLP); 2 = Nucleus dorsalis intermedius ventralis anterior (DIVA). See list of abbreviations, p. 89.

anterior thalami (DIVA) upon the Wulst and from the thalamic n. dorsolateralis posterior upon the transitional area of intermediate and caudal neostriatum (Ni, Nc). However, their pictures of the intratelencephalic connections show some differences. Funke identified a secondary relay area in the hyperstriatum ventrale (HV), receiving input from Ni/Nc and from the rostral Wulst (Fig. 2.3). Wild did not mention this area in HV, but described a reciprocal connection between somatosensory Wulst and Ni/Nc. There is no good explanation for this discrepancy; perhaps the two sets of data should be considered complementary rather than contradictory.

More data are available about the visual part of the Wulst. It has been studied in the pigeon (Karten *et al.* 1973; Miceli *et al.* 1979) and the chicken (Miceli *et al.* 1980; Wilson 1980; Denton 1981), but the owl appears to be particularly well suited for the study of this area (Karten *et*

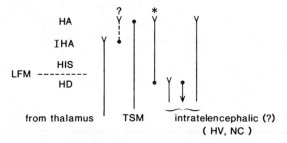

Fig. 2.4 Possible pattern of connections between the layers of the eminentia sagittalis, together with incoming and outgoing fibres. '?' indicates that it is uncertain whether this connection exists. See list of abbreviations, p. 89.

al. 1973). The visual Wulst receives bilateral projections from the dorsal thalamic complex, an important target of retinal afferents. Unlike the situation in mammals, visual information reaching the ipsilateral Wulst has to cross over twice, firstly through the optic chiasma, then back again through the thalamofugal system.

All studies show that IHA is the recipient of visual input and HA the main source of the septomesencephalic tract (TSM; Fig. 2.4). Again, there is some discrepancy in the reports on the pigeon: Reiner and Karten (1983) describe HA as the sole source of TSM, but Bagnoli *et al.* (1980) include a small dorsal part of HIS. No specific data are available about the connections of HIS. HD is a recipient as well as a source of intratelencephalic connections with HV and with the lateral neostriatum and periectostriatal belt (Ritchie, 1979).

Little is known about the intrinsic organization of the visual Wulst. Gusel'nikov *et al.* (1977) found a retinotopic representation in the Wulst of the owl, and Revzin (1969, 1970), recording visual evoked activity, recognized a rough columnar organization in the pigeon. However, there are no firm neuroanatomical data to support their conclusion. Several authors have commented upon the similarity of appearance of the avian visual Wulst and mammalian striate cortex (e.g. Parent 1986) and the significance of this similarity has been the subject of some speculation. Again, the question is, whether this similarity is proof of the homology of the two areas or merely reflects the existence of a common functional role. In 1976 Pettigrew and Konishi already concluded that 'despite its different evolutionary history and its totally crossed primary visual pathway, the owl has a neural basis for binocular depth discrimination directly comparable to that found in cat, monkey, and probably men'. In fact, these authors correlate the specific organization of the visual Wulst and striate cortex and the specific feature of binocular vision.

A more satisfactory functional explanation may be reached, if the functional demands for processing binocular visual information can be

formulated more explicitly. A detailed comparative functional and anatomical analysis of this area in various birds may provide more definite
answers. The anatomical data have little value as criteria for homology:
the number and order of layers differ in visual Wulst and striate cortex.
Even if we accept the homology of the cell populations of these areas, it
does not help much to understand the underlying organizational principles.

Another interesting aspect is the possible lateralization of functions.
Boxer and Stanford (1985) observed an asymmetry of thalamic projections
upon IHA in the chicken: the n. lateralis anterior from both sides project
upon the right IHA, but not upon its left counterpart. This asymmetry,
however, is transient and disappears after day 20 post-hatching (Rogers
and Sink 1988). Moreover, this transient asymmetry has been found in
males, but not in female animals (Adret and Rogers 1989). This phenomenon is discussed in detail in Chapter 20.

A final remark about the TSM is needed. This fibre system splits into a
dorsal and a basal or ventral branch. The available data indicate that HA
of the visual Wulst is the main source of the dorsal branch projecting upon
retinorecipient thalamic cell groups, the ventral geniculate nucleus, pretec-
tal visual nuclei and tectum mesencephali (Bagnoli *et al.* 1980; Miceli and
Repérant 1983; Reiner and Karten 1983; Miceli *et al.* 1987). This pattern
of projections is reminiscent of that from the striate cortex in mammals.
The fibres of the ventral branch originate from the more rostral, somatosensory part of the Wulst and reach the prerubral area, the medial
spiriform nucleus, the medial pontine nucleus and, in the owl, also the n.
ruber and cuneate–gracilis complex (cf. Cohen and Karten 1974).

HIPPOCAMPUS AND AREA PARAHIPPOCAMPALIS

The cortex dorsomedialis forms the most medial and caudal part of the
Wulst. It has been subdivided into an area entorhinalis and area para-
entorhinalis in the atlas of van Tienhoven and Juhasz (1962). More
recently, the names hippocampus (Hp) and area parahippocampalis
(APH) were introduced to indicate these regions (Fig. 2.1). In the chicken
two main layers can be recognized in Golgi preparations (Mollà *et al.*
1986), a plexiform and a granular layer. The latter is occupied by
pyramidal, bipyramidal, and some multipolar cells. The plexiform layer
contains predominantly horizontally orientated neurons. The input of Hp
and APH comes from HA, from the diagonal band of Broca, the n. teniae
and CDL; there are also reciprocal connections between Hp and APH as
well as between the left and right Hp (Casini *et al.* 1986). In addition,
Benowitz and Karten (1976) found that APH receives afferents from the
medial septal nucleus, the lateral hypothalamus, the thalamic n. superfici-
alis parvocellularis, and locus coeruleus.

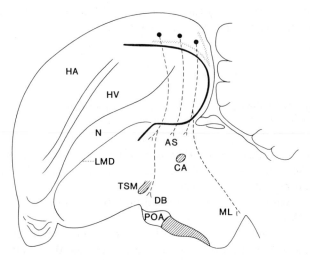

Fig. 2.5 Diagram showing some efferent connections of the avian hippocampus in sagittal section. See list of abbreviations, p. 89.

Efferents from Hp and APH reach the septal nuclei and diagonal band of Broca (Fig. 2.5). Krayniak and Siegel (1978) found no hippocampal projection upon the hypothalamus and considered the efferent hippocampal system to be the equivalent of the precommissural part of the mammalian fornix. Casini *et al.* (1986), however, also report the existence of a small projection upon the hypothalamus disappearing near the lateral n. mammillaris (Fig. 2.5). Other recipients of Hp and APH efferents are the n. teniae and CDL. HD and archistriatum (A) receive an input from APH. Bradley *et al.* (1985), summarizing the sources of afferents to the medial intermediate HV (IMHV), also mention Hp, but this is not supported by the observations of Krayniak and Siegel (1978) or Casini *et al.* (1986).

Comparing the patterns of connections of the avian dorsomedial cortex and the mammalian hippocampus + parahippocampal area, a number of parallels can be recognized. In mammals, efferents from the hippocampus reach through the fornix, the mammillary body in the hypothalamus, the septum, and the band of Broca. Sources of hippocampal and parahippocampal afferents are the medial and lateral entorhinal cortex, the medial septal nuclei, the locus coeruleus, the dorsal and medial raphe nuclei and the supramammillary body (e.g. Segal and Laudis 1974). Even though this comparison leaves some questions unanswered, the many parallels strongly suggest the homology of the avian dorsomedial cortex and the hippocampus and area parahippocampalis in mammals, and thus justify the use of these names in birds. From a functional point of view, the suggestion of

Bingham *et al.* (1984, 1985) can be mentioned that the avian dorsomedial cortex may be involved in spatial recognition.

THE DORSAL VENTRICULAR RIDGE

Already in 1915 Johnston used the term dorsal ventricular ridge (cf. Ariens Kappers *et al.* 1936). It is much later that the pallial nature of the DVR was recognized. Recently, Ulinski (1983) extensively discussed the development and organization of DVR in reptiles and birds and explored the limits of the comparability of the sauropsid and mammalian forebrain. Rather than repeat this discussion, the aim of the present overview is to look for a possible basic organizational pattern of cells and connections in the avian DVR.

So far, four main sensory endstations for ascending fibre systems have been recognized. The most rostral is the nucleus basalis receiving quinto-frontal fibres that convey trigeminal/tactile information; recently, a small auditory component has also been recognized in this cell area of the pigeon (Schall and Delius 1986; Arends and Zeigler 1986). The ectostria-tum (E) is a visual endstation; the part of Ni medial to it is recipient of a second tectofugal visual pathway (Gamlin and Cohen 1986). Field L in the caudal neostriatum (Nc) receives input from the n. ovoidalis and is an auditory centre. The somatosensory area in the transitory area Ni-Nc has already been mentioned (Fig. 2.3). Most of these cell areas can be recognized as distinct entities within the neostriatum (Fig. 2.6). The other parts of the neostriatum and the overlying hyperstriatum ventrale (HV) possess predominantly intratelencephalic connections. All afferent systems enter the telencephalon through the fasciculus lateralis prosencephali (FPL).

The archistriatum (A) is the source of a large extratelencephalic output system, the occipitomesencephalic tract (TOM). The rostral and interme-diate A is a sensorimotor area with connections with many cell groups within the telencephalon as well as in the brainstem (through TOM). The medial and caudal parts have a distinct projection upon the hypothalamus and can be considered the avian equivalent of the amygdalar complex (cf. Zeier and Karten 1971, 1973). Projections from various other parts of DVR upon the palaeostriatal complex have already been mentioned.

Neostriatum and HV can each be subdivided in a number of regions using cell density and myeloarchitecture as criteria (Rehkämper *et al.* 1984, 1985). Associative and co-ordination functions are ascribed to N and HV; parts of these may also form the substrate for learning and memory formation. In the following review, in the first place the pattern of cells and their connections to the 'tactile' basalis system will be considered. The next step will be to see whether this pattern has a more general validity

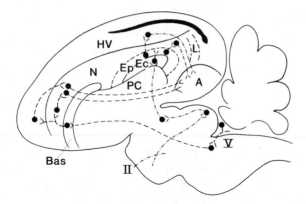

Fig. 2.6 Diagram showing the patterns of connections of the trigeminal/tactile system and the ectostriatal/visual system in the dorsal ventricular ridge of 'the bird'. See list of abbreviations, p. 89.

for DVR, comparing it with those of the ectostriatal visual and auditory field L systems.

Nucleus basalis and its connections

In anseriform birds the n. basalis and overlying parts of neostriatum (Nf) and HV form a multilayered system that is readily accessible to experimental exploration (Veenman and Gottschaldt 1985: goose; Dubbeldam and Visser 1987: duck). Figure 2.7 diagrammatically summarizes the pattern of connections as revealed by the use of tracing techniques. Nucleus basalis receives afferents from the trigeminal principal sensory nucleus (PrV; e.g. Zeigler and Karten 1973: pigeon; Dubbeldam *et al.* 1981: duck) and sends its efferents to the ventral layer of Nf (Nf,v), to the most dorsal layer of Nf bordering the lamina hyperstriatica (LH), and to the ventral zone of HV (HV-LH complex in Fig. 2.7), with a lighter projection upon the most dorsal zone of HV. Nf,v projects upon the dorsal layer of Nf (Nf,d), upon the HV-LH complex, and upon the palaeostriatal complex. The HV-LH complex has reciprocal connections with Bas and Nf,v and a light, but distinct projection upon Nf,d. The latter cell area is the origin of fibres terminating in the rostral and intermediate sensorimotor part of the archistriatum, in the lateral zone of LPO and also in the palaeostriatal complex. It seems likely that the various groups of fibres derive from different populations of cells in Nf,d. The lateral zone of neostriatum seems to be a relay between HV (Nf,l) or Nf,d (Ni,l) and the archistriatum. The anatomical observations are supported partly by electrophysiological data (Gottschaldt *et al.* 1980; Félix and Roesch 1986).

Essentially the same pattern of connections can be recognized in the

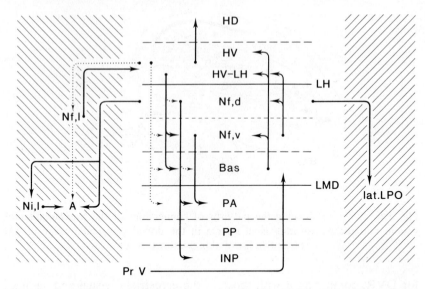

Fig. 2.7   Radial pattern of connections of n. basalis with the frontal neostriatum and HV; efferent connections of the Nf–HV complex project directly or through the lateral neostriatum upon the sensorimotor part of A, upon the palaeostriatal complex and the lateral zone of LPO (modified after Dubbeldam and Visser 1987). See list of abbreviations, p. 89.

pigeon, with the exception of the projection upon the palaeostriatal complex (Wild *et al.* 1985). In this bird n. basalis is a minor cell group compared to that in the anseriform birds. In this respect the chicken is comparable to the pigeon. Comparison between species is hampered because of the large differences in differentiation and in the proportions of the brain parts, which may also be the cause of some nomenclatural differences in the different studies. Nevertheless, in my opinion some generality can be attributed to the scheme depicted in Figure 2.7.

Ectostriatal connections

A comparable scheme of the ectostriatal connections is shown in Fig. 2.8; this is based upon data on the pigeon (Ritchie 1979; also cf. Karten 1979). The ectostriatum is surrounded by Ni; the ectostriatum itself can be subdivided into a core (Ec) and a belt (Ep). The pattern of reciprocal connections of Ec, Ep, Ni and overlying HV is reminiscent of that between Bas, Nf,v, Nf,d and HV. Again, the lateral neostriatum (Ni,l) is a relay between Ni or HV and the archistriatum. Unlike the trigeminal system, the visual system also has an input into the amygdaloid part of A (AV). Figure 2.6 summarizes some of the similarities and differences between

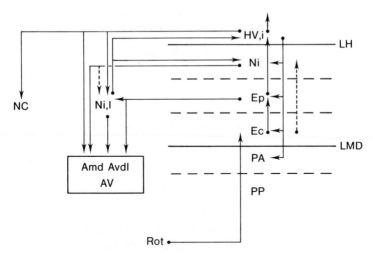

Fig. 2.8   Radial pattern of connections of the ectostriatal system with projections upon the sensorimotor and amygdaloid parts of the archistriatum (based upon Ritchie 1979). See list of abbreviations, p. 89.

the tactile/trigeminal and visual/ectostriatal system in a 'generalized' bird. A specific aspect of the ectostriatal complex is that cells from the rostral Ep project upon HV, from the dorsal Ep upon Ni,l and from the caudal Ep upon Avdl. Such a differentiation has not been recognized in the basalis system, but the possibility cannot be excluded that here, too, different cell populations are the sources of the corresponding projections.

Field L and telencephalic vocalization centres

Field L has long been recognized as the receptive area of auditory ovoidalis efferents (e.g. Cohen and Karten 1974). The results of more recent studies in the guinea fowl (Bonke *et al.* 1979*a*, *b*) suggest that field L can be subdivided into three zones, L1–L3; most ovoidalis fibres project upon the intermediate zone L2. Autoradiographic studies in guinea fowl (Bonke *et al.* 1979*b*) and Golgi studies in the starling (Saini and Leppelsack 1981) suggest the existence of projections upon Nc and HV, with perhaps some fibres extending into the cell group HVc.

   The latter cell group is an important telencephalic centre of the vocalization system (e.g. Nottebohm *et al.* 1976), and a close association with field L has been assumed. Later studies in the canary (Kelley and Nottebohm 1979; Nottebohm *et al.* 1982) and budgerigar (Paton *et al.* 1981) showed that field L projects upon a neostriatal area ventrally bordering the cell group HVc and that HVc receives a direct as well as an indirect projection (through a relay in the neostriatal 'interface nucleus', N,If) from the

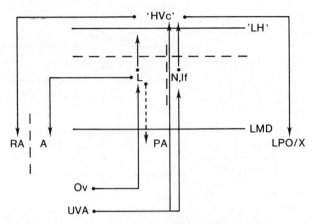

Fig. 2.9   Radial pattern of connections of the auditory and vocalization system. For explanation, see text. See list of abbreviations, p. 89.

thalamic n. uvaeformis (Fig. 2.9). Moreover, though originally described as a cell group in the caudal HV, HVc appears to be a neostriatal rather than a HV cell group. The resulting picture is different from that of the basalis or ectostriatal system, unless neostriatum and hyperstriatum ventrale can be considered to form one system for the processing and storage of information and the initiation and co-ordination of activities.

For all three systems a radial organization seems to prevail in the neostriatum—hyperstriatum ventrale complex: information arrives in a specific patch of cells (within n. basalis or ectostriatum, for example), and is distributed to neurons lying above and below this patch within a radial sector (Ulinski 1986). The pattern of reciprocal connections within such a sector appears to be a general feature, as described in the preceding paragraphs, and this may also be true for the the auditory component of Bas (Delius *et al.* 1979) or the neostriatal somatosensory area. One of the functions of this pattern of reciprocal connections may be the storage of information. At least two regions have already been implicated in the process of memory formation: the medial zone of the intermediate HV (IMHV) for filial imprinting (Chapters 8 and 10) and HVc for auditory imprinting or, perhaps better, learning of vocalizations. Bradley *et al.* (1985) made an inventory of connections of IMHV in the chicken and mentioned afferents from N, HD/HA, other parts of HV and from archistriatum. An archistriatum—HV connection has not been found in the pigeon (Zeier and Karten 1971, 1973), or in the duck (Dubbeldam, unpublished observations). The presence of labelled cells in A after HRP injections in IMHV in the chicken could be due to the interruption of passing fibres.

Only a part of the cells and fibres participate in the radial pattern.

Veenman and Gottschaldt (1985) describe distinct horizontal patterns of connections in the respective layers of Nf and HV of the goose. In a recent Golgi study Tömböl *et al.* (1988) describe two main types of neurons in the HV of the chicken, putative projection neurons and putative local circuit neurons. Our own study in the duck (Dubbeldam and Visser 1987) suggests that only a modest proportion of neostriatal and HV cells project upon the archistriatum and palaeostriatal complex. The lateral zone of the neostriatum, including the area corticoidea dorsolateralis (CDL) and area temperoparieto-occipitalis (TPO), seems to form another important link between the neostriatum—HV complex and the 'output' areas, archistriatum and palaeostriatum.

CONCLUDING REMARKS

From studies of roughly the last 20 years gradually a new picture of avian telencephalic organization has emerged. Now, it has generally been accepted that the palaeostriatal complex represents the avian subpallial component, whereas DVR and Wulst contain the pallial cell groups. Though sometimes there is a tendency in the literature to compare n. basalis with a somatosensory cortex or field L with an auditory cortex, it must be stressed that these areas in birds contain at best neurons comparable to those in layers III and IV of the respective cortical areas. As for the visual system, in birds as well as in mammals at least two ascending visual pathways can be recognized (see Chapter 3). If the avian thalamic–Wulst pathway may be considered the equivalent of the thalamo–striate system in mammal (see above), then the tecto–rotundo–ectostriatal system could comprise the elements corresponding to the mammalian colliculo–thalamo–temporal (visual II) cortex pathway. The ectostriatum and overlying parts of neostriatum and HV might then contain cell populations corresponding to those in the extrastriate cortex. However, even were this to be true, considerable differences in the arrangement of cells and their connections remain in the two groups of animals.

The picture is still incomplete; nevertheless, our survey leads to the suggestion that a basic similar radial organization exists throughout the DVR. This radial organization makes the avian telencephalon a very suitable object for the study of specific brain mechanisms. An intriguing aspect is the subdivision of the pallium into the two large components DVR and Wulst, apparently each with a specific pattern of organization. Specific functional demands may underlie these differences; further comparative studies of the structure and functions of brain regions may help to clarify these differences.

REFERENCES

Adret, P. and Rogers, L. J. (1989). Sex differences in the visual projections of young chicks: a quantitative study of the thalamofugal pathway. *Brain Research*, **478**, 59–73.

Arends, J. J. A. and Zeigler, H. P. (1986). Anatomical identification of an auditory pathway from a nucleus of the lateral lemniscal system to the frontal forebrain (nucleus basalis) of the pigeon. *Brain Research*, **398**, 375–81.

Ariens Kappers, C. U., Huber, G. C., and Crosby, E. C. (1936). *The comparative anatomy of the nervous system of vertebrates, including man.* Hafner, New York.

Bagnoli, P., Grassi, S. and Magni, F. (1980). A direct connection between visual Wulst and tectum opticum in the pigeon (*Columba livia*) demonstrated by horseradish peroxidase. *Archives Italiennes de Biologie*, **118**, 72–88.

Baumel, J. J. (1979). *Nomina anatomica avium. An annotated anatomical dictionary of birds.* Academic Press, London.

Bayon, A., Koda, L., Battenberg, E., Azad, R., and Bloom, F. E. (1980). Regional distribution of endorphin, met5-enkephalin and leu5-enkephalin in the pigeon brain. *Neuroscience Letters*, **16**, 75–80.

Benowitz L. I. (1980). Functional organization of the avian brain. In *Comparative neurology of the telencephalon* (ed. S. O. E. Ebbeson), pp. 389–421. Plenum Press, New York.

Benowitz, L. I. and Karten, H. J. (1976). The tractus infundibuli and other afferents to the parahippocampal region of the pigeon. *Brain Research*, **102**, 174–180.

Bingman, V. P., Bagnoli, P., Ioale, P., and Casini, G. (1984). Homing behavior of pigeons after telencephalic ablations. *Brain, Behavior and Evolution*, **24**, 94–108.

Bingham, V. P., Ioale, P., Casini, G., and Bagnoli, P. (1985). Dorsomedial forebrain ablations and home loft association behavior in homing pigeons. *Brain, Behavior and Evolution*, **26**, 1–9.

Blähser, S. and Dubois, M. P. (1980). Immunocytochemical demonstration of met-enkephalin in the central nervous system of the domestic fowl. *Cell Tissue Research*, **213**, 53–68.

Bonke, B. A., Bonke, D., and Scheich, H. (1979a). Connectivity of the auditory forebrain nuclei in the guinea fowl (*Numida meleagris*). *Cell Tissue Research*, **200**, 101–21.

Bonke, D., Scheich H., and Langner, G. (1979b). Responsiveness of units in the auditory neostriatum of the guinea fowl (*Numida meleagris*) to species-specific calls and synthetic stimuli. I. Tonotopy and functional zones of field L. *Journal of Comparative Physiology*, **A132**, 243–55.

Bons, N. and Olivier, J. (1986). Origin of the afferent connections to the parolfactory lobe in quail shown by retrograde labeling with fluorescent neuron tracers. *Experimental Brain Research*, **63**, 125–34.

Bout, R. G.(1987). Neuroanatomical circuits for proprioceptive and motor control of feeding movements in the mallard (*Anas platyrhynchos*). PhD thesis, Leiden University, The Netherlands.

Boxer, M. I. and Stanford, D. (1985). Projections to the posterior visual hyperstriatum region in the chick—an HRP study. *Experimental Brain Research*, **57**, 494–8.

Bradley, P., Davies, D. C., and Horn, G. (1985). Connections of the hyperstriatum ventrale of the domestic chick (*Gallus domesticus*). *Journal of Anatomy*, **140**, 577–89.

Brauth, S. E., Ferguson, J. L., and Kitt, C. A. (1978). Prosencephalic pathways related to the paleostriatum of the pigeon (*Columba livia*). *Brain Research*, **147**, 205–21.

Brauth, S. E., Kitt, C. A., Reiner, A., and Quirion, R. (1986). Neurotensin binding sites in the forebrain and midbrain of the pigeon. *Journal of Comparative Neurology*, **253**, 358–73.

Campbell, C. B. G. and Hodos, W. (1970). The concept of homology and the evolution of the nervous system. *Brain, Behavior and Evolution*, **3**, 353–67.

Casini, G., Bingman, V. P., and Bagnoli, P. (1986). Connections of the pigeon dorsomedial forebrain studied with WGA- HRP and 3H-proline. *Journal of Comparative Neurology*, **245**, 454–70.

Cohen, D. H. and Karten, H. J. (1974). The structural organization of avian brain: an overview. In *Birds, brain and behavior* (ed. I. J. Goodman and M. W. Schein), pp. 29–73. New York. Academic Press.

Davies D. C., and Horn, G. (1983). Putative cholinergic afferents of the chick hyperstriatum ventrale: a combined acetylcholinesterase and retrograde fluorescence labelling study. *Neuroscience Letters*, **38**, 103–8.

de Lanerolle, N. C., Elde, R. P., Sparber, S. B., and Frick, M. (1981). Distribution of methionine-enkephalin immunoreactivity in the chick brain: an immunohistochemical study. *Journal of Comparative Neurology*, **199**, 513–33.

Delius, J. D. and Bennetto, K. (1972). Cutaneous sensory projections to the avian forebrain. *Brain Research*, **37**, 205–21.

Delius, J. D., Runge, T. E., and Oeckinghaus, H. (1979). Short-latency auditory projection to the frontal telencephalon of the pigeon. *Experimental Neurology*, **63**, 594–603.

Denton, C. J. (1981). Topography of the hyperstriatal visual projection area in the young domestic chicken. *Experimental Neurology*, **74**, 482–98.

Dietl, M. M. and Palacios, J. M. (1988). Neurotransmitter receptors in the avian brain. I. Dopamine receptors. *Brain Research*, **439**, 354–9.

Dietl, M. M., Cortés, R., and Palacios, J. M. (1988). Neurotransmitter receptors in the avian brain. II. Muscarinic cholinergic receptors. III. GABA-benzodiazepine receptors. *Brain Research*, **439**, 360–5; 366–71.

Divac, I. and Mogensen, J. (1985). The prefrontal 'cortex' in the pigeon. Catecholamine histofluorescence. *Neuroscience*, **15**, 677–82.

Divac, I., Mogensen, J., and Björklund, A. (1985). The prefrontal 'cortex' of the pigeon. Biochemical evidence. *Brain Research*, **332**, 365–8.

Divac, I., Mogensen J., and Björklund, A. (1988). Strain differences in catecholamine content of pigeon brains. *Brain Research*, **444**, 371–3.

Domenici, L., Waldvogel, H. J., Matute, C., and Streit, P. (1988). Distribution of GABA-like immunoreactivity in the pigeon brain. *Neuroscience*, **25**, 931–50.

Dubbeldam, J. L., Brauch, C. S. M., Don, A., and Zeilstra S. (1981). Studies on the somatotopy of the trigeminal system in the mallard, *Anas platyrhynchos* L.

III. Afferents and organization of the nucleus basalis. *Journal of Comparative Neurology*, **196**, 391–405.

Dubbeldam, J. L. and Visser, A. M. (1987). The organization of the nucleus basalis-neostriatum complex of the mallard (*Anas platyrhynchos*) and its connections with the archistriatum and the paleostriatum complex. *Neuroscience*, **21**, 487–517.

Félix, B. and Roesch, T. (1986). Telencephalic bill projections in the Landes goose. *Somatosensory Research*, **4**, 141–52.

Funke, K. (1988). Das zentrale somatosensorische System des Vogels. Elektrophysiologische und neuroanatomische Untersuchungen am ZNS der Taube. Inaug. Diss. Bochum.

Gamlin, P. D. R. and Cohen, D. H. (1986). A second ascending visual pathway from the optic tectum to the telencephalon in the pigeon (*Columba livia*). *Journal of Comparative Neurology*, **250**, 296–310.

Gottschaldt, K.-M., Veenman, C. L., and Steindler, D. A. (1980). Projection of tactile beak afferents into the forebrain of the goose. *Proceedings of the International Union of Physiological Sciences*, **14**, 441.

Gusel'nikov, V. I., Morenkov, E. D., and Hunh Do Cong (1977). Responses and properties of receptive fields of neurons in the visual projection zone of the pigeon hyperstriatum. *Neuroscience and Behavioral Physiology*, **8**, 210–15.

Hall, K., Brauth, S. E., and Kitt, C. A. (1984). Retrograde transport of [³H] GABA in the striotegmental system of the pigeon. *Brain Research*, **310**, 157–63.

Källen, B. (1953). On the nuclear differentiation during ontogenesis in the avian forebrain and some notes on the amniote strio-amygdaloid complex. *Acta Anatomica*, **17**, 72–84.

Karten, H. J. (1969). The organization of the avian telencephalon and some speculations on the phylogeny of the amniote telencephalon. *Annals of the New York Academy of Sciences*, **167**, 164–79.

Karten, H. J. (1979). Visual lemniscal pathways in birds. In *Neural mechanisms of behavior in the pigeon* (ed. A. M. Granda, and J. H. Maxwell), pp. 409–30. Plenum Press, New York.

Karten, H. J. and Dubbeldam, J. L. (1973). The organization and the projections of the paleostriatal complex in the pigeon. *Journal of Comparative Neurology*, **148**, 61–90.

Karten, H. J. and Hodos, W. (1967). *A stereotaxic atlas of the brain of the pigeon*. Johns Hopkins, Baltimore.

Karten, H. J., Hodos, W., Nauta, W. J. H., and Revzin, A. M. (1973). Neural connections of the visual Wulst of the avian telencephalon. Experimental studies in the pigeon (*Columba livia*) and the owl (*Speotyto cunicularis*). *Journal of Comparative Neurology*, **150**, 253–78.

Kelley, D. B. and Nottebohm, F. (1979). Projections of a telencephalic auditory nucleus—field L—in the canary. *Journal of Comparative Neurology*, **183**, 455–70.

Kitt, C. A. and Brauth, S. E. (1981). Projections of the paleostriatum upon the midbrain tegmentum in the pigeon. *Neuroscience*, **6**, 1551–66.

Krayniak, P. F. and Siegel, A. (1978). Efferent connections of the hippocampus and adjacent regions in the pigeon. *Brain, Behavior and Evolution*, **15**, 372–88.

Kusunoki, T. (1969). The chemoarchitectonics of the avian brain. *Journal für Hirnforschung*, **11**, 477–97.

Miceli, D., Gioanni, H., Repérant, J., and Peyrichoux, J. (1979). The avian visual Wulst. I. An anatomical study of afferent and efferent pathways. II. An electrophysiological study of the functional properties of single neurons. In *Neural mechanisms of behavior in the pigeon.* (ed. A. M. Granda and J. H. Maxwell,) pp. 223–54. Plenum, New York.

Miceli, D., Peyrichoux, J., Repérant, J., and Weidner, C. (1980). Etude anatomique des afferences du telencephale rostral chez le poussin, *Gallus domesticus L. Journal für Hirnforschung*, **21**, 627–46.

Miceli, D. and Repérant, J. (1983). Hyperstriatal-tectal projections in the pigeon (*Columba livia*) as demonstrated by the retrograde double-label fluorescence technique. *Brain Research*, **276**, 147–53.

Miceli, D., Repérant, J., Villalobos, J., and Dionne, L. (1987). Extratelencephalic projections of the avian visual Wulst. A quantitative autoradiographic study in the pigeon, *Columba livia. Journal für Hirnforschung*, **28**, 45–58.

Mollà, R., Rodriguez, J., Calvet, S., and Garcia-Verdugo, J. M. (1986). Neuronal types of the cerebral cortex of the adult chicken (*Gallus gallus*). A Golgi study. *Journal für Hirnforschung*, **27**, 381–90.

Nauta, W. J. H. and Karten, H. J. (1970). A general profile of the vertebrate brain, with sidelights on the ancestry of cerebral cortex. In *The neurosciences: second study program* (ed. F. O. Schmitt), pp. 7–26. Rockefeller University Press, New York.

Nieuwenhuys, R. (1985). *Chemoarchitecture of the brain.* Springer, Berlin.

Northcutt, R. G. (1981). Evolution of the telencephalon in non-mammals. *Annual Review of Neurosciences*, **4**, 301–50.

Nottebohm, F., Kelley, D. B., and Paton, J. A. (1982). Connections of vocal control nuclei in the canary telencephalon. *Journal of Comparative Neurology*, **207**, 344–57.

Nottebohm, F., Stokes, T. M., and Leonard, C. M. (1976). Central control of song in the canary, *Serinus canarius. Journal of Comparative Neurology*, **165**, 457–86.

Palkovits, M. (1984). Distribution of neuropeptides in the central nervous system: a review of biochemical mapping studies. *Progress in Neurobiology*, **23**, 151–89.

Parent, A. (1986). *Comparative neurobiology of the basal ganglia.* John Wiley, New York.

Parent, A. and Olivier, A. (1970). Comparative histochemical study of the corpus striatum. *Journal für Hirnforschung*, **12**, 73–81.

Paton, J. A., Manogue, K. R., and Nottebohm, F. (1981). Bilateral organization of the vocal control pathway in the budgerigar, *Melopsittacus undulatus. Journal of Neuroscience*, **1**, 1279–88.

Pettigrew, J. D. and Konishi, M. (1976). Neurons selective for orientation and binocular disparity in the visual Wulst of the barn owl (*Tyto alba*). *Science*, **193**, 675–8.

Rehkämper, G., Zilles, K., and Schleicher, A. (1984). A quantitative approach to cytoarchitectonics. IX The areal pattern of the hyperstriatum ventrale in the domestic pigeon, *Columba livia f.d. Anatomy and Embryology*, **169**, 319–27.

Rehkämper, C., Zilles, K., and Schleicher, A. (1985). A quantitative approach to cytoarchitectonics. X. The areal pattern of the neostriatum in the domestic pigeon, *Columba livia f.d.* A cyto- and myeloarchitectonic study. *Anatomy and Embryology*, **171**, 345–55.

Reiner, A., Brauth, S. E., and Karten, H. J. (1984*a*). Evolution of the amniote basal ganglia. *Trends in Neuroscience*, **7**, 320–5.

Reiner, A. and Carraway, R. E. (1987). Immunohistochemical and biochemical studies on Lys[8]-Asn[9]-Neurotensin[8–13] (LANT6)-related peptides in the basal ganglion of pigeons, turtles and hamsters. *Journal of Comparative Neurology*, **257**, 453–76.

Reiner, A., Davis, B. M., Brecha, N. C., and Karten, H. J. (1984*b*). The distribution of enkephalin-like immunoreactivity in the telencephalon of the adult and developing domestic chicken. *Journal of Comparative Neurology*, **228**, 245–62.

Reiner, A. and Karten, H. J. (1983). The laminar source of efferent projections from the avian Wulst. *Brain Research*, **275**, 349–54.

Reiner, A., Karten, H. J., and Solina, A. R. (1983). Substance P: localization within paleostriatal-tegmental pathways in the pigeon. *Neuroscience*, **9**, 61–85.

Revzin, A. M. (1969). A specific visual projection area in the hyperstriatum of the pigeon (*Columba livia*). *Brain Research*, **15**, 246–9.

Revzin, A. M. (1970). Some characteristics of wide-field units in the brain of the pigeon. *Brain, Behavior and Evolution*, **3**, 195–204.

Ritchie, T. L. C. (1979). Intratelencephalic visual connections and their relationship to the archistriatum in the pigeon (*Columba livia*). PhD thesis, University of Virginia.

Rogers, L. J. and Sink, H. S. (1988). Transient asymmetry in the projections of the rostral thalamus to the visual hyperstriatum of the chicken, and reversal of its direction by light exposure. *Experimental Brain Research*, **70**, 378–84.

Saini, K. D. and Leppelsack, H. J. (1977). Neuronal arrangement in the auditory field L of the neostriatum of the starling. *Cell Tissue Research*, **176**, 309–16.

Schall, U. and Delius, J. D. (1986). Sensory inputs to the nucleus basalis prosencephali, a feeding–pecking centre in the pigeon. *Journal of Comparative Physiology*, **A159**, 33–41.

Schall, U., Güntürkün, O., and Delius, J. D. (1986). Sensory projections to the nucleus basalis prosencephali of the pigeon. *Cell Tissue Research*, **245**, 539–46.

Segal, M. and Laudis, S. (1974). Afferents to the hippocampus of the rat studied with the method of retrograde transport of horseradish peroxidase. *Brain Research*, **78**, 1–15.

Stingelin, W. (1958). *Vergleichend-morphologische Untersuchungen am Vorderhirn der Vogel auf cytologischer und cytoarchitektonischer Grundlage.* Helbig und Lichtenhahn, Basel.

Takatsuki, K., Shioseha, S., Inagaki, S., Sakanaka, M., Takagi, H., Senba, E., Matsuzaki, T., and Tohyama, M. (1981). Topographic atlas of somatostatin-containing neuron system in the avian brain in relation to catecholamine-containing neuron system. I.Telencephalon and diencephalon. *Journal of Comparative Neurology*, **202**, 103–13.

van Tienhoven, A. and Juhasz, L. P. (1962). The chicken telencephalon, diencephalon and mesencephalon in stereotaxic coordinates. *Journal of Comparative Neurology*, **118**, 185–97.

Tömböl, T., Csillag, A., and Stewart, M. G. (1988). Cell types of the hyperstriatum ventrale of the domestic chick (*Gallus domesticus*): a Golgi study. *Journal
für Hirnforschung*, **29**, 319–34.
Ulinski, P. S. (1983). *Dorsal ventricular ridge. A treatise on forebrain organization
in reptiles and birds*. John Wiley, New York.
Veening, J. G., Cornelissen, F. M., and Lieven, P. A. J. M. (1980). The topical
organization of the afferents to the caudatoputamen of the rat. A horseradish
peroxidase study. *Neuroscience*, **5**, 1253–68.
Veenman, C. L. and Gottschaldt, K. M. (1985). The organization of the nucleus
basalis-neostriatum complex in the goose (*Anser anser L*). *Advances of Anat-
omy, Embryology and Cell Biology*, **96**, 1–85.
Wächtler, K. (1985). Regional distribution of muscarinic acetylcholine receptors
in the telencephalon of the pigeon (*Columba livia f.domestica*). *Journal für
Hirnforschung*, **26**, 85–90.
Webster, K. E. (1979). Some aspects of the comparative study of the corpus
striatum. In *The neostriatum* (ed. I. Divac and R. G. E. Oberg), pp. 107–26.
Pergamon Press, New York.
Wild, J. M. (1987a). Thalamic projections to the paleostriatum and neostriatum in
the pigeon (*Columba livia*). *Neuroscience*, **20**, 305–27.
Wild, J. M. (1987b). The avian somatosensory system: connections of regions of
body representation in the forebrain of the pigeon. *Brain Research*, **412**, 205–23.
Wild, J. M., Arends, J. J. A., and Zeigler, H. P. (1985). Telencephalic connections
of the trigeminal system in the pigeon (*Columba livia*): a trigeminal sensorimotor
circuit. *Journal of Comparative Neurology*, **234**, 441–64.
Wilson, P. (1980). The organization of the visual striatum of the domestic chick. I.
Topology and topography of the visual projection. II. Receptive field properties
of single units. *Brain Research*, **188**, 319–45.
Youngren, O. M. and Phillips, R. E. (1978). A stereotaxic atlas of the brain of the
three-day-old domestic chick. *Journal of Comparative Neurology*, **181**, 567–600.
Zeier, H. J. and Karten, H. J. (1971). The archistriatum of the pigeon: organiza-
tion of afferent and efferent connections. *Brain Research*, **31**, 313–26.
Zeier, H. J. and Karten, H. J. (1973). Connections of the anterior commissure in
the pigeon (*Columba livia*). *Journal of Comparative Neurology*, **150**, 201–16.
Zeigler, H. P. and Karten, H. J. (1973). Brain mechanisms and feeding behavior
in the pigeon (*Columba livia*). Quintofrontal structures. *Journal of Comparative
Neurology*, **152**, 59–81.

LIST OF ABBREVIATIONS

Nomenclature according to Karten and Hodos (1969) and Baumel (1979).
A   Archistriatum
Amd   A, pars medialis dorsalis
AV   A, pars ventralis
Avdl   A, pars ventralis dorsolateralis
AL   Ansa lenticularis
APH   Area parahippocampalis

AS	Area septalis
B(as)	Nucleus basalis
CA	Commissura rostralis (anterior)
CDL	Area corticoidea dorsolateralis
DA	Tractus dorso-archistriaticus
DB	Fasciculus diagonalis (Brocae)
E	Ectostriatum
Ec	Ectostriatal core
Ep	Peri-ectostriatal belt
FA	Tractus fronto-archistriaticus
FPL	Fasciculus lateralis prosencephali
HA	Hyperstriatum accessorium
HD	Hyperstriatum dorsale
HIS	Hyperstriatum intercalatum supremum
Hp	Hippocampus
HV	Hyperstriatum ventrale
HVc	Caudal auditory area of HV/N
HV,i	HV, pars intermedia
IHA	Nucleus intercalatus of HA
IMHV	Nucleus medialis of HV, i
INP	Nucleus intrapeduncularis
L	Field L in neostriatum, pars caudalis
LFM	Lamina frontalis suprema
LFS	Lamina frontalis superior
LH	Lamina hyperstriatica
LMD	Lamina medullaris dorsalis
LPO	Lobus parolfactorius
LPO,X	Area X in LPO
ML	Nucleus mammilaris lateralis
N	Neostriatum
NC	N, pars caudalis
Nf,d,l,v	N, pars rostralis (frontale), dorsal, lateral, ventral zone
Ni,l	N, pars intermedia, lateral zone
N,If	Nucleus interfacialis
Ov	Nucleus ovoidalis
PA	Palaeostriatum augmentatum
PC	Palaeostriatum complex
POA	Nucleus preopticus anterior
PP	Palaeostriatum primitivum
PrV	Nucleus sensorius principalis, nervi V
RA	Nucleus robustus of A
Rot	Nucleus rotundus
Tn	Nucleus teniae
TPO	Area temporoparieto-occipitalis

TSM   Tractus septomesencephalicus
UVA   Nucleus uvae
Val   Vallecula telencephali
II   Nervus opticus
V   Nervus trigeminus

3

The functional organization of the avian visual system

O. Güntürkün

INTRODUCTION

Rochon-Duvigneaud (1943) coined the phrase that a pigeon is nothing else but two eyes with wings. The more we learn about the visual system of birds, the more we appreciate the truth of this remark. Pigeons are visually able to distinguish between bars differing in length by less than 2 per cent (Schwabl and Delius 1984). Thus the pigeon's length-difference threshold is about half that of humans (Ono 1967). The mean log luminance-difference threshold is 0.1, which corresponds approximately to a luminance difference created by two microscopy coverslips (Hodos *et al.* 1985). Unlike humans, pigeons are able to discern the plane of oscillation of polarized light (Delius *et al.* 1976) and they perform pattern discriminations in the near-ultraviolet (Emmerton 1983*b*). Their maximum critical fusion frequency is 145 Hz, which clearly exceeds the 60–70 Hz temporal resolution of humans (Emmerton 1983*a*). The pentachromatic visual system of pigeons probably enables them to differentiate colour qualities that humans with their trichromatic visual system cannot perceive (Emmerton and Delius 1980). The visual memory of many bird species also has a remarkable capacity. For example, nutcrackers can remember the position of thousands of food hoards (Shettleworth 1983), and pigeons learn to discriminate 100 positive from 625 negative patterns (von Fersen and Delius 1989).

Since birds are classic subjects of the ethologist and behavioural scientist, a large number of studies on avian visually guided behaviour have accumulated over time. This offers the possiblity of combining this wealth of behavioural data with electrophysiological and anatomical results on the ascending visual pathways. Starting with the retina, this review will therefore try to provide a brief account of the functional organization of the avian visual system.

THE RETINA

The avian retina appears to have attracted more attention than have the retinae of other non-mammals. Among the birds studied, the pigeon (*Columba livia*) and the chick (*Gallus domesticus*) are probably the most thoroughly examined species. Both have a central retinal area of enhanced vision, where ganglion cell densities reach up to 41 000 cells per mm² in the pigeon (Hayes *et al*. 1987) and 24 000 cells per mm² in the chick (Ehrlich 1981). The pigeon has an additional area with high ganglion cell densities in the superior-temporal retina where cell densities increase up to 36 000 neurons per mm² (Hayes *et al*. 1987). The area is the so-called red field, which is clearly distinct from the yellow field encompassing the remaining part of the pigeon's retina. The colouring arises from the inclusion in the cone receptor cells of brightly coloured oil-droplets which are differentially distributed throughout the retina. Each kind of oil-droplet is found in both the red and the yellow field. However, in the red field most of the oil-droplets are red or orange, with fewer yellow droplets. In the yellow field, the yellow droplets predominate. Because of their positions, the red fields project binocularly in front of, and below the beak and view objects such as food grains which fall in this visual field. The yellow field projects laterally and monocularly (Martinoya *et al*. 1981; Jahnke 1984, McFadden and Reymond 1985). These two areas are probably functionally equivalent to the foveae of most mammals or many birds, although they lack the formal anatomical properties of foveae (Fite and Rosenfield-Wessels 1975). The two retinal subdivisions also differ in their spectral sensitivities, with a greater sensitivity for short wavelength in the yellow field (Remy and Emmerton 1989*a*). Additionally, function differences between the retinal areas, corresponding to frontal and lateral visual fields, have been established for movement sensitivity (Martinoya *et al*. 1983), and for visual acuity, with pigeons being myopic in the lower half of the visual field, which includes the projection area of the red field (Bloch and Martinoya 1982; Fitzke *et al*. 1985).

The red and the yellow fields of the pigeon retina also seem to differ with respect to their capacity of interocular transfer. This is demonstrated with experiments in which the birds learn a visual discrimination with one eye occluded and are tested for transfer of learning with the stimuli presented to the untrained eye (Watanabe 1986). Mallin and Delius (1983) trained head-fixed pigeons under monocular conditions to discriminate two colours, using mandibulation as an operant. In one group the stimuli were presented in the lateral visual field, in the other group in the frontal one. After reaching criterion the subjects were tested for interocular transfer. They now saw the stimuli at homologous positions with the untrained eye. The transfer of colour discrimination presented frontally was significantly better than that presented laterally. The situation is even more complex when intraocular transfer is tested, that is, the transfer of a visual discrimination from an experienced to an unexperienced locus of one retina. Successful transfer of a visual discrimination occurs only when stimulus presentation is changed from the lateral to the frontal visual field but not vice versa (Remy and Emmerton 1989*b*). This asymmetry in intraocular transfer is probably adaptive for pigeons, since they switch from lateral to frontal vision when they approach food from a distance and then start pecking (Bloch *et al.* 1988).

The axons of the retinal ganglion cells converge to form 2.4 million fibres in the pigeon and 2.4–2.6 million fibres in the chick optic nerve (Binggeli and Paule 1969; Rager and Rager 1978; Ehrlich 1981). Virtually all axons from one eye project to the contralateral halfbrain, where they enter 19 different neuronal structures in the pigeon and 18 in the chick (Repérant 1973; Ehrlich and Mark 1984*a*). The large number of retinorecipient areas in birds, in comparison to other vertebrates, reflects the importance of vision for avian species. Two of these retinorecipient structures, the tectum opticum and the n. opticus principalis thalami (OPT), give rise to separate ascending tectofugal and thalamofugal pathways projecting to the forebrain.

THE FIRST TECTOFUGAL PATHWAY

The axons of the retinal ganglion cells, which constitute the first of the 15 tectal laminae, innervate only the superficial layers 2–5 and 7 (Cajal 1891; Repérant 1973). Visual information is transmitted either directly with axodendritic contacts (Hardy *et al.* 1985) or with interneurons to the cells of layer 13, which project to the n. rotundus in the thalamus. The rotundus itself sends efferent fibres to the ipsilateral ectostriatum, a core portion of the forebrain. Kondo (1933) was the first to discover this pathway in the fowl, but since he published his results in Japanese, western scientists were for a long time not aware of his studies. Karten and coworkers (Revzin and Karten 1966/67; Karten and Hodos 1970; Benowitz and Karten 1976) rediscovered this projection in the pigeon.

Single unit recordings in the optic tectum demonstrated that the visual receptive fields (RF) of neurons in the superficial layers are small (0.5–4 degrees) but increase up to 180 degrees in the deeper laminae (Bilge 1971; Jassik-Gerschenfeld *et al.* 1975; Frost *et al.* 1981). The majority (70 per cent of tectal cells are movement-sensitive, with about 30 per cent of them having directional preferences (Jassik-Gerschenfeld and Guichard 1972). Directionally responsive units are either narrowly tuned or, more commonly, they respond to a wide range of directions, with the majority being inhibited by backward movement (Frost and DiFranco 1976). Tectal cells also respond selectively to the spatial frequency of drifting sine-wave gratings, with most neurons having their optima between 0.45 and 0.6 cycles per degree (Jassik-Gerschenfeld and Hardy 1979). Most of these cells are also more selective to spatial frequency than they are to the width of a single bar stimulus (Jassik-Gerschenfeld and Hardy 1980). Birds therefore appear to be able to perform a Fourier analysis of patterns in visual space.

Rotundal and ectostriatal units share most of the features of deep tectal units. Most of them have large receptive fields of up to 180 degrees (Revzin 1970) and demonstrate movement sensitivity, with a proportion having directional preferences for forward movements (Kimberley *et al.* 1971; Maxwell and Granda 1979; Revzin 1979). Additionally, Yazulla and Granda (1973) found colour-opponent units in the ventral part of the rotundus.

Behavioural studies on the visual system of birds started with the experiments of Rolando (1809) in fowls. He demonstrated that after subtotal bilateral hemispherectomies the animals could avoid obstacles while walking, but had a tendency slightly to displace their pecks during feeding. These results triggered an interest in the optic tectum of birds, since forebrain structures seemed not to be crucial for visually guided behaviour. Flourens (1824) was the first to remove unilaterally the optic tectum in pigeons. He describes the lesioned animal as being blind with its contralateral eye. This result was generally confirmed in several studies, although there were disputes as to whether birds without optic lobes were completely blind or demonstrated only 'psychic blindness' (Schrader 1892). Cohen (1967) was the first to study the optic tectum with modern behavioural techniques using a brightness discrimination task. He showed that small lesions of the optic tectum involving less than 15 per cent structure-volume had only little effect on visual discrimination in pigeons. Jarvis (1974) and Hodos and Karten (1974) studied pigeons with extensive tectal lesions and demonstrated virtually a complete loss of the postoperative discrimination capacity in brightness and pattern discrimination tasks. Most of the animals failed to improve or else required a prolonged reacquisition period with the simpler discrimination tasks, but did not reach criterion on more difficult problems.

Lesion studies on the rotundus demonstrated generally milder impairments. After bilateral ablations of the rotundus in pigeons, the animals relearned the colour discrimination in approximately the same number of trails as required preoperatively (Hodos 1969). The deficits in an intensity and pattern discrimination task were more severe. Postoperatively, the animals relearned the distinction only after 2–3 times the number of preoperative trials (Hodos and Karten 1966).

Tasks which require the discrimination of coarse differences in luminance or geometric patterns are generally not sufficiently sensitive to

detect subtle postoperative deficits in lesion studies. Therefore psychophysical techniques with which sensitivity limits can be determined are
more appropriate to test the postoperative integrity of visual functions.
Hodos and Bonbright (1974) studied intensity difference thresholds of
pigeons with rotundal lesions. The experimental animals showed large
initial threshold elevations, but with extended postoperative training,
these deficits returned to approximately the preoperative baseline. Macko
and Hodos (1984) tested pigeons with rotundal lesions in a visual acuity
task and demonstrated threshold elevations of about 100 per cent. Contrary to the results of the intensity discrimination study, the performance
of the animals did not return to preoperative levels.

Ectostriatal lesions generally result in similar deficits to rotundal lesions.
Pigeons with extensive ablations of the ectostriatum demonstrate a postoperative return to chance levels in a visual intensity and pattern discrimination task; however, they reach preoperative performance after extensive
training (Hodos and Karten 1970). More recent studies using psychophysical methods determined that the pigeons with ectostriatal lesions did not
return completely to the preoperative performance but lost 50–83 per cent
of their preoperative capacity in an intensity discrimination task (Hodos
et al. 1988). Similarly, Hodos et al. (1984) demonstrated that most of the
ectostriatal birds did not return to their preoperative performance in a
visual acuity task.

One of the major problems for the understanding of the function of the
first tectofugal pathway is the discrepancy between the electrophysiological
and the behavioural data. It is surprising that acuity suffers from lesions in
a system, the neurons within which have generally very large receptive
fields. One possible explanation is that, nevertheless, some tectal units are
concerned with fine texture of large stimuli. Jassik-Gerschenfeld and
co-workers (Hardy and Jassik-Gerschenfeld 1979; Jassik-Gerschenfeld and
Hardy 1979) demonstrated that some tectal units perform a Fourier
analysis of patterns in visual space, with some cells being tuned to changes
in temporal frequency. Thus, with an array of neurons encoding different
spatial frequencies the tectofugal pathway could be able to process even
subtle visual details. This interpretation would then overcome the discrepancies of the electrophysiological and behavioural results.

THE SECOND TECTOFUGAL SYSTEM

Recent experiments in pigeons demonstrated that the optic tectum
projects not only to the rotundus, but also to the n. dorsolateralis posterior
thalami (DLP), which itself projects to the ipsilateral forebrain (Gamlin
and Cohen 1986). The telencephalic projection area of the DLP was
defined as a subarea of the neostriatum intermedium (NI) (Gamlin and

Cohen 1986) and the neostriatum caudale (NC), from which visual evoked potentials could be recorded (Güntürkün 1984, 1985). Since the general outline of this projection resembles the first tectofugal pathway, lesion studies were performed to study possible postoperative visual deficits. Hodos *et al.* (1986) and Kertzmann and Hodos (1988) could not reveal deficits in size-difference thresholds after lesions of the DLP or the NI. However, combined lesions of rotundus and DLP or ectostriatum and NI resulted in larger deficits than lesions of rotundus or ectostriatum alone. These results provide at least indirect evidence for a participation of the second tectofugal pathway in visual information processing.

However, recent anatomical and electrophysiological data cast doubt on the assumption that the projection via the DLP constitutes a smaller version of the first tectofugal pathway. Arends *et al.* (1984), Wild (1987), and Korzeniewska and Güntürkün (1989) demonstrated a massive somatosensory projection of the *nuclei gracilis et cuneatus* onto the DLP. Korzeniewska (1987) and Korzeniewska and Güntürkün (1990) showed that 38 per cent of the DLP per cent units responded to somatosensory, 24 per cent to visual, and 9 per cent to auditory stimuli. The remaining 29 per cent of neurons were multimodal and integrated all three modalities.

The studies to reveal the functional importance of the second tectofugal pathway have just begun. Presently, it is difficult to decide to which degree this projection participates in visual analysis. As pointed out by Brauth *et al.* (1987), it could be that the second tectofugal pathway primarily integrates stimuli of different modalities to provide the capacity for supramodal operations. The analysis of visual information would thus be only a part of the functions of this projection.

THE THALAMOFUGAL PATHWAY

As outlined above, the retinal ganglion cells project not only to the optic tectum but also to a complex of nuclei in the dorsolateral thalamus, which themselves send fibres to the ipsilateral and the contralateral Wulst in the forebrain. This complex of nuclei is collectively called the *n. opticus principalis thalami* (OPT) (Karten *et al.* 1973). Electrophysiological studies demonstrated that the receptive fields (RF) of OPT units are generally smaller than those of neurons within the tectofugal pathway. For example Pateromichelakis (1981) estimates an average of 15 degrees for the OPT of chicks and Britten (1987) an average of 16 degrees for the OPT of pigeons. However, all authors agree that there is considerable variation in the receptive field sizes of OPT units reaching from 2 to 180 degrees. With the exception of the study of Jassik-Gerschenfeld *et al.* (1976), all experiments (DeBritto *et al.* 1975; Maxwell and Granda 1979; Pateromichelakis

1981; Britten 1987) demonstrated a majority of movement sensitive cells, with most of them having directional selectivity.

Similar results were obtained for the visual Wulst, the projection area of the OPT. According to Revzin (1969), Gusel'nikov *et al.* (1976), and Miceli *et al.* (1979) the smallest RF in the visual Wulst of pigeons have diameters of about 2 degrees. The estimates for the largest RF reach from 10 degrees (Revzin 1969) to 50 degrees (Miceli *et al.* 1979). According to Wilson (1980*b*) the size of the RF in the chick's visual Wulst are in the range of 10–45 degrees and thus close to the receptive field sizes of Wulst neurons in pigeons. All authors agree that the majority of visually responsive units in the Wulst of pigeons and chicks are movement sensitive, with a small proportion showing directional selectivity.

Remy and Güntürkün (1991) studied the retinal afferents of the OPT in pigeons using microinjections of retrograde tracers into various OPT substructures. They demonstrated that most of the labelled retinal ganglion cells were located in the yellow field, while the number of labelled neurons in the red field was extremely small. As outlined above, the red field is suggested to transmit visual information from the binocular visual field situated mainly below the eye–beak axis. The projection of the red field onto the contralateral OPT, and the bilateral projections of the OPT onto the visual Wulst were thought to establish binocular convergence in the forebrain. This assumption was supported by the results of Pettigrew and Konishi (1976*a*,*b*) and Pettigrew (1979), who demonstrated that a large amount of neurons in the visual Wulst of barn owls possess binocular visual fields with retinal disparity. In accordance with these results, Bravo and Pettigrew (1981) and Bravo and Inzunza (1983) showed that the temporal retina representing the binocular visual field projects heavily onto the OPT in owls and falcons. The study of Remy and Güntürkün (1991) therefore demonstrates a dramatic difference in the properties of the thalamofugal pathway in birds. This is reflected in the electrophysiological data which are available for the thalamofugal pathway of pigeons. Single unit analyses of the pigeon's OPT were performed in six studies. Only one of them (Britten 1987) provides data on the position of the RF in visual space. Britten (1987) recorded from 167 OPT units and demonstrated that only about 15 per cent of them had their RF in the red field projection area. The situation for the Wulst is similar. Miceli *et al.* (1979) recorded from 170 neurons of the Wulst. None of them had their RF in the red field projection area. Thus, the electrophysiological studies of the Wulst and the OPT match the anatomical data, in that the thalamofugal pathway of pigeons seems to be mainly involved in the visual analysis of objects in the monocular visual field.

The situation seems to be different for chicks. Ehrlich and Mark (1984*b*) demonstrated projections from the superiotemporal retina (comparable to the red field of pigeons) to the rostral part of the OPT. Wilson (1980*a*) and Denton (1981) revealed a complete representation of visual space, including the frontal field, onto the visual Wulst of chicks. However, neither author could find a substantial number of binocularly driven units.

Comparing the thalamofugal pathway of chicks, pigeons, and barn owls reveals substantial differences between these three species. The visual Wulst of owls, with its topographical representation of visual space and the large number of binocularly driven units, shows important similarities to the primary visual cortex of mammal. With respect to owls, the thalamofugal pathway of chicks and pigeons appears to be rather undifferentiated. Between these two latter species the main difference seems to be the degree of representation of frontal vision within the thalamofugal pathway. It might be speculated that the occurrence of a retinal red field in pigeons may have initiated a specialization for lateral monocular vision in the thalamofugal and for whole field analysis (including frontal vision) in the tectofugal pathway.

Lesion studies of the thalamofugal system generally showed little or no effects on coarse discrimination tasks. Pritz *et al.* (1970) and Parker and Delius (1980) could not demonstrate any postoperative deficits in a colour discrimination after lesions of the Wulst in pigeons. Lesions of the OPT (Hodos *et al.* 1973; Mulvanny 1979) or the Wulst (Pritz *et al.* 1978; Hodos *et al.* 1973) produced only minor impairments in tasks involving the discrimination of visual intensities, patterns, or line orientations. Using more sophisticated psychophysical procedures, Hodos and coworkers were able to demonstrate more profound deficits after thalamofugal lesions. According to these studies, ablations of the OPT (Hodos and Bonbright 1974) or the Wulst (Pasternak and Hodos 1977) resulted in small but rather stable postoperative threshold elevations of visual intensity differences. In terms of visual acuity, OPT lesions had no effect on the discrimination capacity of pigeons (Macko and Hodos 1984). Wulst-ablated birds suffered initial losses in the same task but regained their previous performance during postoperative training (Hodos *et al.* 1984).

Since thalamofugal lesions did not produce substantial deficits in any of the visual discriminations employed, experimentators began to be interested in other visual tasks, for which lesion deficits could be demonstrated. Weiss and Hodos (1986) trained pigeons to discriminate lateral mirror image patterns and placed lesions either into the ectostriatum or the Wulst. They could only demonstrate an impairment after ectostriatal lesions, but not after ablations of the visual Wulst. Delius and Hollard (1987) were interested in whether Wulst lesions could affect the capacity of birds to recognize rotated patterns. Hollard and Delius (1982) had shown that pigeons are able to solve visual pattern recognition tasks involving rotated forms more efficiently than humans. Therefore Delius and Hollard (1987) trained pigeons to perform a visual orientation invariance task consisting of shape matching-to-sample or oddity-from-sample discriminations where the comparison forms differed in orientation from the sample forms, and the odd comparison forms were always a mirror image of the sample. After reaching criterion the birds received lesions either into the Wulst or, as a control, into the dorsal neostriatum. Both groups of pigeons evinced only minor transient postoperative deficits. Only when novel forms were introduced was the performance of Wulst-ablated animals significantly worse than that of the neostriatal pigeons, but still well above chance.

As outlined above, lesions of the OPT or the Wulst produce only minimal deficits in a large number of different visual tasks, while ablations of the first tectofugal pathway lead to severe visual performance attenuations. Most tasks used so far with pigeons involved frontal presentation. Since the thalamofugal pathway is mainly concerned with the lateral visual field, thalamofugal lesions are likely to produce only minimal deficits when tested with this procedure. Behavioural deficits after thalamofugal ablations could be tested more accurately with other techniques, in which the stimuli are presented in the lateral visual field (Bloch and Martinoya 1982; Mallin and Delius 1983; Remy and Emmerton 1989a). It is conceivable that these experiments might then reveal information about functional differences between the visual pathways of birds which are presently beyond our reach.

REFERENCES

Arends, J. J. A., Woelders-Blok, A., and Dubbeldam, J. L. (1984). The efferent connections of the descending trigeminal tract in the mallard (*Anas platyrhynchos 1.*). Neuroscience, **13**, 797–817.

Benowitz, L. I. and Karten, H. J. (1976). Organization of the tectofugal visual pathway in the pigeon: a retrograde transport study. *Journal of Comparative Neurology*, **167**, 503–20.

Bilge, M. (1971). Electrophysiological investigations on the pigeon's optic tectum. *Quarterly Journal of Experimental Physiology*, **56**, 242–9.

Binggeli, R. L. and Paule, W. J. (1969). The pigeon retina: quantitative aspects of the optic nerve and ganglion cell layer. *Journal of Comparative Neurology*, **137**, 1–18.

Bloch, S. and Martinoya, C. (1982). Comparing frontal and lateral viewing in the pigeon. I. Tachistoscopic visual acuity as a function of distance. *Behavioral Brain Research*, **5**, 231–44.

Bloch, S., Jäger, R., Lemeignan, M., and Martinoya, C. (1988). Correlation between ocular saccades and headmovements in walking pigeons. *Journal of Physiology (London)*, **406**, 173.

Brauth, S. E., McHale, C. M., Brasher, C. A., and Dooling, R. J. (1987).

Auditory pathways in the budgerigar. I. Thalamo-telencephalic projections. *Brain, Behavior and Evolution*, **30**, 174–99.

Bravo, H. and Inzunza, O. (1983). Estudio anatomico en las vias visuales paralelas en falconiformes. *Archivos de Biologia y Medicina Experimentales*, **16**, 283–9.

Bravo, H. and Pettigrew, J. D.(1981). The distribution of neurons projecting from the retina and visual cortex to the thalamus and tectum opticum of the barn owl, *Tyto alba*, and the burrowing owl, *Speotyto cuniculana*. *Journal of Comparative Neurology*, **199**, 419–41.

Britten, K. H. (1987). Receptive fields of neurons of the principal optic nucleus of the pigeon (*Columba livia*). PhD thesis, State University of New York, Stony Brook, NY.

Cajal, S. R. Y. (1891). Sur la fine structure du lobe optique des oiseaux et sur l'origine réelle des nerfs optiques. *Internationale Monatsschrift für Anatomie und Physiologie*, **8**, 347–61.

Cohen, D. H. (1967). Visual intensity discrimination in pigeons following unilateral and bilateral tectal lesions. *Journal of Comparative Physiology and Psychology*, **63**, 172–4.

DeBritto, L. R. G., Bunelli, M., Francesconi, W., and Magni, F. (1975). Visual response pattern of thalamic neurons in the pigeon. *Brain Research*, **97**, 337–43.

Delius, J. D., Perchard, R., and Emmerton, J. (1976). Polarized light discrimination by pigeons and an electroretinographic correlate. *Journal of Comparative Physiology and Psychology*, **90(6)**, 560–71.

Delius, J. D. and Hollard, V. D. (1987). Orientation invariance of shape recognition in forebrain-lesioned pigeons. *Behavioral Brain Research* **23**, 251–9.

Denton, C. J. (1981).Topography of the hyperstriatal visual projection area in the young domestic chicken. *Experimental Neurology*, **74**, 482–98.

Ehrlich, D. (1981). Regional specialization of the chick retina as revealed by the ganglion cell layer. *Journal of Comparative Neurology*, **195**, 643–57.

Ehrlich, D. and Mark, R. (1984*a*). An atlas of the primary visual projections in the brain of the chick *Gallus gallus*. *Journal of Comparative Neurology*, **223**, 592–610.

Ehrlich, D. and Mark, R. (1984*b*). Topography of primary visual centers in the brain of the chick, *Gallus gallus*. *Journal of Comparative Neurology*, **223**, 611–25.

Emmerton, J. (1983*a*). Functional morphology of the visual system. In M. Abs (ed.) *Physiology and behavior of the pigeon* (ed. M. Abs), pp. 221–44. Academic Press, London.

Emmerton, J. (1983*b*). Pattern discrimination in the near ultra-violet by pigeons. *Perceptual Psychophysics*, **34**, 555–9.

Emmerton, J. and Delius, J. D. (1980). Wavelength discrimination in the 'visible' and ultraviolet spectrum by pigeons. *Journal of Comparative Physiology*, **141**, 47–52.

Fite, K. V. and Rosenfield-Wessels, S. (1975). A comparative study of deep avian foveas. *Brain, Behavior and Evolution*, **12**, 97–115.

Fitzke, F. W., Hayes, B. P., Hodos, W., Holden, A. L., and Low, J. C. (1985). Refractive sectors in the visual field of the pigeon eye. *Journal of Physiology*, *(London)*, **369**, 33–44.

Flourens, P. (1824). Recherches experimentales sur les proprietés et les fonctions du systeme nerveux dans les animaux vertebrés. Paris.

Frost, B. and diFranco D. E. (1976). Motion characteristics of single units in the pigeon optic tectum. *Vision Research*, **16**, 1229–34.

Frost, B. J., Scilley, P. L., and Wong, S. C. P. (1981). Moving background patterns reveal double-opponency of directionally specific pigeon tectal neurons. *Experimental Brain Research*, **43**, 173–85.

Gamlin, P. D. R. and Cohen, D. H. (1986). Second ascending visual pathway from the optic tectum to the telencephalon in the pigeon (*Columba livia*). *Journal of Comparative Neurology*, **250**, 296–310.

Güntürkün, O. (1984). Evidence for a third primary visual area in the telencephalon of the pigeon. *Brain Research*, **294**, 247–54.

Güntürkün, O. (1985). Four independent visual pathways to the telencephalon of the pigeon. *Neuroscience Letters Supplement*, **22**, 319.

Gusel'nikov, V. I., Morenkov, E. D., and Do Cong Hunh (1976). Responses and properties of receptive fields of neurons in the visual projection zone of the pigeon hyperstriatum. *Neurofiziologiya*, **8**, 230–6.

Hardy, O. and Jassik-Gerschenfeld, D. (1979). Spatial frequency and temporal frequency of single cells in the pigeon optic tectum. *Vision Research*, **19**, 1001–4.

Hardy, O., Leresche, N., and Jassik-Gerschenfeld, D. (1985). Morphology and laminar distribution of electrophysiologically identified cells in the pigeon's optic tectum: an intracellular study. *Journal of Comparative Neurology*, **233**, 390–404.

Hayes, B. P., Hodos, W., Holden, A. L., and Low, J. C. (1987). The projection of the visual field upon the retina of the pigeon. *Vision Research*, **27**, 31–40.

Hodos, W. (1969). Color discrimination deficits after lesions of the nucleus rotundus in pigeons. *Brain, Behavior and Evolution*, **2**, 185–200.

Hodos, W. and Bonbright, J. C. (1974). Intensity difference threshold in pigeons after lesions of the tectofugal and thalamofugal visual pathways. *Journal of Comparative Physiology and Psychology*, **87**, 1013–31.

Hodos, W. and Karten, H. J. (1966). Brightness and pattern discrimination deficits in the pigeon after lesions of nucleus rotundus. *Experimental Brain Research*, **2**, 151–67.

Hodos, W. and Karten, H. J. (1970). Visual intensity and pattern discrimination deficits after lesions of the ectostriatum in pigeons. *Journal of Comparative Neurology*, **140**, 53–68.

Hodos, W. and Karten, H. J. (1974). Visual intensity and pattern discrimination deficits after lesions of the optic lobe in pigeons. *Brain, Behavior and Evolution*, **9**, 165–94.

Hodos, W., Karten, H. J., and Bonbright, J. C. (1973). Visual intensity and pattern discrimination after lesions of the thalamofugal visual pathways in pigeons. *Journal of Comparative Neurology*, **148**, 447–68.

Hodos, W., Macko, K. A., and Besette, B. B. (1984). Near-field acuity changes after visual system lesions in pigeons. II. Telencephalon. *Behavioural Brain Research*, **13**, 15–30.

Hodos, W., Bessette, B. B., Macko, K. A., and Weiss, S. R. B. (1985). Normative data for pigeon vision. *Vision Research*, **10**, 1525–7.

Hodos, W., Weiss, S. R. B., and Bessette, B. B. (1986). Size threshold changes after lesions of the visual telencephalon in pigeons. *Behavioural Brain Research*, **21**, 203–14.

Hodos, W., Weiss, S. R. B., and Bessette, B. B. (1988). Intensity difference thresholds after lesions of ectostriatum in pigeons, *Behavioural Brain Research*, **30**, 43–53.

Hollard, V. D. and Delius, J. D. (1982). Rotational invariance in visual pattern recognition by pigeons and humans. *Science*, **218**, 804–6.

Jahnke, K. J. (1984). Binocular visual field differences among various breeds of pigeons. *Bird Behaviour*, **5**, 96–102.

Jarvis, C. D. (1974). Visual discrimination and spatial localisation deficits after lesions of the tectofugal pathway in pigeons. *Brain, Behavior and Evolution*, **9**, 195–228.

Jassik-Gerschenfeld, D., Guichard, J., and Tessier, Y. (1975). Localization of directionally selective and movement sensitive cells in the optic tectum of the pigeon. *Vision Research*, **15**, 1037–8.

Jassik-Gerschenfeld, D., Teulon, J., and Ropert, N. (1976). Visual receptive field types in the nucleus dorsolateralis anterior of the pigeon's thalamus. *Brain Research*, **108**, 295–306.

Jassik-Gerschenfeld, D., and Guichard, J. (1972). Visual receptive fields of simple cells in the pigeon's optic tectum. *Brain Research*, **40**, 303–17.

Jassik-Gerschenfeld, D., and Hardy, O. (1979). Single neuron responses to moving sine-wave gratings in the pigeon optic tectum. *Vision Research*, **19**, 993–9.

Jassik-Gerschenfeld, D., and Hardy, O. (1980). Single-cell responses to bar width and to sine-wave grating frequency in the pigeon optic tectum. *Vision Research*, **21**, 715–47.

Karten, H. J. and Hodos, W. (1970). Telencephalic projections of the nucleus rotundus in the pigeon (*Columba livia*). *Journal of Comparative Neurology*, **140**, 35–52.

Karten, H. J., Hodos, W., Nauta, W. J. H., and Revzin, A. L. (1973). Neural connections of the 'visual wulst' of the avian telencephalon. Experimental studies in the pigeon (*Columba livia*) and owl (*Speotyto cunicularia*). *Journal of Comparative Neurology*, **150**, 253–77.

Kertzmann, C. and Hodos, W. (1988). Size-difference threshold after lesions of thalamic visual nuclei in pigeons. *Visual Neuroscience*, **1**, 83–92.

Kimberley, R. P., Holden, A. L., and Bamborough, P. (1971). Response characteristics of pigeon forebrain cells to visual stimulation. *Vision Research*, **11**, 475–8.

Kondo, T. (1933). Über die Verbindung des Sehhügels mit dem Streifenhügel beim Huhn. *Okayama I. Z.*, **45**, 797–817.

Korzeniewska, E. (1987). Multisensory convergence in the thalamus of the pigeon (*Columba livia*). *Neuroscience Letters*, **80**, 55–60.

Korzeniewska, E., and Güntürkün, O. (1990). Sensory properties and afferents of the nucleus dorsolateralis posterior thalami (DLP) of the pigeon. *Journal of Comparative Neurology*, **292**, 457–79.

McFadden, S. A. and Reymond, L. (1985). A further look at the binocular visual field of the pigeon (*Columba livia*). *Vision Research*, **25**, 1741–6.

Macko, K. A., and Hodos, W. (1984). Near field acuity after visual system lesions in pigeons. I. Thalamus. *Behavioural Brain Research*, **13**, 1–14.

Mallin, H. D. and Delius, J. D. (1983). Inter- and intraocular transfer of color discriminations with mandibulation as an operant in the head-fixed pigeon. *Behavioural Analysis Letters*. **3**, 297–309.

Martinoya, C., Bloch, S., and Rivaud, S. (1983). Comparing frontal and lateral viewing in the pigeon. II. Velocity thresholds for movement discrimination. *Behavioural Brain Research*, **8**, 375–85.

Martinoya, C., Rey, J., and Bloch, S. (1981). Limits of the pigeon's binocular field and direction for best binocular viewing. *Vision Research*, **21**, 1197–1200.

Maxwell, J. H. and Granda, A. M. (eds) (1979). Receptive fields of movement sensitive cells in the pigeon thalamus. In *Neural mechanisms of behavior in birds*, Plenum Press, New York.

Miceli, D., Gioanni, H., Repérant, J., and Peyrichoux, J. (1979). The avian visual Wulst: I. an anatomical study of afferent and efferent pathways. II. an electrophysiological study of the functional properties of single neurons. In *Neural mechanisms of behavior in birds* (ed. A. M. Granda and J. H. Maxwell). Plenum Press, New York.

Mulvanny, P. (1979). Discrimination of line orientation by pigeons after lesions of thalamic visual nuclei. In *Neural mechanisms of behavior in birds* (ed. A. M. Granda and J. H. Maxwell). Plenum Press, New York.

Ono, H. (1967). Difference threshold of stimulus length under simultaneous and non-simultaneous viewing conditions. *Perception and Psychophysiology*, **2**, 201–7.

Parker, D. M. and Delius, J. D. (1980). The effect of Wulst lesions on single visual discrimination performance in the pigeon. *Behavioral Proceedings*, **5**, 151–9.

Pasternak, T., and Hodos, W. (1977). Intensity difference thresholds after lesions of the visual Wulst in pigeons. *Journal of Comparative Physiology and Psychology*, **91**, 485–97.

Pateromichelakis, S. (1981). Response properties of visual units in the anterior dorsolateral thalamus of the chick (*Gallus domesticus*). *Experientia*, **37**, 279–80.

Pettigrew, J. D. (1979). Binocular visual processing in the owl's telencephalon. *Proceedings of the Royal Society of London Series B*, **204**, 435–55.

Pettigrew, J. D. and Konishi, M. (1976a). Neurons selective for orientation and binocular disparity in the visual Wulst of the barn owl (*Tyto alba*). *Science*, **193**, 675–8.

Pettigrew, J. D. and Konishi, M. (1976b). Effect of monocular deprivation on binocular neurons in the owl's visual Wulst. *Nature*, **264**, 753–4.

Pritz, M. B., Mead, W. R., and Northcutt, R. G. (1970). The effect of Wulst ablations on color, pattern and brightness discrimination in pigeons (*Columba livia*). *Journal of Comparative Neurology*, **140**, 81–100.

Rager, G. and Rager, U. (1978). Systems-matching by degeneration. *Experimental Brain Research*, **33**, 65–78.

Remy, M. and Emmerton, J. (1989a). Behavioral spectral sensitivities of different retinal areas in pigeons. *Behavioral Neuroscience*, **103**, 170–7.

Remy, M. and Emmerton, J. (1989b). Directional dependence of intraocular transfer of stimulus detection in pigeons (*Columba livia*). (Submitted.)

Remy, M. and Güntürkün, O. (1991). Retinal afferents to the optic tectum and the nucleus opticus principalis thalami in the pigeon. *Journal of Comparative Neurology*. (In press.)

Repérant, J. (1973). Nouvelles données sur les projections visuelles chez le pigeon (*Columba livia*). *Journal für Hirnforschung*, **14**, 151–87.

Revzin, A. M. (1969). A specific visual projection area in the hyperstriatum of the pigeon. *Brain Research*, **15**, 246–9.

Revzin, A. M. (1970). Some characteristics of wide-field units in the brain of the pigeon. *Brain, Behavior and Evolution*, **3**, 195–204.

Revzin, A. M. (1979). Functional localisation in the nucleus rotundus. In *Neural mechanisms of behavior in birds* (ed. A. M. Granda, and J. H. Maxwell). Plenum Press, New York.

Revzin, A. M. and Karten, H. (1966/67). Rostral projections of the optic tectum and the nucleus rotundus in the pigeon. *Brain Research*, **3**, 264–76.

Rochon-Duvigneaud, A. (1943). Les yeux et la vision des vertebrés. Masson, Paris.

Rolando, L. (1823). Saggio sopra la vera struttura del cervetto e sopra le fonzioni del sistema nervoso. Sassari 1809. Translated and reprinted: Expériences sur les Fonctions du Système Nerveux. *Journal de Physiologie Experimental. (Paris)*, **3**, 95–113.

Schrader, M. E. G. (1892). Über die Stellung der Grosshirns im Reflexmechanismus des Centralen Nervensystems der Wirbeltiere. *Archiv für Pathologie und Pharmakologie*, **29**, 55–118.

Schwabl, U. and Delius, J. D. (1984). Visual bar length discrimination threshold in pigeons. *Bird Behaviour*, **5**, 118–21.

Shettleworth, S. J. (1983). Memory in food-hoarding birds. *Scientific American*, **3**, 102–10.

Von Fersen, L. and Delius, J. D. (1989). Longterm retention of many visual patterns by pigeons. *Ethology*, **82**, 141–55.

Watanabe, S. (1986). Interocular transfer of learning in the pigeon: visuo-motor integration and separation of discriminanda and manipulanda. *Behavioural Brain Research*, **19**, 227–32.

Weiss, S. R. B., and Hodos, W. (1986). Discrimination of mirror image stimuli after lesions of the visual system in pigeons. *Brain, Behavior and Evolution*, **29**, 207–22.

Wild, J. M. (1987). The avian somatosensory system: connections of regions of body representation in the forebrain of the pigeon. *Brain Research*, **412**, 205–23.

Wilson, P. (1980a). The organisation of the visual hyperstriatum in the domestic chick. I. Topology of the visual projections. *Brain Research*, **188**, 319–32.

Wilson, P. (1980b). The organisation of the visual hyperstriatum in the domestic chick. II. Receptive field properties of single units. *Brain Research*, **188**, 333–45.

Yazulla, S. and Granda, A. M. (1973). Opponent-color units in the thalamus of the pigeon (*Columba livia*). *Vision Research*, **13**, 1555–63.

PART III

Development

Introduction

R. J. Andrew

It was clear from the inception of work on imprinting that a type of learning had been chosen (for good reasons), which was likely to have special properties. Presumably, this is true to a greater or lesser extent of all behaviour and learning in a very young vertebrate. Rostas (Chapter 7), as a result, raises the question: how far is it safe to extrapolate from a young to an adult nervous system?

Three possibilities can usefully, if crudely, be distinguished.

1. Young and adult animals show the same range of processes, and these are essentially similar in character. The special features of youth merely complicate, or prevent the use of some measures (e.g. because of maturational shifts in baselines: Chapter 7).
2. The same processes of plasticity and learning are present in youth and adulthood, but in markedly different proportions: some may even be present only at certain ages.
3. Not only do the proportions differ, but even apparently similar processes really differ significantly in character at different ages. Which of these three possibilities is nearest to the truth is likely to depend on the processes chosen for study.

Rostas (Chapter 7) shows that changes with age in the relative ease with which different types of protein phosphorylation occur are likely to affect the outcome of changes in the availability of second messengers. The processes potentially affected include ones which are likely to be important in learning: for example, the supply of vesicles to synapses and changes in the shape of dendrites and spines. It remains to be seen whether these effects are best considered as an example of the first or third possibility.

Horn (Chapter 8, and see Rostas, Chapter 7) notes that a number of properties of neurons, which are either known to change, or are likely to change as a result of learning, also change with age. If a property such as the mean length of the postsynaptic density (PSD) reaches an asymptote with age, and yet still continues to be increased in individual neurons as a result of learning (first possibility, above), this means that some opposite compensatory process must occur in the adult. As PSD lengthen on one neuron, they must shorten elsewhere (Horn, Chapter 8). The alternative is that an asymptote is not really reached, but so few neurons are affected at each episode of learning that change ceases to be experimentally measurable.

Processes like neuronal (perhaps even synapse) differentiation and elimination are likely to be much more widespread in the young CNS (Chapters 7 and 11); it may be that they are as a result then more important in plasticity and learning (second and third possibilities).

Such arguments are further complicated by the fact that maturational changes depend in part on experience (Bateson, Chapter 4); the background changes, on which change due to a particular learning task is superimposed, may themselves result to some extent from learning. This holds at a variety of levels: Horn (1985, p. 270 *et seq*) reviews the evidence for effects of experience on visual feature detectors in mammals and raises the possibility of comparable changes in the chick Wulst. Bateson (Chapter 4) models such changes as part of the consequences of imprinting. Since feature detectors are involved in visual analysis in general, changes of this sort are not part of the storage of a specific description of the properties of the imprinting object.

The first occasion on which a visual stimulus is paired with powerful reinforcement, which is clearly contingent on the appearance of the stimulus, might have a variety of central consequences. Thus Horn (Chapter 8) suggests the acceleration by imprinting of the development of brain stem projections: these might be involved in all subsequent reinforced learning (for example), and so again not represent storage of specific information.

Accelerated development can also be viewed as forced maturation when it occurs precociously. A number of important maturational changes are brought about in the chick by relatively non-specific perceptual inputs: examples include asymmetric light input to the late fetus (Rogers, Chapter 20) and locomotor activity after hatching: the latter causes maturation of releasing mechanisms for head features (Johnson and Bolhuis, Chapter 5). Such inputs occur reliably at the right time in normal development. They may have come to play such roles because they help to time the maturational change correctly in relation to other developmental changes. Given prematurely, inputs of this sort may produce precocious maturation. This possibility deserves special attention in the chick, in that chicks are commonly used on days 1 and 2 in tasks which in normal development they might more usually first encounter on later days (Chapter 6).

It thus seems sensible to consider the possibility that learning-induced change in the chick might represent: (i) storage of specific information, (ii) bringing mechanisms into working order which are necessary for learning (but not directly responsible for storage). This question is also considered in Part 4.

All of these features of early learning and plasticity, whether demonstrated or matters of speculation, suggest opportunities for research which would be difficult or impossible in the adult. The same is true at the behavioural level. The special features of imprinting (Johnson and Bolhuis, Chapter 5) are at least partly due to the fact that the visual input from the imprinting object simultaneously induces powerful motivation and provides very novel information to be stored. The intensity and duration of the memory formation which follows is unlikely to be matched in later life. Early learning when pecking potential food objects has the special property of being free of the after effects of ingestion, since the gut is still full of yolk (Chapter 1). As a result, perceptual learning may be available in a purer form.

Finally, the study of the development of plasticity and learning is important in its own right (Bateson, Chapter 4). The chick offers unusually rich material for such study in that several periods of rapid change have now been demonstrated. Two (days 3–5 and days 8–12) are considered in Chapters 6 and 20. Both involve marked and rapid shifts in hemispheric dominance, which may play a part both in causing behavioural change at these times, and also in making possible specialized learning.

4

Making sense of behavioural development in the chick

P. P. G. Bateson

INTRODUCTION

At an early stage in their lives, domestic chicks are capable of highly organized patterns of behaviour. These activities serve requirements that must be met if the animal is to stay alive. The process of hatching involves complex co-ordination of neck and leg movements. Shortly after hatching chicks are able to peck at objects on the ground, scratch the ground prior to pecking, preen themselves and become immobile when the mother calls in a particular way. They search for objects that are suitable as social companions; when they find one, they approach and nestle against it and once familiar with it, escape from dissimilar objects. On the sensory side, chicks have clear predispositions to peck at small objects and also to behave socially towards rather larger ones and in both cases, have marked preferences for particular colours. As well as all these proclivities and predispositions chicks have considerable capacities for learning. The phenomenon of imprinting provides perhaps one of the most famous attributes of precocious birds, including the domestic chick. Chicks are also able to learn in rather similar fashion the characteristics of food to which they have been exposed. They can rapidly learn to avoid pecking at unpalatable objects which they have tasted. They learn to repeat patterns of behaviour that bring them into contact with social companions or sources of heat and are able to use previously neutral events to predict the occurrence of other events that already had significance for them.

The capacities of young animals to show highly organized preferences and motor patterns and also to change their behaviour have both fascinated and teased generations of psychologists and ethologists. Many biologists wrote as if the different systems involved in development were identifiable in the final expression of the modified behaviour. The developmental processes giving rise to predispositions on the one hand and learning processes on the other were supposedly neatly separable in terms of the forms of behaviour they produced. This idea was clearly expressed in the metaphor of 'intercalation' used in the writings of Konrad Lorenz and some of his followers (e.g. Eibl-Eibesfeldt 1970). On this view the instinctive elements have inserted between them the elements acquired by learning. It was supposed that these separate elements could be identified by isolating the animal from opportunities to insert the learned ones. The attacks on this view by Hinde (1969), Lehrman (1970), Schneirla (1956), and many others have been largely successful in changing the thinking about such aspects of development.

While behavioural biologists nowadays are less likely to confuse process with outcome, the discredited instinct versus learning dichotomy of behaviour resurfaces in images which imply the same opposition such as 'hard versus soft-wired circuits' or 'closed versus open programs'. These distinctions probably express the fond hope that simple links will be found between the starting points and the end-points of development. The desire to relate by means of a single chain of events a pattern of behaviour to its origin has not been extinguished. In keeping with such causal arrow approaches, a neural pathway or a pattern of behaviour is commonly referred to as 'genetically determined' or simply as 'genetic'. The implication is that the genes may exclusively influence the outcome of developmental processes. The view that the genes *code* for the behaviour is not easily reconciled with what is known about developmental biology. A small subset of genes and cytoplasmic conditions start the whole process of development off after fertilization of the egg. These starting conditions create products that switch off some active genes, switch on others and bring the developing components into contact with new influences from outside. For such reasons, simple one-to-one correspondences between genes and any network property of the nervous system or any patterning of behaviour do not seem at all plausible. Undoubtedly a certain gene may be crucial for the building of particular neural connections or the expression of particular bits of behaviour. Even so, accepting that a particular gene is a necessary condition for the expression of a given pattern of behaviour is not the same as saying that the gene is all that is needed to determine the outcome.

The growing acceptance of the inadequacies of the causal chain approach to development has brought about a subtle change. Instead of asking whether behaviour is caused by genes or the environment, the question becomes: 'How much is due to each?' In more sophisticated form the question is restated as: 'How much of the variation in a character is due to a particular factor?' When individual differences in behaviour may be attributed to variation in genetic and environmental sources, the nature/nurture controversy appears to be resolved by a neat rephrasing of that misleading old question about where behaviour comes from. The influences on the outcome of development act directly and straightforwardly, adding together but rarely interacting in combinatorial fashion.

Needless to say, there is considerable dissatisfaction with this view and the desire to examine the dynamics of what happens during the

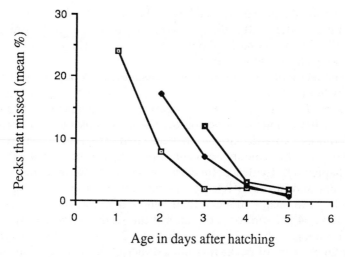

Fig. 4.1 Changes in the accuracy with which chicks pecked at millet seeds. The mean percentage number of misses is shown for three groups, the first receiving its first experience of pecking on day 1, the second on day 2 and the third on day 3. Note that the spontaneous improvement is equal to about half the improvement observed in the group receiving its first experience on the previous day. (From Cruze 1935.)

developmental process has been growing in strength (e.g. ten Cate 1989*a*). Even so, the evidence has been slotted back all too easily and misleadingly, I shall argue, into an additive framework. I shall take examples from the development of pecking in chicks and then deal more extensively with the development of social preferences. Finally, I shall consider whether the examples of plasticity early in development are different from what happens later in life.

PECKING

Cruze (1935) performed a famous experiment, in which he attempted to tease out the ways in which the accuracy of pecking is dependent upon both the experience of previous pecking attempts and the gross development of the animal (Fig. 4.1). The results showed clearly that both a chick's experience and its age affected its ability to hit a seed with its bill. They have commonly been taken as evidence for the interplay between internal and external factors. Even so, about half the improvement in accuracy could be attributed to direct experience of pecking and about half to more general changes such as the ability to maintain a steady posture while pecking (until pecking becomes virtually perfect on the third day after hatching in experienced birds). This result might seem to support an additive model of the development of pecking, with 'learning' and 'maturation' contributing in about equal measure. The conclusion would be far too facile (see Hogan 1988).

The ontogeny of pecking provides classic evidence for the distinctions drawn by Gottlieb (1976) between induction, facilitation and maintenance. An inducing (or initiating) event is required for a change in the behaviour. Without it the change does not occur. Clear examples are the formation of preferences for particular colours associated with food or the avoidance of pecking at other colours associated with unpleasant tasting substances (see Chapter 1). Evidence for facilitation is found in Cruze's (1935) experiment and in the effects of straightforward exposure to light when the chicks were unable to move their heads. In chicks that had been kept in the dark, 54 per cent of pecks missed the seeds; however, exposure to light for 1 hour, with the head restrained for 3–5 hours before testing, led to only 26 per cent of pecks that missed the seeds (Vauclair and Bateson 1975). Finally, an experiment by Padilla (1935) showed that keeping chicks in darkness eventually led to a loss of visually-guided pecking 14 days after hatching. This provides some evidence for the maintenance function of visual experience, although Hogan (1988) has suggested an alternative explanation. He argued that chicks force-fed for the first 2 weeks may not peck when deprived of food because the motor mechanism for pecking has remained independent of the central mechanism for hunger.

I introduced a fourth descriptive category to add to Gottlieb's trio to cover those events that permitted changes in patterns of behaviour but did not themselves produce those changes (Bateson 1983). These are *enabling* events. An example was provided by the experiment performed by Cherfas (1977). He showed that exposure for at least 30 minutes to light enabled chicks to learn to discriminate between two coloured beads, one of which had been coated with a bitter-tasting substance (methylanthranilate). Interestingly, he also showed that exposure to a homogeneous illuminated field while the chicks' heads were restrained did not improve the passive avoidance learning. However, if the field contained brightness contours provided by two black crosses, the chicks subsequently learned to suppress pecks at the colour associated with the bitter substance.

While the importance of the distinctions between initiating, facilitating, maintaining and enabling events should not be exaggerated, these descriptive categories provided a way of organizing the evidence. They also strengthened the hand of those who had been strongly influenced by the writings of Schneirla and Lehrman and who doubted that an element of a behaviour pattern is either due to a direct influence of the genes or to a direct influence of experience. Just how the various developmental influences work has to be studied, but it seems likely that the facilitating and enabling effects of patterned light on pecking (and other visually guided behaviour patterns) operate in the same way by enhancing the efficiency of the feature-detecting mechanisms of the visual system (see also Chapter 20). The main upshot of the work on pecking has been to point to the variety of different factors that can interact in many different ways to affect the behavioural outcome. The evidence from the imprinting literature, which I shall consider next, has been equally unequivocal in pointing in the same direction.

DEVELOPMENT OF SOCIAL PREFERENCES

It has been obvious for a long time that the results of an imprinting experiment depend greatly on the conditions that were used. Many authors reported, for instance, that the character of the stimuli used, both for training and testing the chicks, greatly affected the outcome (e.g. Smith 1962). An early study suggested that the stimulus value of an object might change with age (Gray 1961). Recently, substantial support for this view came from studies in which chicks had either been trained with a flashing, rotating light or with a rotating stuffed jungle fowl and then given a choice between them (Horn and McCabe 1984; Johnson, *et al.* 1985). The artificial and naturalistic stimuli were matched for their effectiveness in eliciting approach from day-old domestic chicks by varying the rate of rotation of the object. Despite the matching, the stuffed jungle fowl became more attractive than the box in untrained birds by the second day after hatching. The shift towards a stronger fowl bias was also apparent in birds that had been imprinted with either a fowl or a box. Finally, the developmental process that led to a strengthening preference for the fowl could be facilitated by accentuating both visual and non-visual experience. Subsequent work has suggested that features of the jungle fowl that make it especially attractive as the predisposition develops are located around the head. However, they are not specific to jungle fowl, since a stuffed rotating Gadwall duck was equally attractive (Johnson and Horn 1988).

The development of the chick's predispositions to respond more strongly to some stimuli than to others already looks complicated. However, the problems for explanation do not end here. The list of the factors that influence whether or not a chick shows a preference for the object with which it has been supposedly imprinted is a long one. Some of the important factors are the following:

a. The characteristics of the object.
b. The stage of the bird's development at which the object was first presented.
c. The length of time for which the object was first presented.

d. The bird's experience prior to first presentation of the object.
e. The bird's experience subsequent to first presentation.

Many other conditions can be added to this list. Obviously, the chick's response will depend on its current state, such as whether it is sleepy, alert, or highly distressed during training and during testing. The precise character of the stimulus presentation is important, such as whether the exposure is continuous, at fixed intervals or unpredictably intermittent (Bolhuis and Johnson 1988). The importance of arousing or potentiating stimuli, such as the natural maternal calls of the mother, have been stressed by Gottlieb (e.g. 1971) for many years. Recently, ten Cate (1989*b*) has shown that in Japanese quail, the posture of the mother has a powerful motivating effect on the response of the chicks to her. Furthermore, we also know that when the bird is developmentally ready, it will actively work to present itself with appropriate forms of stimulation (Bateson and Reese 1969). Even without these additional complications, the list of five major factors draws attention to the type of explanation that will be needed to pull the information together. The explanation will have to refer to internally driven development of preferences and to changes in state. It will have to take account of non-specific enabling and facilitating effects of experience and it will have to show why the conditions of training and testing are so important. When an area of research gets to this point, the commonly used metaphors (such as 'imprinting' itself) and the implicit theory that goes with them tend to become inadequate or simply misleading.

The case for introducing some explicit theory is that a working model brings with it mental discipline and may expose unstated assumptions. It can also serve several other valuable functions. It can show how we are easily misled by the dynamics of development into supposing that the processes are so complicated that they are beyond comprehension. From the point of future empirical research, it can suggest profitable new lines of enquiry. Finally, it bears directly on the general arguments about the interplay between internal and external factors.

CONTROL OF THE CHICK'S BEHAVIOUR

One approach to making explicit how behaviour is controlled is to postulate a flow diagram. I give an example in Fig. 4.2 (from Bateson 1981, 1987). The first step involves detection of features in a stimulus presented to a young bird. Aspects of the stimulus which the bird is predisposed to find attractive are thought to be picked out by analysis at this stage. The second step involves comparison between what has already been experienced and the current input. Of course, before imprinting has

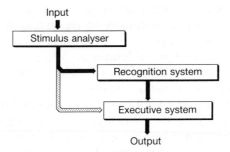

Fig. 4.2 A flow diagram of the stages from input to output involved in filial responses to a mother hen or a substitute imprinting object. In domestic chicks the stimulus analyser is thought to continue developing until the second day after hatching. Plasticity resulting from imprinting occurs both in the recognition system and at the limited access to the executive system controlling filial behaviour. Finally the direct input to the executive system from the stimulus analyser may degenerate or become inhibited with increasing use of the recognition system. (From Bateson 1987.)

taken place, no comparison is involved. Once it has occurred, recognition of what is familiar and what is novel is crucial. Finally, the third stage involves control of the various motor patterns involved in executing filial behaviour. This model is given the acronym ARE, for analysis, recognition, and execution.

Four developmental changes are thought to be involved in the neural mechanisms concerned with filial imprinting in the domestic chick. The first change is relatively non-specific, involving alterations in the stimulus analysing systems—alterations which may continue into the second day after hatching. These changes enhance the efficiency of the feature detection. A second change is specifically related to the characteristics of the imprinting stimulus in the system devoted to recognition. The third involves changes in the access to the executive system from the neural mechanisms concerned with recognition of particular familiar objects. The assumption is that the capacity for plastic change here is limited. By contrast, the capacity of the recognition system is thought to be much greater, so that it is possible for a well-imprinted bird to become familiar with and tame to a repeatedly presented novel object, but it will not behave socially towards this object. Finally, I thought it was necessary to postulate a fourth developmental change in the neural mechanisms, namely a degeneration or inhibition of the direct control of highly effective stimuli on the executive system. The pathway that supposedly loses its function is depicted as a stippled arrow.

The proposal for the developmental changes between the recognition and executive systems is especially relevant to understanding the sensitive period in development to which imprinting seems to be confined. When prior experience influences sensitivity to the long-term effects of novel input, it may pre-empt other types of experience from having the same impact, a proposed mechanism known as 'competitive exclusion' (see Bateson 1987). A number of possible physiological mechanisms might be suggested for competitive exclusion. For instance, suppose that gaining access involves growth of neural connections and that the area available for connections has finite size. When growth has proceeded beyond the half-way point and cannot be reversed easily, the input experienced first will be better able to control the behaviour than other forms of input. In terms of the flow diagram, the competitive exclusion effect is likely to be most pronounced in the access to the executive system because the capacity for change in this system is limited.

Recently, Bolhuis (1989) has proposed a somewhat similar scheme to the one shown in Figure 4.2. However, he separates stimulus analysis into a coarse 'filter' and a 'predisposition system'. He did so because unimprinted chicks can store details of sub-optimal stimuli even at a stage when the predispositions are fully established (Bolhuis *et al.* 1989). His conclusion would follow if stimulus analysis in my scheme were thought of as a simple filter through which input with the wrong characteristics could not pass. As the result of a neural network model that Gabriel Horn and I have been developing, stimulus analysis is not thought of in these terms (Bateson and Horn, in preparation). We regard the stimulus analysing system as decomposing the input into a number of features, such as lines, colours and head shapes. The feature detectors then address the recognition system which stores information about the combination of detectors that were active. The advantage of this approach is that the intensity with which a given feature detector is activated can vary. The characteristics of a sub-optimal stimulus that only weakly activated detectors addressing the recognition system would be stored, but only slowly. With such a scheme a novel stimulus with features that powerfully drove the detectors could prove more attractive than the familiar sub-optimal one. With this form of stimulus analysis, the elaboration proposed by Bolhuis (1989) is unnecessary.

The flow diagram leaves out of account two important features of chicks' behaviour, namely their active searching for suitable objects with which they can then be imprinted and, once learning has occurred, their withdrawal from novel objects. The ARE model may, however, be relatively easily modified, as is shown in Fig. 4.3. Consider a chick that is motivated to respond in filial fashion but cannot as yet see a suitable object. It starts to move about. Its activity brings it into visual contact with a source of stimulation which it is strongly predisposed to approach. Execution of approach inhibits search. However, either the stimulus or the action may strengthen the activities that were performed immediately

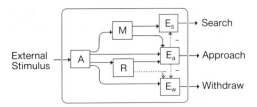

Fig. 4.3 A revised flow diagram of the control of a chick's social behaviour. The proposed systems are abbreviated as follows: A is analysis, R is recognition, E_a is executive for approach, E_s is executive for search, E_w is executive for withdrawal and M is motivation. In this version the chick is thought to search for objects with certain features when it is in a particular motivational state. Some of the features of the objects for which it may search further enhance its motivational state. The effective objects also elicit approach behaviour which simultaneously inhibits search and any tendency to withdraw. Output from the recognition system also inhibits withdrawal directly. As a bird becomes increasingly familiar with an object, the representation of that object gains increasing access to the executive system and displaces direct control by the analysis system. As a consequence the chick may withdraw from novel objects until it has become familiar with them.

prior to the appearance of the attractive object. In this way, pressing a pedal that turns on a highly conspicuous stimulus could rapidly be repeated when the stimulus disappears—as was the case in the experiments of Bateson and Reese (1969).

When a chick has become sufficiently familiar with a particular input, it withdraws from novel objects. The proposed explanation is that withdrawal is no longer inhibited by the execution of approach, because of the loss of effectiveness of the direct connection between the analysis and executive systems. Also, no inhibition of withdrawal is received from the recognition system. The second route of inhibition is proposed because birds that become tame to objects do not necessarily express any social behaviour towards them.

Models with proliferating boxes have not had an especially happy history and in recent years, theorizing has tended to go in two other directions. One fashionable area has been neural nets (see Durbin *et al.* 1989). These may incorporate known features of the nervous system and are particularly attractive when they do so. I have already alluded to a neural net model currently being developed by Gabriel Horn and myself. I shall not say anything more about it here, other than to remark that the ARE model was an important step in developing our thinking.

The other direction for theorizing is towards formalization. The mathematical models are important because the dynamics of a process are much more easily portrayed. Also, the remorseless consequences of the algebra quickly point to confusions of thought. I shall consider here my own attempt to formalize what I believe happens in the case of imprinting. Here again, the development of the ideas was greatly helped by having an explicit flow diagram in mind.

A FORMAL MODEL OF IMPRINTING

As in the flow diagram, the formal model which I shall describe here rests on three stages. The analysis stage picks out the features in the external stimulus and determines the overall input to the recognition system and the direct links to executive systems. The process of storage in the recognition system is thought to occur quickly, so that for purposes of most modelling exercises, the output of the recognition system is the same as its input from the analysis system when the bird is exposed to a familiar object. When it is confronted with a novel object, the output of the recognition system is proportional to the number of features shared with a familiar object. The dynamics of development are most strongly affected by change in access to the executive system. To begin with, a newly formed representation has no access but the access increases rapidly, displacing the direct link from the analysis system. The model assumes the process of growth and displacement occur in tandem. However, this feature is not crucial and inhibition of direct input from the analysis could occur later in development. In the case of imprinting with a second object the upper limit of access is determined by how much access has been captured by the first object. The relation between the input to the executive system and the output which directly affects observed behaviour is thought to be sigmoid. The equations for the model are given in Box 1.

An important feature of the model is that some crucial variables and parameters are multiplied together rather than added. The justification for doing this when dealing with, for example, the interaction between the attractiveness of an object and the bird's motivational state is that, if either is a zero value, nothing happens. If the model were additive, an unmotivated bird would learn the characteristics of things and motivated birds would appear to learn in the absence of anything to learn about.

The constants should be regarded as characteristics of the organism. They refer in the real animal to properties of its nervous system which, of course, also have to develop. These characteristics may or may not be affected by relatively small changes in the conditions of development or by variation in genotype. If and when they can be estimated, they should not be treated as though they were similar to gravitational constants! Sometimes external conditions will have relatively non-specific effects on such features, a point that has been frequently stressed in the literature on behavioural development (e.g. Lehrman 1970; Bateson 1976).

I have given an example of what the model does when a novel object

Box 1. The equations used for withdrawal from or approach to a novel object after imprinting in chicks.

Approach to a novel object is a function of the input to the executive system, i_n.

$$i_n = a_n \, m \, [g_n \, cf \pm (1 - cf)] \tag{1}$$

where a_n is the stimulus value of the novel object. It is a characteristic of the organism based on a prior predisposition (0 to 1);

m is the current motivational state of the bird affecting its readiness to approach (0 to 1);

g_n is the extent of the generalization from the familiar to the novel object (0–1);

cf is the extent to which output from the representation of the familiar object has captured access to the executive system (0–1).

The value for cf is obtained from the following equation:

$$cf = 1 - \exp(-af \, m \, t \, K_c) \tag{2}$$

Where af is the stimulus value of the familiar, imprinting object. It is subject to exactly the same assumptions as the stimulus value of novel objects (0–1);

t is the length of exposure to the imprinting object;

K_c is a constant affecting the rate of capture of the executive system by an output from the recognition system.

The shape of the generalization gradient is assumed to be sigmoid. Progressing from novel to familiar:

$$g_n = 1 - \exp \{K_g \, s_n \, [\exp(-s_n) - 1]\} \tag{3}$$

where s_n is the proportion of features in the familiar shared by the novel (0–1);

K_g is a constant influencing the shape of the generalization gradient.

The function describing the output of the approach executive system, o_a, is assumed to be sigmoid.

$$o_a = 1 - \exp\{i_n \, K_e \, [\exp(-i_n) - 1]\} \tag{4}$$

where K_e is a constant influencing the shape of the response curve and i_n is given by Equation (1).

Withdrawal from a novel object will occur when $a_n \, K_w > o_a$ where K_w is a constant influencing the output of the withdrawal executive system, o_w. As the bird becomes familiar with the novel object, o_w wanes.

(exp refers to an exponent of the natural logarithm, e. Most programming languages and many scientific calculators have a command for obtaining a given value. e^{-t} starts at 1 when t is 0 and drops towards 0 quickly at first and then more slowly as t increases.)

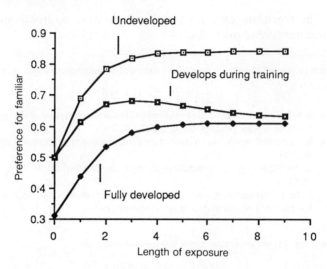

Fig. 4.4 Simulations of changes in the preference for red box in a choice between the box and a unfamiliar jungle fowl. The top curve shows the development of the preference as a function of length of exposure to the box when the predisposition to prefer fowl has not yet developed. The bottom curve shows what happens after the predisposition has already developed. The middle curve shows what happens when the predisposition starts to emerge during the course of the tests as a non-specific result of exposure to the box.

has a higher stimulus value than the familiar object in Fig. 4.4. It was deliberately chosen because of its relevance to those studies in which the stimuli were initially unequal in attractiveness, or became so as the animal developed—as with the jungle fowl and the rotating box. If the same parameter values are used, while varying the length of exposure, the growing preference for a familiar rotating box when compared with a novel stuffed fowl can be simulated. The result is shown in the lower curve in Fig. 4.4. The simulation which produced the lower curve was based on the assumption that the stimulus value of the novel object was fully developed. In the case of the jungle fowl the stimulus value has not usually developed fully immediately after imprinting on the first day, at least when the birds are reared in the dark. If the stimulus value of the novel object is the same as that of the familiar one, then the upper curve is obtained. Perhaps the most interesting case is the middle one, where the training has a specific effect on preference for the familiar and also a non-specific effect on the development of the predisposition for the fowl. In the simulation, the constant affecting the rate of development of the predisposition is one quarter that affecting the development of the preference. In all cases a bird's preference in a test is affected both by how strongly it

Box 2.   A method for calculating the change in motivational state at the onset of the sensitive period.

$$m_t = m_{t-\delta} + (1 - m_{t-\delta}) [1 - \exp(-a_c K_m \delta)]$$

where m_t is the motivational state at time t;

$m_{t-\delta}$ is the motivational state at the previous step;

a_c is the stimulus value of the conditions in which the chick is kept;

δ is the time interval of each successive step;

K_m is a parameter affecting the rate of increase of the motivational state concerned with filial behaviour.

---

is attached to the familiar object and by the stimulus value of the novel object relative to that of the familiar.

In many simulations, the motivational state can be treated as a fixed parameter or as a variable that fluctuates randomly within certain limits, but at the onset of the sensitive period for imprinting, the readiness to learn increases from zero. Once chicks are ready to be affected by particular types of stimulation from the environment, they are also liable to be affected by the conditions around them, however sub-optimal those conditions might be. In the model, then, the rate of increase of the motivational state depends on the character of the stimulation. The process is fast if the birds are kept with members of their own species in the light (conditions that have high stimulus value); it is much slower if they are kept in isolation and slower still if they are kept in a patternless environment (low stimulus value) (see Bateson and Wainwright 1972). The rate of increase of the motivational state can be derived iteratively in a series of small time steps as shown in Box 2.

The model is developed in detail elsewhere (Bateson, in preparation). It is worth mentioning that it considers the specific and non-specific influences on the beginning and ending of sensitive periods. It deals with learning about a second imprinting object. Finally, it goes into generalization from the familiar and the preferences that chicks can express for slight novelty. It suffices to point out here that such a formal model can teach us some useful lessons. When I generated variable toy data by allowing the motivational state to fluctuate randomly from one run to the next so as to represent individual differences in chicks, I could obtain results remarkably similar to those from real experiments involving training with stuffed jungle fowl or rotating boxes (see Fig. 4.5). Despite the non-linear character of the model, the data suggest misleadingly an additive process with an acquired preference for the imprinting object adding to or subtracting from the bias for the fowl. This rang a bell uncomfortably for me.

In a previous publication I presented real data on chicks' preferences

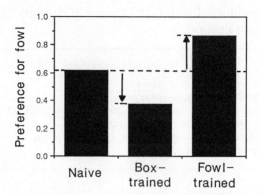

Fig. 4.5 The apparent additive effects of predispositions and imprinting obtained with the multiplicative model shown in Box 1. The first column shows the initial predisposition of naïve birds given a choice between two objects of unequal stimulus values. The second column shows the preference after imprinting with the initially less attractive object and third the preference after imprinting for the same length of time with the more attractive one.

for yellow and red flashing lights in a comparable fashion to that shown in Fig. 4.5 and wrote '. . . in this experiment the preference of experienced birds was determined by the superimposition of the effects of experience on an initial bias.' (Bateson 1978, p. 37). Fortunately for me, I added: 'It is unlikely that the simple additive process suggested by these results will usually operate and experience with the initially less effective stimulus would be expected to leave less impact.' Even so, the implication of the way the data were presented is probably misleading.

Equally alarmingly, analysis of variance suggests that the process generating the data is additive. It is easy to run toy experiments with the model in which the stimulus of training objects and the length of exposure to them are varied. While the conclusion that there is no statistical interaction between predisposition and length of training depends a lot on hows long the training process has been allowed to run, analysis of variance is notoriously insensitive to non-linear interactions (see Wahlsten 1990). In the cases where the toy data suggest no statistical interaction, I *know* that the process generating these data is not additive. This knowledge is salutary, if we had been tempted (as many have been) to use the real data to make statements about the innate and acquired *components* of the bird's preference.

I obviously believe that this model has some merits for work at the behavioural level, otherwise I would not have spent so much time and space describing it. It can be generalized to other cases such as the development of pecking. I suspect that the major advantages of such formalizations are to people doing experiments on behaviour rather than to neuroscientists. The models take some of the mystery out of the seemingly complex dynamics of behavioural development. When critics say: 'You make the whole process of development sound so complicated', it is possible to reply: 'No, the explanatory devices are really very simple.' Importantly, they enable combinations of conditions to be explored systematically, which would take a very long time with live animals. Furthermore, in the process of such explorations, surprises are frequently encountered which then propose experiments with real chicks or re-examination of data not previously analysed.

LINKING LEVELS

The flow diagram of how a chick's behaviour is controlled and the formalization of what happens during development do not explain how the processes of learning work. They do not state whether or not any of them is associative in the sense that an initially neutral and an initially effective set of external events become paired as a result of the process. Even though the imprinting procedure is not explicitly associative, the underlying mechanism could involve the establishment of some associations. Be that as it may, what are the links between analysis of the intact animal and the analysis of mechanism?

The move from a formal behavioural model based on what is known about the character of the system at the level of the whole organism to lower levels of analysis can usefully begin with the simple flow diagram of what might happen from reception of input to the performance of output. The next step is to consider what might happen to neural connectivity on the basis of knowledge of neural components. The speculations about the neural basis of competitive exclusion, considered briefly above, emphasize the need to establish serious links between the systems models derived from behaviour and neurobiology. The links are only likely to become really productive when knowledge of real neurons and the changes in connectivity that can occur between them are incorporated into the models.

As far as formalizations of the type attempted here are concerned, they point to the parameters that are characteristics of the organism as opposed to ones that might be manipulated externally by experiment. One example is the constant affecting the rate at which plastic changes occur. These hypothetical features of the organism, if real, must have some correspondence to underlying neural mechanisms. Here again, theoretical activity primarily designed to provide help at the behavioural level can be of service in guiding work on the neural bases of development.

EARLY AND LATE PLASTICITY

The examples I have considered in this chapter are of learning occurring early in life. Apart from the underlying regularities that give these cases their special flavour, should some extra significance be added because learning occurs when the nervous system is still immature? Preferences acquired early in the life-cycle may develop more rapidly and be more stable than those acquired later, because the interference from previously established preferences and habits is relatively slight. Certainly, the stage at which filial imprinting occurs is one of the first obvious occasions on which initially broad preferences are restricted by experience. As a result of such experience the bird withdraws from novel objects. Such early experience can aid as well as hinder later learning, depending on its relationship to subsequently encountered stimuli. In the case of a developing preference such an effect would presumably enable the animal to learn further details of the preferred objects. Without any necessary changes in the processes of acquisition, the information that can be acquired by them varies with and depends on past experience.

Nearly 30 years ago Vince (1961) reviewed much of the literature on early learning and was tempted to suggest that changes occur in the behavioural mechanisms over and above the storage of information. She wrote: 'In comparing the behaviour of a very young animal or one reared under very restricted conditions with a normal adult of the same species, we may well be dealing with two mechanisms which function rather differently.' (p. 247). The rules of learning might change in ways that could not be attributed to the effects of experience, for instance. At the time it was not obvious how the impact of experience and maturation of learning systems not present in early life might be separated.

This chapter and those by Johnson and Bolhuis and Horn (Chapters 5 and 8) present evidence suggesting that the mechanisms involved in the development of predispositions can be separated usefully from the mechanisms specifically concerned with the development of recognition. Furthermore, the executive systems that are required for the expression of a preference develop at different rates, the most obvious being the one required for filial behaviour and the one required for sexual behaviour. On the other hand, sexual imprinting, which is thought to be completed considerably later in development than filial imprinting (see Bateson 1979), seems to require the same part of the brain for recognition of the imprinting object (Bolhuis *et al.* 1989). Therefore it would seem that the question 'Is early learning different from later learning?' is not going to resolve itself into a simple 'Yes' or 'No'. If the theoretical considerations which I have presented in this chapter are of any value, they suggest that the question has to be greatly refined. Hogan (1988, p. 67) has made essentially this point when he argued that '. . . perceptual, central, and motor mechanisms are the building blocks out of which complex behavior is formed . . .' He went on to argue that '. . . a developmental analysis requires looking for the factors causing the development of the building blocks themselves, as well as for the way connections among those building blocks become established.' Once the connections are made, we have every reason to suppose the properties of the whole system can sometimes change quite radically.

CONCLUSION

On grounds of biological plausibility alone, the notion of genetic and environmental factors adding together to produce their effects should be treated with utmost scepticism. By thinking about the nature of the developmental processes, it is possible to ask rather more interesting questions of the available data than simply proposing linear developmental processes with additive characteristics. Better still, deeper understanding comes from studying the processes in action. Biologists are not alone, of course, in having to deal with properties that are the product of many different factors which often interact in surprising ways. Dynamical systems with non-linear properties are commonplace and well understood by chemists and physicists (e.g. Pippard 1985). Given that the changes occurring in behavioural development are not linear, what should be done about it?

In this chapter I have suggested that, first, we should list the influences on the outcome. In doing so, we should describe the ways in which they are identified and the specificity of their effect. Identifying sources of variation does not in itself help us to pinpoint how development works. Therefore, when we discover that an animal has a predisposition to do something, we are not absolved of a responsibility to carry out analysis of how that feature of the animal develops. We may not be able to do much at the behavioural level, but we should not fall into the old trap of supposing that, if it is not learned, it is 'coded in the genes'.

An important step towards understanding development is uncovering the regularities by studying the process—and by reflecting on what happens. Fashionable methodologies for analysing data will not do the thinking for us. In the case of behavioural development in the chick, I have tried to show that simple components, when put together, can generate surprising and adaptively powerful solutions to the problems that most animals face.

How can a growing understanding of what happens at the behavioural level be linked to the underlying neural mechanisms? The approach can start usefully with flow diagrams that propose ways in which the system might be organized. However, the links only become really productive when knowledge of real neurons and the changes in connectivity that can occur between them become a feature of the models. The explanations are likely to be greatly improved by knowledge of constraints on the neural mechanisms. Even so, in order to understand mechanism, a broad understanding of what is happening to the whole animal is also needed. By analogy, the study of the weather involving measurements of the temperature, pressure, wind speed and so forth at hundreds of stations on the earth's surface has considerable limitations. It certainly provides a lot of data. But if you want to get a sense of the overall pattern, looking at the weather systems in pictures taken from a satellite is hard to beat. The global approach gives us a chance to develop a far better insight into the way the whole system works. For that reason the movement between levels must go both ways.

Finally, how far can the ways in which early learning processes, like imprinting, be regarded as special by virtue of occurring in an immature nervous system? The problem does not resolve itself neatly because early learning can make subsequent learning with the very same mechanisms easier in some cases and more difficult in others. At the same time, other aspects of the neural mechanisms required for the analysis of input or for the execution of the output may develop independently of the specific experience which the animal has had. To proceed further in this type of analysis, the questions have to be refined so that we focus on the development of the sub-systems required in learning and the connections that form between them.

Acknowledgements

I am grateful to Richard Andrew and Johan Bolhuis for their comments on a draft of this chapter.

REFERENCES

Bateson, P. P. G. (1976). Specificity and the origins of behavior. *Advances in the Study of Behavior*, **6**, 1–20.
Bateson, P. P. G. (1978). Early experience and sexual preferences. In *Biological determinants of sexual behaviour* (ed. J. B. Hutchison), pp. 29–53, John Wiley, Chichester.
Bateson, P. (1979). How do sensitive periods arise and what are they for? *Animal Behaviour*, **27**, 470–86.
Bateson, P. (1981). Control of sensitivity to the environment during development. In *Behavioral development* (ed. K. Immelmann, G. W. Barlow, L. Petrinovich, and M. Main), pp. 432–453. Cambridge University Press, Cambridge.
Bateson, P. (1983). Genes, environment and the development of behaviour. In

Animal behaviour Vol.3. Genes, development and learning (ed. T. R. Halliday and P. J. B. Slater), pp. 52–81. Blackwell, Oxford.

Bateson, P. (1987). Imprinting as a process of competitive exclusion. In *Imprinting and cortical plasticity* (ed. J. P. Rauschecker and P. Marler), pp. 151–68. John Wiley, New York.

Bateson, P. P. G. and Reese, E. P. (1969). The reinforcing properties of conspicuous stimuli in the imprinting situation. *Animal Behaviour*, 17, 692–9.

Bateson, P. P. G. and Wainwright, A. A. P. (1972). The effects of prior exposure to light on the imprinting process in domestic chicks. *Behaviour*, 42, 279–90.

Bolhuis, J. J. (1989). The development and stability of filial preferences in the chick. University of Gröningen: Unpublished PhD dissertation.

Bolhuis, J. J. and Johnson, M. H. (1988). Effects of response-contingency and stimulus presentation schedule on imprinting in the chick *(Gallus gallus domesticus)*. *Journal of Comparative Psychology*. 102, 61–5.

Bolhuis, J. J., Johnson, M. H., and Horn, G. (1985). Interaction between acquired preferences and developing predispositions in an imprinting situation. *Animal Behaviour*, 33. 1000–06.

Bolhuis, J. J., Johnson, M. H., and Horn, G. (1989). Interacting mechanisms during the formation of filial preferences: the development of a predisposition does not constrain learning. *Journal of Experimental Psychology: Animal Behaviour Processes*. (In press.)

Cherfas, J. J. (1977). Visual system activation in the chick: one-trial avoidance learning affected by duration and patterning of light exposure. *Behavioral Biology*, 21, 52–65.

Cruze, W. W. (1935). Maturation and learning in chicks. *Journal of Comparative Psychology*, 19, 371–408.

Durbin, R., Miall, C., and Mitchison, G. (eds) (1989). *The computing neuron*. Addison-Wesley, Wokingham, UK.

Eibl-Eibesfeldt, I. (1970). *Ethology: the biology of behaviour*. Holt, Rinehart & Winston, New York.

Gottlieb, G. (1971). *Development of species identification in birds*. University of Chicago Press.

Gottlieb, G. (ed.) (1976). The roles of experience in the development of behavior and the nervous system. In *Neural and behavioral specificity: studies in the development of behavior and the nervous system*, pp. 25–54. Academic Press, New York.

Gray, P. H. (1961). The releasers of imprinting: differential reactions to color as a function of maturation. *Journal of Comparative and Physiological Psychology*, 54, 597–601.

Hinde, R. A. (1969). Dichotomies in the study of development. In *Genetic and environmental influences on behaviour*, (ed. J. M. Thoday and A. S. Parkes). Oliver & Boyd, Edinburgh.

Hogan, J. A. (1988). Cause and function in the development of behavior systems. In *Handbook of behavioral neurobiology. Vol. 9. Developmental psychobiology and behavioral ecology* (ed. M. Blass), pp. 63–106. Plenum Press, New York.

Horn, G and McCabe, B. J. (1984). Predispositions and preferences. Effects on imprinting of lesions to the chick brain. *Animal Behaviour*, 32, 288–92.

Johnson, M. H. and Horn, G. (1988). Development of filial preferences in dark-reared chicks. *Animal Behaviour*, **36**, 675–83.

Johnson, M. H., Bolhuis, J., and Horn, G. (1985). Interaction between acquired preferences and developing predispositions in an imprinting situation. *Animal Behaviour*, **33**, 1000–6.

Lehrman, D. S. (1970). Semantic and conceptual issues in the nature-nurture problem. In *Development and evolution of behavior* (ed. L. R. Aronson, E. Tobach, D. S. Lehrman, and J. S. Rosenblatt), pp. 17–52. Freeman, San Francisco.

Padilla, S. G. (1935). Further studies on the delayed pecking of chicks. *Journal of Comparative Psychology*, **20**, 413–43.

Pippard, A. B. (1985). *Response and stability*. Cambridge University Press.

Schneirla, T. C. (1956). Interrelationships of the 'innate' and the 'acquired' in instinctive behavior. In *L'Instinct dans le comportement des l'homme* (ed. P. Grassé), pp. 387–452. Masson, Paris.

Smith, F. V. (1962). Perceptual aspects of imprinting. *Symposium of the Zoological Society of London*, **8**, 193–8.

ten Cate, C. (1989a). Behavioral development: toward understanding processes. In *Perspectives in ethology*, Vol. 8. *Whither ethology?* (ed. P. P. G. Bateson and P. H. Klopfer), pp. 243–269. Plenum Press, New York.

ten Cate, C. (1989b). Stimulus movement, hen behaviour and filial imprinting in Japanese quail (*Coturnix coturnix japonica*). *Ethology*. (In press.)

Vauclair, J. and Bateson, P. P. G. (1975). Prior exposure to light and pecking accuracy in chicks. *Behaviour*, **52**, 196–201.

Vince, M. A. (1961). Developmental changes in learning capacity. In *Current problems in animal behaviour* (ed. W. H. Thorpe and O. L. Zangwill), pp. 225–47. Cambridge University Press, London.

Wahlsten, D. (1990). Insensitivity of the analysis of variance to heredity-environment interaction. *Behavioral and Brain Sciences*, **13**, 109–61.

5

Imprinting, predispositions, and filial preference in the chick

M. H. Johnson and J. J. Bolhuis

INTRODUCTION

The development of filial preference has been extensively studied in several species of birds with precocial young such as ducklings, goslings and chicks. Hatchlings of such species will initially approach a wide variety of conspicuous objects, but after continued exposure to one object will come to restrict their approach and other filial behaviour to it alone. When close to such an object, a recently hatched domestic chick will often emit contentment twitters and if the object moves away it will attempt to follow. If the object is removed and replaced by another, novel, object the chick will often run away emitting distress calls. From these observations we may infer that the chick or duckling has learned about the visual characteristics of the object concerned. Although a large variety of inanimate objects can serve as mother surrogates in this way, in the natural environment the biologically appropriate mother is normally selected. Attachment to particular auditory stimuli can be demonstrated in a similar way, although a combination of sound and vision may be most effective.

Lorenz (1935, 1937) was one of the first to investigate experimentally the formation of filial attachments in precocial avian species. Lorenz proposed that filial preferences are formed by means of a unique learning process which he called 'Prägung' or imprinting. He argued that the learning process was unique on the basis of two claims; firstly, that once a preference had been acquired it was irreversible and would influence behaviour in later life, and secondly, that there was a sharply defined critical time within which the learning could take place. Both of these claims have subsequently been brought into question. For example, with regard to the latter claim Sluckin and Salzen (1961) and Bateson (1966) have argued that the 'sensitive period' for imprinting is not as circumscribed as Lorenz claimed. Since the sensitive period can be extended by delaying the onset of exposure to a conspicuous object, these authors argue it is better viewed as a self-terminating process.

The first claim is also now disputed. There is abundant evidence that a preference for a particular stimulus can be reversed to a preference for another object as a result of prolonged exposure to the latter (e.g. Salzen and Meyer 1967). A weaker version of Lorenz's original claim of irreversibility, namely that information about the first imprinting object is overridden but not forgotten (Jaynes 1956), has received some support from recent studies (e.g. Cherfas and Scott 1981; Bolhuis and Bateson 1990). The general issue of the uniqueness or otherwise of imprinting is also entwined with the debate about the extent to which it can be accounted for in terms of associative conditioning theory. This debate and that concerning reversibility are addressed in later sections of this chapter.

Filial imprinting as described above is normally distinguished from sexual imprinting, the latter being the process by which birds or other animals come to direct their sexual preferences toward a particular individual or species (see Bateson 1983). However, the relationship between the two remains unclear and may vary between species (for chicks see Vidal 1980; Bolhuis *et al.* 1989*a*). Lorenz (1937) provides one clear example:

A musk drake (*Cairina moschata*) hatched with four siblings by a pair of grey geese, and led by them for seven weeks, subsequently proved to be bound to his siblings, that is, to his own species, in all his social activities. But when his mating reactions awoke the following year, they were focused on the species of the foster parents, to whom he had paid no attention for over ten months.

In the present chapter evidence that the formation of filial preference in the domestic chick is the result, not only of exposure to a particular conspicuous object (i.e. 'imprinting'), but also of the development of a specific predisposition, will be presented. The development of this predisposition is not dependent on exposure to a particular stimulus, but is influenced by non-specific factors.

Imprinting can be reliably reproduced in the laboratory in the following way. Chicks are dark-reared until being exposed to a conspicuous object such as a rotating, illuminated red box, for a period of time, normally several hours. Figure 5.1 shows some typical imprinting objects commonly used in the laboratory. From between two hours and several days later, chicks are given a choice between the object to which they were exposed and a novel object. The extent to which the chick approaches each of the two objects is compared and a preference score calculated.

Throughout this chapter we shall use the term 'imprinting' to describe the learning underlying the formation of filial preference as a result of exposure to an object or objects after hatching. Components of filial preference not attributable to specific experience we shall refer to as predispositions. Predispositions may be further divided into two types: specific and non-specific.

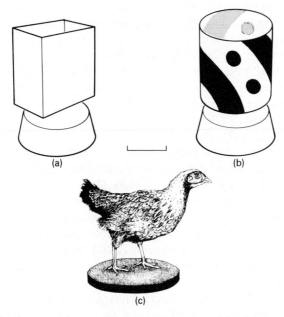

Fig. 5.1 Examples of objects which have been used as imprinting stimuli in various experiments. Stimulus (a) is a rotating box illuminated from within. The two square surfaces of the box were translucent and had coloured filters placed across them. Stimulus (b) is similar to (a) except in shape and pattern. Stimulus (c) was a rotating stuffed jungle fowl illuminated by a spotlight. All stimuli rotated at 28 r.p.m. Scale bar equals 10 cm. (After Horn 1985.)

NON-SPECIFIC VISUAL PREDISPOSITIONS IN THE CHICK

Young chicks and ducklings have predispositions to approach or peck at objects with certain general characteristics (for review see Sluckin 1972; for auditory predispositions see later section). With regard to size, Fabricius and Boyd (1952/53) found that objects below the size of a matchbox tend to be pecked, while objects larger than a matchbox can elicit approach and imprinting in ducklings. Further, Schulman *et al.* (1970) ascertained that circular objects with a diameter of 10–20 cm were approached most readily by chicks. Unfortunately, as yet there are few data available on size constancy with varying distance in the filial preference context.

Other characteristics of larger objects which influence approach in naïve chicks and ducklings include movement, colour, and pattern. Although initially movement of a stimulus toward a chick may be most attractive, eventually movement away from the chick becomes more effective at eliciting approach. With regard to colour, red and blue are often claimed to be most effective and yellow and green amongst the least effective both for approach and imprinting (e.g. Schaefer and Hess 1959; Gray 1961). In a long series of experiments Kovach (1984) has demonstrated that unconditioned colour preferences are susceptible to genetic selection. Although no preferences for the complexity of patterning of a stimulus have been detected in naïve chicks up to two days old (Berryman *et al*. 1971; Johnson and Horn 1988), such preferences have been found in older chicks (Berryman *et al*. 1971; Dutch 1969).

Chicks not only have predispositions to approach particular objects, they are also predisposed to peck at stimuli with particular characteristics. Contrary to the original claims of Hess (1959), the colours which most strongly elicit pecking appear to be the same as those that most strongly elicit approach (Davis and Fischer 1978; Andrew *et al*. 1981; Clifton and Andrew 1983), suggesting a common colour filter for the two responses (see Chapter 1). Clifton and Andrew (1983) discuss a number of possible mechanisms underlying these colour preferences in chicks, and demonstrate that the colour preferences are more apparent with smaller (5 mm) than with larger beads (13–37 mm). Thus, for both pecking and approach, particular combinations of colour, size, and shape may be necessary for maximum elicitation of the response.

Objects that are most optimal for eliciting initial pecking also appear to be those that are learned about most rapidly (Roper and Wistow 1986; Roper and Redston 1987). Whether it is also the case that objects which elicit most initial approach and other filial behavior are also most effective as imprinting stimuli remains to be established.

A SPECIFIC PREDISPOSITION

In the previous section we described various studies which revealed predispositions to respond to particular classes of stimuli in particular ways. Although some authors have suggested that more specific predispositions related to the visual characteristics of the natural mother bird may be operating in filial preference (e.g. Moltz 1960; Hinde 1961), until recently no direct evidence for such a specific predisposition had been obtained.

In many laboratory imprinting experiments only artificial stimuli such as rotating red boxes or swinging blue balls have been used. In more naturalistic studies either real or stuffed models were employed. Rarely, however, have preferences for both types of stimuli been directly compared within the same experiment (Reese *et al*. 1972). One exception to this was a study in which we (Johnson *et al*. 1985) gave trained and

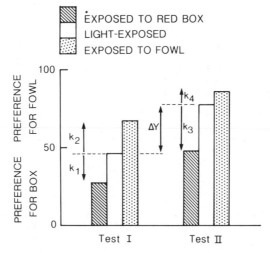

Fig. 5.2 A model of the interaction between acquired preferences and a developing predisposition. Preference score values are taken from the data obtained by Johnson *et al.* (1985). All mean preferences score are expressed as preferences for the stuffed jungle fowl. Broken lines represent baselines at the two testing times set by the respective light control groups. ΔY represents the difference in mean preference score between the light exposed birds in test I and test II. k_1–k_4 represent the effects of prior exposure to the red box or to the jungle fowl.

untrained chicks choice tests involving the simultaneous presentation of a rotating red box and a rotating stuffed fowl (see Fig. 5.1).

One group of chicks was exposed to the red box, another group to the stuffed fowl, and a third group was merely exposed to dim overhead light. The preferences of the chicks were ascertained in a 'railway' choice test (see Chapter 1) either 2 hours or 24 hours after the end of training. The results are shown in Fig. 5.2. When tested 2 hours after training the groups of birds behaved as expected: each of the trained groups showed a significant preference for the object to which they had been exposed, while the untrained group had no preference. When separate groups of birds were tested 24 hours after the end of training it became evident that, although the effects of training were still present, all three groups had shifted their preference toward the stuffed fowl. The group of chicks which had not been exposed to any conspicuous object, but had merely been exposed to dim overhead light, showed a significant preference for the stuffed fowl over the red box at this testing time. Two obvious questions arise: firstly, what are the necessary environmental conditions for the emergence of this predisposition, and secondly, what are the visual characteristics of the stuffed fowl that cause it to be preferred to the red box?

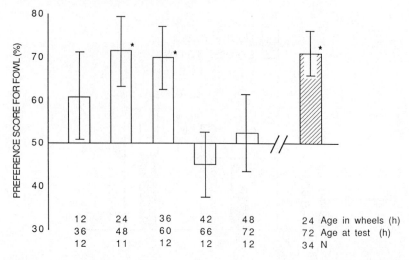

Fig. 5.3 The mean preference scores (±SEM) of groups of chicks placed in running wheels and tested at the various stated times after hatching. Blank bars represent groups of chicks tested 24 hours after being put in the running wheels. The hatched bar represents a group of chicks placed in the running wheel at 24 hours and tested at 72 hours after hatching. A preference score of 100 per cent indicates maximal preference for the stuffed fowl. A score of 0 per cent indicates maximal preference for the red box. Asterisks signify $p < 0.025$. (After Johnson *et al.* 1989).

The first question was addressed in a series of experiments in which it was established that even completely dark-reared birds will come to prefer the stuffed fowl to the red box if allowed a period of time in running wheels (Bolhuis *et al.* 1985). Dark-reared birds which were merely kept in small holders in an incubator did not develop the preference. Although exposure to overhead light was not essential, exposure to patterned light accelerated the emergence of the preference. These results suggested that under conditions likely to be experienced in the natural environment, the opportunity for motor activity and exposure to patterned light, the predisposition will emerge rapidly.

Dark-reared chicks not allowed a period of time in running wheels around 24 hours after hatching do not subsequently show the predisposition. In a recent study Johnson *et al.* (1989) investigated the effects on the emergence of the predisposition of allowing dark-reared chicks a period of time in the running wheels at varying ages after hatching. The results indicated that there is a time window between 12 hours and 36 hours after hatching within which this non-specific experience must occur (Fig. 5.3). Time spent in the running wheels after this age does not result in the subsequent emergence of the predisposition. While it is conceivable that the prolonged deprivation of visual stimulation experienced by birds not put in the running wheels until 36 hours or more posthatch may result in abnormal developmental changes in the visual system, this is unlikely to explain the results, since (1) the activity of these birds during test was not significantly less than that of the birds put in the wheels at an earlier age and (2) birds that are reared under identical conditions until being placed in the wheels 45 hours after hatching are still able to form strong preferences for particular objects to which they are exposed (Davies *et al.* 1985; Bolhuis *et al.* 1989*b*). An alternative explanation is that some aspect of being in the running wheels 'triggers' the emergence of the predisposition, but only within a particular sensitive period. What the particular aspect of the treatment may be remains unclear, although the lack of a significant correlation between activity while in the running wheel and subsequent preference for the fowl (Johnson *et al.* 1989) suggests it is unlikely to be motor activity alone.

The second question relating to the predisposition concerns its specificity, or the characteristics of the stuffed fowl which cause it to be preferred over the red box. One possibility is that the stuffed fowl is more attractive simply because it has greater outline or textural complexity than the box. As mentioned earlier, there is some evidence that older chicks preferentially approach objects of greater visual complexity (Dutch 1969; Berryman *et al.* 1971), and this preference may also be important in younger chicks. Johnson and Horn (1988) compared preference of dark-reared chicks for an intact stuffed fowl with their preference for other 'test' objects, which were constructed by scrambling or degrading a similar stuffed fowl in various ways. In all of the experiments in this series dark-reared chicks were placed in running wheels in darkness 24 hours after hatching. Twenty-four hours after this they were simultaneously presented with an intact stuffed fowl and a second test object, and their preference ascertained.

The first 'test' object to which the intact stuffed jungle fowl was compared was a stuffed jungle fowl which had been partially disarticulated and reassembled in an anatomically unusual way (Fig. 5.4, top left). With this stimulus there was no significant preference for the intact fowl, suggesting that, while both objects had similarly complex outlines (the same number and shape of wings, legs etc. protruding from the body) and were of similar 'textural' complexity (feather patterns, species markings etc.), the fact that one object had an intact fowl outline while the other had jumbled limbs made no difference to their relative attractiveness to the chicks. The next test object investigated was similar to the previous one, except that several of the elements (wings, leg, head etc) were separated from the trunk of the body (Fig. 5.4; top right). Again, the intact fowl was not significantly preferred over this object, reinforcing the earlier conclusion that a fowl-shaped overall outline is not a critical factor for the emerging predisposition: stuffed fowl with 'scrambled' outlines are

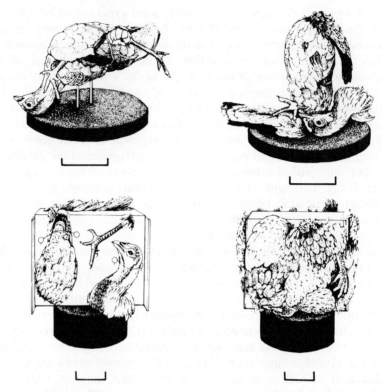

Fig. 5.4 The 'test' stimuli used as alternatives to the intact jungle fowl. Upper left: a stuffed fowl with limbs and head rearranged into anatomically unusual positions. Upper right: a stuffed fowl with limbs and head detached. Lower left: large regions of stuffed fowl mounted on a rotating box. Lower right: a fowl skin 'scrambled' and stuck on to a rotating box. Scale bar 6 cm. Drawing by Priscilla Barrett.

as attractive as an intact jungle fowl. This leaves several other possibilities, for example: (i) the chicks could be responding to some particular features such as the eyes or beak, or to some specific arrangement (configuration) of these features; (ii) the chicks could be responding simply to particular feather patterns or colours.

The next test object was composed of the entire pelt of a jungle fowl (including the head and neck) cut up into small pieces and jumbled up with all the other parts of the body, before being stuck onto the cork sides of a rotating box (Fig. 5.4, bottom right). Using this test object there was a strong preference for the intact jungle fowl. Therefore, this test object did not contain the essential attractive characteristics. Since the test object possessed the 'textural' complexity and colours of the intact fowl, these characteristics do not appear to be critical. Although this test object possessed individual features of the jungle fowl, these features were not always in their correct configuration relative to each other. For example, the eye, beak and neck region were separated. The presence of such clusters of features may be critical for the attractiveness of the object. Another critical factor may have been the greater complexity of the intact fowl outline compared to the simple box outline of the test object. One way to decide which of these two factors is most important is to create a test object which possesses the clusters of features absent in the previous object, but retains the simple box outline. Such a test object can be seen in Fig. 5.4 (bottom left). With this test object there was no significant preference for the intact fowl, despite the fact that the overall outline of the test object was less complex. This evidence suggests that arrangement of particular features may be the important characteristic.

There is some evidence from studies of adult chickens and quail that features of the head and neck are particularly important in the recognition of individuals in a dominance hierarchy (Candland 1969) and for the elicitation of social proximity behaviour (Domjan and Nash 1988). Could it be that features of the head are particularly important for the chicks also? To investigate this possibility all of the clusters of features except those from the head region were removed from the last test object: this resulted in an object that contained only the head region mounted on a rotating box. This test object was slightly preferred over the intact fowl. This suggests that not only is the cluster of features associated with the head an important characteristic, but that the rest of the jungle fowl body may simply act as a 'distractor' from this critical region.

Having established that the cluster of features of the jungle fowl head are critical, the next question investigated was how specific to particular species these features need to be. Although the jungle fowl is a direct ancestor of the domestic chicken (Zeuner 1963), the Gadwall duck (*Anas strepera*) is not. When dark-reared chicks allowed time in running wheels were given a choice between these two species they had no preference, suggesting the critical facial features need not be species specific (Johnson and Horn 1988). Further experiments indicated that the intact fowl was not preferred to a variety of similar sized stuffed mammals such as a polecat (*Mustela putorius*) (Johnson and Horn 1988). This indicates that the configuration of features associated with the head or face region may be more important than the details of the features themselves.

In the natural environment, the specific predisposition just discussed may ensure that the chick attends toward and approaches an appropriate object, normally the chick's own mother, when it emerges from under her for the first time after hatching. The young chick may then learn about the visual characteristics of the adult bird and so come to recognize her. Since features of the head and neck are particularly important for the predisposition, it may be this region about which the chick learns most. As well as this being the region of the adult chicken most likely to vary between individual birds, this would be consistent with the evidence from studies on adult chicken and quail (Candland 1969; Domjan and Nash 1988).

THE INTERACTING SYSTEMS MODEL

The evidence for a specific predisposition just discussed, taken together with the stimulus-dependent effects of lesions on imprinting, led to the proposal (Horn 1985; Johnson *et al.* 1985) that there are two dissociable systems underlying filial preference behaviour in the domestic chick: firstly, a system underlying the specific predisposition just discussed, and secondly a learning system which is engaged by a variety of conspicuous objects early in life. The forebrain region IMHV is essential for the normal functioning of the latter system (see Horn, Chapter 8; Davies, Chapter 12). In the natural situation, the predisposition may serve to orient the chick preferentially toward adult fowl rather than to inanimate objects in its visual environment; the learning system is then engaged by particular objects to which the chick attends, normally the chick's own mother. Several predictions arise from these proposals;

(i) If the two systems are truly dissociable then bilateral ablation of IMHV will not impair the specific predisposition. This prediction was tested by Johnson and Horn (1986). A group of chicks with bilateral IMHV lesions developed the predisposition under the same conditions as groups of intact chicks do. However, chicks with bilateral IMHV lesions are unable to acquire specific information as a result of exposure to an object. As predicted by the proposal, therefore, chicks with bilateral IMHV lesions behave like untrained birds.

(ii) Chicks should be capable of learning to discriminate between individual adult birds. Note that this prediction is in conflict with Lorenz's (1935, 1937) view that imprinting is primarily for the identification of own species. In order to test this prediction, Johnson and Horn (1987) exposed intact two-day-old chicks to one of two individual stuffed fowl for four periods of 50 minutes. Two hours after the end of the last training session the birds were given a simultaneous choice between the two stuffed fowl. The chicks were significantly more likely to start approaching the individual fowl to which they had been exposed previously.

(iii) Bilateral ablation of IMHV should preclude learning about the characteristics of individual adult birds. In order to test this hypothesis chicks with bilateral IMHV lesions and chicks with similar sized lesions to a different part of the forebrain (the visual Wulst) were trained by exposure to individual fowl and tested as described above. Chicks with control lesions, like intact chicks, preferred the individual to which they had previously been exposed. In contrast, chicks with IMHV lesions had no preference (Johnson and Horn 1987). We have recently extended this study to examine the effects of bilateral IMHV lesions on the ability of chickens to recognize individuals in later life (Bolhuis *et al.* 1989*a*). Small social groups of female chickens were raised with single males. When juvenile, the females were allowed to approach the male with which they had been reared, a novel male of the same strain, or a novel male of a novel strain. In accordance with optimal outbreeding theory (Bateson 1980), the intact females preferred the novel male of the same strain over the other two. However, birds which had had bilateral IMHV lesions placed on the first day after hatching had no significant preferences, although they behaved normally in other respects. This result suggests that the impairment in the ability to recognize individual congeners persists into adult life.

Recently, we (Bolhuis *et al.* 1989*b*) have investigated further the interaction between the two systems thought to be involved in the formation of filial preferences. One possibility is that the developing predisposition reflects the maturation of a 'sensory filter' or 'template' (Marler 1976; Staddon 1983) that only allows a certain class of information to be stored, restricting the chicks' ability to learn to those objects resembling conspecifics (see Bolhuis and Johnson, 1990, for further discussion). This possibility was investigated in a series of experiments in which the predisposition was allowed to develop in dark-reared chicks, using the procedure described earlier. In the first experiment such a group of chicks ('wheel/box') was subsequently trained by exposure to the red box for 2 hours. The chicks in a second group ('wheel/light') received the same initial treatment but were not subsequently exposed to the red box. Chicks in a third group ('box') were not placed in running wheels, but kept in a dark incubator until 50 hours old. In this latter group of chicks the predisposition would not have developed (Bolhuis *et al.* 1985). This group of birds was then exposed to the red box at the same age as the 'wheel/box' group. All three groups of chicks had their preference measured in a simultaneous test involving the red box and the stuffed fowl when 56 hours old.

The mean preference scores of the three groups of chicks are shown in Fig. 5.5. The chicks in the wheel/light group developed a significant preference for the stuffed fowl over the red box as predicted. The 'box' group of birds showed a significant preference for the training stimulus, also as expected. The preference of the 'wheel/box' group revealed a significant effect of exposure to the red box compared to the 'wheel/light' controls.

In a second experiment, two groups of chicks in which the predisposition had been allowed to develop were exposed to either a rotating red box or a rotating blue box. The results of the subsequent preference test are

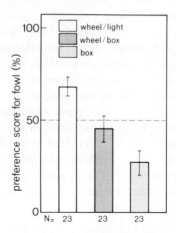

Fig. 5.5 The mean preference scores (±SEM) of the three groups of chicks treated as described in the text. For details of preference scores see legend to Fig. 5.3. All scores are expressed as a preference for the stuffed fowl (*n* = 23 for each group). (After Bolhuis *et al.* 1989*b*.)

shown in Fig. 5.6. Training on either colour results in a significant preference for that colour over the other.

These results show that once the predisposition has developed chicks are still capable of acquiring information about the visual characteristics of imprinting objects to which they are exposed, even when these bear no resemblance to a conspecific. This finding is more consistent with the notion of imprinting as exposure learning (Sluckin 1972) than as a form of template learning (Marler 1976; Staddon 1983).

THE INTERACTING SYSTEMS MODEL AND THE NATURAL
ENVIRONMENT

Evidence was cited in an earlier section that, in order for the predisposition to be expressed, chicks require some experience related to being in running wheels between 12 and 36 hours after hatching. Might this correspond to particular events in the natural rearing environment? Workman *et al.* (Chapter 6; Workman and Andrew 1989) provide some evidence from a semi-natural rearing situation that up to the fourth day after hatching chicks spend most of their time very near or actually under the hen. Initially this observation may appear not to be concordant with our experimental findings. However, three factors should be considered:

1. Guyomarc'h (1975) demonstrated that broods of 2-day-old chicks have short periods of activity (6–7 minutes) every half an hour or so.

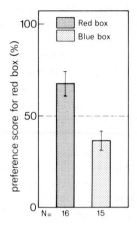

Fig. 5.6 The mean preference scores (±SEM) of two groups of chicks exposed to either a red or a blue box. Scores are expressed as a preference for the red box, i.e. 100 per cent signifies maximum preference for the red box and 0 per cent maximum preference for the blue box (*n* = 16 for red and *n* = 15 for blue) (After Bolhuis *et al.* 1989*b*.)

Obviously, unless sampling occurred during the active phase of the brood cycle, no activity would be recorded.

2. Workman placed hatched chicks under a broody hen. Guyomarc'h (1975) found that normally the activity cycles of the brood are coordinated with those of the hen. However, when younger chicks were placed under a hen, the activity cycles broke down. Thus, it is possible that the normal activity cycles were not present in Workman's observational study.

3. The tactile stimulation of being under the hen may be equivalent in some respect to the experience of being placed in the running wheels (handling by the experimenter, for example). Clearly, more research both in the laboratory and in natural situations is required to resolve these issues.

When a chick emerges from under the hen it will be exposed to a variety of patterned light. We have demonstrated (Bolhuis *et al.* 1985) that exposure to patterned light accelerates the emergence of the preference. Thus, the conditions which a chick encounters shortly after emerging from under its mother, even for brief periods, may ensure the rapid appearance of the specific predisposition. In turn, the presence of the predisposition may ensure that the newly emerged chick will attend toward the head region of the nearest adult bird, normally the mother. Comparatively rapid learning about the characteristics of individual adult birds head may be important for at least two reasons. Firstly, association with one female may prevent attacks from others, and secondly chicks may learn about particular food types by watching or copying what the adult bird pecks (Bartashurnas and Suboski 1984).

In most of the laboratory studies we have described, chicks or ducklings are reared in isolation. However, in the natural situation chicks or ducklings would be reared with siblings. What effect might this social rearing have on the ability to imprint on the hen? In general, rearing chicks with siblings prior to exposure depresses but does not eliminate imprinting on the hen (Guiton 1959; Zajonc *et al.* 1975). Rearing ducklings with siblings during the period of exposure to a stuffed mallard hen also interferes with maternal imprinting (Lickliter and Gottlieb 1986*a*). However, social interaction with conspecific brood mates after a period of maternal imprinting may strengthen or maintain subsequent preference for the mother (Lickliter and Gottlieb 1986*b*, 1988). As yet, little is known about the role of siblings in imprinting on a live hen in the natural situation.

THE REVERSIBILITY OF ACQUIRED PREFERENCES

As mentioned earlier, there is ample evidence to show that a preference for an artificial object can be reversed following prolonged exposure to a second object (e.g. Salzen and Meyer 1967). However, the results of recent experiments indicate that information about the first imprinting object to which a chick is exposed is not forgotten and that, under certain circumstances, the original preference may return or 'resurface'. For instance, Cherfas and Scott (1981) attempted to replicate the experiments of Salzen and Meyer (1967). Domestic chicks were exposed to a coloured ball for a period of three days which resulted in a strong preference for this object in a preference test. When the original stimulus was removed and the chicks exposed to a ball of a different colour for a similar period, there was a significant change in preference score toward the more recently seen object. This finding was in accordance with Salzen and Meyer's previous observation. However, when both objects were removed from the chicks' home cage for a further period of three days, Cherfas and Scott reported a significant change in preference toward the first object (cf. Bolhuis and Bateson 1990).

Boakes and Panter (1985) have reported findings suggesting that under certain conditions filial preferences may not be reversible. They exposed chicks on the first two days after hatching to either a live hen or to a moving artificial object (a toy windmill) for a period of time. During the next three days the animals and a naïve control group were exposed to a moving cup for a similar length of time. This procedure resulted in a significant preference for the cup in the control group. Significant 'secondary imprinting' on the cup was achieved in the 'windmill' group, but not in the group of chicks that had previously been exposed to a live hen. The authors conclude that 'secondary imprinting' is blocked when the first stimulus is a live hen.

The results of a series of experiments by Bolhuis and Trooster (1988) suggest a possible alternative explanation for the findings of Boakes and Panter, that is consistent with the interacting systems model which was outlined earlier. Bolhuis and Trooster (1988) exposed day-old chicks to either a stuffed jungle fowl or a red box for two hours. The chicks in both groups showed a strong preference for the training stimulus in a sub-sequent preference test involving the two objects. The next day the chicks were exposed to the alternative object for two hours, and preferences were tested again. There was a reversal of preference score in the group initially exposed to the box (box-fowl group), but no significant change in preference score in the group of chicks that had been exposed to the stuffed fowl first (fowl-box group). This result was obtained even in an experiment in which the relative attractiveness of the two objects had been manipulated such that the chicks initially trained on the box had a significantly greater preference score than the chicks trained on the stuffed fowl. Bolhuis and Trooster (1988) argued that, in the box-fowl situation, the emerging predisposition and the effects of exposure to the second object would affect the chicks' preferences in the same direction in the second phase of the experiment, resulting in a preference for the fowl. When the chicks were exposed to the stuffed fowl (or the live hen in the experiments of Boakes and Panter) as the first stimulus, both systems would be counteractive in the second phase of the experiment, resulting in a relatively stable preference for the fowl.

IMPRINTING AND ASSOCIATIVE LEARNING

Much of the literature about imprinting has concerned the extent to which the process can be seen as a form of conditioning. Although Lorenz himself was somewhat equivocal on this topic, several authors since have argued strongly that imprinting does not easily fit into a conditioning framework. For example, Hess (1962) deprecated attempts to 'fit the imprinting phenomenon into the association learning framework', and supported this by claiming that (i) unlike association learning, the primacy of experience is more important than the recency: early exposure is more important than recent exposure, and (ii) not only does imprinting not require reinforcement, but it is actually enhanced by punishment. How-ever, as both Hinde (1962) and Sluckin (1972) have pointed out, the evidence in support of these claims is meagre. Other authors have argued more convincingly that imprinting is best viewed as a type of perceptual or exposure learning (Sluckin and Salzen 1961; Sluckin 1972). Sluckin (1972) argues that the young animal becomes familiar with a particular object merely by exposure to it, and Salzen (1962) that during this process a 'neuronal model' is formed. Subsequent stimulus input was thought to be compared to this model. More recently, this idea has been expressed as 'template' learning (Marler 1976; Staddon 1983).

Alternatively, filial imprinting has been interpreted in terms of conditioning theory. In particular, Hoffman and his collaborators (Hoffman *et al.* 1972; Hoffman and Ratner 1973; Hoffman 1987) have formulated a theory of imprinting in terms of classical conditioning in which different characteristics of the object concerned act as CS and UCS, respectively. One difficulty with the conditioning approach to imprinting is identifying what the elements to be associated are. Since a naive chick will approach and follow the first conspicuous object it sees, this object must possess both the conditioned and unconditioned stimulus elements. For Hoffman and Ratner (1973) movement of the object acts as the UCS, whereas characteristics like colour, shape, and pattern act as CS and are initially neutral. However, Eiserer (1980) has shown that movement of an object is not essential for imprinting to occur, and that other attributes of a stimulus can be equally effective in eliciting initial approach.

Recently, Bolhuis, De Vos, and Kruijt (1990) have suggested an approach to this problem, in which it is assumed that certain elements of the imprinting object act as a UCS, without specifying what these elements are. Thus, within a conditioning interpretation of imprinting, it is assumed that when the chick is confronted with an imprinting object, the CS and the UCS occur simultaneously. In such an approach, phenomena that require the separate presentation of CS and UCS, like latent inhibition and extinction, cannot be tested in an imprinting situation. However, the occurrence of phenomena such as blocking and overshadowing can be investigated (see Bolhuis *et al.* 1990, for further discussion). The results of a recent study (De Vos and Bolhuis 1990) suggest that imprinting to a novel object is blocked when it is presented as part of a compound stimulus with a familiar object, but further research is necessary to study the mechanisms that are responsible for these findings.

THE ROLE OF AUDITORY CUES IN FILIAL PREFERENCE

Throughout this chapter we have focused mainly on visual factors in maternal attachment. This is not to deny the importance of the auditory modality in filial attachment. Auditory stimulation plays an important role in the formation of filial preferences in the chick (Gottlieb 1971; Kent 1987; Chapter 6) as well as in ducklings. Gottlieb (1965a) found that both naive mallard ducklings (*Anas platyrhynchos*) and chicks preferred their own species-specific parental call to that of some other species. When mallard ducklings were briefly exposed to a model emitting a wood duck (*Aix sponsa*) parental call, they later preferred that call to that of a chicken in a simultaneous preference test (Gottlieb 1965*a*). However, when these ducklings could choose between a wood duck call and a mallard call in a simultaneous test, they preferred the mallard call. Prolonged exposure to a model emitting a wood duck call reduced the preference for the mallard call, but only to the no-preference level. Thus, the ducklings could 'imprint' on a call, but their behaviour was also strongly affected by a preference for the parental call of their own species, although they had not heard this before.

In subsequent studies, Gottlieb has investigated the possible influence of prenatal experience on postnatal auditory preferences by recording responses of the embryo to different parental calls (Gottlieb 1965*b*). It was found that communally incubated mallard embryos, 12–24 hours before hatching, showed an increased oral response (bill clapping) to the mallard parental call, but not to the calls of the wood duck, the chicken or to sibling calls. When the embryos were incubated in isolation, they were not able to make this auditory discrimination before hatching, but did prefer the mallard parental call in a preference test conducted a day after hatching. Thus, the sub-total auditory deprivation (the animal could still hear its own vocalizations) induced a time lag in the development of species-specific preferences. Subsequent experiments, in which embryos were not only isolated, but also temporarily devocalized, showed that the preference for the species-specific parental call developed in advance of auditory experience (Gottlieb 1979). However, when the embryos were subsequently deprived of hearing their own or sibling vocalizations, the preference became less specific (Gottlieb 1978). It was found that the embryo needed to be exposed to the embryonic 'contact-contentment' call (4 notes per second) in order for the species-specific preference to be maintained until after hatching. Exposure to different rates of the embryonic call was not sufficient for the maintenance of the post-hatch preference.

Recently, Gottlieb (1988) has shown that mallard ducklings can learn the individual mallard maternal calls after only 12 minutes of exposure on the first day after hatching. Similarly, Fält (1981) and Kent (1987) have demonstrated the ability of domestic chicks to develop a preference for the clucking vocalizations of an individual hen (Chapter 6). Kent (1987) found that the preferences were stronger when live hens were presented.

The results of all these experiments taken together reveal interesting parallels between the development of visual and auditory preferences. From Gottlieb's work it is apparent that predispositions to respond to certain auditory stimuli play an important role in the development of preferences and that they interact with the effects of exposure to a particular stimulus (Gottlieb 1965*a*). In the case of auditory preferences in ducklings, the predisposition is more specific than the specific predisposition discussed earlier in this chapter. Furthermore, as was described above, the induction and maintenance (Gottlieb 1980) of the auditory predisposition in ducklings was shown to be dependent upon specific (embryonic) experience. In contrast, the development of the specific visual predisposition is dependent upon comparatively non-specific experience. In both the auditory and the visual specific predispositions in the chick there is evidence for a 'sensitive period' for experience to affect its development. Finally, experiments with both paradigms show that exposure to particular stimuli can lead to recognition of, and a preference for, individual conspecifics (Johnson and Horn 1987; Kent 1987; Gottlieb 1988).

IMPRINTING AND FILIAL PREFERENCE IN MAMMALS

What relevance does the extensive literature on filial preference in precocial birds have for those interested in mammalian behavioural development? Reports of imprinting-like phenomena in the young of various species of mammal, including dogs, sheep, rabbits, guinea pigs, and humans, have been persistent over the past few decades (e.g. Sluckin 1968, 1972). In precocial species imprinting is easily measured by a locomotor approach response. However, as Sluckin (1972) and Horn and Johnson (1989) point out, there is no requirement that the underlying learning process must be tied to a particular type of behavioural response. Similar learning may occur in altricial species, but evidence of it is more difficult to obtain as their responses may be less reproducible and more difficult to quantify. Human infants may be particularly difficult in this regard. Nevertheless, several attempts have been made to extend our knowledge about filial preference in the precocial birds, especially the chick, to human infants:

1. Bowlby (1969) was heavily influenced by Lorenz's original studies in his analysis of the stages of attachment of the human infant to its mother. This approach has suffered both from the attacks on Lorenz's original claims, and from the complexity of the effects of early maternal deprivation on subsequent human development (see Rutter 1972).
2. Several of the pioneers of the study of visual preferences in human infants, including Robert Fantz (e.g. Fantz 1966), based their studies on their earlier work on visual preferences in chicks. Many of the techniques developed by these pioneers are still in use today and have given rise to much of our present knowledge about perceptual and cognitive capacities of young infants.
3. More recently, Johnson and Morton (1990; Johnson 1988; Morton

and Johnson 1989) have attempted to account for apparently contradictory evidence on the development of human face recognition in terms of an interacting systems model similar to that proposed in the present chapter for recognition of mother in the chick.

Goren, Sarty, and Wu (1975) demonstrated that newborn human infants will turn their head and eyes further to keep a moving face pattern in view than to keep a variety of 'scrambled' face patterns in view. This finding challenged the established view that it takes the infant two or three months to learn about the arrangement of features that make a face (see for example, Gibson 1969; Maurer 1985; Nelson and Ludemann 1990), and accordingly came under criticism for methodological reasons. However, the result described by Goren and colleagues has recently been replicated using procedures less susceptible to criticism (Johnson *et al.* 1990).

One way to reconcile these findings in newborns with the view that it takes several months to learn about the arrangement of features that constitutes a face is to interpret the data in terms of two systems analogous to those just described for chicks. Firstly, newborn infants are predisposed to attend to face-like patterns within their visual field, and secondly, a learning system is engaged by those objects to which the infant attends: in this case faces.

With regard to the specific predisposition mentioned earlier, there are some striking similarities between the chick and infant. In both species there is an attraction to the correct arrangement of features associated with an adult conspecific's head. As mentioned earlier, for the chick the period in the running wheel 'triggers' the expression of the predisposition, possibly mediated by a hormonal surge (Bolhuis *et al.* 1985; Horn 1985). In the human infant, the surge of catecholamines associated with normal birth (Lagercrantz and Slotkin 1986) may have a similar 'triggering' effect. Turning to the second (learning) system, the chick is capable of discriminating between individual adult chickens in the first few days (Johnson and Horn 1987). Although it may take the human infant three months to recognize their mother on the basis of the internal features of her face (Bushnell 1982), the infant may be able to use more general visual cues to discriminate her from others by the second or third day after birth (Bushnell *et al.* 1989).

Acknowledgements

We acknowledge financial support from the SERC (UK), MRC (UK), and The European Science Foundation. Thanks are due to Richard Andrew and John Morton for useful comments on a draft of this chapter.

REFERENCES

Andrew R. J., Clifton, P. G., and Gibbs, M. E. (1981). Enhancement of effectiveness of learning by testosterone in domestic chicks. *Journal of Comparative and Physiological Psychology*,**95**, 406–17.

Bartashunas, C. and Suboski, M. D. (1984). Effects of age of chick on social transmission of pecking preferences from hen to chicks. *Developmental Psychobiology*, **17**, 121–7.

Bateson, P. P. G. (1966). The characteristics and context of imprinting. *Biological Reviews*, **41**, 177–220.

Bateson, P. P. G. (1980). Optimal outbreeding and the development of sexual preferences in Japanese quail. *Zeitschrift fur Tierpsychologie*, **53**, 321–44.

Bateson, P. P. G. (ed.) (1983). *Mate choice*. Cambridge University Press.

Berryman, J., Fullerton, C. and Sluckin, W. (1971). Complexity and colour preferences of chicks of different ages. *Quarterly Journal of Experimental Psychology*, **23**, 255–60.

Boakes, R. and Panter, D. (1985). Secondary imprinting in the domestic chick blocked by previous exposure to a live hen. *Animal Behaviour*, **33**, 353–65.

Bolhuis, J. J. and Bateson, P. P. G. (1990). The importance of being first: A primacy effect in filial imprinting. *Animal Behaviour*, **40**, 472–83.

Bolhuis, J. J. and Johnson, M. H. (1990). Sensory templates: mechanism or metaphor? *Behavioral and Brain Sciences*. (In press.)

Bolhuis, J. J. and Trooster, W. J. (1988) Reversibility revisited: stimulus-dependent stability of filial preference in the chick. *Animal Behaviour*, **36**, 668–674.

Bolhuis, J. J., Johnson, M. H., and Horn, G. (1985). Effects of early experience on the development of filial preferences in the domestic chick. *Developmental Psychobiology*, **18**, 299–308.

Bolhuis, J. J., Johnson, M. H., Horn, G., and Bateson, P. (1989a). Long-lasting effects of IMHV lesions on social preferences in the domestic fowl. *Behavioral Neuroscience*, **103**, 438–41.

Bolhuis, J. J., Johnson, M. H., and Horn, G. (1989b). Interacting mechanisms during the formation of filial preferences: the development of a predisposition does not prevent learning. *Journal of Experimental Psychology: Animal Behavior Processes*, **15**, 376–82.

Bolhuis, J. J., de Vos, G. J., and Kruijt, J. P. (1990). Filial imprinting and associative learning. *Quarterly Journal of Experimental Psychology*, **42B**, 313–29.

Bowlby, J. (1969). *Attachment and loss: 1. Attachment*. Hogarth Press, London.

Bushnell, I. W. R. (1982). Discrimination of faces by young infants. *Journal of Experimental Child Psychology*, **33**, 298–308.

Bushnell, I. W. R., Sai, F., and Mullin, J. T. (1989). Neonatal recognition of the mother's face. *British Journal of Developmental Psychology*, **7**, 3–15.

Candland, D. K. (1969). Discrimination of facial regions used by the domestic chick in maintaining the social dominance order. *Journal of Comparative and Physiological Psychology*, **69**, 281–5.

Cherfas, J. and Scott, A. (1981). Impermanent reversal of filial imprinting. *Animal Behaviour*, **30**, 301.

Clifton, P. G. and Andrew, R. J. (1983). The role of stimulus size and colour in the elicitation of testosterone-facilitated aggressive and sexual responses in the domestic chick. *Animal Behaviour*, **31**, 878–901.

Davies, D. C., Horn, G., and McCabe, B. J. (1985). Noradrenaline and learning: the effects of the noradrenergic neurotoxin DSP4 on imprinting in the domestic chick. *Behavioral Neuroscience*, **99**, 652–60.

Davis, S. J. and Fischer, G. J. (1978). Chick colour preferences are altered by cold stress: colour pecking and approach preferences are the same. *Animal Behaviour*, **26**, 259–64.

De Vos, G. J. and Bolhuis, J. J. (1990). An investigation into blocking of filial imprinting during exposure to a compound stimulus. *Quarterly Journal of Experimental Psychology*, **42B**, 289–312.

Domjan, M. and Nash, S. (1988). Stimulus control of social behaviour in male Japanese quail. *Animal Behaviour*, **36**, 1006–15.

Dutch, J. (1969). Visual complexity and stimulus pacing in chicks. *Quarterly Journal of Experimental Psychology*, **64**, 281–5.

Eiserer, L. A. (1980). Development of filial attachment to static visual features of an imprinting object. *Animal Learning and Behavior*, **8**, 159–66.

Fabricius, E. and Boyd, H. (1952/53). Experiments on the following reactions of ducklings. *Wildfowl Trust Annual Report*, **6**, 84–9.

Fält, B. (1981). Development of responsiveness to the individual maternal 'clucking' by domestic chicks. *Behavioural Processes*, **6**, 303–17.

Fantz, R. L. (1966). Pattern vision in newborn infants. *Science*, **151**, 354.

Gibson, E. J. (1969). *Principles of perceptual learning and development*. Appleton-Century-Crofts, New York.

Goren, C. C., Sarty, M., and Wu, P. Y. K. (1975). Visual following and pattern discrimination of face-like stimuli by newborn infants. *Pediatrics*, **56**, 544–9.

Gottlieb, G. (1965a). Imprinting in relation to parental and species identification by avian neonates. *Journal of Comparative and Physiological Psychology*, **59**, 345–56.

Gottlieb, G. (1965b). Prenatal auditory sensitivity in chickens and ducks. *Science*, **147**, 1596–8.

Gottlieb, G. (1971). *The development of species identification in birds*. University of Chicago Press.

Gottlieb, G. (1978). The development of species identification in ducklings: IV. Change in species-specific perception caused by auditory deprivation. *Journal of Comparative and Physiological Psychology*, **92**, 375–87.

Gottlieb, G. (1979). Development of species identification in ducklings: V. Perceptual differentiation in the embryo. *Journal of Comparative and Physiological Psychology*, **93**, 831–54.

Gottlieb, G. (1980). Development of species identification in ducklings: VI. Specific embryonic experience required to maintain species-typical perception in pecking ducklings. *Journal of Comparative and Physiological Psychology*, **94**, 579–87.

Gottlieb, G. (1988). Development of species identification in ducklings XV. Individual auditory recognition. *Developmental Psychobiology*, **21**, 509–22.

Gray, P. H. (1961). The releasers of imprinting: differential reactions to color as a function of maturation. *Journal of Comparative and Physiological Psychology*, **54**, 597–601.

Guiton, P. (1959). Socialisation and imprinting in brown leghorn chicks. *Animal Behaviour*, **7**, 26–34.

Guyomarc'h, J. C. (1975). Les cycles d'activité d'une couvée naturelle de poussins et leur coordination. *Behaviour*, **53**, 31–75.

Hess, E. H. (1959). Imprinting. *Science*, **130**, 133–41.

Hess, E. H. (1962). Ethology: an approach toward the complete analysis of behaviour. In *New directions in psychology* (ed. R. Brown *et al.*) Holt, Rinehart & Winston, New York.

Hinde, R. A. (1961). The establishment of parent-offspring relations in birds, with some mammalian analogies. In *Current problems in animal behaviour* (ed. W. H. Thorpe and O. L. Zangwill), pp. 175–93. Cambridge University Press.

Hinde, R. A. (1962). Some aspects of the imprinting problem. *Symposium of the Zoological Society of London*, **No.8**, 129–38.

Hoffman, H. S. (1987). Imprinting and the critical period for social attachments: some laboratory investigations. In *Sensitive periods in development: interdisciplinary perspectives* (ed. M. H. Bornstein). Lawrence Erlbaum, Hillsdale, NJ.

Hoffman, H. S. and Ratner, A. M. (1973). A reinforcement model of imprinting. *Psychological Reviews*, **80**, 527–44.

Hoffman, H. S., Ratner, A. M., and Eiserer, L. A. (1972). Role of visual imprinting in the emergence of specific filial attachment in ducklings. *Journal of Comparative and Physiological Psychology*, **81**, 399–409.

Horn, G. (1985). *Memory, imprinting, and the brain*. Clarendon Press, Oxford.

Horn, G. and Johnson, M. H. (1989). Memory systems in the chick: dissociations and neuronal analysis. *Neuropsychologia*, **27**, 1–22.

Jaynes, J. (1956). Imprinting: the interaction of learned and innate behaviour. I. Development and generalisation. *Journal of Comparative and Physiological Psychology*, **49**, 200–6.

Johnson, M. H. (1988). Memories of mother. *New Scientist*, **1600**, 60–2.

Johnson, M. H. (1990). Information processing and storage during filial imprinting. In *Kin recognition* (ed. P. G. Hepper). Cambridge University Press.

Johnson, M. H., Bolhuis, J. J., and Horn, G. (1985). Interaction between acquired preferences and developing predispositions during imprinting. *Animal Behaviour*, **33**, 1000–6.

Johnson, M. H., Davies, D. C., and Horn, G. (1989). A sensitive period for the development of filial preferences in dark-reared chicks. *Animal Behaviour*, **37**, 1044–5.

Johnson, M., Dziurawiec, S., Ellis, H. D., and Morton, J. (1990). Newborns, preferential tracking of faces and its subsequent decline. *Cognition* (submitted).

Johnson, M. H. and Horn, G. (1986). Dissociation of recognition memory and associative learning by a restricted lesion of the chick forebrain. *Neuropsychologia*, **24**, 329–40.

Johnson, M. H. and Horn, G. (1987). The role of a restricted lesion of the chick forebrain in the recognition of individual conspecifics. *Behavioral Brain Research*, **23**, 269–75.

Johnson, M. H. and Horn, G. (1988). Development of filial preferences in dark-reared chicks. *Animal Behaviour*, **36**, 675–83.

Johnson, M. H. and Morton, J. (1991). *Biology and Cognitive Development: The case of face recognition*. Blackwell, Oxford. (In press.)

Kent, J. P. (1987). Experiments on the relationship between the hen and chick. *Behaviour*, **102**, 1–14.

Kovach, J. K. (1984). Behavioural genetics and the search for the engram: genes, perceptual preferences and the mediation of stimulus information. In *Behavior genetics, principles and applications II* (ed. J. L. Fuller and E. C. Simmel). Lawrence Erlbaum Associates, Hillsdale, NJ.

Lagercrantz, H. and Slotkin, T. A. (1986). The 'stress' of being born. *Scientific American*, **254**, 92–8.

Lickliter, R. and Gottlieb, G. (1986a). Training ducklings in broods interferes with maternal imprinting. *Developmental Psychobiology*, **19**, 555–66.

Lickliter, R. and Gottlieb, G. (1986b). Visually imprinted maternal preference in ducklings is redirected by social interaction with siblings. *Developmental Psychobiology*, **19**, 265–77.

Lickliter, R. and Gottlieb, G. (1988). Social specificity: interaction with own species is necessary to foster species-specific maternal preference in ducklings. *Developmental Psychobiology*, **21**, 311–21.

Lorenz, K. (1935). Der Kumpan in der Umwelt des Vogels. *Journal für Ornithologie*, **83**, 137–213, 289–413.

Lorenz, K. (1937). The companion in the bird's world. *Auk*, **54**: 245–73.

Marler, P. (1976). Sensory templates in species specific behaviour. In *Simpler networks and behaviour*, (ed. J. C. Fentress). Sinauer, Sunderland, Mass.

Maurer, D. (1985). Infants' perception of facedness. In *Social perception in infants* (ed. T. N. Field and N. Fox). Ablex, New Jersey.

Morton, J. and Johnson, M. H. (1989). Four ways for faces to be 'special'. In *Handbook of research on face processing* (ed. A. W. Young and H. D. Ellis). North Holland, Amsterdam.

Moltz, H. (1960). Imprinting: empirical basis and theoretical significance. *Psychology Bulletin*, **57**, 291–314.

Nelson, C. A. and Ludemann, P. M. (1990). Past, current, and future trends in infant face perception research. *Canadian Journal of Psychology*. (In press.)

Reese, E. P., Schotte, C. S., Bechtold, R. E., and Cowley, V. L. (1972). Initial preference of chicks from five rearing conditions for a hen or a rotating light. *Journal of Comparative and Physiological Psychology*, **81**, 76–83.

Roper, T. J. and Redston, S. (1987). Conspicuousness of distasteful prey affects the strength and durability of one-trial avoidance learning. *Animal Behaviour*, **35**, 739–47.

Roper, T. J. and Wistow, R. (1986). Aposematic colouration and avoidance learning in chicks. *Quarterly Journal of Experimental Psychology*, **38B**, 141–9.

Rutter, M. (1972). *Maternal deprivation reassessed*. Penguin Books, Harmondsworth.

Salzen, E. A. (1962). Imprinting and fear. *Symposium of the Zoological Society of London*, No. 8, 197–217.

Salzen, E. A. and Meyer, C. C. (1967). Imprinting: reversal of a preference established during the critical period. *Nature*, **215**, 785–6.

Schaefer, H. R. and Hess, E. H. (1959). Color preferences in imprinting objects. *Zeitschrift für Tierpsychologie*, **16**, 161–72.

Schulman, A. H., Hale, A. H., and Graves, H. B. (1970). Visual stimulus characteristics for initial approach response in chicks. *Animal Behaviour*, **18**, 461–6.

Sluckin, W. (1968). Imprinting in guinea pigs. *Nature*, **220**, 1148.

Sluckin, W. (1972). *Imprinting and early learning* (2nd edn). Methuen, London.

Sluckin, W. and Salzen, E. A. (1961). Imprinting and perceptual learning. *Quarterly Journal of Experimental Psychology*, **13**, 65–77.

Staddon, J. E. R. (1983). *Adaptive behaviour and learning*. Cambridge University Press.

Vidal, J-M, (1980). The relations between filial and sexual imprinting in the domestic fowl: effects of age and social experience. *Animal Behaviour*, **28**, 880–91.

Workman, L. and Andrew, R. J. (1989). Simultaneous changes in behaviour and in lateralisation during the development of male and female domestic chicks. *Animal Behaviour*, **38**, 596–605.

Zajonc, R. B., Wilson, W. R., and Rajecki, D. W. (1975). Affiliation and social discrimination produced by brief exposure in day-old domestic chicks. *Animal Behaviour*, **23**, 131–8.

Zeuner, F. E. (1963). *A history of domesticated animals*. Hutchison, London.

6

Development of behaviour in the chick

GENERAL ISSUES
P. P. G. Bateson

Behavioural development can be studied by cross-sectional research, which involves measuring different individuals at each age, or by longitudinal research, which involves measuring the same individuals repeatedly. One problem with longitudinal studies is that age-related developmental changes and experience of the test situation are inevitably confounded if the same subjects are repeatedly tested as they grow older. For example, testing a young animal's responsiveness to a stimulus can influence its development and thereby affect its behaviour in subsequent tests of responsiveness. Thus the general problem of repeated testing of the same subjects (known as an order effect) is particularly important in developmental studies).

Cross-sectional measurements are not subject to order effects, but do have a number of other drawbacks. First, individuals of two different ages may differ from each other in ways that are not merely due to differences in age and the experience obtained between the two ages at which measurements are made. Unless there is careful balancing of separate age groups between and within batches, they may differ systematically in some property established prior to the age when the first group was tested. This could arise, for instance, if fetal development were dependent on atmospheric pressure (e.g. Bateson 1974), or other factors which may vary between batches.

Another problem is that cross-sectional measurement necessarily averages the scores of individuals that may be developing in markedly different ways. If a measure increase sharply over a narrow age-range, but the timing of this increases varies between individuals, a cross-sectional study, which measured different subjects at each age, would show an apparently gradual increase in the measure, a pattern of development that would not represent any individual. For instance, if recognition of a familiar object after imprinting was either present or absent and birds took a variable amount of time to learn, the apparent gradual increase in ability to recognize revealed by average scores would be misleading.

It will be apparent that both cross-sectional and longitudinal approaches have their advantages and both raise different problems of practice and interpretation. Ideally, both methods should be used, as exemplified by

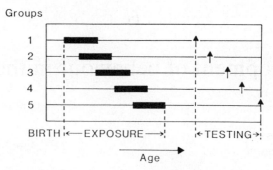

Fig. 6.1 An illustration of the methods used in measuring a sensitive period. Exposure to a stimulus, such as an imprinting object, is denoted by the thick horizontal bars and subsequent testing is denoted by the vertical arrows. In this example, five different groups of subjects are exposed to the stimulus, starting at different ages. The duration of exposure is the same for all five groups, as is the interval between the end of exposure and testing. However, this procedure means that the groups are tested at different ages. If the age of testing is kept constant, the time from the end of exposure to testing must vary.

the study of the development of pecking in domestic chicks by Cruze (1935). He kept the chicks in the dark from when they hatched and fed them by hand. Starting at different ages, he tested the accuracy with which the chicks pecked at seeds. Once a chick had been tested, it was retested on subsequent days of its life. In this way Cruze was able to obtain cross-sectional data on chicks that were first tested at a given age, and longitudinal data on chicks that were retested each day. Not surprisingly, he found that both a chick's age and its prior experience of pecking at seeds affected its accuracy.

A sensitive period in development is an age-range when particular events are especially likely to affect the individual's development (see Bateson and Hinde 1987). The experimental procedures needed to establish an influence at one age and not at others are shown in Fig. 6.1. The age-range when a group of subjects is exposed to the condition is shown by the heavy line. If the exposure were started at different ages and ended at the same age, then the age at first exposure would be confounded with duration of exposure. Thus, any observed effect could have arisen because the individuals that were exposed at an earlier age were also exposed for longer. (Unfortunately, this possibility is not hypothetical; many examples of the ambiguity can be found in the literature.)

A more subtle difficulty is raised by the time of testing. If the time from the end of exposure to testing is not kept constant, then some of the differences between groups could have arisen because the effects of exposure had more time in which to decline in the groups first exposed at the younger ages. However, if time from exposure to testing is kept constant (as shown in Fig. 6.1), the ages and intervening experiences of the groups at testing are necessarily different. Here again, the counsel of perfection is to use both methods for fixing the time for testing.

When experiments are not feasible, the existence of sensitive periods may sometimes be suggested by correlational methods. One approach is to study development retrospectively, looking backwards in time to what may have been important events in development. In contrast, a prospective approach identifies all the individuals that have had a particular experience and examines what subsequently happens to them. Even if a certain type of experience is strongly associated with a particular outcome later in life, a retrospective study cannot detect individuals who received the same early experience but showed no subsequent effect.

NATURAL BROODS
L. Workman, J. P. Kent, and R. J. Andrew

Brückner (1933) described three discrete phases in the development of social contact between brood and hen.

1. Total concentration (hatching to day 3 or 4). The hen remains on or very close to nest, and the chicks are nearly always very close to her, never being further away than 1 metre (at the very most).
2. 'Fluctuating contact' (day 4 or 5 to day 10 or 11). The chicks occasionally travel to 2 or 3 metres but regularly return to close to the hen.
3. 'Dispersion stage' (day 10 or 11 to weaning). Chicks do not keep continuously in close contact but do return to the hen.

A recent study of the behaviour of standard broods living under semi-natural conditions (Workman 1986; Workman and Andrew 1989) has broadly confirmed the existence of these phases. The proportion of time spent beneath the hen during the day time falls from about two thirds to one tenth between day 4 and day 6. Between day 5 and day 6, marked changes occur in measures based both on hen and on chicks. Hen locomotion rises very sharply as does the mean distance between chicks and hens (Fig. 6.2). Since all moves are initiated by the hen at this time, it seems likely at first sight that it is mainly the increase in hen locomotion that causes chicks to find themselves at a greater distance from her. However, there is evidence of changes at this time in chicks reared without a mother (below).

Between day 9 and day 10 the mean distance between chicks and hen rises markedly again to a sharp peak on day 10 (Fig. 6.2). Here there is no

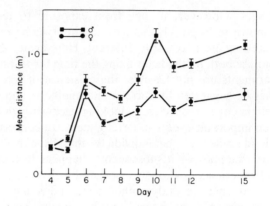

Fig. 6.2 The mean distance (averaged over 30 scores/chick) between a chick and the hen is shown for each day. There was significant variation with age ($F_{9,151} =$ 83.60, $p < 0.001$), which was largely due to a rise at two transitions: days 5/6 ($F_{1,14}$ = 119.58, $p < 0.001$) and days 9/10 ($F_{1,18}$ = 26.84, $p < 0.001$). The fall after day 10 was also significant (days 10/11, $F_{1,18}$ = 4.44, $p = 0.049$). Males were consistently further from the hen than females ($F_{1,18}$ = 65.47, $p < 0.001$), and the male scores rose more at each step (Sex × Day, $F_{9,51}$ = 3.43, $p < 0.001$). (Reproduced from Workman and Andrew, 1989, *Animal Behaviour*, **38**, 596–605.)

accompanying rise in locomotion by the hen, and it seems clear that it is the behaviour of the chicks which changes. This is confirmed by direct observation: thus on day 10 for the first time chicks begin to initiate locomotion by the hen and the rest of the brood by running ahead of the hen Fig. 6.3). This behaviour not only appears on day 10 but peaks on that day and on day 11.

Transitions in chick behaviour are thus markedly sharper, and more constant in timing across individuals and broods than Brückner's description suggests. The clearest example is the transition between day 9 and day 10: up to day 9 chicks follow their mother as though tied to her heels by elastic strings, but then on day 10 they suddenly begin to move independently of her, as well. However, it is clear that division into three phases does not adequately describe the development of behaviour in broods of chicks. At least one other sharply timed change occurs. On day 8, chicks suddenly begin to fixate the human observer and adult fowl other than their mother. The change is abrupt: up to day 7, chicks completely ignore such objects, whereas on day 8 they will stand and stare at them. Such behaviour both appears and peaks on day 8. The period from day 8 to day 12 is then a complex one which is broken up (at least) into day 8, day 9, days 10 and 11, and day 12 onwards.

Other change probably follows with almost equally sharp timing. 'Frolicking at other chicks', when a chick suddenly runs with wings raised

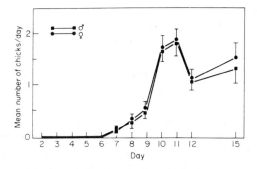

Fig. 6.3 The number of observation points (maximum 60) at which a chick runs ahead of the hen is shown as a mean score/chick. There was significant variation with age ($F_{11,387} = 326.91$, $p < 0.001$), which was largely due to a marked rise between days 9 and 10 ($F_{1,33} = 162.49$, $p < 0.001$) and a fall after day 11 (days 11–15, $F_{2,66} = 27.36$, $p < 0.001$). The Sex by Day interaction was significant ($F_{2,66} = 3.50$, $p = 0.036$), largely because the male curve fell below the female on day 15. (Reproduced from Workman and Andrew, 1989, *Animal Behaviour*, **38**, 596–605).

(and often flapping) directly at, and sometimes collides with another chick, appears between days 10 and 12. Sparring, in which the two chicks become erect, chest to chest, becomes common as a result of such collision by day 15; it represents incipient fighting.

Other behaviour appears more gradually: perching on elevated objects and ground scratching both increase in frequency continuously from about day 5 to day 15 (the last day of observation).

This picture can be filled in from other studies. Workman (unpublished), studying a small colony of feral fowl (descendants of birds from Northwest Island off the east coast of Australia: McBride *et al.* 1969), found that broody hens (two, each with six chicks) remained virtually motionless on days 1 and 2. Locomotion appeared gradually thereafter, with a sudden increase between days 4 and 6. Tidbitting (calling the chicks to food items) was common (about one quarter of all observation points) until day 6, after which it fell away sharply. Both timings were exactly what was found in the hens studied by Workman and Andrew (above), except that tidbitting fell in the latter study between days 7 and 8. The chicks remained almost continuously under the hen on day 1; the time spent under her fell most markedly between day 4 and 6. Again, the same was true in the earlier larger study.

Wood-Gush *et al.* (1978), also working in the field, gave mean distances between hen and most distant chick averaged over a number of days. Between day 2 and day 7 this was about 1 metre; by day 16 it had reached 7 metres; in weeks 6 and 7 values were as high as 20 metres.

Finally, Guyomarc'h (1975), using continuous recording of activity, found that chicks begin to appear from under the hen on day 2 or day 3. Activity, and resting under the hen alternate in cycles of roughly 30 minutes. Periods of activity are quite brief on the first days (6–7 minutes) but increase rapidly in duration: immediately following day 10 they are about 20 minutes long. Since the cycles change little in periodicity, resting periods show corresponding shortening.

The results reported by Guyomarc'h suggest that chicks see little or nothing of the hen until about day 2. Opportunity to see the hen on day 2 is also suggested by Bateson (1963); this study found that the proportion of chicks which were 2 feet and more from the hen at points of observation was 0 per cent on day 1, but had already risen to 15 per cent by day 2. By day 11, the value was 60 per cent. It should also be noted that following the hen is likely to be rare or even absent until day 4; it did not become common until day 5 in the study by Workman and Andrew (1989). Broom (1968) provides complementary evidence, since here the chicks raised in the absence of a hen. All of the 11 behaviours which were measured increased in frequency between day 2 and 10; in particular, there was a marked increase in four behaviours between days 5 and 6. Broom suggested that all four (locomotion, groundpecking, twittering and preening) are related directly or indirectly to an increase in feeding. Twittering is usual during vigorous feeding, although completely undisturbed chicks will feed in complete silence (Andrew and de Lanerolle 1974). However, an association of feeding and preening must have a more indirect cause, perhaps because of increased preening in states of satiation following feeding.

The timing of the change is striking: it coincides precisely with the first increase in distance between chicks and hen reported by Workman and Andrew (1989). In that study, it was argued that this increase was probably due to the hen, whose locomotion increased sharply at this time. A rise in chick locomotion in the absence of a hen suggests a more complex causation, with changing chick behaviour perhaps driving, as well as responding to an increase in locomotion in the hen. The other important conclusion to be drawn from Broom's paper is that the changes in chick behaviour between day 5 and day 6 may stem largely from an increase in the need to feed. Yolk reserves fall from 10 per cent of body weight at hatching to 1 per cent by day 5 (Schilling and Bleecker 1928). Hogan (1971) also picks out day 5 as the day by which feeding preferences must be established if the chick is to survive.

Other evidence suggests that feeding may begin to be important on day 3 or 4. Body weight falls off following hatching to reach a trough at the beginning of day 3 in both domestic (Latimer 1924) and feral fowl (Workman, unpublished). Drinking is also infrequent for the first 36 hours in both Red Jungle Fowl (Kruijt 1964) and domestic birds (Broom 1968).

In natural broods, then, the hen and chicks probably would tend to move together away from the vicinity of the nest on day 5, exactly when feeding (as opposed to exploratory pecks, with some feeding thrown in) becomes essential to the chick. It is interesting to note the marked fall in tidbitting by the hen between days 7 and 8 (above) from a high plateau to continuing very low values, meaning that instruction by the mother in what is, and is not food begins as soon as the chicks are able to watch her pecking and continues for the first 3 days of intensive feeding. Both the tidbitting call and the head movements during pecking at a food item are potent and specific releasers of feeding. Naïve chicks will choose the type of particle at which a model is pecking behind glass from amongst a range of stimuli accessible to them (Turner 1963; Suboski and Bartashunas 1984).

The sudden disappearance of tidbitting on day 8 provides a second example of co-ordinated changes in chicks and hen. Here, too, the changes in chick behaviour (appearance of fixation of humans and conspecifics: above) might have been interpreted as entirely driven by changes in the hen (disappearance of tidbitting), were it not for a variety of evidence (pp. 116 *et seq.*) of similar change on day 8 in chicks growing up without a mother. One crucial consequence of the changes in both hen and chick is that on day 8 chicks are likely to shift from learning a great deal about types of food (and non-food) to learning about other features of the world.

Broodiness can be induced in hens by the presentation of young chicks, even if there has been no incubation (Saeki and Tanabe 1955), and can be maintained by replacement of older chicks by young ones (Guhl 1962). This makes clear how strongly hens are affected by stimuli provided by chicks. An important question for future research is the nature of the links between the behaviour of chick and hen. Is there endogenous timing of changes in the hen as well as the chick? If not, how do changes in chick behaviour on day 8 bring about the reduction of tidbitting by the hen?

It should be noted that there is little doubt that the physiological state of a broody hen does directly affect her behaviour in dramatic ways. Even though hens may lose as much as a third of their body weight during incubation, feeding remains strongly inhibited during tidbitting. Behaviour such as preening is relatively rare until about day 10 (feral fowl: Workman, unpublished). However, what is at issue is whether the sharp timing of some changes in hen behaviour is entirely driven by changes in the chicks.

A variety of different changes accompany and underpin the behavioural changes shown by chicks during development. Some are physiological: the ability to maintain body temperatures in a relatively cool environment increases rapidly as inactive periods under the hen shorten (Sherry 1981). Changes in the CNS are discussed at length elsewhere in this book (e.g. Chapter 7). There is thus an embarassment of choice in the search for causes of changes in behaviour. Nevertheless, one very important cause seems to be abrupt changes in hemispheric dominance (Andrew 1988; Workman and Andrew 1989; Chapter 19). Day 8 is a day of uniquely marked control by the left hemisphere and days 10 and 11 are marked by right hemisphere control. All indices of chick behaviour point to a sudden increase in interest in distant features of the environment on days 10 and 11: the peak in running ahead of the mother (Fig. 6.3) is one such index. This agrees well with evidence of right hemisphere advantages in the use of topographical features in orientation (Rashid and Andrew 1989). It is less clear why left hemisphere control should lead to fixation of objects like the human observer, but the coincidence of the two phenomena in time is striking and has been confirmed in chicks reared in isolation (Workman and Andrew 1989).

Auditory stimuli

The first 2 or 3 days of life, when chicks are continuously or almost continuously under their mother, are dominated by auditory responses. These begin to be important in the late fetus. Two types of sound are emitted in the period before hatching. The first is a click (produced on each breath), such as has been shown to synchronize hatching in the Bobwhite quail (*Colinus virginianus*) by Vince (1964a, b); in this species late developing chicks are accelerated and precocious ones delayed in their hatching. These effects are certainly less marked in chicks of the domestic fowl (Vince 1969) which do not synchronize their hatching whether in incubators or under a hen (Vince 1970). However, prenatal exposure of domestic chicks to artificial clicks advanced the mean time of hatching (Vince *et al.* 1970); there was no evidence of retardation. Clicks were shown to be more effective than clucks or white noise by White (1984).

The relative asynchrony of hatching in the fowl makes it unlikely that the time of hatching is itself of great importance as a starting point for the sequence of changes which occur on particular days in subsequent development. It is much more likely that these are related to circadian cycles, themselves phase-locked to external changes. It should be noted that vocal interaction between hen and late fetus (below) may make it possible for such phase-locking to begin before hatching.

Such interaction is likely to involve much the same range of calls as chicks give after hatching. Gottlieb and Vandenbergh (1968) describe three types of fetal calls: longer calls corresponding to peeps ('distress calls'), shorter twitters ('pleasure calls') and bursts of short calls which may correspond to chick warbles, given when drowsy (cf. Collias and Joos 1953; Andrew 1964). Calling begins on day 19 of incubation. External stimulation such as warming or cooling, or shifts in position will induce calling (Collias 1952). Maternal calls also increase the rate of calling (and of bill clapping) on the day before hatching (Gottlieb 1965). Effects of chick calling on the hen were demonstrated by Tuculescu and Griswold (1983): the hen vocalizes and/or moves on the nest in response to distress calls from within an egg. The fetus in turn responds by falling silent or emitting pleasure calls.

Comparable interactions occur after hatching; as the brood becomes more mobile they involve chicks which are separated from the hen. Peeps attract the hen, which clucks as it approaches, sometimes causing the peeps to cease (Brückner 1933; Collias 1952; McBride *et al.* 1969). Clucks allow social contact to be maintained when in dense cover; chicks actively approach the sound of clucks (Graves 1970; Kent 1987).

Chicks specifically attach to the sound of the clucks of their mother. Brückner (1933) and Collias (1952) showed that when two broods were put together in the dark, in the presence of two broody hens, the chicks tended to go to their own mother, using only the sound of her calls. It is likely that acoustic imprinting begins before hatching. Grier *et al.* (1967) showed chicks to prefer the particular simple artificial sound to which they had been exposed in the egg. Guyomarc'h (1974) presented one of two recorded clucks during the last 2 days of incubation and showed that in choice tests, after hatching, chicks approached the cluck to which they had earlier been exposed.

However, an interesting complication is introduced by evidence that incubating hens use a special call which is longer and lower than the brood cluck (Kent, personal observation), and is probably commoner during incubation than the latter, particularly when on the nest (rather than feeding beside it). It appears to correspond to the 'mew' incubation call described by Bailey (1983) in pheasants; Tuculescu and Griswold (1983) mention an 'intermediate' call in broody hens, in addition to the cluck. Hess (1972) notes a perhaps corresponding change in the calls of mallards from 'clucks' before and during hatching, to quacks after the ducklings have left the nest. It is thus possible that different properties of the maternal calls are normally learned before and after hatching.

Kent (1987), using natural broods, confirmed that in tests on days 4–8 of life chicks will choose to approach recordings of the clucks of their own mother. Interestingly, such choice disappears after a separation of 4 hours (although it is still present after 30 minutes' separation).

This loss of choice occurred even though the two hens could be seen as well as heard at test. Strange broody hens nearly always adopted chicks; after 3 days with the foster mother, chicks chose her rather than the original mother. It thus seems that long-term memory does not provide an adequate basis for individual recognition, at least when differences are rather subtle. It is likely that both visual and auditory cues contribute to the ability to choose the mother rather than a very similar hen: choice is significantly clearer when the hens can be seen as well as heard. Changes in the information available to recall during memory formation are discussed in Chapters 17 and 19.

The cluck varies markedly between hens, but is relatively constant in any one individual over the period of broodiness (Kent 1989). The other common call directed at chicks by the broody hen, the food call, varies much more within an individual, suggesting that the cluck may be of special importance in recognition of the mother (Kent 1989). Food calls are certainly attractive: naïve chicks approach them in preference to adult distress calls (Snapp 1969). This is likely to be an expression of a general tendency to approach short repetitive low-pitched sounds (Collias and Joos 1953).

It will be seen that there is a close parallel between attachment to parental clucks and later visual imprinting. Early exposure in the egg can lead to attachment to artificial sounds, just as exposure on day 1 to simple artificial visual stimuli can cause attachment (Chapter 5). On the other hand, chicks which have lived with a broody hen show clear preferences for both her clucks and her visual appearance when choosing between her and a very similar hen.

In normal development, visual attachment is likely to be guided and facilitated by the fact that the first moving object consistently seen by the chick (other than siblings) will be the head of the mother, emitting the clucks to which the chick is already attached.

A TIMETABLE OF DEVELOPMENT
R. J. Andrew and M. Dharmaretnam

Guhl (1962), writing about chicks, notes that 'there is much variability among individuals in the age at which certain behaviour patterns appear', and stresses that this variability begins with marked variation in the time of hatching. This eminently reasonable position agrees with what is usually found in studies of the development of behaviour. More specifically, in the chick as well, it is often only a minority of individuals which show a particular behaviour pattern on the day on which it is first recorded. More exhaustive observations and ideal conditions for the evocation of the behaviour would no doubt increase the proportion of individuals showing the behaviour, but by how much remains a matter for speculation.

However, the previous section will have made clear that, whatever the apparent variation between individuals, there is an underlying timetable of change, which is remarkably constant. The aim of this section is to try to establish what is the most likely form of this timetable, and briefly to consider more general implications of its existence and properties. Evidence of sharply timed changes in behaviour during development under semi-natural conditions has been given in the previous section. To this must be added evidence from laboratory studies.

Between day 1 and day 2 releasing mechanisms for visual properties of the mother's head mature (Chapter 5). Between day 2 and day 3 there develops the ability to associate the visual properties of objects at which pecks are directed with physiological consequences of digesting and absorbing food (Hogan 1973; Hale and Leonard 1988).

Information about later events comes from studies of shifts in laterali- zation during development. The first evidence for such shifts, based on changes in sensitivity to injected cycloheximide, was provided by Drennen (1977; see also Rogers and Ehrlich 1983) working in the laboratory of Rogers, who presents the most up-to-date time-course in Chapter 21. The time-course for shifts of lateralization is now clearly established, for the period from days 6 or 7 to days 13 and 14. Briefly, injection of cyclohex- imide into one or other of the cerebral hemispheres produces long term disturbance of performance in a visual learning task. In male chicks, on day 8 only left hemisphere, and on days 10 and 11 only right hemisphere injection is effective; on days 7, 9, 12 and 14, all injection is ineffective (there are no data for days 6 and 13).

Behavioural tests (Dharmaretnam 1989) agree with these timings. They show unusual bias to left hemisphere control on day 8 and to right hemisphere control on days 10 and 11 (probably peaking on day 11). In addition to these age-dependent shifts in control, there is bias associated with the nature of the stimulus or task. In the first time-course shown here, this latter effect is apparently minimal. The test consisted of simultaneous presentation of two similar dead *Tenebrio* beetles, one in each lateral visual field. The first to be pecked gave an indication of the side to which there was bias: on day 8 the beetle on the right was pecked, whereas from day 10 onwards, that on the left was pecked (Fig. 6.4). Some task-specific bias is suggested by the fact that leftward choice remained the rule on days 14 and 15.

A second task showed marked bias to the right. Female chicks were allowed to view a hen (for the first time). They tended to use the lateral visual field of one or other eye. The right eye was preferred in general, this being most marked on day 8. However, on day 11, as predicted there was a marked shift to use of the left eye (Fig. 6.5).

A third task measured head position just before the chick approached the sound of a broody hen clucking; the chicks had been exposed to the cluck on day 1 before test, and were tested repeatedly on successive days, so that they were familiar with, and probably attached to the cluck. Two time-courses are shown, one for males (Fig. 6.6a) and one for females (Fig. 6.6b), because (i) repeated testing of the same chicks makes it impossible to separate effects of prior testing from effects of age without comparing between time-courses with differing distribution of tests, (ii) time-courses

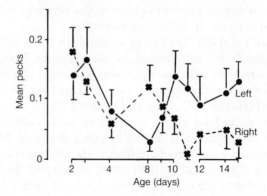

Fig. 6.4 The mean number of pecks directed by male chicks to the right and to the left are shown, for a test in which a pair of mealworm beetles appeared simultaneously, one in each lateral visual field (see text). Each point is for a separate batch of chicks. There is overall heterogeneity with age ($F_{9,661} = 2.24$, $p = 0.018$). On day 8 right side bias, and on days 10 and 11 left side bias was expected from earlier work; significant such bias was obtained (day 8: $F_{1,68} = 4.38$, $p = 0.040$; day 11 $F_{1,72} = 7.77$, $p = 0.007$).

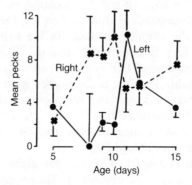

Fig. 6.5 The mean time spent in viewing a hen, seen for the first time, and placed at a distance of about 50 cm, is shown separately for right and left eyes in female chicks. Chicks put their head through a hole in order to view but were under no other constraint. Under such conditions a chick holds its head nearly all the time in one of a number of precisely defined positions (30–39° to right or left, 60–69° to right or left, facing straight forward). Only the 30–39° and 60–69° sectors are considered here, in order to exclude possible brief periods of viewing other features of the environment. All points are for separate batches of chicks. The ANOVA was carried out on (duration of viewing by right eye minus duration of viewing by left eye). There was significant variation in the relative use of the two eyes with age ($F_{6,197} = 3.89$, $p = 0.001$). This was largely due to preponderant use of the right eye on days 8–10, and of the left eye on day 11.

for this test (unlike viewing a hen: above) can be established from day 1 to day 11; they are thus well suited to show that males and females follow the same timecourse. Over the period from day 8 onwards, there is probably a general bias towards turning the left side of the head to the sound: there is only a slight preponderance of use of the right side on day 8, but the shift to marked preference for the left side on days 9, 10, and 11 is clear. On days 6 and 7 there is roughly equal use of either side, but just before this there is evidence for a new transition; the right side is used on day 3, and the left on day 4. It is likely that head position in this test was chiefly related to listening to the sound, since little or nothing could be seen (legend, Fig 6.6); however, attempts to see cannot be excluded, and so the neutral term 'side' is used.

Further behavioural evidence for these shifts is provided by tests of ability to orient by topographical cues (Rashid and Andrew 1989). Here chicks using only the left eye, normally have a marked advantage. (This holds for both sexes: data for females, Rashid 1989). However, on day 8 (and only on that day) they perform badly, apparently because of interference from the left hemisphere (which tends to control behaviour on day 8, and is here attempting to do so, despite little or no direct visual input: see Chapter 21). Uniquely on day 8 right-eyed chicks are able to orient well, but do so by using local rather than distant cues.

The picture for the period up to day 5 is less clear, partly because there are fewer data, and partly because of apparent disagreements between what are available. The beetle test shows chicks to be highly responsive, but to choose apparently at random; the first eye to catch sight of a beetle probably initiates response. Chicks show little interest in viewing distant objects like a hen seen for the first time up to day 5, at least under our condition of test, when sustained viewing has to begin within the first 30 seconds, if it is to be scored.

Head position during response to clucks in this period is most simply explained as reflecting a general moderate bias to presentation of the right side, but with two exceptions. In both sexes on day 4 the left side is markedly preferred, whilst on day 3 preference is for the right side. In males the latter is true on day 1, but interpretation here is complicated by the fact that day 1 is also the day of first experience of the clucks; the effects of progressive experience of clucks on head orientation on day 1 will be considered elsewhere.

The evidence from sensitivity to cycloheximide is rather different. Visual learning is sensitive to bilateral hemispheric injection on days 1 and 2 but not 3 (Rogers *et al.* 1974); on day 2 left hemisphere injection is effective but not right hemisphere (Rogers and Anson 1979).

Little can be gained at present by comparing this evidence in detail with that from head position. Sensitivity of visual learning mechanisms does not seem to show changes between days 4 and 5, unlike head position

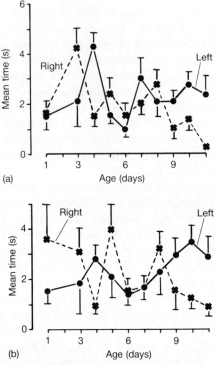

Fig. 6.6 Clucks of a broody hen were played to a chick in a small pool of dim light in the centre of a darkened arena. A circular curtain (82 cm diameter) hung to within 12 cm of the floor to reduce echo and further to restrict view; it is likely that nothing but darkness could be seen outside the pool of light, but attempts to view cannot be excluded. Chicks were repeatedly tested. In this situation no standard head position was taken up. The side to which the head was turned during the last 15 s before approach to the sound source was measured; mean durations are shown. Female (a) and male (b) curves are shown separately. The ANOVA was carried out on (duration of right side minus duration of left side). There was no hint of difference between the sexes (Sex, $F_{1,204} = 0.00$; Age × Sex, $F_{1,8} = 0.62$). Variation with age was significant ($F_{8,204} = 13.25$, $p < 0.001$). This was partly due to the predicted shift towards left side use beginning after day 8; note that under these conditions such shift begins earlier than when viewing the hen. If the male curve is used to predict the shape of the female curve, then days 3,4,5 and 8–10 are picked out as points where significant bias and its direction may be predicted. On days 3,4,9,10,11 such bias was found ($p = 0.036$, $p = 0.022$, $p = 0.017$, $p = 0.048$, $p = 0.017$, Wilcoxon).

when listening to clucks. If it is assumed that the latter measure is affected over the first 5 days only by properties of acoustic lateralization and that these change independently of, and differently from visual lateralization over this period, then the discrepancy disappears. However, other explanations are possible.

For our present purposes, the important thing is that it now seems likely that virtually each new day of a chick's life over the first 2 weeks brings changes which are surprisingly constant across populations and strains of chicks (see also Chapter 20). These are summarized below for normal development, breaking the two weeks into five main periods.

Under hen

Day 1. Interaction with the mother by calls is the main behaviour, probably continuing from the last day of incubation (previous section). Visual learning mechanisms are insensitive to cycloheximide; releasing mechanisms for features of maternal head have not yet matured. These features, together with the fact that the chick spends all or nearly all of the time in the dark under the mother, suggests that visual learning is relatively unimportant in normal development. Acoustic learning is important and may have special features: predominant involvement in this of the right hemisphere is suggested by head posture, but this still requires confirmation.

Day 2. Behaviour is much as on day 1, except that chicks may emerge from under the mother for short periods; only the mother's head is likely to be seen in motion. Acoustic learning is still important (sensitivity evidence). However, visual releasing mechanisms mature and visual learning mechanisms become sensitive to cycloheximide. This presumably represents preparation for visual learning (on days 3 and 4).

Day 3. The chick begins to spend time beside, as well as under the hen. This presumably makes more likely visual learning of the features of the mother's head, moving near the ground (tidbitting and pecking) or clucking from a more raised position. Since the sound of the calls is already familiar, the obvious relationship between sounds and visual appearance may be important. Pecking at potential food, often directed by the tidbitting behaviour of the mother, is likely to become more common.

Transition

Day 4. The chicks spend yet more time active beside the hen, but the hen does not yet commonly lead them or move any distance from the nest. Learning about food is probably important, although ingestion and experience is presumably limited by the small area available to be searched. The bias towards use of the left side of the head in the listening test suggests that acoustic stimuli (or some categories of acoustic stimuli) are important on this day. One possibility is that it is important to learn the properties of common environmental sounds before following begins in earnest on day 5.

Following hen; feeding and drinking essential

Day 5. This is the first day of this period; it may have special properties because of this. Sensitivity of visual learning mechanisms to cycloheximide in the left hemisphere continues but ceases either on day 6 (no data) or day 7. Listening data suggest that preference for the right side of the head becomes more marked on day 5. Predominance of left hemisphere control is thus suggested; it may be associated with intensive learning about food objects, or with the first periods of extensive following. Against the latter possibility, responsiveness at first presentation of an imprinting object declines sharply on day 5 (Bateson 1963).

Days 6 and 7. As on day 5, following the mother and feeding are the dominant activities.

Preparation for independence

Day 8. Unique bias to control by the left hemisphere, together with left hemisphere sensitivity to cycloheximide, suggests a period of special learning. Following and feeding remain the main behaviour but interest (without approach) in conspecifics, and probably other moving or moveable objects, may allow categories like 'conspecific', 'predator' to be established before the chicks move away from mother. Note that the calls of the mother (e.g. warning of predators) will give relevant information, so that acoustic mechanisms could also be involved. A fall in tidbitting means that instruction in feeding by the mother is much reduced; chicks may as a result learn more about foraging themselves.

Day 9. Shift towards right hemisphere control has begun but no more. The special features of day 8 reduce or disappear: absence of cycloheximide sensitivity suggests a day without special preparations for specific learning.

Development of independence

Day 10. The sudden appearance of locomotion which is independent of the mother presumably leads both to greater independence in foraging and to learning about features of the environment and their layout. This is coupled with, and perhaps caused by shifts to right hemisphere control. Cycloheximide sensitivity also suggests specific learning.

Day 11. The features of day 10 continue.

Day 12. The disappearance of cycloheximide sensitivity and the reduction in behavioural measures of independent movement suggest the end of a period of specific learning.

Days 13–15. Appearance of social responses (previous section).

The most obvious and immediate conclusion to be drawn from the timetable which has just been presented is that age of chicks is a crucial experimental variable. The first question in applying the timetable is clearly how to measure age in chicks held under a variety of regimes. The data considered in this chapter are drawn, at one extreme, from broods living under natural alternation of day and night with associated changes in maternal behaviour, and at the other from chicks held under continuous light, and living in visual isolation from each other (e.g. Fig. 6.1–6.4). In fact, behavioural rhythms of 24 hour duration, which are locked to environmental changes, are well established for chicks living under the latter conditions. Reymond and Rogers (1981) found that such chicks showed excellent discrimination of food from pebbles in morning tests, but almost no differential pecking in the evenings. Food was available *ad libitum*; sound cues are the most likely source of locking to environmental change, perhaps coupled with visual cues from human caretakers.

The time of hatching is so variable across batches of chicks (Chapter 1) that the most likely starting point for the day-by-day changes is the first period of sustained rest (i.e. the first night) after the day following hatching. However, evidence is lacking on this issue.

There are clearly advantages to be obtained by carefully choosing the age appropriate to a particular type of experiment (e.g. when a particular type of learning or a particular ability is likely to be maximal or minimal). However, at present it is probably more important to stress the dangers which might arise from ignoring age. It is unsafe to try to establish the consequences of an important manipulation such as a specific brain lesion, or an amnestic drug, by assembling evidence from different tasks carried out on different days. This is a useful intermediate step, but it must be followed by studies in which all the critical tests are carried out on birds of the same age.

Sex differences are also pervasive (Chapters 20, 21) and must be borne in mind when designing experiments; however, the time courses given here strongly suggest that the basic timetable of development is similar in male and female chicks.

REFERENCES

Andrew, R. J. (1988). The development of visual lateralisation in the domestic chick. *Behavioural Brain Research*, **29**, 201–9.
Andrew, R. J. and de Lanerolle, N. (1974). The effects of muting lesions on

emotional behaviour and behaviour normally associated with calling. *Brain, Behaviour and Evolution*, **10**, 377–98.

Bailey, E. D. (1983). Influence of incubation calls on post-hatching repertoire in pheasant chicks. *Condor*, **85**, 43–9.

Bateson, P. P. G. (1963). The development of filial and avoidance behaviour in the domestic chicken. Ph.D. thesis, Cambridge.

Bateson, P. P. G. (1974). Atmospheric pressure during incubation and post-hatch behaviour in chicks. *Nature*, **348**, 805–7.

Bateson, P. and Hinde, R. A. (1987). Development changes in sensitivity to experience. In *Sensitive periods in development* (ed. by M. H. Bornstein), pp. 19–34. Erlbaum, Hillsdale, NJ.

Broom, D. M. (1968). Behaviour of undisturbed 1 to 10-day-old chicks in different rearing conditions. *Developmental Psychobiology*, **1**, 287–95.

Brückner, G. H. (1933). Untersuchungen zur Tiersoziologie inbesondere zur Auflösung der Familie. *Zeitschrift für Psychologie*, **128**, 1–105.

Collias, N. E. (1952). The development of social behaviour in birds. *Auk*, **69**, 127–59.

Collias, N. E. and Joos, M. (1953). The spectrographic analysis of the sound signals of the domestic fowl. *Behaviour*, **5**, 175–88.

Cruze, W. W. (1935). Maturation and learning in chicks. *Journal of Comparative Psychology*, **19**, 371–408.

Dharmaretnam, M. (1989). Lateralization of viewing and other functions in the domestic chick. D. Phil thesis, University of Sussex.

Drennen, H. D. (1977). Behavioural effects of controlled visual experience on chickens under the influence of cycloheximide. D. Phil. thesis, Australian National University.

Gottlieb, G. (1965). Prenatal auditory sensitivity in chicks and geese. *Science*, **147**, 1596–8.

Gottlieb, G. and Vandenbergh, J. G. (1968). Ontogeny of vocalization in duck and chick embryos. *Journal of experimental Zoology*, **168**, 307–26.

Graves, H. B. (1970). Comparative ethology of imprinting: field and laboratory studies of wild turkeys, jungle fowl and domestic fowl. *American Zoologist*, **10**, 483.

Grier, J. B., Counter, S. A., and Sheaver, W. M. (1967). Parental auditory imprinting in chickens. *Science*, **155**, 1692–3.

Guhl, A. M. (1962). The behaviour of chickens. In *The behaviour of domestic animals* (ed. E. S. E. Hafez), pp. 491–530. Ballière, Tindall and Cox, London.

Guyomarc'h J. C. (1974). L'empreinte auditive prenatale chez le poussin domestique. *Revue de la Compartement Animal*, **8**, 3–6.

Guyomarc'h J. C. (1975). Les cycles d'activité d'une couvée naturelle de poussins et leur coordination. *Behaviour*, **53**, 31–75.

Hale, C. and Leonard, G. (1988). Effects of early ingestional experiences on the acquisition of appropriate food selection by young chicks. *Animal Behaviour*, **36**, 211–24.

Hess, E. H. (1972). Imprinting in a natural laboratory. *Scientific American*, **227**, 24–31.

Hogan, J. A. (1971). The development of a hunger system in young chicks. *Behaviour*, **39**, 128–201.

Hogan, J. A. (1973). Development of food recognition in young chicks: II Learned association over long delays. *Journal of Comparative and Physiological Psychology*, **83**, 367–73.

Kent, J. P. (1987). Experiments on the relationship between the hen and chick (*Gallus gallus*) : the role of the auditory mode in recognition and the effects of maternal separation. *Behaviour*, **102**, 1–14.

Kent, J.P. (1989). On the acoustic basis of recognition of the other hen by the chick in the domestic fowl (*Gallus gallus*). *Behaviour*, **108**, 1–9.

Kruijt, J. P. (1964). Ontogeny of social behaviour in Burmese Red Jungle Fowl. *Behaviour* supplement, **12**.

Latimer, H. B. (1924). Postnatal growth of the body, systems and organs of the single-comb White Leghorn chicken. *Journal of Agricultural Research*, **29**, 363–97.

McBride, G., Parer, I. P., and Foenander, F. (1969). The social organization and behaviour of the domestic fowl. *Animal Behaviour*, **2**, 125–81.

Rashid, N. (1989). Lateralization of topographical learning and other abilities in the chick. D. Phil. thesis, University of Sussex.

Rashid, N. and Andrew, R. J. (1989). Right hemisphere advantage for topographical orientation in the domestic chick. *Neuropsychologia*, **27**, 937–48.

Reymond, E. and Rogers, L. J. (1981). Diurnal variations in learning performance in chickens. *Animal Behaviour*, **29**, 241–8.

Rogers, L. J. and Anson, J. M. (1979). Lateralization of function in the chicken forebrain. *Pharmacology and Biochemistry of Behaviour*, **10**, 679–86.

Rogers, L. J., Drennen, H. D., and Mark, R. F. (1974). Inhibition of memory formation in the imprinting period: irreversible action of cycloheximide in young chickens. *Brain Research*, **79**, 213–33.

Rogers, L. J. and Ehrlich, D. (1983). Asymmetry in the chicken forebrain during development and possible involvement of the supraoptic decussation. *Neuroscience Letters*, **37**, 123–7.

Saeki, Y and Tanabe Y. (1955). Changes in prolactin content of fowl pituitary during broody periods and some experiments on the induction of broodiness, *Poultry Science*, **34**, 909–19.

Schilling, S. J. and Bleecker, W. L. (1928). The absorption rate of the reserve yolk in baby chicks. *Journal of the American Veterinary Association*, **25**, 618–26.

Sherry, D. F. (1981). Parental care and the development of thermoregulation in Red Jungle Fowl. *Behaviour*, **76**, 250–80.

Snapp, B. D. (1969). Recognition of maternal calls by parentally naive *Gallus gallus* chicks. *Animal Behaviour*, **17**, 440–5.

Suboski, M. D. and Bartashunas, C. (1984). Mechanisms for social transmission of pecking preferences to neonatal chicks. *Journal of Experimental Psychology*, **10**, 182–92.

Tuculescu, R. A. and Griswold, J. G. (1983). Pre-hatching interactions in domestic chickens. *Animal Behaviour*, **31**, 1–10.

Turner, E. R. A. (1963). Social feeding in birds. *Behaviour*, **24**, 1–45.

Vince, M. A.(1964a). Social facilitation of hatching in the Bob-White Quail. *Animal Behaviour*, **12**, 531–4.

Vince, M. A. (1964b). Synchronisation of hatching in American Bob-White Quail (*Colinus virginianus*). *Nature*, **203**, 1192–3.

Vince, M. A. (1969). Embryonic communication, respiration and the synchronisation of hatching. In *Bird vocalization* (ed. R. A. Hinde), pp. 233–60. Cambridge University Press.

Vince, M. A., Green, J., and Chinn, S. (1970). Acceleration of hatching in the domestic fowl. *British Poultry Science*, **11**, 483–8.

White, N. R. (1984). Effects of embryonic auditory stimulation on hatch time in the domestic chick. *Bird Behaviour*, **5**, 122–6.

Wood-Gush, D. G. M., Duncan, I. J. H., and Savory, C. J. (1978). Observations on the social behaviour of domestic fowl in the wild. *Biology of Behaviour*, **3**, 193–205.

Workman, L. (1986). Lateralization of brain function and behavioural ontogeny in the chick under natural conditions. D. Phil. thesis, University of Sussex.

Workman, L. and Andrew R. J. (1989). Simultaneous change in behaviour and in lateralisation during the development of male and female domestic chicks. *Animal Behaviour*, **38**, 596–605.

7

Molecular mechanisms of neuronal maturation: a model for synaptic plasticity

J. A. P. Rostas

The plasticity of the adult nervous system allows it to learn new things and remember them, to adapt to change and to recover from injury. It is believed that all these processes ultimately depend upon the appropriate modification and regulation of individual synapses and synaptic networks at two levels. At a structural ('coarse') level, new synaptic connections are formed either in response to injury or as part of a cyclic turnover which is occurring continually (Cotman and Nieto-Sampedro 1984, Carlin and Siekevitz 1983). At a 'fine' level, plasticity occurs within a fixed number of nerve cells and synapses by local modulation of the efficacy of synapses.

The technical problem facing those wishing to identify molecular changes underlying plasticity is to obtain sufficient tissue undergoing plastic change to make biochemical investigation possible. This chapter describes a developmental approach to this problem based on the premise that the maturational events of normal brain development offer an experimental model for the study of synaptic plasticity.

NEURONAL MATURATION AS A MODEL FOR SYNAPTIC PLASTICITY (Fig. 7.1)

The many events involved in normal synaptogenesis can be divided into at least two broad phases: synapse formation and synapse maturation.* Synapse formation encompasses all of the events which convert a growing neurite into a neuronal process making contact with another cell via a differentiated structure which looks and functions like a synapse. This phase produces a net increase in synapses in a cellular environment which is peculiar to developing brain and is usually not found in adult brain.

---

* Despite the fact that the names of both phases refer specifically to the synapse, both phases involve changes occurring throughout the entire neuron.

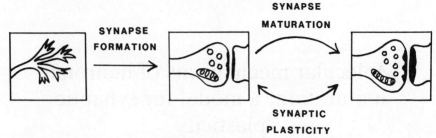

Fig. 7.1   Schematic representation of the synapse formation and synapse maturation phases of synaptogenesis.

Synapse maturation encompasses all the changes that convert the immature but functional synaptic networks into synaptic networks with properties like those found in adult brain. This phase produces no net increase in
synapses (in some systems it may produce a net decrease) and occurs
within functional networks of neurons in a cellular environment similar to
that in the adult. Therefore, all the changes in the maturation phase are
potentially enhanceable or reversible, and those that result in a functional
change in the properties of the synaptic networks may be similar or
identical to the changes responsible for plasticity in the adult. Thus, I
believe that the maturation phase of normal brain development can be
used as an experimental model system for the identification and study of
molecular mechanisms responsible for synaptic plasticity. Because synapses in the brain develop asynchronously, studies of the maturation
process require a system in which the maturation phase is long relative to
the formation phase. The developing chicken forebrain is such a system.

THE POSTSYNAPTIC DENSITY

The postsynaptic density (PSD) is a protein-rich specialization on the
cytoplasmic surface of the postsynaptic membrane at most synapses
irrespective of neurotransmitter type. The PSD has been much studied
morphologically, since it is easy to identify by electron microscopy and
can be selectively stained (Bloom and Aghajanian 1966). It can also be
isolated by subcellular fractionation techniques in good yield and purity,
allowing extensive biochemical analysis (Fig. 7.3a) (Cotman and Kelly
1980; Gurd 1982). The PSD is mostly composed of cytoskeletal proteins
(Cotman and Kelly 1980; Gurd 1982; Rostas *et al.* 1986; Sedman *et al.*
1986), is contiguous with the postsynaptic cytoskeletal matrix, and may
develop, initially, as a specialization of it (Gulley and Reese 1981). The
PSD appears to be tightly bound to protein components of the postsynaptic
membrane, many of which, including neurotransmitter receptors and ion

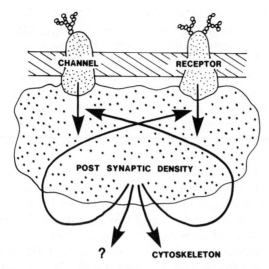

Fig. 7.2 Schematic diagram of the postsynaptic density (PSD) and its proposed role in modulating the postsynaptic response to receptor activation. Activation of receptors and ion channels linked to the PSD result in some changes in proteins of the PSD. These changes can alter the subsequent responsiveness of the postsynaptic element by modifying the ion channels or the receptor via one of the PSD proteins (a direct effect) or by affecting the cytoskeleton or some other cellular structure (an indirect effect).

channels (Matus et al. 1981; Carlin and Siekevitz 1984; Fagg and Matus 1984; Wu *et al.* 1985, 1986*a,b*; Monaghan and Cotman 1986), protrude into the synaptic cleft (Gurd 1989). The PSD is thought to regulate synaptic function and may do so by modifying receptors and ion channels directly and/or modulating the consequences of receptor activation by affecting the postsynaptic cytoskeleton and so altering the shape of the membrane surface or the dendritic spine (Fig. 7.2). Thus, the PSD is thought to be a critical structure, and ideal control point, which acts as a link between the cellular apparatus for the reception and propagation of synaptic signals. There is considerable evidence that the PSD is a dynamic structure which, in adult brain, can undergo morphological and biochemical changes under conditions known to alter synaptic activity (reviewed in Siekevitz 1985; see also pp. 192–4). It has been proposed that these changes in the PSD are in fact an index of the changing properties of the synapse (Nieto-Sampedro *et al.* 1982; Carlin and Siekevitz 1983).

The proposal that maturation is a distinct phase of synaptic development was initially based on biochemical and morphological studies of PSDs in developing forebrain. The first suggestions came from studies in rat brain which showed that the most rapid increase in the concentration of the major PSD protein (mPSDp), which is now known to be one form of the α subunit of calmodulin stimulated protein kinase II (Kennedy *et al.* 1983*a*; Goldenring *et al.* 1984*b*; Kelly *et al.* 1984; Sahyoun *et al.* 1984), occurred in the third postnatal week (Fu *et al.* 1981; Kelly and Cotman 1981; Kelly and Vernon 1985; Weinberger and Rostas 1986). Since the most rapid rate of synapse formation occurred in the second week, the increase in the α subunit of calmodulin stimulated protein kinase II (α CMK II) was interpreted as representing a maturation of the synapses which had formed previously. However, there is a considerable variation in PSD thickness (Colonnier 1968) and α CMK II concentration (Walaas *et al.* 1983*a,b*; Ouimet *et al.* 1984; Erondu and Kennedy 1985) from region to region in brain, neurons establish synapses at slightly different rates and times in each region, and synapse formation in the rat forebrain as a whole is not complete until about postnatal day 30 (Aghajanian and Bloom 1967; Wolff 1976, 1978; Blue and Parnavelas 1983; Markus *et al.* 1987), by which time both PSD morphology (Markus *et al.* 1987) and α CMK II concentration (Weinberger and Rostas 1986) are also mature. Hence, differential rates of development of the neurons with thick and thin postsynaptic densities would also have been able to explain the data. Clear evidence that synapse maturation is indeed a separate phase of neuronal development came with the observation that, in chicken forebrain, the changes in PSD protein composition and morphology occurred over a protracted period well after synapse formation was complete.

THE DEVELOPING CHICKEN FOREBRAIN AS A MODEL SYSTEM FOR THE STUDY OF SYNAPSE MATURATION

Even though young chickens are precocious in some aspects of their behaviour, there is clear evidence from biochemical (Jerusalinsky *et al.* 1986; Tehrain and Barnes 1986) and morphological (Corner *et al.* 1977; Bradley 1985) studies that, in the forebrain as a whole, synapse formation is still occurring rapidly at hatching and is not complete until about 1–2 weeks post-hatch. Quantitative electron microscopy of synapses in the forebrain of newly hatched chickens shows the postsynaptic densities are much thinner than in the adult (Rostas *et al.* 1984). Comparison of the protein compositions of subcellular fractions enriched in PSDs from newly hatched and adult chicken brain reveals a striking result: there is a dramatic increase in the concentration of α CMK II measured either by protein stain (Rostas and Jeffrey 1981; Fig. 7.3b) or the rate of autophosphorylation (Rostas *et al.* 1983; Fig. 7.3c), although the concentrations of the other major proteins do not change. This increase in α CMK II is accompanied by an increase in the thickness of the postsynaptic density (Rostas *et al.* 1984). Both changes occur slowly and do not reach maturity until 8–10 weeks post-hatch (Rostas and Jeffrey 1981; Fig. 7.4). These changes in the postsynaptic density occur after synapse formation is complete and are thus maturational changes.

Figure 7.4 shows a comparison of the developmental patterns of change in rat and chicken forebrain, illustrating the unique advantages provided by the chicken forebrain as an experimental system for studying synaptic maturation because of the clear temporal separation of the synapse formation and synapse maturation phases of neuronal development. Comparable parameters of neuronal development are shown for both species. The marker for synapse formation is the increase in the concentration of Thy-1 in forebrain (small filled circles). Thy-1 is a developmentally regulated cell surface glycoprotein which is present, but not enriched, in synaptic membranes; however, the time at which there is a great increase in expression of Thy-1 in neurons correlates with synapse formation in a number of systems (Barclay 1979; Morris 1985; Sinclair *et al.* 1987). Synapse maturation is identified by increases in the thickness of the postsynaptic density (large speckled circles) and the concentration of α CMK II in the postsynaptic density. We have found that all the developmental changes observed in chicken forebrain also occur in rat forebrain but much more rapidly, so that it is not possible to determine which changes specifically relate to the formation phase and which to the maturation phase, because the two overlap to such a degree. In contrast, by measuring the changes at appropriate ages (e.g. 2 days, 8 days, 21 days, and adult) it is possible to ascribe changes clearly to one phase or another using the chicken system.

DEVELOPMENTAL CHANGES IN PROTEIN PHOSPHORYLATION SYSTEMS

We have compared the developmental changes in the cAMP stimulated and Ca^{2+}/calmodulin stimulated protein phosphorylation systems in chicken forebrain. Before describing these developmental changes in protein phosphorylation, it is important to give some background information about the properties of the enzyme CMK II, which appears to play such a central role in the maturation changes.

CMK II, also known as the multifunctional Ca^{2+}/calmodulin/stimulated protein kinase, is a protein kinase with a broad substrate specificity (Fukunaga *et al.* 1982; Bennett *et al.* 1983; McGuinness *et al.* 1983; Kuret and Schulman 1984) which appears to be responsible for the majority of the calmodulin stimulated protein phosphorylation in brain (Weinberger and Rostas 1986, 1988*b*). The enzyme is found throughout neurons in both soluble and particulate forms (Schulman 1988) but it is most concentrated in the PSD (Grab *et al.* 1981; Kennedy *et al.* 1983*a*; Sahyoun *et al.* 1984;

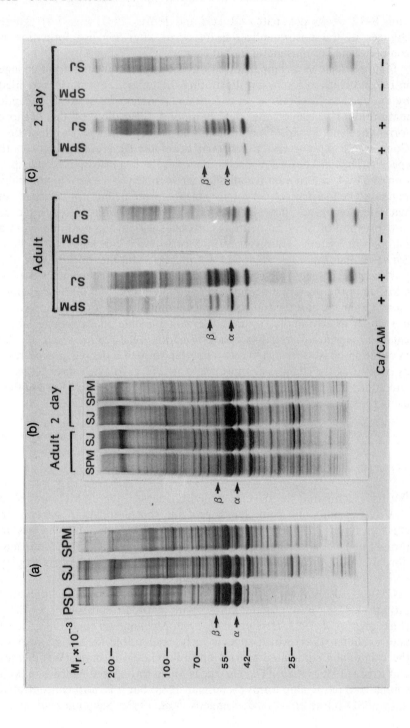

Fig. 7.3 Protein composition of PSD enriched subcellular fractions from 2-day and adult chicken forebrain. (a) Protein stain of synaptic plasma membrane (SPM), synaptic junction (SJ) and post-synaptic density (PSD) fractions prepared from adult chicken brain. α and β indicate the positions of the α and β subunits of calmodulin stimulated protein kinase II (CMK II); the α-CMK II in the PSD used to be called the major PSD protein (mPSDp) and is progressively enriched in fractions as they become more enriched in PSDs. (b) Comparison of the protein content of SPM and SJ fractions from 2-day and adult chicken forebrain. The concentration of α-CMK II increases dramatically, whereas the concentrations of the other major proteins do not change. (c) Autoradiogram of SPM and SJ fractions from 2-day and adult chicken forebrain phosphorylated in the presence or absence of Ca^{2+} calmodulin. α and β indicate the positions of the autophosphorylated α- and β-subunits of CMK II.

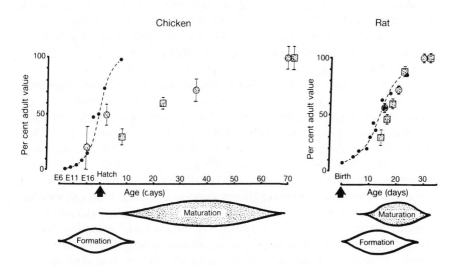

Fig. 7.4 Comparison of the time course of the synapse formation and synapse maturation phases of neuronal development in chicken and rat forebrain. The upper part of the figure shows experimental results obtained for the time of increase in expression of Thy-1 (a marker for synapse formation) and the thickness of PSD and α-CMK II content of PSDs (markers for synapse maturation). The lower part of the figure shows a schematic representation of synapse formation and synapse maturation in chicken and rat: the length and position of the shapes show the period during which the phases occur and the width of the shape indicates how rapidly the changes are occurring during the phase. Thy-1 concentration in brain (small filled circles): Jeffrey, Greig, and Rostas, unpublished (chicken); Barclay (1979) (rat). PSD thickness (large speckled circles): Rostas *et al.* (1984) and Rostas and Guldner, unpublished (chicken); Markus *et al.* (1987) (rat). α CMK II concentration in the PSD (speckled squares): measured by autophosphorylation in chicken (Rostas *et al.* 1987*a*) and protein stain in isolated synaptic junction fractions from rat forebrain (Weinberger and Rostas 1986).

Kelly *et al.* 1984; Kelly and Vernon 1985; Rostas *et al.* 1986) and the cytoskeleton (Job *et al.* 1983; Goldenring *et al.* 1984*a*; Sahyoun *et al.* 1985*a*; Larson *et al.* 1985 Vallano *et al.* 1985*a,b*). It is a member of a family of calmodulin-stimulated protein kinases found in many different tissues, all of which have subunits between 50 and 60 kDa molecular weight (Schulman 1988). The neuronal enzyme is much more abundant than related enzymes in non-neural tissues and has three subunits called α, β and β', whose molecular weights are 50 kDa, 60 kDa, and 58 kDa, respectively. The concentration of the enzymes varies more than 20-fold between different brain regions, being most concentrated in the 'higher' areas such as the hippocampus where it can constitute as much as 2 per cent of total protein (Erondu and Kennedy 1985). Thus, it is most likely to have both a structural and regulatory role at certain intracellular locations. The metabolic turnover of the PSD-associated α subunit in anaesthetized chickens was found to be very slow ($t_{1/2} \approx 25$ days), which is consistent with a structural role (Sedman *et al.* 1986). The enzyme from young and old chicken brain has been purified and characterized (Rostas *et al.* 1989) and shown to be very similar to that in rat brain.

Molecular cloning of the α (Hanley *et al.* 1987; Lin *et al.* 1987; Bulleit *et al.* 1988) and β and β' (Bennett and Kennedy 1987) subunits from rat brain revealed extensive homologies between them, as predicted by earlier peptide mapping experiments (Bennett *et al.* 1983; Goldenring *et al.* 1983; Kuret and Schulman 1984; McGuinness *et al.* 1985; Miller and Kennedy 1985). The deduced amino acid sequences also revealed a common structure containing three domains for all the subunits: an N-terminal catalytic domain, a central regulatory domain containing the calmodulin-binding site and potential phosphorylation sites and an association, or binding, domain at the C terminal which contains several potential phosphorylation sites and has no strong sequence homology to any other known proteins. The autophosphorylation activity which is possessed by all the subunits has attracted much attention and has been shown to have a number of effects, including making the enzyme independent of calcium (Miller and Kennedy 1986; Lai *et al.* 1986; Lou *et al.* 1986; Rostas *et al.* 1987*b*; Schworer *et al.* 1986). The relative abundance of the subunits varies greatly between brain regions (Miller and Kennedy 1985; McGuinness *et al.* 1985), cell type (Walaas *et al.* 1988), and development (Sahyoun *et al.* 1985*b*; Weinberger and Rostas 1986, 1988*b*; Kelly *et al.* 1987), and it has been suggested that the subunits may in fact be independent enzymes selectively expressed by different neurons or at different times during development (Rostas *et al.* 1988). The existence of multiple forms of CMK raises the possibility of multiple genes for each subunit and/or post-translation modification of the subunits, but there is no compelling evidence for either possibility. There appears to be only one copy of the gene for the β subunit and the mRNA for the β' subunit is probably produced by alternative splicing of the mRNA for the β subunit (Bulleit *et al.* 1988). The number of genes for the α subunit has not been established but, in both rat and chicken, all the mRNA molecules for α CMK II are of the same size.* Despite the extensive differences in properties of the enzyme in different cellular locations, once it has been solubilized and purified, the biochemical properties of the enzyme from soluble and particulate sources are indistinguishable (Bennett *et al.* 1983; Kennedy *et al.* 1983*b*; McGuinness *et al.* 1985; Miller and Kennedy 1985). Thus, the differences in properties must be due to reversible modifications such as autophosphorylation or the allosteric changes due to binding to other proteins.

Capitalizing on the fact that the α subunit of CMK II is the only calmodulin stimulated phosphoprotein at that molecular weight in all subcellular fractions of forebrain examined so far (Weinberger and Rostas 1986, 1988*b*), we examined the changes in the concentration of α CMK II by measuring the autophosphorylation of the subunit under conditions where the rate of autophosphorylation is proportional to the concentration of the enzyme (Rostas *et al.* 1987*b*, 1988, 1989; Weinberger and Rostas 1988*b*). Fig. 7.5 shows the results for three subcellular fractions: S3, a cytosol fraction; P2M, a crude synaptic plasma membrane fraction; P2S, an occluded cytosol fraction mainly from presynaptic cytoplasm. It can be seen from Fig. 7.5 that the concentration and distribution of α CMK II varies markedly during development. During the synapse formation phase there is an increase in the concentration of CMK II in all subcellular fractions (Fig. 7.5a) and the relative distribution of the enzyme between the subcellular fractions remains roughly constant, with the majority being soluble (Fig 7.5b). During the maturation period, and particularly after 3 weeks post-hatch, there is a major redistribution of α CMK II in that the amount of membrane bound enzyme continues to rise but the amount of soluble enzyme falls so that the majority of the enzyme in the adult is particulate. In other experiments we have shown that α CMK II accumulation at PSDs accounts for the majority of the increase in membrane bound α CMK II (Rostas *et al.* 1986, 1987*a*; Dunkley *et al.* 1988) and that a parallel increase occurs in a detergent insoluble cytoskeletal fraction prepared from whole brain (Koszka *et al.* 1991). By contrast, the amount of α CMK II which can be polymerized with microtubules decreases during maturation, showing that α CMK II is also changing its relative distribution between different compartments of the cytoskeleton (Koszka *et al.* 1991).

An analysis of the pattern of calmodulin-stimulated phosphorylation of

* Despite earlier suggestions (Hanley *et al.*1987) that there were two populations of mRNA (7.2 and 4.3. kb) for α CMK II in chicken forebrain, recent work (Rostas, Jeffrey, Gunning, Dowsing, Sentry, and Kelly, unpublished) has shown that in Northern blots only the 7.2 kb mRNA species hybridizes under conditions of high stringency; this suggests that the 4.3 kb band was due to cross reactivity of the probe with the mRNA for β CMK II.

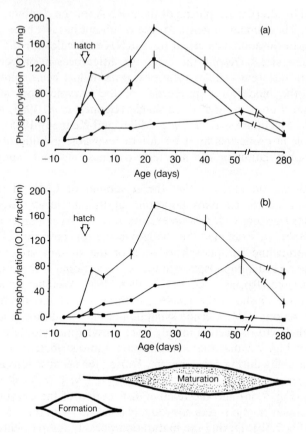

Fig. 7.5 Changes in the concentration and distribution of CMK II during development in chicken forebrain as measured by the initial rate of autophosphorylation of the α subunit. a: concentration of α CMK II in arbitrary optical density units per mg protein; b: total amount of α CMK II in subcellular fraction from one brain (arbitrary optical density units per fraction). ▲ Cytosol (S3); ■ occluded (mainly presynaptic) cytosol (P2S); ● Crude synaptic membranes (P2M). The durations and rates of change in the synapse formation and maturation phases are shown by the shapes below the graph (see Fig. 7.4 for explanation). Adapted from Weinberger and Rostas (1988*b*).

endogenous protein substrates in the subcellular fractions (which is mostly due to the action of CMK II) indicated that most of the changes in endogenous protein substrate phosphorylation occur during the synapse formation period and that the phosphorylation of these proteins by CMK II appears to be mainly limited by the amount of the enzyme in the subcellular fraction. As expected, the addition of extra soluble enzyme to subcellular fractions resulted in an increase in the phosphorylation of endogenous proteins (Rostas, unpublished). Thus, paradoxically, this unusual and most abundant of protein kinases seems to be present in limiting concentrations as far as its ability to phosphorylate endogenous protein substrates is concerned, at least *in vitro*.

The developmental pattern observed for the cyclic AMP-stimulated protein kinase (PKA) was completely different. The concentration and the subcellular distribution of PKA determined by an exogenous peptide phosphorylation assay did not change during either synapse formation or synapse maturation (Weinberger and Rostas 1988*a*). By contrast, the pattern of cyclic AMP-stimulated phosphorylation of endogenous protein substrates in both soluble and membrane fractions showed dramatic changes. Virtually all of these changes were finished by the end of the synapse formation phase (Weinberger and Rostas 1988*a*). Thus, in contrast to CMK II, the cyclic AMP-stimulated phosphorylation system appears to have excess enzyme and to be governed primarily by changes in the concentrations of endogenous protein substrates. This concept was first suggested by Holmes and Rodnight (1981) based on studies of membrane fractions from developing rat brain.

Since the concentration of CMK II appears to be limiting, the change in the subcellular localization of CMK II during the maturation period means that a unit rise in intracellular Ca^{2+} should result in a different degree of Ca^{2+}/calmodulin stimulated kinase activity in the various subcellular compartments. By contrast, the kinase activity produced by a unit rise in intracellular cAMP should change little if at all. This reasoning led to the following hypothesis: that, during maturation, any cellular stimulus producing an elevation in both intracellular cAMP and Ca^{2+} would produce a different pattern and degree of phosphorylation of substrates labelled by both kinases. This implies that, since protein phosphorylation is a regulatory event (i.e. produces a change in some property of the protein being phosphorylated) certain cellular functions will change their relative sensitivities to cAMP and Ca^{2+} during maturation.

We have tested this hypothesis *in vitro* by examining the phosphorylation of identified endogenous protein substrates which are known to be phosphorylated by PKA and CMK II. The first such substrate we examined was synapsin I, an acid soluble neuronal phosphoprotein which is associated with synaptic vesicles (DeCamilli *et al.* 1983*a,b*) and cytoskeletal structures (Goldenring *et al.* 1986; Bahler and Greengard 1987) and whose developmental expression in brain has been shown in other systems to correlate with synapse formation (De Gennaro *et al.* 1983; Wallace *et al.* 1985). There is a chicken counterpart of synapsin I (Goelz *et al.* 1985). It is a single phosphoprotein of 75 000 daltons (Sorensen and Babitch 1984; Weinberger and Rostas 1988*c*) which reaches adult levels by day 6 and does not significantly change its concentration throughout the maturation period (Weinberger and Rostas, in preparation).

Cyclic AMP-stimulated protein kinase and CMK II are known to

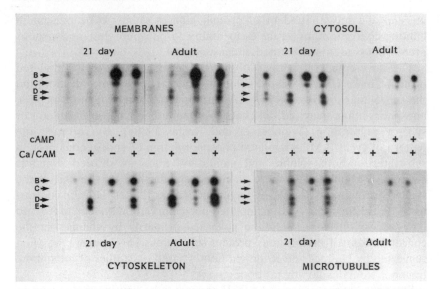

Fig. 7.6 Maturation changes in phosphorylation of the chicken synapsin-I protein by CMK II and PKA in four subcellular fractions: crude synaptic plasma membranes, detergent insoluble cytoskeleton, cytosol and taxol polymerized microtubules. The figure shows autoradiograms of radioactive phosphopeptide fragments from synapsin I which contain the sites specifically phosphorylated by CMK II (D and E) and PKA (B and C). The results were obtained as follows: the four subcellular fractions from 21-day and adult chicken forebrain were phosphorylated in the presence or absence of cyclic AMP, calcium/calmodulin (Ca/CAM) or both as indicated by the symbols in the centre of the figure; the chicken synapsin I was separated from the other proteins by electrophoresis and partially digested with staphylococcus V8 protease to yield peptides which were resolved by electrophoresis and detected by autoradiography.

phosphorylate synapsin I at distinct sites at opposite ends of the molecule (Huttner *et al.* 1981; Czernik *et al.* 1987). Our hypothesis predicted that there would be no change in the phosphorylation at the cAMP-stimulated site during the maturation period but that the phosphorylation at the CMK II site would change in parallel with the change in subcellular distribution of CMK II. It is possible to measure the phosphorylation of synapsin I at these individual sites by digestion of the protein with a suitable protease and separation by electrophoresis of the peptides containing the phosphorylation sites. Figure 7.6 shows the results from such an experiment in which crude synaptic plasma membranes, cytosol, detergent insoluble cytoskeleton, and taxol polymerized microtubules from 21-day-old and adult chickens were phosphorylated in the absence of exogenous activators, or the presence of cAMP or Ca^{2+}/calmodulin, or both. The 75 kDa protein band was excised after SDS-PAGE, partially digested with

Staphylococcus aureus V8 protease, and the resulting phosphopeptides separated by SDS-PAGE and detected by autoradiography. Previous experiments had established that peptides B and C contained the cAMP-stimulated site, whereas peptides D and E contained the Ca^{2+}/calmodulin-stimulated sites. In both synaptic membranes and detergent insoluble cytoskeleton, where there was an increase in CMK II during maturation, there was also an increase in the phosphorylation of the Ca^{2+}/calmodulin-stimulated sites relative to the cAMP-stimulated sites in a way which was proportional to the change in CMK II concentrations. Similarly, in both cytosol and taxol polymerized microtubules, where there is a decrease in CMK II during maturation, there was a decrease in the phosphorylation of the Ca^{2+}/calmodulin-stimulated site relative to the cAMP-stimulated site in a way which was proportional to the change in CMK II concentration. These results are entirely in agreement with the hypothesis.

A second endogenous protein substrate we have examined is MAP-2 (microtubule associated protein-2), a 280 kDa protein which regulates the rate of polymerization and stability of microtubules and is phosphorylated at multiple sites by several protein kinases including PKA and CMK II (Olmsted 1986; Matus 1988). Because MAP-2 is a major protein in the cytosol and microtubules, the concentration of this protein can be determined directly from protein staining on SDS polyacrylamide gels. However, unlike synapsin I, the individual sites of phosphorylation on MAP-2 cannot be identified by one-dimensional peptide mapping. We found that the concentration of MAP-2 in the cytosol increased during both the synapse formation and synapse maturation phases. Nevertheless, Fig. 7.7 shows that, as predicted, the cyclic AMP stimulated phosphorylation per mole of MAP-2 was constant during the maturation phase, whereas the calmodulin stimulated phosphorylation decreased in proportion to the decrease in the amount of CMK II as determined by the autophosphorylation of α CMK II.

WHAT ARE THE FUNCTIONAL SIGNIFICANCES OF THESE CHANGES IN PHOSPHORYLATION?

Although the functional effect of such changes in the phosphorylation of synapsin I and MAP-2 are not known, it is possible to speculate along the following lines. Synapsin I is an elongated asymmetrical protein with its PKA and CMK II phosphorylation sites located at the structurally different and opposite sends of the molecule (Czernik *et al.* 1987). The molecule is believed to function as a cross-link between intracellular structures, and both the binding of synapsin I to synaptic vesicles and its ability to bundle actin filaments are very sensitive to phosphorylation (Huttner *et al.* 1983; Schiebler *et al.* 1983; Bahler and Greengard 1987). Thus, a change in the

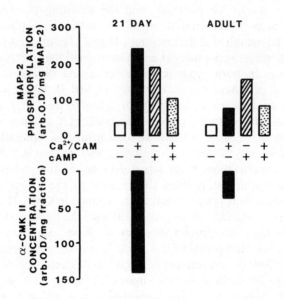

Fig. 7.7   Phosphorylation of MAP-2 and autophosphorylation of α-CMK II in the cytosolic fraction from 21-day and adult chicken forebrain. The radioactivity incorporated into MAP-2 (upper panel) after phosphorylation in the presence or absence of cyclic AMP, calcium/calmodulin or both (as indicated by the symbols in the centre of the figure) is compared with the radioactivity incorporated into the α subunit of CMK II by autophosphorylation (lower panel) in the presence of calcium/calmodulin alone. Proteins labelled under the same conditions are indicated by bars of the same shading.

phosphorylation of one end relative to the other would be expected to have significant functional consequences. It has been shown that changing the relative proportion of phospho and dephospho synapsin I in the presynaptic terminal of the squid giant axon has a dramatic effect on the ability of the terminal to release neurotransmitter (Llinas *et al.* 1985), although the precise mechanism of the change is not known.

MAP-2 is one of a number of microtubule associated proteins which is differentially distributed within and between neurons (Matus 1988). MAP-2 is known to regulate the rate of polymerization of microtubules and the properties of this molecule are in turn regulated by multisite phosphorylation by multiple protein kinases including PKA, CMK II, and the calcium/phospholipid-stimulated protein kinase (Olmsted 1986). Microtubules are involved in a variety of intracellular functions including intracellular movement of organelles, the elongation of cellular processes and the maintenance of cell shape. MAP-2 is particularly concentrated in dendrites and dendritic spines (Caceres *et al.* 1983, 1984) where, it is reasonable to assume, the polymerization of microtubules could alter the shape and diameter of spines and dendrites, which in turn would affect their electrical conduction properties and thereby regulate the postsynaptic response of a neuron to neurotransmitter receptor activation. Since CMK II is a structural as well as a regulatory component of detergent insoluble cytoskeleton and microtubules, the opposite changes in the two cytoskeletal compartments may produçe changes in cell shape or changes in the ability of cells to modify their shape in response to stimuli.

All of our phosphorylation results have been obtained with subcellular fractions *in vitro* and it remains to be established whether all the changes we see during development also occur *in vivo*. Nevertheless, if we assume that the general pattern of change does occur *in vivo*, the consequences of this type of change would be to alter the responsiveness of certain intracellular processes to changes in the concentrations of intracellular second messengers. Many receptor activated events produce a change in more than one second messenger system inside cells. A redistribution of CMK II would produce local changes in the amount of available active enzyme. Thus, the maturational changes in the relative balance of PKA and CMK II mean that the cellular consequences of the same change in intracellular second messengers may be different in immature and mature neurons, and that this change in response to receptor activation can be produced independent of any change in receptor properties. It may be expected that, under normal conditions of synaptic transmission, the transient change in the concentration of intracellular second messengers would not be large enough to fully activate all the available protein kinase molecules. Therefore, under conditions of low frequency synaptic activity, the changes in levels of PKA and CMK II may not become apparent. However, under conditions of repetitive or high frequency stimulation, intracellular second messenger levels may be high enough to fully activate both sets of kinases (thus mimicking the *in vitro* assay conditions) so that the changes in relative kinase activities described above would become manifest.

The fact that the maturational changes in the PSD are mainly due to changes in CMK II may have implications for the differences in effect of high and low frequency synaptic activity. Because calmodulin is present in high concentrations in the PSD (Grab *et al.* 1980; Wood *et al.* 1980) the initial activation of CMK II in the PSD is probably primarily controlled by changes in local intracellular calcium concentrations which will be regulated by synaptic activity. When CMK II is activated and phosphorylates its substrates it also phosphorylates itself at several different sites. The best characterized autophosphorylation effect is that due to the phosphorylation of the threonine immediately N-terminal to the calmodulin binding site (α-286 and β-287) which abolishes the calcium requirement of the enzyme without decreasing its activity (Lickteig *et al.* 1988; Miller *et al.* 1988; Thiel *et al.* 1988; Lou and Schulman 1989). In this way the activity of the enzyme could be maintained after intracellular calcium concentrations had returned to normal (Miller and Kennedy 1986). Autophosphorylation at different sites, which occurs under certain conditions, results in either inhibition (Hashimoto *et al.* 1987; Lou and Schulman 1989) or stimulation (Lickteig *et al.* 1988) of the kinase. The association of CMK II with other proteins may also be affected by autophosphorylation, as suggested by studies of the *Aplysia* and *Drosophila* counterparts of CMK II which undergo translocation (Saitoh and Schwartz 1985), or the potential for translocation (Willmund *et al.* 1986), from particulate to soluble fractions following autophosphorylation.

The effects of autophosphorylation can be reversed by endogenous phosphatases and the extent to which the autophosphorylation-induced changes in CMK II will be manifested in a cell will be determined by the relative rates of autophosphorylation and dephosphorylation. At a given postsynaptic site where, in the short term, the relative concentrations of phosphatases and CMK II do not change, the principal determinant of the balance of these two activities will be synaptic firing rate: low frequency activity might favour the phosphatases so that little autophosphorylated CMK II will be produced; high frequency stimulation will lead to the activation of slow voltage dependent Ca^{2+} channels (Herron *et al.* 1986), producing a prolonged rise in intracellular Ca^{2+} which will favour the kinase and lead to a conversion of a large proportion of the CMK II into its autophosphorylated form. It has been suggested (Lisman 1985) that the latter situation could lead to a self-sustaining change in the state of phosphorylation of a group of CMK II molecules that would persist beyond the lifetime of individual molecules within the group and provide a stable, long term storage of graded information about patterns of cellular activity (Lisman and Goldring 1988).

ARE THE MATURATION CHANGES PLASTIC?

A major assumption inherent in the hypothesis that the maturation changes can be used as a model for synaptic plasticity is that at least some of the maturation changes alter synaptic efficacy and can be enhanced or reversed in the adult brain and during development. Studies which provide both direct and indirect support for this assumption have shown:

1. That changes in synaptic activity can alter PSD morphology and CMK II distribution or activity.
2. That synapses known to have undergone a change in efficacy show changes in PSD morphology or CMK II activity or distribution.

3. That the pattern of change during normal development can be modified by exogenous influences.
4. That alterations in the amount of CMK II can alter synaptic efficacy.

These studies were done in a number of systems which yielded results which, though not identical, are nevertheless consistent. The experiments relating to points 1–4 above are described in turn in the following paragraphs.

In the mature visual and auditory systems of the rat a change in sensory stimulation has been shown to produce a change in PSD thickness without a change in PSD length at the primary afferent terminals (Guldner and Ingham 1979, 1980; Rees *et al.* 1985) even in senescent rats (Guldner and Phillips 1988). An increase in sensory stimulation resulted in a thinner PSD and a decrease in sensory stimulation resulted in a thicker PSD. Furthermore, it has been suggested that the rate at which these changes in the PSD occur depends on the intrinsic firing rate of the afferent neuron (Rees *et al.* 1985). In a much more complex paradigm, electrical stimulation of undercut cerebral cortex has been shown to have many effects on synaptic morphology, including an increase in PSD length and an increase in the proportion of symmetric synaptic contacts (Rutledge 1978). Because normal maturation involves a decrease in soluble and an increase in particulate CMK II accompanying an increase in PSD thickness and PSD associated CMK II, it is reasonable to suggest that in all these cases the change in synaptic activity induced a translocation of CMK II which was responsible for the change in PSD size. There is direct evidence to support such a possibility in *Aplysia*, where depolarization induced both autophosphorylation of CMK II and a release of particulate CMK II into a soluble form (Saitoh and Schwartz 1985).

PSD morphology and CMK II have also been examined in a number of adult systems where the efficacy of synapses is known to have changed. When long-term potentiation is induced in hippocampal neurons resulting in a marked increase in the efficacy of certain synapses, a number of morphological changes occur at these synapses, including an increase in PSD length (reviewed in Desmond and Levy 1988). Unfortunately PSD thickness was not measured in these studies, so it is not clear whether the increased junctional area was produced by a redistribution of existing PSD material or an increased assembly of PSD components. In 'kindled' synapses, which show a decreased threshold to normally subconvulsive levels of neuronal stimulation, there was a marked decrease in the $Ca^{2+}/$calmodulin-stimulated phosphorylation of synaptic membrane proteins and particularly in the autophosphorylation of α and β CMK II (Wasterlain and Farber 1982, 1984; Goldenring *et al.* 1986). The time-course and extent of the phosphorylation change mimicked the physiological change: it could be inhibited by pretreatment of the animals with diazepam (which also inhibited the seizures), and the change persisted for at least 2 months. A similar change in phosphorylation was produced by prolonged, bicucul-line-induced epileptic seizures (Bronstein *et al.* 1988). Since most of the synaptic membrane bound CMK II is associated with the PSD, this could be due to either a loss of CMK II from the PSD or an inhibition of the CMK II in the PSD. Training *Drosophila* in a visual adaptation task results in a change in the autophosphorylation state of the CMK II counterpart in this system and change in the ease with which it can be released from a particulate fraction of *Drosophila* brain (Willmund *et al.* 1986). It is also important that this change in CMK II persisted as long as the behavioural change persisted.

The range of PSD thickness at adult synapses, even within one region, varies widely (Colonnier 1968), as does the overall concentration, subunit composition, and soluble versus particulate distribution of CMK II (see above). Presumably, both endogenous (genetic) and exogenous factors during development combine to produce this range of mature states. The demonstration that hippocampal pyramidal cells in tissue culture can mimic some of the developmental changes in CMK II (Scholz *et al.* 1988) and that the maturational changes in CMK II are relatively resistant to modification by a number of treatments that affect brain development such as sympathec-tomy, castration, and hypothyroidism (Rostas, Weinberger, and Wang, unpublished results) show that endogenous factors are important. However, the effect of monocular deprivation during development on CMK II distri-bution among the ocular dominance columns in the visual cortex demon-strates that the endogenously determined development pattern is modifiable by exogenous factors in some neurons at least (Hendry and Kennedy 1986).

Finally, the question of whether a change in intracellular CMK II concen-tration can lead to a change in synaptic efficacy has been addressed directly. Injection of CMK II into the presynaptic terminals of the squid giant axon led to an increased quantal release following nerve stimulation (Llinas *et al.* 1985). Introduction into synaptosomes of CMK II which had been autoacti-vated by thiophosphorylation increased the rate of release of both glutamate and noradrenaline, whereas introduction of a selective peptide inhibitor of CMK II inhibited the rate of release of glutamate (Nichols *et al.* 1990).

ARE THE MATURATION CHANGES THE SAME IN ALL NEURONS?

Experiments using whole forebrain give results which are population averages heavily biased towards the changes occurring in the most abun-dant cell types. Our studies of the regional distribution of CMK II in chicken brain have shown that CMK II is most concentrated in the cortical areas of the forebrain, with a distribution which is analogous to that which has been reported in rat (Rostas *et al.* 1987*c*). Therefore one might expect variations in the maturational changes with this enzyme in different regions of forebrain. We have carried out two types of experiment in order to investigate the degree to which changes observed in whole forebrain were common to all neurons.

The first series of experiments was to compare CMK II concentration and calmodulin-stimulated phosphoprotein patterns among different regions of chicken brain from 2-day and adult animals. The results of one such experiment are shown in Fig. 7.8, where four regions of forebrain are compared. In general, the developmental pattern and change from 2 days to adult which is observed in whole forebrain was reproduced in each region: α CMK II was primarily soluble at 2 days, there was an increase in the concentration of α CMK II in the crude synaptic plasma membrane fraction (P2M), and there was a decrease in the concentration of α CMK II in the soluble fraction (S3). However, the degree of change varied from region to region, particularly in the cytoplasmic fractions: the decrease observed in soluble α CMK II in hyperstriatum accessorium (HA) and hippocampus, parahippocampalis and adjacent cortex (HIP) was about the same as that seen in whole brain but the decrease in the neostriatum caudale (NC) and, particularly, hyperstriatum ventrale (HV) was much more pronounced. We have not determined the detailed time course of these changes in the different regions but we would predict that synapse formation would be completed in some regions earlier than others and that the time taken for the maturation phase may also be different. At the level of gross regions of forebrain we have not detected any lateral asymmetries in phosphoprotein patterns.

In a second group of experiments we have tried to examine a single population of synapses using morphological techniques. For these studies we have chosen the synapses of the superior cervical ganglion (SCG). The exact time course of synapse formation in the SCG in chickens is not known but it is expected to be finished by hatching, so that a comparison between 2-day and adult chicken SCG should be looking only at the maturational changes. The results of these experiments are shown in Table 7.1, where they are compared with previous measurements made on forebrain synaptosomes. The postsynaptic densities in the forebrain showed a large change in thickness between 2-day and adult but no change in length. An increase in PSD length was observed during late embryonic development in the synapse formation phase but this was much less marked than the increase in thickness. By contrast, the length of the PSDs in the SCG increased by 80 per cent between 2 days and adult whereas there was only an 11 per cent increase in their thickness.* When the sites

* The PSDs in the SCG were both thicker and longer than the PSDs in forebrain. Studies in both chicken (compare Rostas *et al.* 1984 with Horn *et al.* 1985 and Bradley 1985) and rat (compare Dunkley *et al.* 1986 with Markus *et al.* 1987) have shown that, under appropriate disruption conditions, the morphology of forebrain PSDs is essentially unchanged by homogenization. Therefore, the difference in size is unlikely to be due to the fact that the

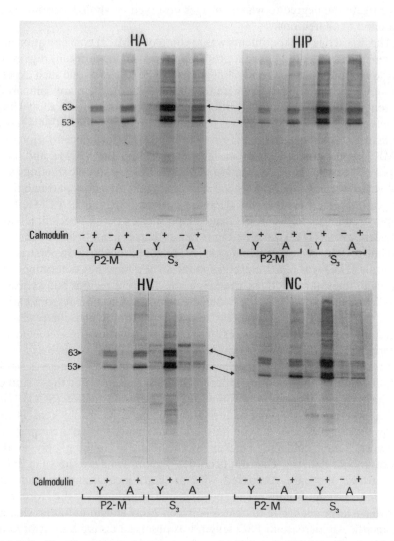

Fig. 7.8 Developmental changes in the subcellular distribution of calmodulin stimulated protein phosphorylation in four regions of chicken forebrain. Crude synaptic plasma membranes (P2-M) and cytosol (S₃) were prepared from hyperstriatum accessorium (HA), hippocampus, parahippocampalis, and adjacent cortex (HIP), hyperstriatum ventrale (HV) and neostriatum caudale (NC) dissected from 2-day (Y) and adult (A) chicken forebrains, phosphorylated in the presence and absence of calcium/calmodulin, separated by SDS-PAGE and visualized by autoradiography. The positions of the autophosphorylated α and β subunits of CMK II are indicated by the apparent molecular weight markers 53 and 63, respectively.

Table 7.1 Developmental changes in the morphology of postsynaptic densities in chicken forebrain and superior cervical ganglion

	Length (nm)	Thickness (nm)
*Forebrain**		
16-day embryo ($n = 55/5$)	170 ± 110	8.3 ± 7.8
2-day ($n = 121/5$)	298 ± 86	20.0 ± 5.3
Adult ($n = 192/5$)	304 ± 39	38.6 ± 5.5
*Superior cervical ganglion***		
2-day ($n = 172/4$)	407 ± 17	49.2 ± 1.1
Adult ($n = 204/4$)	734 ± 32	55.4 ± 1.2

Results are given as means ± SEM. Thickness of the postsynaptic density was measured as maximum thickness; length was measured as sector lengths of a straight line joining the two ends of the PSD.
  * Rostas *et al.* (1984).
 ** Heath, Glenfield, and Rostas (in preparation).

of the SCG synapses in 2-day and adult ganglia were compared there was a decrease in the proportion of synapses on dendritic spines and cell bodies and an increase in the proportion of synapses on dendritic shafts and axons (Heath, Glenfield, and Rostas, unpublished). Clearly, different sets of neurons are capable of different patterns of maturational change.

WHAT IS THE SIGNIFICANCE OF THE DIFFERENCES IN NEURONAL MATURATION?

We have shown that most of the increase in CMK II in the P2M fraction occurs in the PSDs and that, in the forebrain as a whole, this is manifested as an increase in the thickness of the postsynaptic density with no change in its length (this may not be true of every individual synapse—see above) and that there is also a progressive increase in the cytoskeletal CMK II. The decrease in the cytoplasmic (S3) CMK II means that structures such as microtubules, which can be assembled from cytoplasmic components, will contain less CMK II in the adult than in the young (Koszka *et al.* 1991). Since CMK II plays both a structural and a regulatory role in these structures, this would be expected to alter their properties. The regional differences in the extent of redistribution of CMK II suggests that such changes in intracellular structures and the functional consequences of changes in the balance of kinase activities will vary between different types of neurons. Unfortunately, from such biochemical studies alone, it is not possible to

---

SCG synapses were measured on intact tissue and the forebrain PSDs were measured on isolated, intact synaptosomes.

say whether those areas where a greater degree of soluble CMK II is retained possess a greater or lesser degree of plasticity.

The significance of the increase in length versus thickness of the postsynaptic density is not clear but some guesses can be made. If we assume that there are no changes in receptor or ion channel density in the postsynaptic membrane, an increase in the length of the postsynaptic density may imply an increased number of receptors. Since PSD length is usually correlated with increased junctional length, such a change might also produce an increase in the number of release sites presynaptically. Overall, such a change should increase the likelihood of transmission occurring for a given presynaptic depolarization. By contrast, an increase in the thickness of the postsynaptic density may increase the regulatory role of the PSD on the functional components in the postsynaptic membrane overlying it and the part of the dendrite with which it comes into contact; shafts and spines would be expected to be most affected. This change in regulatory function might take the form of increased cross-linking of membrane proteins (such as receptors and ion channels), or increased inter-linking of the PSD with cytoskeletal structures.

In the absence of any detailed understanding of the molecular mechanisms by which the PSD exerts its control, it is not yet possible to predict whether an increase in PSD thickness would increase or decrease the postsynaptic response to synaptic stimulation. In both optic nerve terminals in the suprachiasmatic nucleus (Guldner and Ingham 1979) and auditory nerve terminals in the cochlear nucleus (Rees *et al.* 1985) an increase in synaptic firing rate produced a decrease in PSD thickness. If these changes are assumed to be homeostatic this suggests that, in these two sensory systems, a decrease in PSD thickness may represent desensitization; therefore an increase in PSD thickness may represent a more sensitized state. If the regulatory function of the PSD is partly related to the ability of components within the PSD, or attached to it, to become phosphorylated by the PSD-associated CMK II, then the effects of the change in PSD thickness may be different at different synapses, since phosphorylation of protein can result in either activation or inactivation, depending on the protein.

IMPLICATIONS FOR STUDIES ON THE MECHANISMS OF LEARNING AND MEMORY

These results show that mature neuronal circuitry is achieved only slowly in chicken forebrain. In the forebrain as a whole, new synapses and neuronal circuits are rapidly being formed in the first few days after hatching and the synapse formation phase is not complete until some time in the second week posthatch. At that stage the synapses have structural and biochemical features very different from those in the adult and maturational changes occur for another 6–8 weeks.

It is certain that there will be more biochemical changes occurring during the synapse maturation phase of development than have been described here. Considering protein phosphorylation alone, we have only described two kinase systems and none of the phosphatases or their regulators. A recent report by Anthony *et al.* (1988) that postsynaptic densities from young chicken brain contained very little calcineurin (a calmodulin-stimulated protein phosphatase) whereas calcineurin was concentrated at postsynaptic densities in adult mouse brain (Wood *et al.* 1980) suggests that a change in the distribution of at least one phosphatase may also be occurring during maturation. Therefore, the changing balances in activities of kinases or substrates and effects of Ca on the autophosphory-lation of CMK II are likely to be more complicated and subtle than those described so far. It is difficult to believe that such profound changes do not affect behaviour.

Although the times of synapse formation and the rates of synapse maturation undoubtedly vary in different parts of the brain, most experiments on learning and memory are conducted using young chickens at an age when the majority of their forebrain is undergoing rapid synapse formation. This raises both practical problems for experimentation and theoretical problems of interpretation. The practical problems stem from the fact that the cellular and physiological 'baseline' is rapidly changing during the first week post-hatch. This has been recognized by some workers who have shown that even in the IMHV, one part of the forebrain implicated in learning processes in young chickens, there is a rapid increase in synaptic connectivity over the period used for such experiments (Bradley 1985; Horn *et al.* 1985). Thus, learning tasks need to be chosen so that the training and testing periods and the interval between them is as short as possible in order to minimize the effects of the developmental changes in behavioural capacity. Also, careful control groups need to be included to establish which of the observed changes are due to the learning task and which are due to normal development. Some of the strategies that can be used for doing this have been discussed by Horn (1985).

The theoretical question that arises with regard to the interpretation of learning-induced neuronal changes observed in young chicks is whether these changes represent mechanisms of learning that are the same or fundamentally different from those employed in an adult brain. The simplest assumption is that the basic mechanisms of plasticity, learning and memory are likely to be the same at all ages. Alternatively, it may be argued that mechanisms underlying learning tasks, which are largely restricted to young chicks, may use different mechanisms from those used in the adult because these changes are occurring in an immature nervous system which is still undergoing active synapse formation. No decision can yet be made between these two alternatives and the decision may well depend upon the learning task. However, the difference between these two alternatives may in some cases be more apparent than real.

For instance, one could hypothesize that if a certain effective experience occurred during a period of rapid synapse formation (or elimination), these could influence the rate, extent, or site of synaptic connectivity, thus producing a learning mechanism which is restricted to a rapidly developing system. Indeed, the synapse selection hypothesis of imprinting (Scheich 1987; Wallhauser and Scheich 1987) is based on such an interpretation of neuronal changes following acoustic imprinting. If, however, in the 'plastic' areas of normal mature brain synaptic connectivity is continually changed by synapse turnover (Cotman and Nieto-Sampedro 1984) or division (Carlin and Seikevitz 1983), similar mechanisms could operate in the adult and the difference between young and old may only be a matter of degree.

Similarly, it is not necessarily the case that a behavioural task which is characteristic of a particular early developmental time window involves cellular and molecular changes responsible for learning which are different from those in the adult. A variety of developmental changes in synaptic networks could occur in a system which would change behaviour, and would effectively restrict a particular behaviour to an early developmental period, without changing the mechanisms responsible for the behaviour at the level of the individual synapse or neuron. At a structural ('coarse') level the later development of synaptic inputs whose activity opposes the activity of an earlier established network (which was responsible for eliciting the behavioural change) would effectively limit the performance of the behaviour to an early developmental period. At a 'fine' level, the change in the relative concentration of key regulatory molecules (such as the different kinase systems described in the chapter, or pairs of molecules, such as an enzyme and its inhibitor, whose activities oppose each other) would be expected to make immature and mature synapses differentially sensitive to stimuli. Therefore, the same behavioural stimulus may be more effective at one age than at another, even though the molecular mechanisms responsible for whatever learning does take place are the same at both ages.

If we assume that the basic mechanisms are the same at all ages and that, as I have argued in this chapter, the maturation changes are plastic and at least some are involved in plasticity in the adult, then the learning-induced neuronal changes in young chickens may be seen as a selective acceleration or inhibition of maturational events. This idea could be tested by examining the normal developmental changes in biochemical and cellular parameters which have already been shown to change in learning experiments and by looking for learning-induced changes in parameters which have been measured during the maturation phase of development. Very few such comparisons have been made.

Morphological studies in quail chicks of the dendrites of large neurons in the MNH (an auditory area in the rostromedial neostriatum and hyperstriatum ventrale) revealed that auditory imprinting produced a decrease in dendritic spine number which varied with the imprinting stimulus (Wallhauser and Scheich 1987). The same measurements have not been made in maturing or adult chickens, but a very similar change was observed during maturation in the dendrites of the neurons in the speech control nucleus (hyperstriatum ventrale, pars caudale) of the mynah bird (Rausch and Scheich 1982). A partial comparison is possible between various studies on the morphology of the postsynaptic density. Rostas *et al.* (1984) measured PSD length and thickness, but no other morphological parameters, in synapses from whole forebrain. They showed that the largest change in the PSD was an increase in their mean thickness, which occurred mainly during the synapse maturation phase, but also during the synapse formation phase. There was also a relatively small increase in the mean length of the PSDs which was confined to the synapse formation phase. Learning-induced changes in a number of morphological features of synapses in the IMHV have been measured after visual imprinting (Bradley *et al.* 1981; Horn *et al.* 1985) and passive avoidance training (Stewart *et al.* 1984). In both cases a lateralized increase in PSD length in the left IMHV following training was found but the thickness of the postsynaptic density was not measured.

It is interesting that Horn *et al.* (1985) found that the change in the mean length of the PSD in the IMHV following a visual imprinting task was much more pronounced in chickens trained on day 1 than those trained on day 2. This could be interpreted in at least two ways. The first is that this is a learning mechanism restricted to developing brain and this change in PSD length only occurs in the first few days post-hatch. The second is that the decreased effect of learning on the PSD length with age is an artefact of the need to use mean PSD length, since the individual synapses being affected in the IMHV are not known. If the individual PSD length remains plastic in the adult, the fact that the mean PSD length in the adult is stable implies that a learning-induced increase in PSD length in one set of synapses must be balanced by a decrease in PSD length in another set (see Chapter 8). Thus, learning-induced changes which occur in both mature and immature brain may be detected more easily in young chickens specifically because the brain is immature and has not yet reached a steady state (this view, proposed to me by Horn, is discussed further in Chapter 8). The unambiguous decision between these two alternatives would require the identification of the individual synapses in the IMHV which change as a result of the learning task.

CONCLUSION

The developing chicken forebrain offers a powerful experimental model system with which to investigate cellular mechanisms potentially involved in synaptic plasticity by studying changes during the synapse maturation stage of neuronal development. Because the processes involved in synapse maturation occur over a protracted period well after synapse formation is complete, molecular mechanisms involved in neuronal maturation can be studied without the confounding effects of net increases or decreases in the number of synapses or neurons. In addition, if the basic cellular and molecular mechanisms responsible for learning and memory do not change during development, it may be easier to identify these mechanisms in an immature system which has not yet reached a stable steady state.

Acknowledgements

I am grateful to Ron Weinberger, Christiane Koszka, Peter Dunkley, John Heath, Vicki Brent, Christine Baker, Fritz Guldner, and Peter Jeffrey for their collaboration on various aspects of the work described in this chapter. I thank Geoffrey Kellerman, Sally McFadden, Richard Andrew, Gabriel Horn, Richard Rodnight, and Jim Gurd for their comments on parts of this manuscript and Ena Mawer for typing it. This work was supported by grants from the National Health and Medical Research Council of Australia.

REFERENCES

Aghajanian, G. N. and Bloom, F. E. (1967). The formation of synaptic junctions in developing rat brain: a quantitative electron microscopic study. *Brain Research*, **6**, 716–27.

Anthony, F. A., Winkler, M. A., Edwards, H. H., and Cheung, W. Y. (1988). Quantitative subcellular localisation of calmodulin-dependent phosphatase in chick forebrain. *Journal of Neuroscience*, **8**, 1245–53.

Bahler, M. and Greengard, P. (1987). Synapsin I bundles F-actin in a phosphorylation dependent manner. *Nature*, **326**, 704–07.

Barclay, A. N. (1979). Localisation of the Thy-1 antigen in the cerebellar cortex of rat brain by immunofluorescence during postnatal development. *Journal of Neurochemistry*, **32**, 1249–59.

Bennett, M. W., Erondu, N. E., and Kennedy, M. B. (1983). Purification and characterisation of a calmodulin-dependent kinase that is highly concentrated in brain. *Journal of Biological Chemistry*, **258**, 12735–44.

Bennett, N. K. and Kennedy, M. B. (1987). Deduced primary structure of the β subunit of brain type II Ca^{2+}/calmodulin-dependent protein kinase determined by molecular cloning. *Proceedings of the National Academy of Sciences (USA)*, **84**, 1794–8.

Bloom, F. E. and Aghajanian, G. K. (1966). Cytochemistry of synapses: selective staining for electron microscopy. *Science*, **154**, 1575–77.

Blue, M. E. and Parnavelas, J. G. (1983). The formation and maturation of synapses in the visual cortex of the rat. II quantitative analysis. *Journal of Neurocytology*, **12**, 697–712.

Bradley, P., Horn, G., and Bateson, P. (1981). Imprinting: an electron microscopic study of chick hyperstriatum ventrale. *Experimental Brain Research*, **41**, 115–20.

Bradley, P. (1985). A light and electron microscopic study of the development of two regions of the chicken forebrain. *Developmental Brain Research*, **20**, 83–8.

Bronstein, J., Farber, D., and Wasterlain, C. (1988). Decreased calmodulin kinase activity after status epilepticus. *Neurochemical Research*, **13**, 83–6.

Bulleit, R. F., Bennett, M. K., Molloy, S. S., Hurley, J. B., and Kennedy, M. B. (1988). Conserved and variable regions in the subunit of brain type II $Ca^{2+}/$ calmodulin-dependent protein kinase. *Neuron*, **1**, 63–72.

Caceres, A., Binder, L. I., Payne, M. R., Bender, P., Rebhun, L., and Steward, O. (1984). Differential subcellular localisation of tubulin and the microtubule-associated protein MAP-2 in brain tissue as revealed by immunocytochemistry with monoclonal hybridoma antibodies. *Journal of Neuroscience*, **4**, 394–410.

Caceres, A., Payne, M. R., Binder, L. I., and Steward, O. (1983). Immunocyto-chemical localisation of actin and microtubule-associated protein MAP-2 in dendritic spines. *Proceedings of the National Academy of Sciences (USA)*, **80**, 1738–42.

Carlin, R. K., Grab, D. J., and Siekevitz, P. (1981). Function of calmodulin in post-synaptic densities III. Calmodulin binding proteins at the post-synaptic density. *Journal of Cell Biology*, **89**, 449–55.

Carlin, R. K. and Siekevitz, P. (1983). Plasticity in the central nervous system: do synapses divide? *Proceedings of the National Academy of Sciences (USA)*, **80**, 3517–21.

Carlin, R. K. and Siekevitz, P. (1984). Characterisation of Na^+-independent GABA and flunitrazepam binding sites in preparations of synaptic membranes and postsynaptic densities isolated from canine cerebral cortex and cerebellum. *Journal of Neurochemistry*, **43**, 1011–17.

Colonnier, M. (1968). Synaptic patterns of different cell types in the different laminae of the visual cortex. An electron microscopic study. *Brain Research*, **9**, 268–87.

Corner, M. A., Romjin, H. J., and Richter, A. P. J. (1977). Synaptogenesis in the cerebral hemisphere accessory hyperstriatum in the chick embryo. *Neuroscience Letters*, **4**, 15–19.

Cotman, C. W. and Nieto-Sampedro, M. (1984). Cell biology of synaptic plasticity. *Science*, **225**, 1287–94.

Cotman, C. W. and Kelly, P. T. (1980). Macromolecular architecture of CNS synapses. In *The cell surface and neuronal function* (ed. C. W. Cotman, G. Poste, and G. L. Nicolson), pp. 505–33. Elsevier, North-Holland Biomedical Press, Amsterdam.

Czernik, A. J., Pang, D. T., and Greengard, P. (1987). Amino acid sequences surrounding the cAMP-dependent and calcium/calmodulin-dependent phosphorylation sites in rat and bovine synapsin I. *Proceedings of the National Academy of Sciences (USA)*, **84**, 7518–22.

DeCamilli, P., Cameron, R., and Greengard, P. (1983*a*). Synapsin I (protein I) a nerve terminal specific phosphoprotein. I. Its general distribution in synapses at the central and peripheral nervous system demonstrated by immunofluorescence in frozen and plastic section. *Journal of Cell Biology*, **96**, 1337–54.

DeCamilli, P., Harris, S. M. Jr, Huttner, W. B., and Greengard, P. (1983*b*). Synapsin I (protein I) a nerve terminal specific phosphoprotein, 2. Its specific association with synaptic vesicles demonstrated by immunocytochemistry in agarose embedded synaptosomes. *Journal of Cell Biology*, **96**, 1355–73.

DeGennaro, L. J., Kanazor, S. D., Wallace, W. C., Lewis, R. M., and Greengard, P. (1983). Neuron-specific phosphoproteins as models for neuronal gene expression. *Cold Spring Harbor Symposium on Quantitative Biology*, **43**, 337–45.

Desmond, N. L. and Levy, W. V. (1988). The anatomy of associative long-term synaptic modification. In *Long-term potentiation: from biophysics to behaviour* (ed. P. W. Landfield and S. A. Deadwyler), pp. 265–306. Liss, New York.

Dunkley, P. R., Jarvie, P. E., and Rostas, J. A. P. (1988). Distribution of calmodulin- and cyclic AMP-stimulated protein kinases in synaptosomes. *Journal of Neurochemistry*, **51**, 57–68.

Dunkley, P. R., Jarvie, P. E., Heath, J. W., Kidd, G., and Rostas, J. A. P. (1986). A rapid method for isolation of synaptosomes on Percoll gradients. *Brain Research*, **372**, 115–29.

Erondu, N. E. and Kennedy, M. B. (1985). Regional distribution of type II calcium $^{2+}$/calmodulin dependent protein kinase in rat brain. *Journal of Neuroscience*, **5**, 3270–7.

Fagg, G. E. and Matus, A. (1984). Selective association of N-methylaspartate and quisqualate types of L-glutamate receptor with brain postsynaptic densities. *Proceedings of the National Academy of Sciences (USA)*, **81**, 6876–80.

Fu, S. C., Cruz, T. F., and Gurd, J. W. (1981). Development of synaptic glycoproteins: effect of postnatal age on the synthesis and concentration of synaptic membrane and synaptic junctional fucosyl and sialyl glycoproteins. *Journal of Neurochemistry*, **36**, 1338–51.

Fukunaga, K., Yammamoto, H., Matsui, K., Higashi, K., and Miyamoto, E. (1982). Purification and characterisation of a Ca^{2+} and calmodulin-dependent protein kinase from rat brain. *Journal of Neurochemistry*, **39**, 1607–17.

Goelz, S. E., Nestler, E. J., and Greengard, P. (1985). Phylogenetic survey of proteins related to synapsin I and biochemical analysis of four such proteins from fish brain. *Journal of Nerochemistry*, **45**, 63–72.

Goldenring, J. R., Gonzalez, B., McGuire, J. S., and DeLorenzo, R. J. (1983). Purification and characterisation of a calcium-dependent kinase from rat brain cytosol able to phosphorylate tubulin and microtubule-associated proteins. *Journal of Biological Chemistry*, **258**, 12632–40.

Goldenring, J. R., Casanova, J. E., and DeLorenzo, R. J. (1984*a*). Tubulin-associated calmodulin-dependent kinase: evidence for an endogenous complex of tubulin with a calcium/calmodulin-dependent kinase. *Journal of Neurochemistry*, **43**, 1669–79.

Goldenring, J. R., McGuire, J. S., and DeLorenzo, R. J. (1984*b*). Identification of the major post-synaptic density protein as homologous with the major calmodulin-binding subunit of a calmodulin-dependent protein kinase. *Journal of Neurochemistry*, **42**, 1077–84.

Goldenring, J. R., Lasher, R. S., Vallano, M. L., Veda, T., Naito, S., Sternberger, N. H., Sternberger, L. A., and DeLorenzo, R. J. (1986). Association of synapsin I with neuronal cytoskeleton: identification in cytoskeletal preparations *in vitro* and immunocytochemical localization in brain. *Journal of Biological Chemistry*, **261**, 8495–504.

Grab, D. J., Berzins, K., Cohen, R. S., and Seikevitz, P. (1980). Presence of calmodulin in post-synaptic densities isolated from canine cerebral cortex. *Journal of Biological Chemistry*, **254**, 8690–6.

Grab, D. J., Carlin, R. K., and Siekevitz, P. (1981). Function of calmodulin in post-synaptic densities II: presence of a calmodulin-activatable protein kinase activity. *Journal of Cell Biology*, **89**, 440–8.

Guldner, F. H. and Ingham, C. A. (1979). Plasticity in synaptic apposition of optic nerve afferents under different lighting conditions. *Neuroscience Letters*, **14**, 235–40.

Guldner, F. H. and Ingham, C. A. (1980). Increase in post-synaptic density material in optic target neurons of the rat suprachiasmatic nucleus after bilateral enucleation. *Neuroscience Letters*, **17**, 27–31.

Guldner, F. H. and Phillips, S. C. (1988). Plasticity of postsynaptic density material in optic synapses of the suprachiasmatic nucleus in the senescent rat. *Mechanism of Ageing and Development*, **44**, 169–174.

Gulley, R. L. and Reese, T. S. (1981). Cytoskeletal organisation at the postsynaptic complex. *Journal of Cell Biology*, **91**, 298–302.

Gurd, J. W. (1982). Molecular characterisation of synapses in the central nervous system. In *Molecular approaches to neurobiology* (ed. J. R. Brown), pp. 99–130. Academic Press, New York.

Gurd, J. W. (1989). Glycoproteins of the synapse. In *Neurobiology of Glycoconjugates*, (ed. R. K. Margolis and R. U. Margolis), pp. 219–42. Plenum Press, New York.

Hanley, R. M., Means, A. R., Ono, T., Kemp, B. E., Burgin, K. E., Waxham, N., and Kelly, P. T. (1987). Functional analysis of a complementary DNA for the 50-kilodalton subunit of calmodulin kinase II. *Science*, **237**, 293–7.

Hashimoto, Y., Schworer, C. N., Colbran, R. J., and Soderling, T. R. (1987). Autophosphorylation of Ca^{2+}/calmodulin-dependent protein kinase II. Effects on total and Ca^{2+}-independent activities and kinetic parameters. *Journal of Biological Chemistry*, **262**, 8051–5.

Hendry, S. H. C. and Kennedy, M. B. (1986). Immunoreactivity for a calmodulin-dependent protein kinase is selectively increased in macaque striate cortex after monocular deprivation. *Proceedings of the National Academy of Sciences (USA)*, **83**, 1536–40.

Herron, C. E., Lester, R. A. J., Coan, E. J., and Collingridge, G. L. (1986). Frequency dependent involvement of NMDA receptors in the hippocampus: a novel synaptic mechanism. *Nature*, **322**, 265–68.

Holmes, H. and Rodnight, R. (1981). Ontogeny of membrane bound protein phosphorylating systems in the rat. *Developmental Neuroscience*, **4**, 79–88.

Horn, G., Bradley, P., and McCabe, B. J. (1985). Changes in the structure of synapses associated with learning. *Journal of Neuroscience*, **5**, 3161–8.

Horn, G. (1985). *Memory, imprinting, and the brain*. Clarendon Press, Oxford.

Huttner, W. B., Schiebler, W., Greengard, P., and DeCamilli, P. (1983). Synapsin I (protein I) a nerve terminal specific phosphoprotein. 3. Its association with synaptic vesicles studied in a highly purified synaptic vesicle preparation. *Journal of Cell Biology*, **96**, 1374–88.

Huttner, W. B., DeGennaro, L. J., and Greengard, P. (1981). Differential phosphorylation of multiple sites in purified protein I by cyclic AMP-dependent and calcium-dependent protein kinases. *Journal of Biological Chemistry*, **256**, 1482–8.

Jerusalinsky, D., Aguitar, J. S., Bresco, A., and DeRobertis, E. (1981). Ontogenesis of muscarinic receptors and acetylcholinesterase activity in various areas of chick brain. *Journal of Neurochemistry*, **37**, 1517–22.

Job, D., Rouch, C. T., Fischer, E. H., and Margolis, R. L. (1983). Regulation of microtubule cold stability by calmodulin-dependent and -independent phosphorylation. *Proceedings of the National Academy of Sciences (USA)*, **80**, 3894–8.

Jong, Y. J., Thampy, G., and Barnes, E. M. (1986). Ontogeny of GABA-ergic neurons in chick brain: Studies *in vivo* and *in vitro*. *Developmental Brain Research*, **25**, 83–90.

Kelly, P., McGuinness, T., and Greengard, P. (1984). Evidence that the major postsynaptic density protein is a component of a Ca^{2+}/calmodulin-dependent protein kinase. *Proceedings of the National Academy of Sciences (USA)*, **81**, 945–9.

Kelly, P. T. and Cotman, C. W. (1981). Developmental changes in morphology and molecular composition of isolated synaptic junctional structures. *Brain Research*, **206**, 251–71.

Kelly, P. T. and Vernon, P. (1985). Changes in subcellular distribution of calmodulin kinase II during brain development. *Developmental Brain Research*, **18**, 211–24.

Kelly, P. T., Shields, S., Conway, K., Yip, R., and Burgin, K. (1987). Developmental changes in calmodulin-kinase II activity at brain synaptic junctions: alterations in holoenzyme composition. *Journal of Neurochemistry*, **49**, 1927–40.

Kennedy, M. B., Bennett, M. K., and Erondu, N. E. (1983a). Biochemical and immunochemical evidence that the major postsynaptic density protein is a subunit of a calmodulin-dependent protein kinase. *Proceedings of the National Academy of Sciences (USA)*, **80**, 7457–61.

Kennedy, M. B., McGuinness, T. L., and Greengard, P. (1983b). A calcium/calmodulin-dependent protein kinase from mammalian brain that phosphorylates synapsin I: Partial purification and characterisation. *Journal of Neuroscience*, **3**, 818–31.

Koszka, C., Brent, V., and Rostas, J. A. P. (1991). Developmental changes in phosphorylation of MAP-2 and synapsin I in cytosol and taxol polymerized microtubules from chicken brain. *Neurochemical Research*. (In press.)

Kuret, J. and Schulman, H. (1984). Purification and characterisation of a Ca^{2+}/calmodulin-dependent protein kinase from rat brain. *Biochemistry*, **23**, 5495–504.

Kuret, J. and Schulman, H. (1985). Mechanism of autophosphorylation of the multifunctional Ca^{2+}/calmodulin-dependent protein kinase. *Journal of Biological Chemistry*, **260**, 6429–33.

Lai, Y., Nairn, A. C., and Greengard, P. (1986). Autophosphorylation reversibly regulates the Ca^{2+}/calmodulin-dependence of Ca^{2+}/calmodulin-dependent protein kinase II. *Proceedings of the National Academy of Science (USA)*, **83**, 4253–7.

Lai, Y., Nairn, A. C., Gorelick, F., and Greengard, P. (1987). Ca^{2+}/calmodulin-dependent protein kinase II: Identification of the autophosphorylation sites responsible for the generation of Ca^{2+}/calmodulin-independence. *Proceedings of the National Academy of Science (USA)*, **84**, 5710–14.

Larson, R. E., Goldenring, J. R., Vallano, M. L., and DeLorenzo, J. R. (1985). Identification of endogenous calmodulin-dependent kinase and calmodulin-binding proteins in cold-stable microtubule preparations from rat brain. *Journal of Neurochemistry*, **44**, 1566–74.

LeVine, H. III., Sahyoun, N. E., and Cuatrecasas, P. (1985). Calmodulin binding to the cytoskeletal neuronal calmodulin-dependent protein kinase is regulated by autophosphorylation. *Proceedings of the National Academy of Sciences (USA)*, **82**, 287–91.

Lickteig, R., Shenolikar, S., Denner, L., and Kelly, P. T. (1988). Regulation of a Ca^{2+}/calmodulin dependent protein kinase II by Ca^{2+}/calmodulin-independent autophosphorylation. *Journal of Biological Chemistry*, **263**, 19232–9.

Lin, C. R., Kapiloff, M. S., Durgerian, S., Tatemoto, K., Russo, A. F., Hanson, P., Schulman, H., and Rosenfeld, M. G. (1987). Molecular cloning of a brain-specific calcium/calmodulin-dependent protein kinase. *Proceedings of the National Academy of Sciences (USA)*, **84**, 5962–6.

Lisman, J. E. (1985). A mechnism for memory storage insensitive to molecular turnover: a bistable autophosphorylating kinase. *Proceedings of the National Academy of Science (USA)*, **82**, 3055–7.

Lisman, J. E. and Goldring, M. A. (1988). Feasibility of long term storage of graded information by the Ca^{2+}/calmodulin-dependent protein kinase molecules of the postsynaptic density. *Proceedings of the National Academy of Sciences (USA)*, **85**, 5320–4.

Llinas, R., McGuinness, T. L., Leonard, C. S., Sugimori, M., and Greengard, P. (1985). Intraterminal injection of synapsin I or calcium/calmodulin dependent kinase II alters neurotransmitter release at the squid giant synapse. *Proceedings of the National Academy of Science (USA)*, **82**, 3035–9.

Lou, L. L., Lloyd, S. J., and Schulman, H. (1986). Activation of the multifunctional Ca^{2+}/calmodulin dependent protein kinase by autophosphorylation: ATP modulates production of an autonomous enzyme. *Proceedings of the National Academy of Science (USA)*, **83**, 9497–501.

Lou, L. L. and Schulman, H. (1989). Distinct autophosphorylation sites sequentially produce autonomy and inhibition of the multifunctional Ca^{2+}/calmodulin-dependent protein kinase. *Journal of Neuroscience*, **9**, 2020–32.

McGuinness, T. L., Lai, Y., Greengard, P., Woodgett, J. R., and Cohen, P. (1983). A multifunctional calmodulin dependent protein kinase (similarities between skeletal muscle, glycogen synthase and brain synapsin I kinase). *Federation of European Biochemical Societies' Letters*, **163**, 329–33.

208   J. A. P. Rostas

McGuinness, T. L., Lai, Y., and Greengard, P. (1985). Ca^{2+}/calmodulin-dependent protein kinase II. Isoenzymic forms from rat forebrain and cerebellum. *Journal of Biological Chemistry*, **260**, 1696–704.

Markus, E. J., Petit, T. L., and LeBoutillier, J. B. (1987). Synaptic structural changes during development and ageing. *Developmental Brain Research*, **35**, 239–48.

Matus, A., Pehling, G., and Wilkinson, D. (1981). Gamma-aminobutyric acid receptors in brain postsynaptic densities. *Journal of Neurobiology*, **12**, 67–73.

Matus, A. (1988). Microtubule associated proteins: their potential role in determining neuronal morphology. *Annual Reviews of Neuroscience*, **11**, 29–44.

Miller, S. G., Patton, B.L., and Kennedy, M. B. (1988). Sequences of autophosphorylation sites in neuronal type II CaM kinase that control Ca^{2+}-independent activity. *Neuron*, **1**, 593-604.

Miller, S. G. and Kennedy, M. B. (1985). Distinct forebrain and cerebellar isozymes of type II Ca^{2+}/calmodulin-dependent protein kinase associate differently with the post-synaptic density fraction. *Journal of Biological Chemistry*, **260**, 9039–46.

Miller, S. G. and Kennedy, M. B. (1986). Regulation of brain type II Ca^{2+}/calmodulin-dependent protein kinase by autophosphorylation: A Ca^{2+}-triggered molecular switch. *Cell*, **44**, 861–70.

Monaghan, D. T. and Cotman, C. W. (1986). Identification and properties of N-methyl-D-aspartate receptors in rat brain synaptic plasma membranes *Proceedings of the National Academy of Sciences (USA)*, **83**, 7532–6.

Morris, R. J. (1985). Thy-1 in developing nervous tissue. *Developmental Neuroscience*, **7**, 133–60.

Nichols, R. A., Sihra, T. S., Czernik, A. J., Nairn, A. C., and Greengard, P. (1990). Calcium/calmodulin-dependent protein kinase II increases glutamate and noradrenaline release from synaptosomes. *Nature*, **343**, 647–51.

Nieto-Sampedro, M., Hoff, S. F., and Cotman, C. W. (1982). Perforated postsynaptic densities: probable intermediates in synapse turnover. *Proceedings of the National Academy of Sciences (USA)*, **79**, 5718–22.

Olmsted, J. B. (1986). Microtubule associated proteins. *Annual Review of Cell Biology*, **2**, 421–57.

Ouimet, C. C., McGuinness, T. L., and Greengard, P. (1984). Immunocytochemical localisation of calcium/calmodulin dependent protein kinase II in rat brain. *Proceedings of the National Academy of Sciences (USA)*, **81**, 5604–8.

Rausch, G., and Scheich, H. (1982). Dendritic spine loss and enlargement during maturation of the speech control system of the Mynah bird (*Gracula religiosa*). *Neuroscience Letters*, **29**, 129–33.

Rees, S., Guldner, F. H., and Aitkin, L. (1985). Activity dependent plasticity of post-synaptic density structure in the ventral cochlear nucleus of the rat. *Brain Research*, **325**, 370–4.

Rostas, J. A. P., Brent, V. A., and Guldner, F. H. (1984). The maturation of postsynaptic densities in chicken forebrain. *Neuroscience Letters*, **45**, 297–304.

Rostas, J. A. P., Brent, V., Seccombe, M., Weinberger, R. P., and Dunkley, P. R. (1989). Purification and characterisation of calmodulin stimulated protein kinase II for 2 day and adult chicken forebrain. *Journal of Molecular Neuroscience*, **1**, 93–104.

Rostas, J. A. P., Seccombe, M., and Weinberger, R. P. (1988). Two developmentally regulated isoenzyme forms of calmodulin kinase II in rat forebrain. *Journal of Neurochemistry*, **50**, 945–53.

Rostas, J. A. P. and Jeffrey, P. L. (1981). Maturation of synapses in chicken forebrain. *Neuroscience Letters,* **25**, 299–304.

Rostas, J. A. P. Weinberger, R. P., and Dunkley, P. R. (1986). Multiple pools and multiple forms of calmodulin stimulated protein kinase during development: relationship to postsynaptic densities. *Progress in Brain Research*, **69**, 355–71.

Rostas, J. A. P., Brent, V., Guldner, F. H., and Dunkley, P. R. (1983). Maturation of post-synaptic densities in chicken forebrain. In *Molecular pathology and nerve and muscle: noxious agents and genetic lesions* (ed. A. D. Kidman, J. K. Tomkins, N. A. Cooper, and C. Morris), pp. 67–79. Humana Press, New Jersey.

Rostas, J. A. P., Brent, V. A., Heath, J. W., Neame, R. L. B., Powis, D. A., Weinberger, R. P., and Dunkley, P. R. (1986). The subcellular distribution of a membrane-bound calmodulin-stimulated protein kinase. *Neurochemical Research*, **11**, 253–68.

Rostas, J. A. P., Baker, C. M., Weinberger, R. P., and Dunkley, P. R. (1987*a*). Changes in the pre- and post-synaptic calmodulin stimulated protein kinase II during development in chicken forebrain. *Journal of Neurochemistry*, **48**, 515A.

Rostas, J. A. P., Brent, V., and Dunkley, P. R. (1987*b*). The effect of calmodulin and autophosphorylation on the activity of calmodulin-stimulated protein kinase II. *Neuroscience Research Communications*, **1**, 3–8.

Rostas, J., Weinberger, R., Seccombe, M., Brent, V., Baker, C., and Dunkley, P. (1987*c*). Identification, purification and characterisation of calmodulin stimulated protein kinase II in chicken brain. *Neuroscience Letters Supplement*, **27**, S117.

Sahyoun, N., LeVine, H. III, and Cuatrecasas, P. (1984). Calcium/calmodulin-dependent protein kinases from the neuronal nuclear matrix and post-synaptic density are structurally related. *Proceedings of the National Academy of Sciences (USA)*, **81**, 4311–15.

Sahyoun, N., LeVine, H. III, Bronson, D., Siegel-Greenstein, F., and Cuatrecasas, P. (1985*a*). Cytoskeletal calmodulin-dependent protein kinase. Characterisation, solubilisation and purification from rat brain. *Journal of Biological Chemistry*, **260**, 1230–7.

Sahyoun, N., LeVine, H. III, Burgess, S. K., Blanchard, S., Chang, K. J., and Cuatrecasas, P. (1985*b*). Early postnatal development of calmodulin-dependent protein kinase II in rat brain. *Biochemical and Biophysical Research Communications*, **132**, 878–84.

Saitoh, T. and Schwartz, J. H. (1985). Phosphorylation-dependent subcellular translocation of a Ca^{2+}/calmodulin-dependent protein kinase produces an autonomous enzyme in *Aplysia* neurons. *Journal of Cell Biology*, **100**, 835–42.

Schiebler, W., Jahn, R., Doucet, J-P, Rothlein, J., and Greengard, P. (1986). Characterisation of synapsin I binding to small synaptic vesicles. *Journal of Biological Chemistry*, **261**, 8383–90.

Scheich, H. (1987). Neural correlates of auditory filial imprinting. *Journal of Comparative Physiology A*, **161**, 605–19.

Scholz, W. K., Baitinger, C., Schulman, H., and Kelly, P. T. (1988). Developmental changes in Ca^{2+}/calmodulin-dependent protein kinase II in cultures of hippocampal parametal neurons and astrocytes. *Journal of Neuroscience*, **8**, 1039–51.

210   J. A. P. Rostas

Schulman, H. (1988). The multifunctional Ca^{2+}/calmodulin-dependent protein kinase. *Advances in Second Messenger and Phosphoprotein Research*, **22**, 39–112.

Schworer, C. M., Colbran, R. J., and Soderling, T. T. (1986). Reversible generation of a Ca^{2+}-independent form of Ca^{2+} (calmodulin)-dependent protein kinase II by autophosphorylation mechanism. *Journal of Biological Chemistry*, **261**, 8581–4.

Sedman, G. L., Jeffrey, P. L., Austin, L., and Rostas, J. A. P. (1986). The metabolic turnover of the major proteins of the postsynaptic density. *Molecular Brain Research*, **1**, 221–30.

Siekevitz, P. (1985). The postsynaptic density: a possible role in long lasting effects in the central nervous system. *Proceedings of the National Academy of Sciences (USA)*, **82**, 3494–8.

Sinclair, C. M., Greig, D. I., and Jeffrey, P. L. (1987). Developmental appearance of Thy-1 antigen in the avian nervous system. *Developmental Brain Research*, **35**, 43–53.

Sorensen, R. G. and Babitch, J. A. (1984). Identification and comparison of protein I and chick and rat forebrain. *Journal of Neurochemistry*, **42**, 705–10.

Stewart, M. G., Rose, S. P. R., King, T. S., Gabbott, P. L. A., and Bourne, R. (1984). Hemispheric asymmetry of synapses in chick medial hyperstriatum ventrale following passive avoidance training: a stereological investigation. *Developmental Brain Research*, **12**, 261–9.

Tehrain, M. J. and Barnes, E. M. (1986). Ontogeny of the GABA receptor complex in chick brain: studies *in vivo* and *in vitro*. *Developmental Brain Research*, **25**, 91–8.

Thiel, G., Czernik, A. J., Gorelick, F., Nairn, A. C., and Greengard, P. (1988). Ca^{2+}/calmodulin-dependent protein kinase II: Identification of threonine-286 as the autophosphorylation site in the α subunit associated with the generation of Ca^{2+}-independent activity. *Proceedings of the National Academy of Sciences (USA)*, **85**, 6337–41.

Vallano, M. L., Buckholz, T. M., and DeLorenzo, R. J. (1985a). Phosphorylation of neurofilament proteins by endogenous calcium/calmodulin-dependent protein kinase. *Biochemical and Biophysical Research Communications*, **130**, 957–63.

Vallano, M. L., Goldenring, J. R., Larson, R. E., and DeLorenzo, R. J. (1985b). Separation of endogenous calmodulin and cAMP-dependent kinases from microtubule preparations. *Proceedings of the National Academy of Sciences (USA)*, **82**, 3202–6.

Walaas, S. I., Nairn, A. C., and Greengard, P. (1983a). Regional distribution of calcium and cyclic AMP regulated protein phosphorylation systems in mammalian brain I: Particulate systems. *Journal of Neuroscience*, **3**, 291–301.

Walaas, S. I., Nairn, A. C., and Greengard, P. (1983b). Regional distribution of calcium and cyclic AMP regulated protein phosphorylation systems in mammalian brain II: Soluble systems. *Journal of Neuroscience*, **3**, 302–11.

Walaas, S. I., Lai, Y., Gorelick, F. S., DeCamilli, P., Moretti, M., and Greengard, P. (1988). Cell specific localisation of a α-subunit of the calcium/calmodulin-dependent protein kinase II in Purkinje cells in rodent cerebellum. *Molecular Brain Research*, **4**, 233–42.

Wallace, W. C., Lewis, R. M., Kanazir, S., DeGennaro, C. J., and Greengard, P.

(1985). In *Gene expression in the brain* (ed. W. A. Wallace and C. Zomzely-Neurath), pp. 99–124. John Wiley, New York.

Wallhauser, E. and Scheich, H. (1987). Auditory imprinting leads to differential 2-deoxyglucose uptake and dendritic spine loss in the chick rostral forebrain. *Developmental Brain Research*, **31**, 29–44.

Wasterlain, C. G. and Farber, D. B. (1984). Kindling alters the calcium/calmodulin-dependent phosphorylation of synaptic plasma membrane proteins in rat hippocampus. *Proceedings of the National Academy of Science (USA)*, **81**, 1253–7.

Wasterlain, C. G. and Farber, D. B. (1982). A lasting change in protein phosphorylation associated with septal kindling. *Brain Research*, **247**, 191–4.

Weinberger, R. P. and Rostas, J. A. P. (1986). Subcellular distribution of a calmodulin dependent protein kinase activity in rat cerebral cortex during development. *Developmental Brain Research*, **29**, 37–50.

Weinberger, R. P. and Rostas, J. A. P. (1988*a*)., Developmental changes in protein phosphorylation in chicken forebrain I: Cyclic AMP stimulated protein phosphorylation. *Development Brain Research*, **43**, 249–57.

Weinberger, R.P. and Rostas, J. A. P. (1988*b*). Developmental changes in protein phosphorylation in chicken forebrain II: Calmodulin stimulated phosphorylation. *Developmental Brain Research*, **43**, 259–72.

Weinberger, R. P. and Rostas, J. A. P. (1988*c*). Phosphorylation of synapsin I by cAMP and calmodulin stimulated protein kinases in chicken brain during development. *Neuroscience Letter Supplement*, **30**, S139.

Willmund, R., Mitschulat, H., and Schneider, K. (1986). Long term modulation of Ca^{2+} stimulated autophosphorylation and subcellular distribution of the Ca^{2+}/calmodulin-dependent protein kinase in the brain of *Drosophila*. *Proceedings of the National Academy of Sciences (USA)*, **83**, 9789–93.

Wolff, J. R. (1976). Quantitative analysis of topography and development of synapses in the visual cortex. *Experimental Brain Research Supplement*, **1**, 259–63.

Wolff, J. R. (1978). Ontogenic aspects of cortical architecture: lamination. In *Architectonics of the cerebral cortex* (ed. M. A. B. Brazier and H. J. Petch), pp. 159–73. Raven Press, New York.

Wood, J. G. Wallace, R.W., Whitaker, J. N., and Cheung, W. Y. (1980). Immunocytochemical localization of calmodulin and a heat-labile calmodulin-binding protein ($CaM-BP_{80}$) in basal ganglia of mouse brain. *Journal of Cell Biology*, **84**, 66–76.

Wu, K., Carlin, R. K., Sachs, L., and Siekevitz, P. (1985). Existence of a Ca^{2+}-dependent K^+ channel in synaptic membrane and postsynaptic density fractions isolated from canine cerebral cortex and cerebellum, as determined by apamin binding. *Brain Research*, **360**, 183–94.

Wu, K., Carlin, R. K., and Siekevitz, P. (1986*a*). Binding of L-[³H]-glutamate to fresh or frozen synaptic membrane and postsynaptic density fractions isolated from cerebral cortex and cerebellum of fresh or frozen canine brain. *Journal of Neurochemistry*, **46**, 831–41.

Wu, K., Sachs, L., Carlin, R. K., and Siekevitz, P. (1986*b*). Characteristics of a Ca^{2+}/calmodulin-dependent binding of the Ca^{2+} channel antagonist nitrendipine to a postsynaptic density fraction isolated from canine cerebral cortex. *Molecular Brain Research*, **1**, 167–84.

PART IV

Physical basis of learning and memory

Introduction

R. J. Andrew

The evidence that learning induces specific molecular and structural change in certain structures of the chick brain (which are also unusually active during learning) is compelling. Such changes have been shown to occur only if the opportunity to learn is given, to correlate with the degree of learning, and to be blocked if amnesia is induced after learning (Chapters 8, 10). A wide range of controls for general effects, which might be associated with the learning situation and which might change neuronal properties, have been carried out.

It is thus possible to begin to study the chain of events which leads to the establishment of a permanent memory in the chick. It is true that the story may turn out to be far more complicated than the sketches which are at present possible. Several brain structures are certainly affected by the bead task (Chapters 10, 11); no doubt more remain to be identified for both tasks. Plasticity of neuronal functions may follow different routes in different structures, or during different ways of processing information. Horn (Chapter 8) notes that changes within one structure, the IMHV, seem to differ after different tasks.

A crucial distinction is drawn by Rose (Chapter 10; see also Bateson, Chapter 4) between changes which 'enable' the later processes which lead, through protein synthesis, to the permanent storage of information, but which are not themselves accessible to retrieval mechanisms, and the changes which do allow retrieval during the earlier parts of memory formation. It would be possible for enabling changes to be quite independent of the substrate for early memory: the two might even be held in separate populations of neurons in separate brain structures. Conversely, the two might be tightly coupled, so that each stage on the way to the production of the substrate for permanent memory might itself be responsible for current memory: neurons affected by enabling changes would also be labelled for retrieval. The issue is considered more fully in Part V.

Key events in the route to permanent memory which are already demonstrated in the chick may begin with up-regulation of transmitter receptors (e.g. cholinergic or NMDA: Chapters 8, 10). An early event which has been shown to be essential for permanent memory formation, in that its blockage results in amnesia, is presynaptic change in the phosphorylation of a specific protein (Chapter 10). By 30 minutes an increase in both a particular gene message, and in RNA polymerase marks the earliest steps leading to protein synthesis (which involves both glyco-proteins and tubulin); again, blockage of these steps has been shown to produce amnesia (Chapter 10).

It seems very probable (see also Chapter 7) that such protein synthesis leads to the structural changes which have also been shown to be learning induced. These include both synaptic changes and changes in spine density and shape (Horn, Chapter 8; Stewart, Chapter 11), which can at least partly be understood as facilitating transmission (Chapter 11).

The IMHV has been independently identified as crucial in two very different learning tasks. The possible anatomical correspondence between the HV, of which it is part, and parts of cortical areas such as prefrontal, orbitofrontal, cingulate, and temporal (Section 2; Horn 1985) makes understanding the functioning of the IMHV in learning and memory a matter of great importance. Studies in which the IMHV was lesioned, reviewed here by McCabe (Chapter 9) and Davies (Chapter 12), have led to a model by which, after imprinting, the left IMHV holds permanent memory in the left hemisphere, but the right IMHV acts as a buffer store, establishing permanent memory elsewhere (S^1) in the right hemisphere, after a substantial delay (c. 6 hours). This agrees entirely with the extensive evidence that learning-induced change occurs predominantly in the left IMHV. It explains such a variety of evidence from lesion studies that it must clearly be the preferred hypothesis.

However, the model continues to be extended and changed. Both Davies and McCabe (Chapters 9 and 12) note that unilateral lesions of the left IMHV before training prevent either acquisition or retention of the aversive bead task; lesions of the right IMHV have no effect. They conclude that in this task learning involves only the left IMHV (unlike imprinting, where either IMHV by itself suffices for acquisition; note that brain structures other than the IMHV are likely to be involved in both hemispheres in the aversive bead task). It is thus of great interest that bilateral IMHV lesions only 1 hour after the bead task have no effect on retention. Clearly this implies, on the hypothesis under discussion, that the left IMHV has here acted as a buffer store, and after 1 hour has set up a permanent store elsewhere. One possibility is that this permanent store (S'?) is in the left hemisphere; this idea has the attraction that it would imply that memory formation is similarly organized in the two hemi-spheres, except that it takes far longer to establish S' in the left hemi-sphere. Another possibility is suggested by the hypothesis (McCabe, Chapter 9) that the left IMHV causes the establishment of S' in the right hemisphere: it might do this by transferring information to the right hemisphere.

The idea that in both hemispheres the IMHV functions predominantly as a buffer store meets an obvious and perhaps insurmountable obstacle in the striking concentration of learning-induced change in the left IMHV;

in the case of the bead task, both Rose and Stewart (Chapters 10, 11) stress the surprising scale of such change at both molecular and structural levels. It is worth noting, however, that permanent learning-induced change in the young chick could have a number of functions. These range from: (i) a detailed record of training as a unique experience ('episodic' memory); (ii) a record of key features of the experience, selected after comparison with records of relevant earlier experiences, and their association over time with unpleasant taste. Such 'mediational' memory (Horn, Chapter 8) or 'semantic' memory, is necessary to allow subsequent control of behaviour; (iii) changes in perceptual mechanisms (e.g. the development of complex feature detectors: Chapter 4); (iv) changes in mechanisms necessary for learning (e.g. the establishment of functional connections between reinforcing and other mechanisms; maturation of inputs from arousal mechanisms: Chapter 8). It is possible that a structure which is predominantly used as a buffer store might show permanent changes in categories (iii) and (iv), when it is used for the first time in learning.

It is possible that the description of the IMHV as a buffer store only covers part of its functions. Horn (Chapter 8) compares chicks in which the IMHV have been lesioned with human beings who have become amnesic due to medial temporal lobe/diencephalic damage. Such amnesics are not only able to make use of past learning but also continue to learn, particularly when comparable experiences recur repeatedly; what they lack (or at least deny that they possess) is the ability to recollect specific events. In chicks, bilateral lesions of the IMHV do not affect retention of either imprinting or the bead tast, so long as lesioning occurs sufficiently long after learning. Acquisition of the same tasks is, however, blocked; in contrast, a discrimination task involving unambiguous and repeated pairing of one stimulus with reinforcement and another with its absence can be learned. It is possible that this involves learning comparable with the acquisition of new information by human amnesics as a result of repetitive experience. However, it is also possible that effects of age may be important. Both imprinting and the bead task have been studied in the first 2 days of life, whereas the discrimination tasks used older chicks. Some learning is certainly possible in young chicks with bilateral lesions of the IMHV: they will learn to move on to a pedal to see an imprinting object (Chapters 8 and 12). Nevertheless, it might be interesting to carry out a wide range of tasks in lesioned chicks which are all of the same age.

A final striking feature of learning-induced change in the chick is its asymmetry. In general before training, the biochemical and structural features which change due to training are less well developed in the left IMHV (and probably the left LPO and PA), and training reduces or abolishes this asymmetry by causing the left hemisphere to catch up (Chapters 8, 9, 11). There is increased metabolic and neural activity in right hemisphere structures associated with learning (IMHV, LPO, PA), and all show some more permanent change (Chapter 10), so that they are certainly involved to some extent in both imprinting and the bead task.

Two features of cerebral lateralization in the chick offer potential explanations for such asymmetry. The first is the differing specialization of the two hemispheres for the processing of information (Chapter 21). The right hemisphere appears to be especially concerned with, and good at analysing and storing detailed records of experiences. The left hemisphere is apparently more concerned with the categorization of stimuli for purposes of response. It is likely that categorization is only possible after a certain amount of perceptual learning, based on single stimuli and experiences, has been completed. The more advanced state in the right hemisphere of structures central to learning processes could then be understood in two ways (which are complementary rather than mutually exclusive). Perceptual learning of a variety of types before training might bring about the more advanced state. On the other hand, the advanced state might be a preparation for such learning, rather than a consequence of experience.

The second feature of chick lateralization which may be relevant is that cerebral dominance appears to change with age and task (Chapters 6, 20, 21). If, for either reason, the left hemisphere were predominantly responsible for the processing of information and the control of behaviour in young chicks during imprinting or the aversive bead task, this might explain the asymmetry in learning-induced change. These issues are considered further in later sections.

8

Imprinting and recognition memory; a review of neural mechanisms

G. Horn

INTRODUCTION

Human and non-human animals acquire information about the world through the process of learning, and store that information as memory. Yet, central as the storage process is to adaptive behaviour, progress in understanding its neural bases has been slow and has only recently shown clear signs of being successful. Some of the reasons for this tardiness have been discussed elsewhere (see Lashley 1950; Horn *et al.* 1973*b*; Horn 1981) and include difficulties in identifying changes in the nervous system which are necessary for and specific to the storage of information about particular events or contingencies, and of distinguishing such changes from side-effects of the training procedure. For example, many different brain regions are engaged when new visual information is acquired (see e.g. Horn 1965; Roland and Friberg 1985), so how are we to identify those brain regions, and those neural events which are specifically engaged in the storage process? Another difficulty that besets the field is that the term memory is used in diverse ways. Sometimes it is used in a general sense to refer to effects that depend on past occurrences. In this usage the refractory period that follows a nerve impulse, or the scar tissue which forms in the skin after it has been incised are 'memories' of the antecedent events. Memories of this kind, even if they occur in neural tissue, may have nothing to do with the storage of information acquired through learning. Even in the context of learning it is still necessary to be cautious about the use of the word memory: it is becoming increasingly clear that there are several kinds of learning which may involve different neural circuits and accordingly may involve different memory systems and neural mechanisms.

In 1950 Karl Lashley published a paper entitled 'In search of the engram'. He gave an account of the work that had gone into the search, and of its ultimate failure. He ended the account with the ironic conclusion that, '. . . learning just is not possible' (Lashley p. 478, 1950). Since 1950 many new techniques have been introduced into neurobiology, but the questions raised by Lashley's search must still be answered.

What criteria should be used to decide whether an engram, or even a brain region in which engrams are stored has been discovered? How can one be confident that a given change in the nervous system observed during or after learning reflects the store of information? These questions require answers whether the experimenter is investigating the nervous system of a vertebrate or the relatively small nervous systems of some invertebrates [compare for example Hawkins *et al.* (1983) on the one hand with Colebrook and Lukowiak (1988), Wu *et al.* (1988), Leonard *et al.* (1989) and Morris (1989) on the other hand].

Over the past few years my colleagues and I have attempted to address these questions when studying the learning process of imprinting in the domestic chick (*Gallus gallus domesticus*). Since much of the work has been published it is not necessary to describe it in detail. However, it has become clear over the years that no single experiment has been able to answer any one of the questions. The answers are based on a series of experiments; and the extent to which the answers are convincing depends on considering together the results of those experiments.

NEURAL CHANGES SPECIFIC TO LEARNING?

Behavioural aspects of imprinting

Young, visually naïve chicks will approach a wide range of conspicuous objects. If the chicks continue to be exposed to a particular object they learn its characteristics. If their preferences are subsequently tested the chicks selectively approach the 'training' or 'imprinting' object and may not approach, or may actively avoid a novel object. If the imprinting object is moving the chicks follow it, and when they are near it they emit contentment calls and tend to peck at small particles on the ground. When the chicks are separated from the familiar object they emit distress calls (Spalding 1873; Andrew 1964; Bateson 1966). This pattern of behaviour is taken to signify a filial attachment to the imprinting stimulus. In the usual course of events the attachment is to the chicks' natural mother, although a variety of artificial stimuli, especially if they are moving, will substitute for the mother. The narrowing down of a chick's preference to the object to which it has been exposed implies that the chick recognizes the imprinting object. Accordingly, the strength of imprinting must be measured by some kind of recognition or preference test (see, e.g. Sluckin 1972). However, certain experimental situations may preclude the application of such a test after training. If the experimenter wishes to infer that chicks trained in this way have learned something about the stimulus it is necessary, at the very least, to provide evidence based on other studies that chicks trained on the same regime will, on an average, selectively approach the imprinting object in a test of preference.

Imprinting involves a number of processes, including recognition and selective approach to the familiar object. Whilst the motor component has a sensitive period, there is no reason to suppose that the learning and recognition processes have: an adult fowl recognizes other birds in the flock (Candland 1969), but does not necessarily follow them (see Horn 1985, p. 273). Because imprinting is usually measured by a locomotor approach response, this form of learning has most extensively been studied in precocial species—those whose young show well-co-ordinated locomotor activity within a few hours of birth or hatching. There is, however, no requirement that the underlying learning process must be tied to a locomotor response. Klopfer and Hailman (1964), for example, exposed domestic Vantress-cross chicks to models of life-sized mallard duck decoys. Those chicks which did not follow the decoy during training but sat watching it, showed the same subsequent preference as the 'initial followers', although not as strongly (see also Baer and Gray 1960). Sluckin (1972) considered the evidence to be against the view that imprinting depends on the act of following. Sluckin and Salzen (1961) argued that imprinting is an example of perceptual learning, though Sluckin later came to prefer the expression 'exposure learning' since it 'refers unambiguously to the perceptual registration by the organism of the environment to which it is exposed' (Sluckin 1972). Perceptual registration may occur passively, but the strength of registration may be enhanced if there is active interaction between the observer and that which is observed and if the level of vigilance is high (see for example Klopfer and Hailman 1964; Butler 1953; ten Cate 1986; Bolhuis and Johnson 1988). Such learning is not restricted to birds but occurs in a wide range of animals (see for example Hinde 1962; Sluckin 1972); and far from being a specialized form of learning it may be a very common form of learning.

In many of the studies of imprinting described below chicks were trained by exposing them to a visually conspicuous object. Most experiments employed the following procedures (see McCabe *et al.* 1982; Chapter 1). After hatching, chicks were reared in individual compartments in a dark incubator until they were between 15 and 30 hours old. The chicks were then placed individually in a running wheel, the centre of which stands some 50 cm from the imprinting stimulus. The whole apparatus was contained within a large black box. The chicks were exposed to the stimulus for between 1 and 4 hours, depending on the experiment. A chick's preference was subsequently measured using either a sequential test or a simultaneous choice test. In the sequential test a chick is placed in a running wheel and exposed to the familiar object and to a novel object in succession and in balanced order. The ratio of approach counts (the rotations of the wheel) to the familiar object, to total approach in the test, provides a measure or score of the chick's preference. The sequential test resembles the 'yes or no' test often used to study recognition memory in humans (e.g. Huppert and Piercy 1976). In the simultaneous choice test the training and novel objects are present at the same time. Such a test resembles the delayed matching-to-sample test also used to study recognition memory in humans and other animals (e.g. Freed *et al.* 1987; Aggleton *et al.* 1988).

The first series of experiments were designed to enquire whether biochemical changes occur in the chick brain after imprinting, and if so, whether they are specific to the learning process. The experiments were correlative, in the sense that they involved relating biochemical changes to behavioural changes without interfering with the functioning of the brain except in one case (Horn *et al.* 1971, 1973b). All biochemical analyses were conducted 'blind', that is without knowledge of the chicks' previous behavioural treatment or performance.

Correlative studies

It has often been proposed (James 1890; Tanzi 1893; Cajal 1911; Konorski 1948; Hebb 1949) that learning leads to changes in the connections made between neurons, and that specific changes in connections 'represent' specific memories. If the storage process underlying imprinting involves such changes then alterations in protein and RNA metabolism may be expected in those brain regions in which storage takes place. To examine this possibility one group of chicks was exposed to a conspicuous object, one group was exposed to diffuse light from an overhead lamp and one group was maintained in darkness. Training was found to be associated with an increase in the incorporation of radioactive lysine into protein and of radioactive uracil into RNA in the dorsal part (forebrain roof) of the cerebral hemispheres (Bateson *et al.* 1969, 1972). This regional increase is unlikely to be a simple side-effect of training because (i) when sensory input was restricted to one cerebral hemisphere by monocular occlusion and commissurotomy, incorporation was higher in the forebrain roof of the 'trained' hemisphere than in that of the 'untrained' hemisphere (Horn *et al.* 1971, 1973b), (ii) the magnitude of incorporation was positively correlated with a measure of how much the chicks had learned (Bateson *et al.* 1975), and (iii) the increase associated with training could not be ascribed to short-lasting effects of sensory stimulation (Bateson *et al.* 1973). Of course, the experiments do not exclude all possible side-effects of training; but they do exclude, or reduce the probability that several side-effects can account for the biochemical changes observed in the various studies. To this extent, therefore, we failed to reject the hypothesis that some at least of these changes are closely related to the learning process.

The way in which further analysis could proceed depended on whether or not the biochemical changes were localized to restricted regions of the brain. Using an autoradiographic technique (Horn and McCabe 1978), an increased incorporation of radioactive uracil into RNA was found in a part of the hyperstriatum ventrale close to the mid-line (Horn *et al.* 1979; see Fig. 8, 1*a,b,c*). Accordingly, the region was referred to as the medial hyperstriatum ventrale (MHV). However, the term was misleading. The medial component of the hyperstriatum ventrale extends the whole length of the hyperstriatum ventrale in the antero-posterior plane, whereas the changes associated with imprinting were found in the intermediate part of the structure (see Fig. 8. 1*a,b* and p. 44). The region was subsequently referred to as the intermediate part of the medial hyperstriatum ventrale and abbreviated to IMHV (Horn 1981). Subsequently, the same region and an adjacent part of the medial hyperstriatum ventrale have been reported by other research groups to be involved in visual (Kohsaka *et al.* 1979; Takamatsu and Tsukada 1985) and auditory imprinting (Maier and Scheich 1983), as well as in passive avoidance learning (Rose and Csillag 1985; Davies *et al.* 1988; Chapters 9 to 12). It is perhaps worth emphasizing that in the autoradiographic study of Horn *et al.* (1979) a manually operated microdensitometer was used to measure the optical density of the autoradiographs; as a result it was impracticable to take measurements from all brain areas. Of the areas which were sampled, only in IMHV was a difference found which was attributable to training. It hardly seemed necessary to state when describing that result (Horn *et al.* 1979) that we could not exclude an effect in areas that had *not* been sampled! Certainly there was a suspicion that an area of the medial neostriatum, subjacent to IMHV, was involved (see Fig. 3 of Horn *et al.* 1979), but we had no quantitative evidence to support this suspicion (cf. area MNH of Maier and Scheich 1983).

The results of the correlative studies described in this section were consistent with the view that IMHV stores information, but such studies do not provide evidence that IMHV is necessary for this process. If information storage is indeed a function of IMHV then behaviours which are dependent on storage should be disturbed appropriately if this brain region is destroyed.

DO SPECIFIC BRAIN REGIONS STORE INFORMATION DURING LEARNING?

Intervention studies. Lesions of IMHV

If IMHV is necessary for the storage of information during imprinting, then destruction of the region before training should prevent the acquisition of a preference, and destruction after training should impair retention.

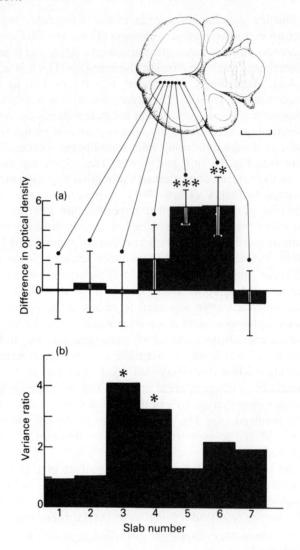

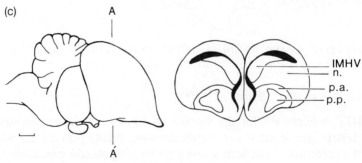

Fig. 8.1 Results of an autoradiographic study. (a) Mean differences ± SEM (undertrained minus overtrained) in standardized optical density at sampling sites within the medial hyperstriatum ventrale. The approximate locations of the sampling sites are shown on the diagram of a chick brain viewed from above, the dorsal surface having been removed (scale bar 4 mm). $**p < 0.01$; $***p < 0.001$. (b) Variance ratios calculated from the standardized data for each of the seven slabs within the medial hyperstriatum ventrale. The ordinate indicates variance of the data from undertrained chicks divided by the variance of the data from the overtrained chicks. $*p < 0.05$. (After Horn *et al.* 1979.) (c) Outline drawings of the chick brain. (After Horn and Johnson 1989.) The vertical lines *AA'* above and below the drawing of the lateral aspect (*left*) indicate the plane of the coronal section outline (*right*) of the brain. Abbreviations: IMHV., the intermediate and medial part of the hyperstriatum ventrale; *n.*, neostriatum; *p.a.*, palaeostriatum augmentatum; *p.p.*, palaeostriatum primitivum. Scale bar: 2 mm.

Both of these predictions were confirmed in a number of lesion studies which involved the bilateral destruction of IMHV (McCabe *et al.* 1981, 1982; Takamatsu and Tsukada 1985). Similar lesions to other brain regions had no effects on acquisition (Johnson and Horn 1987) or retention (McCabe *et al.* 1982).

The poor performance of the IMHV-lesioned chicks in the sequential preference test of recognition used by McCabe *et al.* (1981, 1982) could be accounted for if, for example, some sensory or motor functions were impaired by the lesion, or if the chicks lacked the motivation to approach the training object. Such explanations are implausible for several reasons. Chicks with lesions of IMHV peck small beads or millet seeds as accurately as sham-operated controls, and when allowed to move about freely, lesioned and control chicks could not be distinguished from each other. Lesioned birds are also successfully able to discriminate between different visual patterns (McCabe *et al.* 1982) and different objects (see pp. 247–8). Furthermore, IMHV-lesioned chicks may approach an imprinting object yet perform at chance in a recognition test (Johnson and Horn 1986); this result is inconsistent with a 'motivational' explanation for the chick's behaviour in the test. In the experiments of Johnson and Horn (1986) visually naive chicks were trained on an operant (associative learning) task. Such chicks quickly learn to press a pedal in order to be presented with either a red or a blue rotating illuminated box (Bateson and Reese 1969). As a chick learns to associate the pedal press with the presentation of the reinforcing object, the chick also learns the visual characteristics of this object. When subsequently given a choice between the reinforcing object and another object, the chick will preferentially approach the former. Thus the two processes of imprinting and associative learning develop concurrently. Chicks with bilateral lesions of IMHV learned to perform the operant task as quickly as the sham-operated controls. However, whereas the control chicks preferred the object which had been used as the reinforcer, the chicks with bilateral lesions to IMHV performed at chance. The lesioned chicks were no less active during training or testing than their controls, but unlike the controls the lesioned birds did not direct their movements selectively towards the object they had previously seen; they performed at chance, behaving as if they did not recognize the object.

The lesion studies described in this section (see also Chapters 9 and 12) served to test predictions based on the correlative biochemical studies, and the predictions were met. Other predictions arise if, instead of removing the region, it is artificially excited.

Intervention studies. Electrical stimulation of IMHV

A study was designed (McCabe *et al.* 1979) to investigate the possibility of introducing information directly into IMHV by artificial means to see whether this procedure influenced the chicks' preferences; if the procedure was successful, the result would provide further evidence for the involvement of IMHV in imprinting. Chicks are able to distinguish between lights flashing at 4.5 and 1.5 Hz. In the experiments demonstrating this ability, the flashing effect was achieved by means of a rotating cylinder. It was found that chicks must be exposed to one of these frequencies for 5 hours for a preference to be established. In another series of experiments chicks were not trained by exposing them to the flashing light. Instead IMHV was bilaterally stimulated electrically at one or other of these frequencies, through electrodes which had previously been implanted under surgical anaesthesia. During the 5 hour period of electrical stimulation, a chick was placed in a running wheel and IMHV excited by trains of electrical pulses delivered at the rate of either 1.5 or 4.5 trains of shocks per second. After this period of 'training', electrical stimulation was stopped and the chicks' preferences measured in a test which involved the simultaneous presentation of two lights. One light flashed at 4.5 Hz and the other at 1.5 Hz. The chicks separated themselves out into two clear groups (Fig. 8. 2). Those chicks which had received IMHV stimulation at 1.5 Hz preferred the light flashing at 1.5 Hz; conversely, those chicks which had received IMHV stimulation at 4.5 Hz preferred the light flashing at 4.5 Hz.

When the human visual cortex is electrically stimulated the patient reports seeing flashes of light (Foerster 1929; Penfield and Rasmussen 1952; Brindley and Lewin 1968). These flashes are known as phosphenes. It is possible that the chicks also experienced phosphenes when IMHV was electrically stimulated so that, in effect, the chicks experienced light flashes at 4.5 Hz or 1.5 Hz. It seems unlikely that this explanation alone is sufficient to account for the effects of IMHV stimulation on chicks' subsequent preferences. If electrical stimulation of IMHV generated phosphenes then, by analogy with humans, electrical stimulation of the

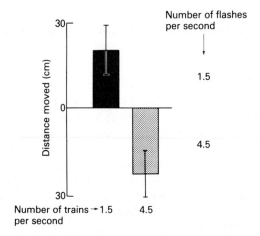

Fig. 8.2 Preferences of chicks stimulated in the IMHV (mean ± SEM). The maximum distance moved by the trolley from the midpoint of the railway in 10 minutes was taken as the chick's preference (Bateson and Wainwright 1972). The horizontal line on the ordinate indicates no preference. Twelve chicks were stimulated at 1.5 trains per second and 13 chicks were stimulated at 4.5 trains per second (after McCabe *et al.* 1979).

visual pathways might also be expected to have generated phosphenes. Yet electrical stimulation of two visual areas respectively, each connected to IMHV (Bradley *et al.* 1985; Horn 1985, pp. 231–5), failed to influence the chicks' preferences, whereas direct stimulation of IMHV did so. The results together suggest that (i) input to the IMHV from visual pathways alone is not sufficient for chicks to use, in subsequent behavioural tests, the temporal information contained within that input and (ii) for information to be used in this way input from at least one other system is necessary. Such a system might, for example, mediate impulse activity associated with the chicks' attentive state. It is conceivable that signals arriving in IMHV from the sensory pathways are more likely to be stored if the chick attends to the stimulus which generates these signals than if it does not attend. Thus attention might serve to gate sensory signals in IMHV and so influence the probability of these signals being stored. Presumably electrical stimulation of IMHV activated the two proposed systems and/or directly activated the postsynaptic elements in IMHV on which these two inputs converge. Whatever may be the physiological significance of the results of the brain stimulation experiments, these results together with those of the lesion studies and the earlier biochemical studies strongly support the view that IMHV is involved in, and may itself be a site of storage for the recognition memory of imprinting.

CELLULAR AND MOLECULAR FOUNDATIONS OF RECOGNITION
MEMORY?

Electron microscope studies

The hypothesis that provided the rationale for the first (Bateson *et al.*
1969, 1972) of our experiments was that learning leads to changes in the
connections made between neurons, and that specific changes in the
connections represent specific memories (see Hebb 1949). Given the
crucial role of IMHV in imprinting, an obvious question to ask is whether
learning leads to changes in synaptic connections in IMHV. The second
question, contingent on the answer to the first, is whether specific groups
of neurons, the 'cell assembly' of Hebb (1949), became interconnected to
'represent' a specific stimulus. The second question has not yet been
addressed experimentally.

In a series of electron microscope studies (Bradley *et al.* 1979, 1981;
Horn *et al.* 1985) quantitative sampling techniques were used to measure
various aspects of synapse structure, including the number of synapses per
unit volume of brain tissue and the mean size of axonal terminal swellings,
the synaptic boutons, in the right and left IMHV. At chemical synapses,
in which transmission is mediated by a neurotransmitter, pre-and postsynaptic elements are separated by a narrow cleft. At vertebrate synapses
part of the postsynaptic membrane is thickened and is known as the
postsynaptic density (PSD); the mean length of this structure was also
determined for each IMHV. Imprinting was associated with an increase in
the mean length of the postsynaptic density in left IMHV synapses. There
were no other effects of training on left IMHV synapses and no changes
in any measure of synapse structure were found in the right IMHV.
Synapses on dendrites occur in two forms, axodendritic and axospinous.
Axodendritic synapses are found on the shafts of dendrites; axospinous
synapses are found on small balloon-shaped structures, the dendritic
spines. The effects of training were restricted to axospinous synapses. The
sampling techniques used to estimate the dimensions of the synaptic
structures did not allow us to determine whether a particular subset of
axospinous synapses were selectively affected by training.

The mean length of the postsynaptic density increases with age and then
stabilizes (e.g. Rostas *et al.* 1984; Bradley 1985). This stabilization may
impose constraints on our ability to detect learning-related changes in
PSD length in adult brains. To clarify the point, suppose that learning in
adults leads to an increase in the length of the postsynaptic density of
some synapses. Such a change is likely to be accompanied by a decrease in
PSD length of other synapses. If this were not the case, every time an
animal learned something new, there would be a small increase in mean

postsynaptic density length, which would go on increasing with age for so long as the animal continued to learn. The quantitative techniques used to measure different aspects of synapse structure from electron micrographs combine measurements from a relatively large number of synapses (see for example Weibel and Bolender 1973). If learning leads to an increase in PSD lengths of some synapses in the sample and to a decrease in length of others, then on average no differences in PSD length would be found between animals that had learned and controls which had not. Such a result might lead to the conclusion, which *ex hypothesi* is false, that learning is without effect on these structures. The view that both decremental and incremental processes affect postsynaptic density lengths has some experimental support from studies of the chick brain (see Bradley *et al.* 1979, 1981; Horn *et al.* 1985; Stewart, Chapter 11) and the rat brain (Desmond and Levy 1986). Since the mean length of the postsynaptic density of synapses in IMHV increases during the first few weeks of life (Bradley 1985), it would seem that incremental changes exceed any decremental changes that may be present during this time. If this is the case it may be that success in finding electron microscope evidence of changes associated with learning derives from using young animals whose brains are continuing to develop.

Stewart *et al.* (1984; Chapter 11) studied the effects of another form of learning on the structure of synapses in IMHV. Young chicks will peck at a wide variety of small objects when presented to them, including small beads. If such a bead is coated with water the great majority of chicks will peck it, and will peck it again when it is presented several hours later. In contrast, if the bead is coated with methylanthranilate (MeA), a liquid which to a human has an unpleasant taste and smell, approximately 75 per cent of chicks refrain from pecking when the bead is presented again (Lee Teng and Sherman 1966). That is, MeA-coated beads are negatively reinforcing. This task is known as one-trial passive avoidance learning or one-trial peck avoidance learning (PAL), and training involves allowing the chicks to peck at the MeA or at the water-coated bead. After PAL the pattern of change in length of the postsynaptic density of synapses in the left and right IMHV was similar to that found after imprinting (see Bradley *et al.* 1979, 1981). Stewart *et al.* (1984) did not sub-divide synapses into axospinous or axodendritic, as was later done for imprinting (Horn *et al.* 1985). Bradley and Galal (1987, 1988) trained chicks on a similar task to that used by Stewart *et al.* Bradley and Galal subdivided synapses into two groups. In one group (asymmetrical synapses) the postsynaptic density is thicker than the corresponding area of the presynaptic membrane; in the other group (symmetrical synapses) the thickenings are similar. In chicks which showed retention (Bradley and Galal 1988), there was an increase in length of the postsynaptic densities of symmetrical synapses; the lengths of the postsynaptic densities of asymmetrical synapses were not significantly different between the chicks which showed retention and those which did not. Asymmetrical synapses are considered to be excitatory in general, whereas symmetrical synapses are considered to be inhibitory. Although symmetrical synapses are occasionally found on dendritic spines, such synapses are relatively rare in this location; axospinous synapses are most commonly of the asymmetrical variety both in the mammalian cerebral cortex (see Peters *et al.* 1976) and in the IMHV of chicks (Bradley, Davies, and Horn, unpublished observations). Thus passive avoidance learning, which is expressed as a *suppression* of a peck response, appears to influence a class of synapses (symmetrical, inhibitory) which is different from that class of synapses (axospinous, excitatory) which is influenced by imprinting, in which the approach response to the training stimulus is *enhanced*.

There are several different types of neuron in IMHV distinguishable on the basis of their morphology (Bradley and Horn 1982; Tömböl *et al.* 1988). No distinction was made between these neuron types in the studies described above. It is possible, therefore, that changes in one direction (e.g. an increase in a synapse measure) may have occurred in some neurons, and in the other direction in other neurons. If this happened, then the electron microscope studies may have failed to reveal a significant effect on that measure (see pp. 228–9). Patel and Stewart (1988), in a light microscope study, used the Golgi technique to examine cells in IMHV. They reported a large change in the number—almost a doubling—of dendritic spines per unit length of dendrite, as well as changes in measures of the shape of the spines on one class of cell in the left IMHV after passive avoidance learning. In a later study Patel *et al.* (1988) trained chicks and subsequently gave one group of them subconvulsive transcranial electroshock. About half the chicks that received this treatment avoided the bead when it was re-presented (the 'recall' group), whereas the remaining chicks pecked the bead ('amnesic group'). Control chicks were allowed to peck beads which had been dipped in water. Sections of IMHV were prepared and neurons visualized with the Golgi stain. There were no significant differences between the three groups of chicks in measures of the shape of the dendritic spines. The number of spines per unit length of dendrite was higher in the left IMHV of birds that avoided the bead (the recall group) than in the group that pecked the bead (amnesic) and in the water control group. The difference, however, was considerably smaller than in the previous study. The results taken together suggest that the dendritic spines of at least one class of cells in IMHV are highly dynamic structures. Some of the changes they undergo are induced by training; but not all of the changes they undergo are related to learning.

The increase in spine number described by Patel *et al.* (1988) following PAL contrasts with the results described by Wallhäusser and Scheich (1987) following the exposure of chicks to an auditory imprinting stimulus. These authors reported a loss of dendritic spines in a region which Scheich and his colleagues (Maier and Scheich 1983; Wallhäusser and Scheich 1987) have implicated in this form of learning. The region, the medial neostriatum/hyperstriatum ventrale (MNH), appears to include the anterior limits of IMHV (see also pp. 223–4). Wallhäusser and Scheich (1987) concluded that auditory imprinting leads to degenerative changes in dendritic spines on the basis of a Golgi study of ten cells from the MNH region of each of 14 chicks. Seven chicks served as controls, five chicks were imprinted to a hen on a farm and two chicks were exposed to bursts of 400 Hz tone. This tone was delivered continually from day 14 of incubation until hatching; and on the next two days post-hatch for 1 hour twice per day. Spine frequency measures were based on spine counts from various segments of dendrites. Wallhäusser and Scheich (1987, p. 37) state that 'With the exception of the basal dendritic segments in naturally and acoustically imprinted chicks, spine frequency differences in all other segments were found to be highly significant ($p < 0.0001$) between all three groups (one-tailed Mann–Whitney U test)'. It is proper to use a one-tailed test when there is a prior expectation of the direction of a change. Wallhäusser and Scheich (1987) make no statement of such prior expectation. Given the stated probability level ($p < 0.0001$), doubling it for a two-tailed test would of course still yield a highly significant p value, so the criticism might seem trivial. However, a Mann–Whitney U test applied to data from two animals (the tone-exposed chicks) and seven controls yields a two-sided p value of 0.056. For a comparison of data from the two tone-exposed chicks and the five chicks imprinted to the hen the two-tailed p value is 0.096. Neither is statistically significant, so the stated p value of < 0.0001 is perplexing (but see Machlis *et al.* 1985). These considerations suggest that the question of whether or not auditory imprinting leads to degenerative changes in dendritic structure is still an open one. However this issue is resolved, it is also important to study the effects on the developing brain, especially the auditory system, of continuously exposing the egg to the acoustic imprinting stimulus at a relatively high intensity (80 dB SPL) throughout the last 7 days of incubation (see Wallhäusser and Scheich 1987).

Molecular changes

When neurotransmitter molecules are liberated from the presynaptic bouton they diffuse into the synaptic cleft and bind to receptors which are present in the postsynaptic density (Fagg and Matus 1984). A consequence of the interaction between neurotransmitter and receptor proteins is that ion channels may open. If the synapse is excitatory, the net ion flux will depolarize the postsynaptic cell membrane and may lead to the discharge of an impulse along the axon. There is strong evidence that at least some excitatory axospinous synapses in the mammalian central nervous system possess receptors for the excitatory amino acid L-glutamate (Nafstad 1967; Errington et al. 1987). Membranes with these receptors bind the radioactive isotope L-[^{3}H]glutamate. If imprinting leads to an increased number of receptors for this amino acid, the membranes prepared from the left IMHV of trained chicks should bind more L-[^{3}H]glutamate than corresponding membranes from dark-reared chicks. McCabe and Horn (1988) trained chicks by exposing them to a rotating red box for 140 minutes. After training all chicks were assigned codes and held individually in darkness for at least 7 hours before being killed together with their dark-reared controls. The left IMHV was then removed, membranes prepared and incubated with L-[^{3}H]glutamate. Imprinting was associated with a significant increase, of approximately 20 per cent, of L-[^{3}H]glutamate binding compared with that in dark-reared controls.

There are several sub-types of receptors for L-glutamate, three of which are defined by the action of selective agonists. One of these is N-methyl-D-aspartate (NMDA). McCabe and Horn (1988) enquired whether at least some of the increased binding of L-[^{3}H]glutamate was to receptors of this type. Chicks were treated as described above and the effects of training on NMDA-sensitive binding to membranes prepared from the IMHV determined. There was a significant increase in NMDA-sensitive binding in the left IMHV of trained chicks compared with that in dark-reared controls; there was no such difference in right IMHV binding.

Whilst these results are consistent with the results of the electron microscope studies of IMHV described above (Bradley et al. 1979, 1981; Horn et al. 1985), there remain many ambiguities in the interpretation of the data. The trained birds were visually experienced, the dark-reared birds were not, so that the differences in NMDA-sensitive binding could be a result of these, and other, consequential differences. To clarify these ambiguities, a group of chicks was exposed to the training stimulus and given a preference test immediately before being killed. The strength of the chick's preference for the familiar object relative to a novel object was measured and expressed as a preference score (McCabe et al. 1982). There was a significant positive correlation between preference score and NMDA-sensitive binding in the left IMHV ($r = 0.38$; 34 df; $p < 0.025$). The corresponding correlation coefficient for NMDA-sensitive binding in the right IMHV was not significant ($r = 0.10$; 30 df). Bateson and Jaeckel (1976) found that approach activity during training is correlated with preference score. It is therefore possible that the observed correlation between NMDA-sensitive binding and preference score reflects a relation between binding and locomotor activity during training. McCabe and Horn (1988) therefore corrected binding and preference score for training approach activity, using the method of partial correlation (training approach activity was measured as the number of revolutions made by the running wheel as a chick attempted to approach the red box during training). There was a positive partial correlation between NMDA-sensitive binding in the left IMHV and preference score ($r_{xy.z} = 0.41$; 34 *df*; $p < 0.02$). The 36 values that contributed to this correlation were divided into three groups of equal size according to their ranked corrected preference scores. The lowest mean corrected preference score (for group 1) was not significantly different from 50, and the corresponding mean binding for this group was not significantly different from that in the left IMHV of the dark-reared chicks of the previous experiments (McCabe and Horn 1988). The highest mean corrected preference score (for group 3) was significantly ($p < 0.001$) greater than 50, and the values of mean corrected binding of groups 1 and 3 were significantly ($p < 0.05$) different from each other. There was no significant partial correlation between NMDA-sensitive binding in the right IMHV and preference score ($r_{xy.z} = 0.09$; 29 *df*).

There is strong evidence that under the incubation conditions used in the above study the NMDA-sensitive binding corresponds to physiological receptors, and there is good reason to suppose that the increase in binding in the left IMHV is due to an increase in the number of receptors (McCabe and Horn 1988). There are several reasons why this increase cannot simply be attributed to side-effects of the training procedure. (i) The studies that led to the localization of IMHV and to the demonstration of the crucial role of this region, especially of the left IMHV (Cipolla-Neto *et al.* 1982), in information storage had controlled for these and other side effects of training (see Horn 1985 for review). (ii) in the present study a general effect of arousal would be expected to affect both right and left IMHV. This was not found in either of the two experiments in which measurements of both left and right IMHV were made. An effect of arousal would also be expected to be expressed in behaviour: the more aroused the chicks, the more vigorously would they be expected to approach the red box during training. However, the partial correlation coefficient between NMDA-sensitive binding and preference score was significant when the effect of approach activity during training was held constant. This latter finding also demonstrates that differences in locomotor activity during training cannot account for the correlation between binding and corrected preference score. (iii) Light exposure *per se* does not account for the findings, since the corrected mean left IMHV binding in chicks that had been exposed to the red box for 140 minutes, but had not developed a preference for it, was closely similar to the mean left IMHV binding of dark-reared chicks. This similarity suggests that this level of binding is the floor level of binding in unimprinted chicks, whether dark-reared or visually experienced. Considerations (ii) and (iii) indicate that NMDA-sensitive binding in the left IMHV is not influenced by arousal, light exposure or locomotor activity *per se*. Instead, the results suggest either (a) that the birds with larger numbers of NMDA receptors learn better than birds with fewer NMDA receptors or (b) that binding increases as the chicks learn about the imprinting object and so form a preference for it. Certain considerations make it possible to distinguish between these hypotheses. The dark-reared birds were not selected for their learning abilities. It is reasonable to suppose, therefore, that this group contained poor learners, which would if trained achieve a low preference score, as well as good learners, which would if trained achieve a high preference score. Hence if hypothesis (a) is correct the variance of NMDA-sensitive binding in the left IMHV of dark-reared chicks should be higher than that of both the poor learners and the good learners since the latter two groups, *ex hypothesi*, are sub-groups of the unselected dark-reared chicks. The variances for left IMHV binding from four groups of chicks, two dark-reared groups, the poor and good learners were not significantly different (Bartlett's test, ($\chi^2 = 5.59$; $df = 3$; $p > 0.1$). Therefore hypothesis (a) may be rejected in favour of the view that learning leads to an increase in the number of NMDA-type receptors in the left IMHV.

The increase in number of NMDA receptors does not occur immediately after training, and indeed is delayed for several hours (Horn and McCabe 1990; McCabe and Horn 1990). These findings imply that the increase in NMDA receptor numbers observed in the left IMHV after imprinting cannot support a preference when it is tested, say, 2 hours after training, since there is no such increase; clearly a different mechanism must be invoked to account for the neural basis of preference measured soon after training. The possibility that at least two mechanisms are involved in memory is not wholly surprising: different pharmacological agents have been found to disrupt retention when given at different times after training (for review see Andrew 1980; see also Chapters 13–17, and 19). A clue as to what might be happening comes from studies of long-term potentiation in the hippocampus (for reviews see Collingridge and Bliss 1987; Teyler and DiScenna 1987). The early phase of the potentiation appears to depend upon an increased liberation of transmitter from the presynaptic terminal when it is invaded by a nerve impulse. The later phase of potentiation involves the postsynaptic cell, possibly an increase in number and/or affinity of L-glutamate receptors of the quisqualate type (Davies *et al.* 1989). Long-term potentiation in the rat dentate gyrus also leads to morphological changes in axospinous synapses (Desmond and Levy 1986). These changes include an increase in length of the postsynaptic density on certain dendritic spines.

The postsynaptic changes associated with hippocampal long-term potentiation thus have some rather general similarities with those described in this and the previous section for imprinting. Is it possible that there are other similarities, and that the early phase of memory in imprinting is sustained by presynaptic events, as is the early phase of long-term potentiation? Although there is no direct evidence for this possibility in the case of imprinting, there is some evidence that presynaptic (as well as postsynaptic) elements are involved in passive avoidance learning in the domestic chick. Stewart *et al.* (1984) found that training was associated with a substantial and highly significant increase in the mean number of vesicles per synaptic bouton in the left IMHV. Such an increase would be consistent with an increased mobilization of transmitter as a consequence of training, and raises the possibility that when such terminals are invaded by a nerve impulse more transmitter is liberated after training than before.

The consequences of an increased number of NMDA receptors are likely to be subtle in several ways:-

(i) Although L-glutamate activates these receptors, the associated ion channels may remain closed, being blocked by magnesium ions (Nowak *et al.* 1981). This block is removed if the membrane of the postsynaptic cell is depolarized. Thus the ion channels associated with the NMDA receptors will pass current only under certain conditions: the receptors must be activated by their neurotransmitter and the postsynaptic cell must be excited through ion channels associated with other receptors. At the behavioural level, such an arrangement could have interesting consequences. For example, the presentation of a familiar object may activate the afferent fibres to the synapses which, through training, have an increased number of NMDA receptors. The activated afferent fibres may release L-glutamate, which binds to these receptors. The postsynaptic cell may not respond to the presynaptic signal unless the cell is depolarized by some other input. This input may be generated by, for example, neurons whose activity is controlled by the attentional state of the animal (see p. 227); that is, attentional mechanisms may exercise some control of the flow of signals through the memory systems of the brain (Horn 1970). Other controlling inputs may be from neural systems underlying affective states of the animal or from neuronal assemblies representing other memories.

(ii) Calcium ions flow inwards through NMDA channels (MacDermot *et al.* 1986). This influx may lead to and maintain changes in the structure of the postsynaptic density and influence its interactions with proteins in the cytoskeleton of the dendritic spine. If this view proves to be correct it may be that prolonged inactivity of a previously modified synapse may lead to a regression of the modification and so to a corresponding loss of the specific memory with which these synapses are involved.

It is clear that many questions remain to be answered in addition to those which are implicit in the considerations outlined in the above paragraph. For example, do the structural changes in axospinous synapses, and the changes in NMDA receptors occur at the same synapses; are there changes in non-NMDA L-glutamate receptors; are all axospinous synapses in the left IMHV affected by training or are the changes restricted to a sub-population of them; and are the changed synapses interconnected as in a Hebbian cell-assembly (Hebb 1949)? It should also be borne in mind that while a change in number of NMDA receptors might functionally weight the synapses to form a basis of recognition memory (cf. Horn 1962); other possibilities exist and need to be explored. For example, the increase in NMDA receptors may play only a 'permissive' role in the cellular mechanisms of memory: the increase might permit a relatively large influx of calcium into the cell to initiate other changes—so far undetected—for example, in synapse structure, after which NMDA receptor numbers may return to lower levels (cf. Wenk *et al.* 1989).

NMDA receptors have been implicated in the processes that control certain forms of plasticity in the developing nervous system (Cline *et al.* 1987; Kleinschmidt *et al.* 1987; Rauschecker and Hahn 1987), in hippocampal long-term potentiation (Collingridge *et al.* 1983; Errington *et al.* 1987), and in the acquisition of place-learning in rats (Morris *et al.* 1986; see also Mondadori *et al.* 1989; Wenk *et al.* 1989). Furthermore, a plausible case has been made that over-activation of NMDA receptors may trigger events which lead to neuronal death, so that these receptors may be involved, at least in part, in a variety of neurodegenerative conditions such as Huntington's chorea and Alzheimer's disease (see for example Maragos *et al.* 1987; Rothman and Olney 1987). If these views prove to be correct then the receptors which play a role in the formation of memory may, paradoxically, also play a role in its destruction. However, the implied link between development processes and learning is not wholly unexpected. Changes occur in the morphological and functional properties of neurons during the course of ontogeny. In some systems the direction of these changes is such that neurons largely lose their capacity for plastic change as their synaptic connections become stabilized in the course of development and maturation (Hubel and Wiesel 1971; Olson and Freeman 1980; Knudsen and Knudsen 1986). A similar direction of change may occur as a result of learning in neural circuits specialized for storage. Thus Horn *et al.* (1973a) suggested that neurons within the memory systems of the brain may remain plastic until they become engaged in the storage process associated with a specific learning experience. Thereafter the synaptic connections may become stabilized, or 'functionally validated' (Horn 1985) although, as suggested above, this stabilization may require active maintenance.

Certain developments in molecular neurobiology afford an opportunity to explore these views. As axons grow after injury or in the course of development there is a high level of synthesis of at least one growth-associated protein, referred to as GAP-43. The apparent molecular mass of this protein is approximately 50 kDa. As synaptic relationships become defined the synthesis of this protein declines (see Skene 1984; Jacobson *et al.* 1986; Benowitz and Routtenberg 1987). Ali *et al.* (1988) studied protein phosphorylation at synapses in chick forebrain. They found a significant decrease in phosphorylation of a 52 kDa component of the synaptic plasma membranes after passive avoidance learning. The membranes were prepared from whole forebrains, so it would be of the greatest interest to know whether such changes are also found in samples of IMHV. Brown and Horn (1990) described the results of experiments designed to investigate changes in protein synthesis associated with imprinting. Slices of IMHV, of the neostriatum and of the visual Wulst, respectively, were removed from the left cerebral hemisphere of chicks which had been trained by exposing them to the rotating red box. The chicks' approach activity during training was measured. The samples were incubated with [^{35}S]methionine, processed for SDS slab gel electrophoresis, and autoradiographs prepared. The optical densities of various bands were measured. There was a negative correlation between the optical density of the *circa* 50 kDa band and approach activity during training ($p < 0.01$; Fig. 8.3*a*). That is, the more chicks ran to the red box during training the lower was the synthesis of proteins with molecular mass of *circa* 50 kDa. In addition to this finding there was a positive correlation between training approach activity and the optical density of a *circa* 80 kDa band ($p < 0.001$; Fig. 8.3*b*). These results suggest that training is associated with both an increase and a reduction in protein synthesis. No training-related changes were observed in gels prepared from the two other samples of the left cerebral hemisphere. Approach activity during training is only a weak predictor of the strength of preference for the training object (Bateson and Jaeckel 1976); whether the changes in protein synthesis are related to a more direct measure of learning and whether the changes in optical density represent changes in the synthesis of only one or more than one protein of molecular mass *circa* 50 kDa and *circa* 80 kDa, respectively, are questions that remain to be answered. However, if growth associated proteins are involved in imprinting, then there may indeed be substance in the suggestion (Horn *et al.* 1973*a*) that there are continuities at the cellular and molecular levels between the development of neurons and the changes that underlie memory.

Neurophysiological studies of the hyperstriatum ventrale

Response properties

There have been relatively few studies designed to characterize the response properties of neurons in the hyperstriatum ventrale. In the guinea fowl, the most caudal part of the medial hyperstriatum ventrale, posterior to IMHV (see Fig. 8.1), has strong reciprocal connections with

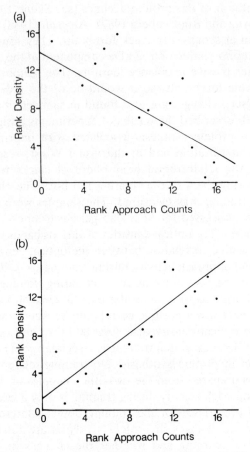

Fig. 8.3 Correlations between rank order approach counts and rank order optical density measures of the autoradiographs for (a) the *circa* 50 kDa and (b) the *circa* 80 kDa bands (after Brown and Horn 1990).

the auditory projection area field L (Bonke *et al.* 1979). Müller and Leppelseck (1985) recorded from the caudal part of the hyperstriatum ventrale of unanaesthetized starlings and found that units within the region responded to auditory stimuli. Margoliash (1986) recorded from neurons in a nucleus referred to as hyperstriatum ventrale pars caudale (HVc). Within this nucleus, of both anaesthetized and unanaesthetized white crowned sparrows, units responded to the bird's own song. It is not clear however whether HVc is a part of the hyperstriatum ventrale (see Konishi 1985), nor is it clear that there is a counterpart of this nucleus in the brain of the domestic chick.

Visual responses may be evoked in the medial part of the hyperstriatum ventrale, though the conditions under which such responses may be elicited are not yet clear. Morenkov and Khun (1977) recorded from the hyperstriatum ventrale of unanaesthetized, immobilized grey crows. Some of the microelectrode penetrations passed through part of the region which, on topographical grounds, corresponds to IMHV. The units possessed large visual receptive fields, reaching diameters of 30–50° of visual angle. These neurons responded to stimuli moving in particular directions, that is the neurons were directionally selective. Gusel'nikov *et al.* (1976) recorded from the hyperstriatum ventrale of unanaesthetized, immobilized adult pigeons. The responses of units in this region were not described in any detail, although it is clear from the text figures that directionally selective units with localized receptive fields were recorded in the anterior part of the hyperstriatum ventrale. No electrode penetrations were made through the region corresponding anatomically to IMHV. In contrast to these positive results, Wilson (1980) failed to detect any visually evoked activity in the hyperstriatum ventrale of 5-week-old domestic chicks anaesthetized with nitrous oxide. Wilson's stimuli were stationary or moving spots of light or moving edges or bars. The part of the hyperstriatum ventrale explored by Wilson (1980) lay deep to the hyperstriatum accessorium and therefore did not include the IMHV. However, Brown, and Horn (1979) recorded from the IMHV of anaesthetized chicks. They found a small number of units which responded weakly to diffuse flashes of light, but were unable to find units with localized visual receptive fields.

The diverse results of experiments designed to study visual evoked responses in the hyperstriatum ventrale are puzzling, though the discrepancies may be more apparent than real. The two studies which were successful in recording from units with discrete receptive fields were conducted on adult pigeons and crows. The two studies which failed to find units with such fields were conducted on young domestic chicks. The two former studies were carried out on unanaesthetized birds whereas in the latter two studies the birds were anaesthetized. This difference may be of some importance. Neuronal responses to sensory stimulations are not difficult to detect in the major sensory pathways of anaesthetized animals, especially if the recorded region is only a few synapses distant from the sensory receptors. In contrast, anaesthetic agents often have a profound depressant effect on transmission in multisynaptic pathways (see Brazier 1961; Clutton-Brock 1961; Brown and Horn 1977). For this reason anaesthetics tend not to be used when attempting to characterize the response properties of neurons in regions that are synaptically remote from the sense organs. There is another reason why it is sometimes necessary to abandon anaesthetics when recording from certain regions of the brain. These agents abolish virtually all interesting aspects of behaviour such as attention, learning, and motor acts of a complex—or even of a quite simple—kind. It is reasonable to infer therefore that anaesthetics affect those brain regions that integrate the neuronal events on which these functions depend. It is not surprising that recent electrophysiological studies of such brain regions were conducted on unanaesthetized, behaving animals (see, for example, Wurtz and Goldberg 1971; Horn and Wiesenfeld 1974; Mountcastle 1976; Mora *et al.* 1976; Brown and Horn 1978; Wurtz *et al.* 1980; Perrett *et al.* 1985; Kendrick and Baldwin 1987).

'Spontaneous' impulse activity and behaviour

Neurons in the IMHV of anaesthetized chicks discharge spontaneously, in the absence of deliberate sensory stimulation (Brown and Horn 1979). As a first step in analysing the physiological changes in IMHV associated with imprinting, this discharge was recorded from chicks which had been exposed to a training stimulus (Payne and Horn 1982, 1984). Recordings were also made from a visual projection area, the hyperstriatum accessorium.

Thirty-six chicks were exposed to an imprinting stimulus, the rotating, flashing red box, for a total of 2 hours on the day of hatching and for a further 1 hour on the following day. Each chick was in a running wheel during the 3-hour period of training. The number of rotations made by the wheel was recorded and used as a measure of approach activity ('approach counts'). Approximately 1 hour after the end of training each chick was anaesthetized. Two microelectrodes were introduced into the left hemisphere of the brain. One microelectrode penetrated vertically into the hyperstriatum accessorium, the other penetrated vertically and at the same time through IMHV. Each electrode was advanced in steps of 250 μm. At the end of each step the spontaneous discharge of multiple units was recorded for 1 minute. At least three such recordings were made in a penetration. After these penetrations had been completed, no further penetrations into the brain were made. The mean firing rate of units in each penetration was calculated.

There was a significant correlation between the total number of approach counts made during the 3-hour training period and the mean spontaneous firing rate of neurons in IMHV. The correlation was negative; that is, the more chicks ran towards the box the lower was the mean firing rate of neurons in IMHV (Fig. 8.4*a*). A different result was found for recordings made simultaneously in the hyperstriatum accessorium of the same chicks. There was no significant correlation between spontaneous impulse activity and total approach counts (Fig. 8.4*b*). This correlation coefficient was significantly different from the corresponding correlation coefficient for IMHV. Thus the relationship between neuronal activity and approach counts during training was regionally specific.

In spite of the fact that the chicks were anaesthetized, the results described above show that spontaneous impulse activity in neurons in IMHV is correlated with, and presumably affected by, prior behavioural activity. The physiological significance of the changed activity is not clear,

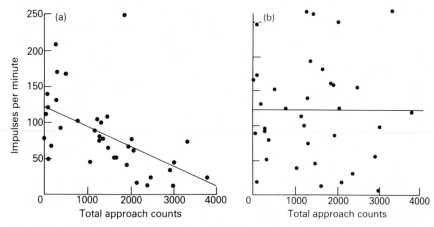

Fig. 8.4 Relationship between neuronal firing rate and approach activity during training for chicks exposed to the red box. Mean spontaneous firing rates are plotted against total approach activity during the 3 hour training period. The lines were fitted by the method of least squares. The recording electrodes simultaneously penetrated the IMHV and the hyperstriatum accessorium respectively in each of the 36 chicks. (a) IMHV. The correlation coefficient was significant ($r = -0.54$, df 34, $p < 0.01$. (b) Hyperstriatum accessorium. There was not a significant correlation between the two variables ($r = -0.02$, df 34). The two correlation coefficients are significantly different ($p < 0.05$) (after Payne and Horn 1984).

however. One possibility is that the lower discharge rate reflects a higher level of inhibitory activity impingeing on the recorded neurons. If such an inhibitory effect were selective, it might serve to exclude from IMHV activity evoked by novel objects whilst allowing the region to be accessible to activity evoked by the familiar object.

Using similar electrophysiological techniques Davey and Horn (in preparation) (see Davey 1988) recorded simultaneously from the right and left IMHV. This work was undertaken to see whether any neurophysiol-ogical evidence of hemispheric asymmetry could be found, as had been found in studies of synaptic organization in IMHV (see pp. 228–33). In the study of Davey and Horn chicks were exposed to the rotating red box for a total of 120 minutes beginning when the chicks were approximately 20 hours old. The trained chicks were then divided into two groups. Chicks in one group were anaesthetized immediately after training (0 hour group, $n = 8$), the other group of chicks was returned to the dark incubator and anaesthetized 6 hours after the end of training (6 hour group, $n = 8$). Sixteen dark-reared chicks of comparable ages served as controls. All recordings were performed without knowledge of the previous experience of the chick.

One electrode penetration was made through the left IMHV and one through the right IMHV. The mean spontaneous firing rate for each penetration was calculated (see above). The mean firing for the multiple unit discharges in the right IMHV (R) was expressed as a ratio of the corresponding mean activity in the left IMHV (L). The ratio (R/R+L) was calculated for each bird. For birds studied directly after training (0 hour) the mean ratio was not significantly different from that of dark-reared controls. For birds studied 6 hours after training the ratio was significantly lower than that of the dark-reared controls. These findings suggest that training alters the balance of firing between right and left IMHV, the alterations being expressed 6 hours after the end of the period of exposure to the red box.

Mason and Rose (1987, 1988; and see Chapter 10) have given an account of multiple unit spontaneous activity in penetrations through the anterior part of IMHV after PAL. They studied the effects of training on patterns of bursting activity (400–450 spikes per second) of units which they classified as being relatively large (200–450 μV peak-to-peak). Training was associated with a trebling of the occurrence of bursts both in the left IMHV and in the right. Such high frequency bursts occurred extremely rarely in the studies of Davey and Horn (4 bursts observed in records from 297 recording sites in IMHV). A more commonly occurring burst in these experiments contained $\geqslant 3$ spikes with an interspike interval of $\leqslant 10$ milliseconds. The frequency with which bursts occurred in the left and right IMHV did not differ significantly; accordingly, burst data from the two sides were combined. There were no significant differences in the mean number of bursts per minute between 0 hour trained chicks and the dark-reared controls. But, compared with these controls, the mean number of bursts per minute was significantly *lower* in the 6 hour trained chicks. An electrode penetration was made through the left hyperstriatum accessorium immediately after the IMHV recordings were complete. The bursting rate in this region was also significantly lower after training, the reduction being present both for the 0 hour and the 6 hour groups of chicks.

Until further experimental work is done the physiological significance of these changes in burst frequency will remain obscure. The changes are, however, reminiscent of the changes in burst activity observed in various parts of the mammalian brain in the transition from sleep to wakefulness. During sleep, especially the phase referred to on the basis of the electroencephalogram as slow-wave sleep, spikes discharge in clusters (for review see Evarts 1967; McCormick 1989). In the waking state spike discharges tend to be regular with few bursts. In mammals the bursting is thought to reflect rhythmic activity in thalamocortical circuits. As an animal wakes up activity arising in the brainstem abolishes this rhythmicity. It is thus possible, if similar mechanisms operate in the chick, that one effect of the imprinting experience is, in effect, to 'waken' the brain by, say, accelerating the development of the brainstem projection systems. One of these systems, originating from cell bodies in and around the locus coeruleus, contains catecholamines, probably noradrenalin (Dubé and Parent 1971; Kitt and Brauth 1986). Exposure to an imprinting stimulus leads to an increase in noradrenalin levels in several areas of the chick brain (Davies *et al.* 1983). In the study of Davey and Horn the reduction in bursting activity appeared in the left hyperstriatum accessorium immediately after training, and persisted since the reduction was present both in the 0 hour and the 6 hour groups. It was found only in the 6 hour group for the recordings from IMHV. If the hypothesis is correct—that the imprinting experience accelerates the development of one or more brainstem projection systems—it is not clear why units in the hyperstriatum accessorium should be affected 0 hour after training, but units in the IMHV affected only 6 hours after training. Perhaps neurons in IMHV acquire, only slowly after training, the receptor/second messenger systems that allow them to be affected by the putative changes in the brainstem projection system. Parenthetically, it is of interest that changes in NMDA receptors occur approximately 8.5 hours after the end of training (Horn and McCabe 1990; McCabe and Horn 1991); the electrophysiological changes in IMHV occur approximately 6 hours after the end of training. Whether the two changes are related is, however, an open question.

It is tempting to suppose that the different patterns of results obtained after imprinting, from those obtained after passive avoidance learning, imply different physiological processes. It is also possible that Mason and Rose (1987, 1988) were sampling a different or a wider population of neurons from those sampled in the studies of imprinting (Brown and Horn 1978; Payne and Horn 1982, 1984; Payne *et al.* 1984; Davey 1988; Davey and Horn, in preparation). In the imprinting studies the mean firing rates of multiple unit discharges in IMHV were within the range of 1–3 spikes per second and the firing rates of units in the hyperstriatum accessorium were *higher* than those in IMHV; in contrast Mason and Rose (1987) reported IMHV firing rates of 70–75 spikes per second and found that the rate of discharge of units in the hyperstriatum accessorium was *lower* than that in IMHV.

The studies described above of spontaneous neuronal impulse activity and its relation to exposure training have disclosed a number of interesting findings: the changes in this activity correlate with a measure of behaviour recorded when the chicks were exposed to the imprinting object, a hemispheric asymmetry in neuronal firing gradually develops after training and, through a study of bursting activity, the studies have provided a hint—no more than that—that training may accelerate the development of one or more brainstem projection systems. What is perhaps most remarkable is that all of these results have been obtained in anaesthetized chicks. The findings, whilst posing numerous questions for experimental analysis, do not help to answer one of the questions originally posed in this chapter (p. 220) concerning the nature of an engram. If some of the various cellular and molecular changes described on pp. 228–37 are directly related to the formation of a memory trace, it is important to know how the activity of neurons in that trace respond to the presentation of the imprinting stimulus. Experiments designed to answer this question are now under way (McLennan and Horn, in preparation).

ASYMMETRY OF FUNCTION

Well over 100 years have elapsed since Broca (1865) first published his work relating left hemisphere damage to aphasia, yet the first widely accepted evidence of a morphological asymmetry in the human cerebral cortex was published barely two decades ago (Geschwind and Levitsky 1968). Given that these studies related to language, it is perhaps not surprising that there was relatively little interest in enquiring whether there is evidence of an asymmetry in the structure of non-human brains. Recently, however, it has become known that such asymmetries exist in several species of non-human mammal and in some species of bird (Denenberg 1981; Andrew 1983; Jason *et al.* 1984; Heffner and Heffner 1986; Rogers 1986). A variety of asymmetries between the right and left IMHV regions have been described in the preceding sections of this chapter. The functional significance of some of these asymmetries is discussed at length by McCabe (Chapter 9; see also Chapters 10, 11, 19, 20, 21). Briefly, and on the basis of a series of studies of imprinting, it has been proposed that (i) the left IMHV acts as a long-term store, (ii) the right IMHV acts as a temporary or buffer store, and (iii) the right IMHV passes information on to another long-term store (S′) over a period of several hours (Cipolla-Neto *et al.* 1982; Davey *et al.* 1987). We still do not know whether the left IMHV and S′ serve different functions in recognition memory. For example (see Horn 1985, pp. 143–7) if one region has the larger capacity, then it may store information which is contextually rich and which, more effectively than information stored in the other region, may be modified or extended through subsequent experience, and be used more flexibly, as in transferring experience gained in one situation to solving problems in another situation. Clearly further work is needed to clarify these issues. Further work may also clarify whether hemispheric asymmetries for topographical cues (Rashid and Andrew 1989; Chapters 19 and 21) relate to the functions of the left IMHV and S′.

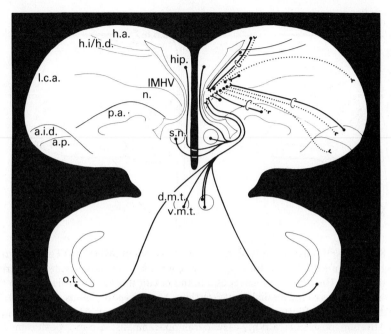

Fig. 8.5 Summary diagram of the connections of the IMHV. Afferent pathways are represented as continuous lines, efferent pathways as dotted lines. Many of the structures shown in the drawing do not lie in the same plane and the routes taken by the pathways do not all correspond to the actual route: the drawing is diagrammatic. Abbreviations: a.i.d., dorsal part of archistriatum intermedium; a.p., archistriatum posterior; d.m.t., dorsomedial thalamus; h.a., hyperstriatum accessorium; h.i./h.d., hyperstriatum intercalatum/hyperstriatum dorsale; hip., hippocampus; l.c.a., lateral cerebral area; n., neostriatum; o.t., optic tectum; p.a., paleostriatum augmentatum; s.n., septal nuclei; v.m.t., ventromedial thalamus (based on Bradley *et al*. 1985).

ANATOMICAL CONSIDERATIONS

The anatomical connections of the IMHV region of the domestic chick were investigated by Bradley *et al.* (1985) and by Davies and Horn (1983). A diagram summarizing the results of these studies is given in Fig. 8.5. As referred to above, IMHV receives projections from most telencephalic sensory receiving areas. The region projects to the archistriatum interme-dialis pars dorsalis. In pigeons the axons of perikarya in this nucleus project to the brainstem and spinal cord (Zeier and Karten 1971) so that this nucleus probably plays a major role in the forebrain control of motor function. Mishkin (1982) has suggested that in primates the hippocampal-amygdaloid complex plays an important part in memory functions. He has

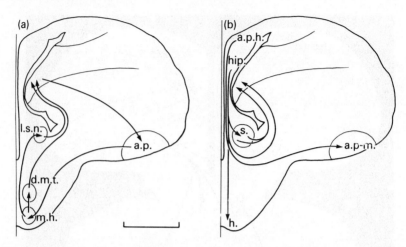

Fig. 8.6 Possible circuit involved in memory functions of IMHV. (a) The structures which are connected may form a circuit controlling various viscero-endocrine functions. (b) The hippocampus feeds into this circuit through its projections to the lateral (as well as to the medial) septal nucleus, to the hypothalamus and to IMHV. For the purposes of illustration only the left forebrain is drawn. Abbreviations: a.p., archistriatum posterior; a.p.h., area parahippocampalis; a.p-m., posteromedial aspect of archistriatum; d.m.t., dorsomedial thalamic nucleus; h, hypothalamus; hip, hippocampus; m.h., medial hypothalamus; l.s.n., lateral septal nucleus; s., medial and lateral septal nuclei. Scale bar 2 mm. (After Horn 1985.)

suggested a possible neural circuit through which this function is achieved. It is possible that a similar circuit exists in the avian brain (Fig. 8.6*a*,*b*). IMHV projects to the archistriatum (archistriatum posterior) which, together with the medial nucleus of this complex, is considered by Zeier and Karten (1971) to correspond to the mammalian amygdala (see Chapter 2). In the pigeon the posterior nucleus of the archistriatum projects to the hypothalamus (Zeier and Karten 1971). The medial part of the hypothalamus is connected to the lateral septal nucleus and the the dorsomedial nucleus of the thalamus (Berk and Butler 1981). In the chick both of these nuclei project to IMHV, so that if all the other connections are present, a 'circuit' is completed. Whether or not this is a functional circuit in the sense of having a specific role in cerebral function, perhaps in memory, is still to be investigated.

The connections of IMHV in the chick are strikingly similar to the connections described by Wallhäusser (personal communication) for MNH, strongly supporting the suggestion made above that at least the MH component of the MNH region is indeed part of IMHV.

The internal organization of IMHV as shown by a Golgi preparation has been the subject of several studies (Bradley and Horn 1982; Tomböl *et al.* 1988). A variety of cell types are present, but they are not organized into laminae as are, say, cells in the optic tectum or mammalian cerebral cortex, and immunocytochemical evidence suggests that inhibition and disinhibition may play important roles in the functioning of the region (Watson *et al.* 1990).

LEARNING AND PREDISPOSITIONS

In the course of a series of lesion studies chicks were trained by exposing them to a rotating red box or a stuffed jungle fowl. The chicks' preferences were measured in a test in which these two objects were presented in sequence (see p. 221 above). It was found that lesions to IMHV impaired the chicks' preferences irrespective of the training object used. However, the effect of the lesion on the preferences of box-trained chicks was very severe and they performed at chance in the preference test. The effects of the lesion on the preference of fowl-trained chicks was less severe: the fowl-trained chicks with IMHV lesions preferred the fowl to the box, though less strongly than did their sham-operated controls (Horn and McCabe 1984). A similar pattern of results was found after chicks had been given the neurotoxic drug DSP4 prior to training (Davies *et al.* 1985). This drug *inter alia* lowers forebrain noradrenalin levels. A different pattern of results was found when chicks were given an injection of testosterone before training. There was a correlation between plasma testosterone levels and preference score in chicks which had been trained by exposure to the fowl. There was no such correlation in the box-trained chicks (Bolhuis *et al.* 1986). These results taken together suggest that some of the neural systems which are engaged when chicks are trained to the fowl are different from those engaged when chicks are trained to the box. Horn and McCabe (1984) suggested that a region outside IMHV may respond to some general features possessed by conspecifics, but that IMHV is involved in learning the specific features of individuals—just as it is involved in learning to recognize artificial objects such as the box. Evidence to support this hypothesis has gradually accumulated and is reviewed by Johnson and Bolhuis in Chapter 5 (see also Johnson *et al.* 1985; Johnson and Horn 1988; Bolhuis *et al.* 1989*a, b*; Johnson *et al.* 1989). The predisposition may simply serve to draw the chick's attention to certain features of the head and neck of a parent, ensuring that the young chick learns to recognize the conspecific which will be important for the young bird's survival. Such learning in turn disposes the chick to act in one way rather than another—to follow the familiar conspecific object rather than an unfamiliar one. The situations to which the young bird is exposed and about which it learns will be different according to which object it follows, such choice necessarily limiting the range of the chick's subsequent experiences. Hence predispositions and dispositions, subtle though they may be, may profoundly affect the kind of information the bird acquires about the world. These constraints on learning are most unlikely to be restricted to birds (see, e.g. Hinde and Stevenson-Hinde 1973).

IMHV, EXPOSURE LEARNING AND ASSOCIATIVE LEARNING

When certain regions of the human brain, especially the medial temporal lobe/diencephalic areas are damaged, the patient may become amnesic, especially for events occurring after the lesion (Milner et al. 1968; Zola-Morgan et al. 1986). One of the features of the amnesic syndrome is that the patients perform poorly in tests involving recognition (Baddeley 1982) and they appear to be unfamiliar with objects and situations which they have previously experienced (Milner 1966; Milner 1989). This lesion-sensitive memory has variously been described as episodic (Tulving 1972), declarative (Cohen and Squire 1980), autobiographical (Jacoby and Dallas 1981), and mediational (Warrington and Weiskrantz 1982). The latter authors refer to a mediational memory system as one '. . . in which the memoranda can be manipulated, inter-related and stored in a continually changing record of events.' Some memories, however, are relatively insensitive to brain damage since the patients have various residual learning abilities. For example, they can acquire and retain simple visual discriminations (Sidman et al. 1968), they can learn to perform new skills (see Milner 1962; Milner et al. 1968) and they can be classically conditioned (Weiskrantz and Warrington 1979). The memories that underlie these residual learning abilities have been lumped together, by exclusion, as non-mediational (Horn 1985) or non-declarative (Squire 1987) memory or habit memory (James 1880; Malamut et al. 1984). In normal human subjects the mediational and non-mediational memory sytems may be presumed to interact: humans are not only able to learn, for example, new skills or discriminations but they are familiar with having done so (see, e.g. Milner et al. 1968; Schacter et al. 1988; Milner 1989). These consider-ations suggest that in intact human subjects, storage occurs in *both* habit memory and mediational memory, so that neuronal changes should occur in both systems. However, damage to the medial temporal lobe appears to make the mediational memory system inaccessible to information acquired after the lesion has occurred (Warrington and Weiskrantz 1982). There appear to be cases in which brain lesions have almost the converse effect, impairing habit memory without affecting mediational memory. Lesions in the posterior left hemisphere may be associated with apraxia in which there is a disturbance of purposeful movements not attributable *inter alia* to weakness, sensory loss or comprehension. In ideomotorapraxia the patient is unable to perform correctly skilled movements which had been learned prior to the onset of the pathology. It has been suggested that the lesion destroys the memory (habit memory) for the movements (for review see Heilman *et al.* 1987).

Whilst medial temporal lobe/diencephalic lesions impair some memories and spare others, the issue of defining precisely which are spared and which are not is far from being resolved; the answers depend much on the experimenters' ingenuity in devising tests of learning and retention, and much on the size and location(s) of the lesion (Weiskrantz 1982; Morton 1985; Squire and Shimamura 1986).

In the light of the difficulty in defining the residual learning abilities of human organic amnesics, it may come as no surprise that similar difficulties arise in defining the learning abilities of chicks with lesions of IMHV. Evidence that some dissociations occur has been given above (pp. 225–6); but there is also good evidence, some of which has been referred to in earlier sections of this chapter, that this brain region, in addition to its role in the recognition memory of imprinting, is also involved in passive avoidance learning (see also Chapters 9–12). IMHV is not the only region implicated in PAL, since metabolic changes associated with PAL were found in two other brain regions, the lobus paraolfactorius and the paleostriatum augmentatum (Kossut and Rose 1984; Rose and Csillag 1985). The evidence suggests that IMHV plays a necessary role in the acquisition of this task. Davies *et al.* (1988) placed bilateral electolytic lesions in IMHV and subsequently trained chicks on the peck-avoidance task. Sham-operated chicks and chicks with lesions placed outside IMHV avoided the bead when it was presented in the test; the IMHV-lesioned chicks, on average, did not do so and behaved as if they were amnesic. Patterson *et al.* (1990) have shown that it is sufficient to place a lesion unilaterally, in the left IMHV, before training to impair the ability of chicks to learn and retain the avoidance task. Patterson *et al.* (1990) went on to show that bilateral IMHV lesions placed either 1 or 6 hours after the training trial did not impair retention. These are very interesting findings since structural changes in IMHV are present as much as 24 hours after passive avoidance training (Stewart *et al.* 1984; Patel *et al.* 1988). If these changes reflect a long-term memory function for IMHV in passive avoidance learning then, considered together with the results of these lesion studies, they suggest that PAL involves more than one storage system (see p. 224 and Chapter 9). Recent work by Rose and his colleagues points to the lobus paraolfactorius as a second store for PAL (Rose, personal communication).

We are, however, still left with the puzzle that the acquisition of some associative learning tasks are not affected by IMHV lesions, whereas PAL is. In learning to perform this task, the chicks presumably associate the MeA-coated bead with an aversive taste; and when the bead is presented again they are reluctant to peck it. After lesions have been placed in IMHV and the birds trained with the MeA-coated bead, they show little reluctance to peck it again (Davies *et al.* 1988; Patterson *et al.* 1990). In this associative learning task there was only one training trial. In the associative learning tasks, the acquisition of which appeared to be unaffected by IMHV lesions, the chicks reached criterion after approximately 15 (McCabe *et al.* 1982) or approximately 30 (Johnson and Horn 1986) trials. It would be worth enquiring whether IMHV-lesioned chicks allowed to peck the MeA-coated bead repeatedly gradually cease to do so. Repetition may establish a habit, a simple stimulus–response relationship (see James 1890) whether of approach (McCabe *et al.* 1972; Johnson and Horn 1986) or avoidance (Davies *et al.* 1988; Patterson *et al.* 1990), in the absence of IMHV. In this connection it is of interest that Mishkin and his collaborators (Bechevalier and Mishkin 1984; Malamut *et al.* 1984) in their studies of the effects of brain lesions on the memories underlying various associative learning tasks, using rhesus monkeys, distinguished between the memory underlying habits established through multiple trials and the memory for trial-unique stimuli requiring one-trial learning. The memory underlying the latter form of learning they considered to be mediated by the limbic system, whereas the memory underlying habit was considered by them to be mediated by non-limbic structures (see Malamut *et al.* 1984, and Horn 1985, pp. 122–6 for further discussion). The limbic system-dependent memory probably involves the frontal lobes (see Warrington and Weiskrantz 1982; Janowsky *et al.* 1989) and the avian IMHV bears some—albeit tenuous—anatomical similarities with this region of the primate brain (Horn 1985, pp. 250–4). In the case of passive avoidance learning the lobus paraolfactorius may be implicated in the habit memory. The habit memory and the mediation memory system may lie in parallel, so that damage to the mediational system may have little effect on habit memory. However, damage to the mediational system may become apparent in at least two ways, (i) if the newly acquired information is to be used in a different learning task, or in a different context, and (ii) if the habit or skill to be acquired is particularly difficult or complex. In the latter case the mediational memory system may interact with the habit memory system whilst both are forming. Once the habit has been established the habit memory alone may be sufficient to support the skill. An anecdotal example is the acquisition and retention of the skill required to ride a bicycle. It is very difficult to acquire this competence, but once acquired riding a bicycle is very easy and indeed becomes 'automatic'. Here acquisition of the skill may draw on previous experiences and skills and so involve mediational memory. Retention of the skill, however, may depend only on habit memory until, say, a bicycle with a quite different set of gears is used, when mediational memory may once again be engaged.

CONCLUSION

Work on the neural basis of imprinting in chicks set out to continue Lashley's search for an engram. The search has had some modest success, at least in identifying a brain region in which, the evidence suggests, storage takes place, and in throwing light on the factors which influence storage (e.g. catecholamine levels, predispositions). However, the extent to which the evidence is convincing depends on the extent to which all the evidence is taken into account. It has for long been obvious that no single experiment can account for all the side-effects of training: one experiment controls for one set of side-effects, another experiment for another set. And so the sequence of investigations goes on, each result advancing knowledge on the shoulders of previous results. Within IMHV cellular and molecular changes occur after imprinting. There is evidence that some of the changes (e.g. in NMDA-sensitive binding) are closely tied to learning. The evidence for a close link with certain other changes is not so strong; it is necessary to gather further data to determine whether or not the link strengthens or weakens. However, even if a change is closely tied to learning it is still not clear precisely how the change relates to a memory trace itself. We are still not able to say whether Hebb's (1949) idea of a cell assembly as a '. . . representative process (image or idea)' (Hebb, p. 60) is correct or not; and if it is correct, to demonstrate the assembly either anatomically or functionally. Whilst computer models of neural networks successfully make use of similar representations to those of Hebb (for review see Rumelhart *et al.* 1986) for information storage, and are heuristically valuable, computers are not biological brains. If one is interested in the neural basis of learning and memory, there is no alternative to continuing the search for an engram in real nervous systems. I am optimistic that the resolution of these issues is within our grasp.

REFERENCES

Aggleton, J. P., Nicol, R. M., Huston, A. E., and Fairbairn, A. F. (1988). The performance of amnesic subjects on tests of experimental amnesia in animals: delayed matching to sample and concurrent learning. *Neuropsychologia*, **26**, 265–72.

Ali, S. M., Bullock, S., and Rose, S. P. R. (1988). Phosphorylation of synaptic proteins in chick forebrain: changes with development and passive avoidance training. *Journal of Neurochemistry*, **50**, 1579–88.

Andrew, R. J. (1964). Vocalization in chicks and the concept of 'stimulus' contrast. *Animal Behaviour*, **12**, 64–76.

Andrew, R. J. (1980). The functional organisation of phases of memory consolidation. *Advances in the Study of Behavior*, **11**, 337–67.

Andrew, R. J. (1983). Lateralisation of emotional and cognitive function in higher vertebrates, with special reference to the domestic chick. In *Advances in vertebrate neuroethology* (ed. J.-P. Ewert and D. J. Ingle). Plenum, New York.

Bachevalier, J. and Mishkin, M. (1984). An early and late developing system for learning and retention in infant monkeys. *Behavioral Neuroscience*, **98**, 770–8.

Baddeley, A. D. (1982). Implications of neuropsychological evidence for theories of normal memory. *Philosophical Transactions of the Royal Society of London Series B*, **298**, 59–72.

Baer, D. M. and Gray, P. H. (1960). Imprinting to different species without overt following. *Perceptual Motor Skills*, **10**, 171–4.

Bateson, P. P. G. (1966). The characteristics and context of imprinting. *Biological Reviews*, **41**, 177–220.

Bateson, P. P. G., Horn, G., and Rose, S. P. R. (1969). The effects of an imprinting procedure on regional incorporation of tritiated lysine into protein of chick brain. *Nature*, **223**, 534–5.

Bateson, P. P. G., Horn, G., and Rose, S. P. R. (1972). Effects of early experience on regional incorporation of precursors into RNA and protein in the chick brain. *Brain Research*, **39**, 449–65.

Bateson, P. P. G., Horn, G., and Rose, S. P. R. (1975). Imprinting: Correlations between behaviour and incorporation of [^{14}C]Uracil into chick brain. *Brain Research*, **84**, 207–20.

Bateson, P. P. G., Rose, S. P. R., and Horn, G. (1973). Imprinting: lasting effects on uracil incorporation into chick brain. *Science*, **181**, 576–8.

Bateson, P. P. G., and Jaeckel, J. B. (1976). Chick's preferences for familiar and novel conspicuous objects after different periods of exposure. *Animal Behaviour*, **24**, 386–90.

Bateson, P. P. G. and Reese, E. P. (1969). The reinforcing properties of conspicuous stimuli in the imprinting situation. *Animal Behaviour*, **17**, 692–9.

Benowitz, L. I. and Routtenberg, A. (1987). A membrane phosphoprotein associated with neural development, axonal regeneration, phospholipid metabolism, and snaptic plasticity. *Trends in Neuroscience*, **10**, 527–32.

Berk, M. and Butler, A. B. (1981). Efferent projections of the medial preoptic nucleus and medial hypothalamus in the pigeon. *Journal of Comparative Neurology*, **203**, 379–99.

Bolhuis, J. J. and Johnson, M. H. (1988). Effects of response-contingency and stimulus presentation schedule on imprinting in the chick (*Gallus gallus domesticus*). *Journal of Comparative Psychology*, **102**, 61–5.

Bolhuis, J. J., Johnson, M. H., and Horn, G. (1985). Effects of early experience on the development of filial preferences in the domestic chick. *Developmental Psychobiology*, **18**, 299–308.

Bolhuis, J. J. Johnson, M. H., and Horn, G. (1989*a*). Interacting mechanisms during the formation of filial preferences: the development of a predisposition does not prevent learning. *Journal of Experimental Psychology: Animal Behavior processes*, **15**, 376–82.

Bolhuis, J. J., Johnson, M., Horn, G., and Bateson, P. (1989*b*). Long-lasting effects of IMHV lesions on social preferences in domestic fowl. *Behavioral Neuroscience*, **103**, 438–41.

Bonke, B. A., Bonke, D., and Scheich, H. (1979). Connectivity in the auditory forebrain nuclei in the guinea fowl (*Numida meleagris*). *Cell Tissue Research*, **200**, 101–21.

Bradley, P. (1985). A light and electron microscopic study of the development of two regions of the chick forebrain. *Developmental Brain Research*, **20**, 83–8.

Bradley, P., Davies, D. C., and Horn, G. (1985). Connections of hyperstriatum ventrale in the domestic chick (*Gallus domesticus*). *Journal of Anatomy*, **140**, 577–89.

Bradley, P. and Horn, G. (1982). A Golgi analysis of the hyperstriatum ventrale in the chick. *Journal of Anatomy (London)*, **134**, 599–600.

Bradley, P., Horn, G., and Bateson, P. (1981). Imprinting: an electron microscopic study of chick hyperstriatum ventrale. *Experimental Brain Research*, **41**, 115–20.

Bradley, P., Horn, G., and Bateson, P. P. G. (1979). Morphological correlates of imprinting in the chick brain. *Neurosciences Letters Supplement*, **3**, S84.

Bradley, P. M., and Galal, K. M. (1987). The effects of protein synthesis inhibition on structural changes associated with learning in the chick. *Developmental Brain Research*, **37**, 267–76.

Bradley, P. M., and Galal, K. M. (1988). State-dependent recall can be induced by protein synthesis inhibition: behavioural and morphological observations. *Developmental Brain Research*, **40**, 243–51.

Brazier, M. A. B. (1961). Some effects of anaesthesia on the brain. *British Journal of Anaesthesia*, **33**, 194–204.

Brindley, G. S. and Lewin, W. S. (1968). The sensations produced by electrical stimulation of the visual cortex. *Journal of Physiology*, **196**, 479–93.

Broca, P. (1865). Sur la faculté du language articulé. *Bulletin du Societé d'Anthropologie (Paris)*, **6**, 337–93.

Brown, M. W. and Horn, G. (1977). Responsiveness of neurons in the hippocampal region of anaesthetised and unanaesthetised cats to stimulation of sensory pathways. *Brain Research*, **123**, 241–59.

Brown, M. W. and Horn, G. (1978). Context dependent neuronal responses recorded from hippocampal region of trained monkeys. *Journal of Physiology*, **282**, 15–16P.

Brown, M. W. and Horn, G. (1979). Neuronal plasticity in the chick brain: electrophysiological effects of visual experience on hyperstriatal neurons. *Brain Research*, **162**, 142–7.

Brown, M. W. and Horn, G. (1990). Are specific proteins implicated in the learning process of imprinting? *Developmental Brain Research*, **52**, 294–7.

Butler, R. A. (1953). Discrimination learning by rhesus monkeys to visual exploration stimulation. *Journal of Comparative Physiology and Psychology*, **46**, 95–8.

Cajal, S. R. (1911). *Histologie du système nerveux de l'homme et des vertebrés*, Vol. 2, Maloine, Paris.

Candland, D. K. (1969). Discriminability of facial regions used by the domestic chicken in maintaining the social dominance order. *Journal of Comparative Physiology and Psychology*, **69**, 281–5.

Cipolla-Neto, J., Horn, G., and McCabe, B. J. (1982). Hemispheric asymmetry and imprinting: the effect of sequential lesions to the hyperstriatum ventrale. *Experimental Brain Research*, **48**, 22–7.

Cline, H. T., Debski, E. A., and Constantine-Paton, M. (1987). N-methyl-D-aspartate receptor antagonist desegregates eye-specific stripes. *Proceedings of the National Academy of Sciences of the USA*, **84**, 4342–5.

Clutton-Brock, J. (1961). The importance of the central nervous effects of anaesthetic agents. *British Journal of Anaesthesia*, **33**, 214–18.

Cohen, N. J. and Squire, L. R. (1980). Preserved learning and retention of pattern analyzing skill in amnesia: dissociation of knowing how and knowing that. *Science*, **210**, 207–209.

Colebrook, E. and Lukowiak, K. (1988). Learning by the *Aplysia* model system: lack of correlation between gill and motor neuron responses. *Journal of Experimental Biology*, **135**, 411–29.

Collingridge, G. L. and Bliss, T. V. P. (1987). NMDA receptors—their role in long-term potentiation. *Trends in Neuroscience*, **10**, 288–93.

Collingridge, G. L., Kehl, S. J., and McLennan, H. (1983). Excitatory amino acids in synaptic transmission in the Schaffer collateral-commissural pathway of the rat hippocampus. *Journal of Physiology*, **334**, 33–46.

Davey, J. (1988). Imprinting and spontaneous activity in the hyperstriatum ventrale of the chick: a developing asymmetry. *Neuroscience Letters Supplement*, **32**, S46.

Davey, J., McCabe, B. J., and Horn, G. (1987). Mechanism of information storage after imprinting in the domestic chick. *Behavioral Brain Research*, **26**, 209–10.

Davies, D. C. and Horn, G. (1983). Putative cholinergic afferents of the chick hyperstriatum ventrale: a combined acetylcholinesterase and retrograde fluorescence labelling study. *Neuroscience Letters*, **38**, 103–7.

Davies, D. C., Horn, G., and McCabe, B. J. (1983). Changes in telencephalic catecholamine levels in the domestic chick. Effects of age and visual experience. *Developmental Brain Research*, **10**, 251–5.

Davies, D. C., Horn, G., and McCabe, B. J. (1985). Noradrenaline and learning: the effects of the noradrenergic neurotoxin DSP4 on imprinting in the domestic chick. *Behavioral Neuroscience*, **100**, 51–6.

Davies, D. C., Taylor, D. A., and Johnson, M. H. (1988). The effects of hyperstriatal lesions on one-trial passive-avoidance learning in the chick. *Journal of Neuroscience*, **8**, 4662–6.

Davies, S. N., Lester, A. J., Reyman, K. G., and Collingridge, G. L. (1989). Temporally distinct pre- and postsynaptic mechanisms maintain long-term potentiation. *Nature*, **338**, 500–3.

Denenberg, V. H. (1981). Hemispheric laterality in animals and the effects of early experience. *Behavioral and Brain Sciences*, **4**, 1-49.

Desmond, N. L. and Levy, W. B. (1986). Changes in the postsynaptic density with long-term potentiation in the dentate gyrus. *Journal of Comparative Neurology*, **253**, 476–82.

Dubé, L. and Parent, A. (1981). The monoamine-containing neurons in the avian brain: 1. A study of the brain stem of the chicken (*Gallus domesticus*) by means of fluorescence and acetylcholinesterase histochemistry. *Journal of Comparative Neurology*, **196**, 695–708.

Errington, M. L., Lynch, M. A., and Bliss, T. V. P. (1987). Long-term potentiation in the dentate gyrus: induction and increased glutamate release are blocked by D(-)aminophonovalerate. *Neuroscience*, **20**, 279–94.

Evarts, E. V. (1967). Unit activity in sleep and wakefulness. In *The neurosciences. A study program.* (ed. G. C. Quarton, T. Melnechuk, and F. O. Schmit), pp. 545–56. The Rockefeller University Press, New York.

Fagg, G. E. and Matus, A. (1984). Selective association of N-methyl aspartate and quisqualate types of L-glutamate receptor with postsynaptic densities. *Proceedings of the National Academy of Sciences of the USA*, **81**, 6876–80.

Foerster, O. (1929). Beiträge zur Pathophysiologie der Sehbahn under der Sehsphäre. *Journal of Psychology and Neurology of Leipzig*, **39**, 463–85.

Freed, D. M., Corkin, S., and Cohen, N. J. (1987). Forgetting in H.M.: a second look. *Neuropsychologia*, **25**, 461–71.

Geschwind, N. and Levitsky, W. (1968). Human brain: left-right asymmetries in temporal speech region. *Science*, **161**, 186–7.

Gusel'nikov, V. I., Morenkov, E. D., and Khun, D. C. (1976). Responses and properties of receptive fields of neurons in the visual projection zone of the pigeon hyperstriatum. *Neirofiziologiya*, **8**, 230–6.

Hawkins, R. D., Abrams, T. W., Carew, T. J., and Kandel, E. R. (1983). A cellular mechanism of classical conditioning in *Aplysia*: activity-dependent amplication of presynaptic facilitation. *Science*, **219**, 400–5.

Hebb, D. O. (1949). *The organization of behavior.* Wiley, New York.

Heffner, H. E. and Heffner, R. S. (1986). Effect of unilateral and bilateral auditory cortex lesions on the discrimination of vocalizations by Japanese macaques. *Journal of Neurophysiology*, **56**, 683–701.

Heilman, K. M., Rothi, L. J. G., and Watson, R. T. (1987). Apraxia: disorders of skilled movement. In *Clinical neurology* (ed. M. Swash and J. Oxbury). Churchill Livingstone, Edinburgh.

Hinde, R. A. (1962). Some aspects of the imprinting problem. In *Evolutionary aspects of animal communications: imprinting and early learning*, pp. 129–38. Symposium of the Zoological Society of London, London.

Hinde, R. A. and Stevenson-Hinde, J. (ed.) (1973). *Constraints on learning.* Academic Press, London.

Horn, G. (1962). Some neural correlates of perception. In *Viewpoints in biology* (ed. J. D. Carthy and C. L. Duddington), pp. 242–85. Butterworths, London.

Horn, G. (1965). Physiological and psychological aspects of selective perception. In *Advances in the study of behavior*, (ed. D. Lehrman, R. A. Hinde, and E. Shaw), Vol. 1, pp. 155–215. Academic Press, New York.

Horn, G. (1970). Changes in neuronal activity and their relationship to behaviour. In *Short-term changes in neural activity and behaviour* (ed. G. Horn and R. A. Hinde), pp. 567–606. Cambridge University Press.

Horn, G. (1981). Neural mechanisms of learning: an analysis of imprinting in the domestic chick. *Proceedings of the Royal Society of London Series B*, **213**, 101–37.

Horn, G. (1985). *Memory, imprinting, and the brain.* Clarendon Press, Oxford.

Horn, G., Bradley, P., and McCabe, B. J. (1985). Changes in the structure of synapses associated with learning. *Journal of Neuroscience*, **5**, 3161–8.

Horn, G., Horn, A. D., Bateson, P. P. G., and Rose, S. P. R. (1971). Effects of imprinting on uracil incorporation into brain RNA in the 'split-brain' chick. *Nature*, **229**, 131–2.

Horn, G. and McCabe, B. J. (1978). An autoradiographic method for studying the incorporation of uracil into acid-insoluble compounds in the brain. *Journal of Physiology*, **275**, 2–3P.

Horn, G. and McCabe, B. J. (1984). Predispositions and preferences. Effects on imprinting of lesions to the chick brain. *Animal Behaviour*, **32**, 288–92.

Horn, G. and McCabe, B. J. (1990). The time course of N-methyl-D-aspartate (NMDA) receptor binding in chick brain after imprinting. *Journal of Physiology*, **423**, 92P.

Horn, G., McCabe, B. J., and Bateson, P. P. G. (1979). An autoradiographic study of the chick brain after imprinting. *Brain Research*, **168**, 361–73.

Horn, G., Rose, S. P. R., and Bateson, P. P. G. (1973a). Monocular imprinting and regional incorporation of tritiated uracil into the brains of intact and 'split-brain' chicks. *Brain Research*, **56**, 227–37.

Horn, G., Rose, S. P. R., and Bateson, P. P. G. (1973b). Experience and plasticity in the central nervous system. *Science*, **181**, 506–14.

Horn, G. and Wiesenfield, Z. (1974). Attentive behaviour in the cat: electrophysiological and behavioural studies. *Experimental Brain Research*, **21**, 67–82.

Hubel, D. H. and Wiesel, T. N. (1970). The period of susceptibility to the physiological effects of unilateral eye closure in kittens. *Journal of Physiology*, **206**, 419–36.

Jacobson, R. D., Virág, I., and Skene, J. H. P. (1986). A protein associated with axon growth, GAP-43, is widely distributed and developmentally regulated in rat CNS. *Journal of Neuroscience*, **6**, 1843–55.

Jacoby, L. L. and Dallas, M. (1981). On the relationship between autobiographical memory and perceptual learning. *Journal of Experimental Psychology*, **3**, 306–40.

James, W. J. (1880). *The principles of psychology*. Henry Holt, New York.

Jankowsky, J. S., Shimamura, A. P., and Squire, L. R. (1989). Source memory impairment in patients with frontal lobe lesions. *Neuropsychologia*, **27**, 1043–56.

Jason, G. W., Cowey, A., and Weiskrantz, L. (1984). Hemispheric asymmetry for a visuo-spatial task in monkeys. *Neuropsychologia*, **22**, 777–84.

Johnson, M. H., Bolhuis, J. and Horn, G. (1985). Interaction between acquired preferences and developing predispositions during imprinting. *Animal Behaviour*, **33**, 1000–6.

Johnson, M. H., Davies, D. C., and Horn, G. (1989). A sensitive period for the development of a predisposition in dark-reared chicks. *Animal Behaviour*, **37**, 1044–5.

Johnson, M. H. and Horn, G. (1986). Dissociation of recognition memory and associative learning by a restricted lesion of the chick forebrain. *Neuropsychologia*, **24**, 329–40.

Johnson, M. H. and Horn, G. (1987). The role of a restricted region of the chick forebrain in the recognition of individual conspecifics. *Behavioral Brain Research*, **23**, 269–75.

Johnson, M. H. and Horn, G. (1988). Development of filial preferences in dark-reared chicks. *Animal Behaviour*, **36**, 675–83.

Kendrick, K. M., and Baldwin, B. A. (1987). Cells in temporal cortex of conscious sheep can respond preferentially to the sight of faces. *Science*, **236**, 448–50.

Kitt, C. A. and Brauth, S. E. (1986). Telencephalic projections from midbrain and isthmal cell groups in the pigeon. II The nigral complex. *Journal of Comparative Neurology*, **247**, 92–110.

Kleinschmidt, A., Bear, M. F., and Singer, W. (1987). Blockade of 'NMDA' receptors disrupts experience-dependent plasticity of kitten striate cortex. *Science*, **238**, 355–8.

Klopfer, P., and Hailman, J. P. (1964). Perceptual preferences and imprinting in chicks. *Science*, **145**, 1333–4.

Knudsen, E. I. and Knudsen, P. F. (1986). The sensitive period for auditory localisation in barn owls is limited by age, not by experience. *Journal of Neuroscience*, **6**, 1918–24.

Kohsaka, S.-I., Takamatsu, K., Aoki, E., and Tsukada, Y. (1979). Metabolic mapping of chick brain after imprinting using [^{14}C]2-deoxyglucose. *Brain Research*, **172**, 539–44.

Konishi, M. (1985). Birdsong: from behavior to neuron. *Annual Review of Neuroscience*, **8**, 125–70.

Konorski, J. (1948). *Conditioned reflexes and neuron organization*. Cambridge University Press.

Kossut, M. and Rose, S. P. R. (1984). Differential 2-deoxyglucose uptake into chick brain structures during passive avoidance training. *Neuroscience*, **12**, 971–7.

Lashley, K. S. (1950). In search of the engram. *Symposia of the Society for Experimental Biology*, **4**, 454–82.

Lee Teng, E. and Sherman, S. M. (1966). Memory consolidation of one-trial learning in chicks. *Proceedings of the National Academy of Sciences of the USA*, **56**, 926–31.

Leonard, J. L., Edstron, J. E. and Lukowiak, K. (1989). Re-examination of the gill withdrawal reflex of *Aplysia california* Cooper (Gastropoda; Opisthobranchia). *Behavioral Neuroscience*, **103**, 585–604.

MacDermot, A. B., Mayer, M. L., Westbrook, G. L., Smith, F. J., and Barker, J. L. (1986). NMDA-receptor adrenalin increased cytoplasmic calcium concentration in cultured spine neurons. *Nature*, **321**, 519–22.

Machlis, L., Dodd, P. W. D., and Fentress, J. C. (1985). The pooling fallacy: problems arising when individuals contribute more than one observation to the data set. *Zeitschrift für Tierpsychologie*, **68**, 201–14.

Maier, V., and Scheich, H. (1983). Acoustic imprinting leads to differential 2-deoxy-D-glucose uptake in the chick forebrain. *Proceedings of the National Academy of Sciences of the USA*, **80**, 3860–4.

Malamut, B. L., Saunders, R. C., and Mishkin, M. (1984). Monkeys with combined amygdalo-hippocampal lesions succeed in object discrimination learning despite 24-hour intertrial intervals. *Behavioral Neuroscience*, **98**, 659–69.

Maragos, W. F., Greenamyre, J.-T., Penney Jr, J. B., and Young, A. B. (1987). Glutamate dysfunction in Alzheimer's disease: an hypothesis. *Trends in Neuroscience*, **10**, 65–8.

Margoliash, D. (1986). Preference for autogenous song by auditory neurons in a

258   G. Horn

song system nucleus of the white crowned sparrow. *Journal of Neuroscience*, **6**, 1643–61.

McCabe, B. J., Cipolla-Neto, J., Horn, G., and Bateson, P. P. G. (1982). Amnesic effects of bilateral lesions placed in the hyperstriatum ventrale of the chick after imprinting. *Experimental Brain Research*, **48**, 13–21.

McCabe, B. J. and Horn, G. (1988). Learning and memory: regional changes in N-methyl-D-aspartate receptors in the chick brain after imprinting. *Proceedings of the National Academy of Sciences of the USA*, **85**, 2849–53.

McCabe, B. J. and Horn, G. (1991). Synaptic transmission and recognition memory: time course of changes in *N*-methyl-D-aspartate receptors after imprinting. *Behavioral Neuroscience*. (In press.)

McCabe, B. J., Horn, G., and Bateson, P. P. G (1981). Effects of restricted lesions of the chick forebrain on the acquisition of filial preferences during imprinting. *Brain Research*, **205**, 29–37.

McCabe, B. J., Horn, G., and Bateson, P. P. G. (1979). Effects of rhythmic hyperstriatal stimulation on chicks' preferences for visual flicker. *Physiology and Behavior*, **23**, 137–40.

McCormick, D. A. (1989). Cholinergic and noradrenergic modulation of thalamocortical processing. *Trends in Neuroscience*, **12**, 215–21.

McLennan, J. G. and Horn, G. (1990). Stimulus-dependent modification of response properties of neurons in IMHV after imprinting. In preparation.

Milner, B. (1966). Amnesia following operation on the temporal lobes. In *Amnesia*. (ed. C. W. M. Whitty and O. L. Zangwill). Butterworths, London.

Milner, B. (1962). Les troubles de la mémoire accompagnant des lésions hippo-campiques bilatérales. In *Physiologié de l'Hippocampe*, pp. 257–72. CNRS Colloques Internationaux No 107, Paris.

Milner, B., Corkin, S., and Teuber, H. L. (1968). Further analysis of the hippocampal amnesia syndrome: 14-year follow-up study of H.M. *Neuropsychologia*, **6**, 215–34.

Milner, P. M. (1989). A cell assembly theory of hippocampal amnesia. *Neuropsychologia*, **27**, 23–30.

Mishkin, M. (1982). A memory system in the monkey. In *The Neuropsychology of cognitive function* (ed. D. E. Broadbent and L. Weiskrantz), pp. 85–96. The Royal Society, London.

Mondadori, C., Weiskrantz, L., Buerki, H., Petschke, F., and Fagg, G. E. (1989). NMDA receptor antagonists can enhance or impair learning performance in animals. *Experimental Brain Research*, **75**, 449–56.

Mora, R., Rolls, E. T., and Burton, M. J. (1976). Modulation during learning of the responses of neurons in the hypothalamus to the sight of food. *Experimental Neurology*, **53**, 508–19.

Morenkov, E. D. and Khun, D. K. (1977). Neuronal responses to visual stimulation in the hyperstriatal area of the brain of the crow *Corvus corone*. *Journal of Evolutionary Biochemistry and Physiology*, **13**, 51–5.

Morris, R. G., Anderson, E., Lynch, G. S., and Baudry, M. (1986). Selective impairment of learning and blockade of long-term potentiation by an N-methyl-D-aspartate receptor antagonist, APS. *Nature*, **319**, 774–6.

Morris, R. G. M. (1989). Synaptic plasticity, neural architecture, and forms of memory. In *Brain organization and memory: cells, systems, and circuits* (ed. J.

L. McGaugh, N. M. Weinberger, and G. Lynch). Oxford University Press, New York.

Mountcastle, V. B. (1976). The world around us: neural command functions for selective attention. *Neurosciences Research Program Bulletin*, **14**, Supplement.

Müller, C. M. and Leppelseck, H. -J. (1985). Feature extraction and tonotopic organisation in the avian auditory forebrain. *Experimental Brain Research*, **59**, 587–99.

Nafstad, P. H. J. (1967). An electron microscopy study of the termination of the perforant path fibers in the hippocampus and the fascia dentata. *Zeitschrift für Zellforschung*, **307**, 532–42.

Nowak, L., Bregestovski, P., Ascher, P., Herbert, A., and Prochiantz, A. (1984). Magnesium gates glutamate-activated channels in mouse central neurons. *Nature*, **307**, 462–5.

Olson, C. R. and Freeman, R. D. (1980). Profile of the sensitive period for monocular deprivation in kittens. *Experimental Brain Research*, **39**, 17–21.

Patel, S. N., Rose, S. P. R., and Stewart, M. G. (1988). Training induced dendritic spine density changes are specifically related to memory formation processes in the chick, *Gallus domesticus. Brain Research*, **463**, 168–73.

Patel, S. N. and Stewart, M. G. (1988). Changes in the number and structure of dendritic spines 25 hours after passive avoidance training in the domestic chick, *Gallus domesticus. Brain Research*, **449**, 34–46.

Patterson, T. A., Gilbert, D. B., and Rose, S. P. R. (1990). Pre- and post-training lesions of the intermediate medial hyperstriatum ventrale and passive avoidance learning in the chick. *Experimental Brain Research*, **80**, 189–95.

Payne, J. K. and Horn, G. (1982). Differential effects of exposure to an imprinting stimulus on 'spontaneous' neuronal activity in two regions of the chick brain. *Brain Research*, **232**, 191–3.

Payne, J. K. and Horn, G. (1984). Long-term consequences of exposure to an imprinting stimulus on 'spontaneous' impulse activity in the chick brain. *Behavioural Brain Research*, **13**, 155–62.

Payne, J. K., Horn, G., and Brown, M. W. (1984). Modifiability of responsiveness in a visual projection area of the chick brain: visual experience is only one of several factors involved. *Behavioural Brain Research*, **13**, 163–72.

Penfield, W. and Rasmussen, T. (1952). *The cerebral cortex of man.* Macmillan, New York.

Perrett, D., Smith, P. A. J., Potter, D. D., Mistlin, A. J., Head, A. S., Milner, A. D., and Jeeves, M. A. (1985). Visual cells in the temporal cortex sensitive to face view and gaze direction. *Proceedings of the Royal Society of London, Series B*, **223**, 293–317.

Peters, A., Palary, S. L., and Webster, H. de F. (1976). *The fine structure of the nervous system.* Saunders, Philadelphia, Penn.

Rashid, N. and Andrew, R. J. (1989). Right hemisphere advantage for topographical orientation in the domestic chick. *Neuropsychologia*, **27**, 937–48.

Rauschecker, J. P. and Hahn, S. (1987). Ketamine-xylazine anaesthesia blocks consolidation of ocular dominance. *Nature*, **326**, 183–5.

Rogers, L. J. (1986). Lateralization of learning in chicks. *Advances in the Study of Behavior*, **16**, 147–89.

Roland, P. E. and Friberg, L. (1985). Localization of cortical areas activated by thinking. *Journal of Neurophysiology*, **53**, 1219–43.

Rose, S. P. R. and Csillag, A. (1985). Passive avoidance training results in lasting changes in deoxyglucose metabolism in left hemisphere regions of chick brain. *Behavioral and Neural Biology*, **44**, 315–24.

Rostas, J. A. P., Brent, V. A., and Guldner, F. H. (1984). The maturation of postsynaptic densities in chick forebrain. *Neuroscience Letters*, **45**, 297–304.

Rothman, S. M. and Olney, J. W. (1987). Excitotoxicity and the NMDA receptor. *Trends in Neuroscience*, **10**, 299–302.

Rumelhart, D. E., McClelland, J. L., and the PDP Research Group (1986). *Parallel distributed processing: exploration and the microstructure of cognition*, Vols I and II. MIT Press. Cambridge, Mass.

Schacter, D. L., McAndrews, M. P., and Moscovitch, M. (1988). Access to consciousness: dissociations between implicit and explicit knowledge in neuropsychological syndrome. In *Thought without language* (ed. L. Weiskrantz). Clarendon Press, Oxford.

Sidman, M., Stoddard, L. T., and Mohr, J. P. (1968). Some additional quantitative observations of immediate memory in a patient with bilateral hippocampal lesions. *Neuropsychologia*, **6**, 245–54.

Skene, J. H. P. (1984). Growth associated proteins and the curious dichotomies of nerve regeneration. *Cell*, **37**, 697–700.

Sluckin, W. (1972). *Imprinting and early learning*. Methuen, London.

Sluckin, W. and Salzen, E. A. (1961). Imprinting and perceptual learning. *Quarterly Journal of Experimental Psychology*, **13**, 65–77.

Spalding, D. A. (1983). Instinct, with original observations on young animals. *Macmillan's Magazine*, **27**, 282–93. Reprinted in 1954 in *British Journal of Animal Behaviour*, **2**, 2–11.

Squire, L. R. (1987). *Memory and brain*. Oxford University Press, New York.

Squire, L. R. and Shimamura, A. P. (1986). Characterizing amnesic patients for neurobehavioural study. *Behavioral Neuroscience*, **100**, 866–7.

Stewart, M. G., Rose, S. P. R., King, T. S., Gabbott, P. L. A., and Bourne, R. (1984). Hemispheric asymmetry of synapses in chick medial hyperstriatum ventrale following passive avoidance training: a stereological investigation. *Developmental Brain Research*, **12**, 261–9.

Takamatsu, K. and Tsukada, Y. (1985). Neurobiological bases of imprinting in chick and duckling. In *Perspectives on neuroscience. From molecule to mind* (ed. Y. Tsukada). University Tokyo Press.

Tanzi, E. (1893). I fatti e le induzioni nell' odierna istologia del sistema nervoso. *Riv. sper. Freniat. Med. leg Alien. ment*, **19**, 419–72.

ten Cate, C. (1986). Does behaviour contingent stimulus movement enhance filial imprinting in Japanese quail? *Developmental Psychobiology*, **19**, 607–14.

Teyler, T. J. and DiScenna, P. (1987). Long-term potentiation. *Annual Review of Neuroscience*, **10**, 131–61.

Tömböl, T., Csillag, A., and Stewart, M. G. (1988). Cell types of the hyperstriatum ventral of the domestic chicken (*Gallus domesticus*): a Golgi study. *Journal für Hirnforschung*, **3**, 319–34.

Tulving, E. (1972). Episodic and semantic memory. In *Organisation of memory*. (ed. E. Tulving and W. Donaldson), pp. 382–403. Academic Press, New York.

Wallhäusser, E. and Scheich, H. (1987). Auditory imprinting leads to differential 2-deoxyglucose uptake and dendritic spine loss in the chick rostral forebrain. *Developmental Brain Research*, **31**, 29–44.

Warrington, E. K. and Weiskrantz, L. (1982). Amnesia: a disconnection syndrome? *Neuropsychologia*, **20**, 233–48.

Watson, A., McCabe, B. J., and Horn, G. (1990). A quantitative analysis of the distribution of GABA-like immunoreactivity in the intermediate and medial part of the hyperstriatum ventrale of the chick. *Journal of Neurocytology* (in press).

Weibel, E. R. and Bolender, R. P. (1973). Stereological techniques for electron microscopic morphometry. In *Principles and techniques of electron microscopy, biological applications*, Vol. 3, (ed. M. A. Hayat), pp. 237–96. Van Nostrand Reinhold, London.

Weiskrantz, L. (1982). Comparative aspects of amnesia. *Philosophical Transactions of the Royal Society of London Series B*, **298**, 97–109.

Weiskrantz, L. and Warrington, E. K. (1979). Conditioning in amnesic patients. *Neuropsychologia*, **17**, 187–94.

Wenk, G. L., Grey, C. M., Ingram, D. K., Spangler, E. L., and Olton, D. S.(1989). Retention performance inversely correlates with *N*-methyl-D-Aspartate receptor number in hippocampus and frontal neocortex in the rat. *Behavioral Neuroscience*, **103**, 688–90.

Wilson, P. (1980). The organisation of the visual hyperstriatum in the domestic chick. II. Receptive field properties of single units. *Brain Research*, **188**, 333–45.

Wu, J., London, J. A., Zecevic, D., Höpp, H. -P., Cohen, L. B., and Xiao, C. (1988). Optical monitoring of activity of many neurons in invertebrate ganglia during behaviors. *Experientia*, **44**, 369–76.

Wurtz, R. H., Goldberg, M. E., and Robinson, D. L. (1980). Behavioural modulation of visual responses in the monkey: stimulus selection for attention and movement. In *Progress in psychobiology and physiological psychology*, Vol. 9 (ed. J. M. Sprague and A. N. Epstein), pp. 43–83. Academic Press, New York.

Zeier, H. and Karten, H. J. (1971). The archistriatum of the pigeon: organization of afferent and efferent connections. *Brain Research*, **31**, 313–26.

Zola-Morgan, S., Squire, L. R., and Amaral, D. G. (1986). Human amnesia and the medial temporal region: enduring memory impairment following a bilateral lesion limited to field CA1 of the hippocampus. *Journal of Neuroscience*, **6**, 2950–67.

9

Hemispheric asymmetry of learning-induced changes

B. J. McCabe

B. J. McCabe

INTRODUCTION

Other chapters in this book describe changes that occur in the brain of the chick when learning takes place, and there is strong evidence that some of these changes are specifically related to memory. It is now clear that some of the changes implicated in memory do not occur equally in the left and right sides of the brain; indeed some may only be detected unilaterally. These considerations suggest that, for some brain regions, one side has a role in learning and/or memory different from that of its contralateral counterpart. Why should there be these hemispheric asymmetries? Are they common to different types of learning in the chick? Are their neural bases common to other vertebrates?

Before attempting to answer these questions, it is useful to discuss the criteria by which one may judge whether hemispheric asymmetry in a learning-related change is present. It is of course important to determine whether a particular change in the brain is specific to learning; this matter is discussed in depth elsewhere in this volume (Chapters 8 and 10) and will further be referred to below. Once evidence of such specificity has been obtained, how does one determine whether an effect of training exhibits hemispheric asymmetry? The most reasonable criterion is that the change in the left hemisphere should be significantly different from that in the right hemisphere or, equivalently, that there should be a significant interaction between the training factor and the hemisphere factor. Generally speaking, statistical tests for an interaction in a factorial experiment are less sensitive than tests for a corresponding main effect because their associated standard errors are larger (Snedecor and Cochran 1982). Such is the variability in results from experiments relating neural events to behaviour that samples often need to be quite large before a treatment x hemisphere interaction can be detected. If there is no significant interaction one may be able to draw the still useful conclusion that there is evidence for an effect in at least one hemisphere.

One may detect asymmetric changes following learning directly by making localised morphological, biochemical or physiological measurements.

Alternatively, lateralization may be revealed by measuring the susceptibility of behaviour to small lesions or to locally applied drugs. Finally, taking advantage of the completely crossed optic chiasm, knowledge of the anatomy of the sensory pathways and behavioural evidence of asymmetric use of the eyes, one can 'instruct' or 'interrogate' systems presumed to reside in different sides of the brain by restricting sensory input to one side during training and/or testing. The chapter by Andrew (19) discusses the grounds for inferring unilateral information processing when one eye is occluded. There are usually considerable advantages in using a combination of the above approaches rather than any one alone. I shall first discuss changes which occur in the brain of the chick following imprinting, changes which are closely associated with learning and which are lateralized. Second, the way in which these results were followed up using lesioning techniques will be described, illustrating the advantages of combining complementary techniques. Third, a comparison will be made between the results from imprinting and those obtained in studies of other types of learning, in an attempt to define the similarities and differences between them. Particular attention will be given to passive avoidance learning (PAL). Fourth, these results will be considered in relation to studies of PAL in which information about lateralization has been sought by training and/or testing with one eye occluded. One important principle which emerges from these considerations is that hemispheric asymmetry can be dynamic: the manifestations of right and left hemisphere function are likely to change separately with time.

HEMISPHERIC ASYMMETRY IN THE INTERMEDIATE AND MEDIAL PART OF THE HYPERSTRIATUM VENTRALE (IMHV) IN RELATION TO IMPRINTING

There is strong evidence to suggest that the IMHV plays a crucial role in the learning process of imprinting and is a site of information storage (see Horn 1985; Chapter 8). A series of quantitative electron microscope studies were undertaken to determine whether morphological changes in synapses occur as a result of imprinting. Imprinting was found to be associated with a significant increase in the mean length of the profiles of postsynaptic densities (PSDs) of axospinous synapses in the left IMHV. There was no significant effect of training on mean PSD length in the right IMHV and there was a significant interaction between training condition and hemisphere (Bradley *et al.* 1979, 1981; Horn *et al.* 1985). A hemispheric asymmetry was thus found in IMHV following imprinting, in a morphological feature likely to reflect synaptic function.

Since at least some axospinous synapses in the vertebrate central nervous system bear glutamate receptors (see, e.g. Nafstad 1967; Erring-ton *et al.* 1987), the binding of L-[^{3}H]glutamate to membranes from IMHV was studied (McCabe and Horn 1988; see Chaper 8). The conditions of the binding assay were chosen so as to be conducive to the labelling of synaptic receptors. Imprinting was found to be associated with a 59 per cent increase in presumed NMDA receptor number in the left IMHV, and the amount of this binding was significantly correlated with the behavioural index used as a measure of the strength of imprinting. In the right IMHV there was no significant effect of training on binding, and no significant correlation between this binding and the strength of imprinting. The results of these experiments implicate the IMHV even more strongly in processes critical for learning and/or memory, parallel the results from the quantitative electron microscope study and provide another example of lateralization in IMHV.

LESION EXPERIMENTS SHOWING A HEMISPHERIC ASYMMETRY IN IMHV

Since the changes in synaptic morphology and L-[^{3}H]glutamate binding following imprinting were found only in the left IMHV, is it just the left IMHV which is important for imprinting? This matter was investigated by making localized lesions in either or both sides of IMHV by electrocoagu-lation. In each experiment, chicks were trained by being exposed to an imprinting stimulus: half of the chicks in each batch were exposed to a rotating red box and the remaining chicks were exposed to a rotating stuffed jungle fowl. The strength of imprinting was measured by sub-sequently giving each chick a preference test, in which the chick was exposed sequentially to each stimulus. A preference score was then derived thus:

$$\frac{\text{Approach to training stimulus} \times 100}{\text{Approach to training stimulus} + \text{Approach to alternative stimulus}}$$

The balanced experimental design permitted one to infer that learning had occurred if the preference scores for box-trained and fowl-trained chicks did not differ significantly from each other and, when combined, were significantly greater than 50. This was the case for sham-operated chicks in all experiments. If the preference scores of lesioned chicks were significantly lower than those of their corresponding shams and not significantly different from 50, the lesioned chicks were inferred to be amnesic.

Bilateral ablation of IMHV before training (i.e. exposure to an imprinting stimulus) was found to prevent imprinting, while having no detectable effect on measures of visuomotor co-ordination, or the acquisition of certain associative tasks (McCabe *et al.* 1981; McCabe *et al* 1982; Johnson and Horn 1986). Bilateral ablation less than 3 hours after training was found to render the chicks apparently amnesic for the training stimulus (McCabe *et al.* 1982); see Fig. 9.1*a*. Bilateral lesions to the forebrain visual projection area hyperstriatum accessorium (HA) were without effect on acquisition (Johnson and Horn 1987) or retention (McCabe *et al.* 1982) of a preference acquired through imprinting. One or both sides of IMHV are therefore critical for acquisition and retention.

THE EFFECTS OF SEQUENTIAL UNILATERAL ABLATION OF IMHV

A simple explanation which is consistent with the results described so far is that only the left IMHV is involved in storage. One would predict from this hypothesis that ablation of the left IMHV after training should result in amnesia and that ablation of the right IMHV after training should not. This hypothesis was tested in a series of experiments in which the right and left IMHVs were ablated sequentially after training (Cipolla-Neto *et al.* 1982). It was found that if the right IMHV was destroyed < 3 hours after training, the animal showed retention. After the remaining left IMHV was destroyed, the chicks were amnesic. This result (Fig. 9.1*b*) is consistent with the simple hypothesis outlined above. However, when the left IMHV was lesioned < 3 hours after training, there was no amnesia; and if the remaining right IMHV was lesioned after the left, the chicks continued to show retention (Fig. 9.1*c*).

Thus, although in all experimental chicks the IMHV had been destroyed bilaterally by the end of the experiment, the ability of chicks to retain a preference depended on the order in which the left and right sides of the IMHV had been ablated. Two principal conclusions were drawn from these results. First, since bilateral destruction of IMHV < 3 hours after training evidently gives rise to amnesia whereas destruction of the left IMHV alone at this time does not, presumably the right IMHV can support retention. Second, the results revealed a functional asymmetry in IMHV, an asymmetry in which both the left and the right IMHV participate in retention. Clearly the simple hypothesis is insufficient.

A model was developed in order to account for these results (Fig. 9.2). The available evidence indicates strongly that IMHV is a site of information storage for imprinting (Horn 1985). Since the morphological results (and, as is now known, the receptor binding effects) were restricted to the left IMHV, the left IMHV was proposed to be a site of storage of information about the training stimulus. It was also suggested that the

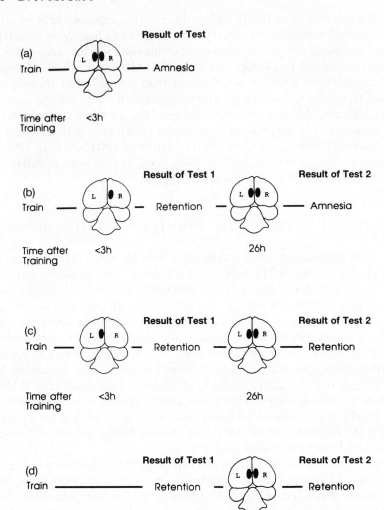

Fig. 9.1 Here and in Fig. 9.3, time progresses from left to right; the surgical procedure is shown on a diagram of the chick brain, the left and right forebrain hemispheres being denoted by L and R, respectively. Lesions to IMHV are shown in black. Below the diagram is given the average time in hours, after the end of training, that the lesions were made. The result of the preference test, conducted approximately 18 hours after surgery, is also given. (a) The effects on retention of bilateral ablation of IMHV < 3 hours after training. (b) The effects of lesioning first the right and then the left IMHV. (c) The effects of performing the unilateral lesions in reverse order. (d) The effect of lesioning both the right and left IMHV 26 hours after training.

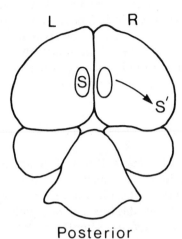

Posterior

Fig. 9.2 Model derived from the experiments in which IMHV was lesioned unilaterally after training. It is proposed that long-term storage occurs in the left IMHV (S). The right IMHV acts as a buffer store and, additionally, is necessary for storage to occur outside IMHV in an as yet unidentified region termed S'. S' is capable of sustaining retention > 6 hours after training but not before this time.

right IMHV acts as a store, but one different in nature from the left, perhaps a temporary or buffer store. It was further proposed that the right IMHV is necessary for storage to occur in a further region (S'), outside IMHV, during the 26 hours following training (Cipolla-Neto *et al.* 1982). This model accounts for the results of the unilateral lesion experiments, since destruction of the right IMHV < 3 hours after training should, according to the model, prevent storage in S' and retention should then become critically dependent on the left IMHV. This was found to be the case (Fig. 9.1*b*). If, however, the right IMHV were allowed to remain intact for 26 hours after training, S' should be able to support retention and the left IMHV would not then be critical. This was also found to be the case (Fig. 9.1*c*).

DOES STORAGE IN S' DEPEND ON THE ABSENCE OF THE LEFT IMHV
OR ON THE PRESENCE OF THE RIGHT IMHV?

There was evidence of storage in S' when the right IMHV was intact for 26 hours after training and the left IMHV had been destroyed. This result could have been due to storage in S' being dependent either on the integrity of the right IMHV, or alternatively on the absence of the left IMHV. The left side might, for example, inhibit storage in S'. In order to resolve this issue, chicks were trained and left in darkness for 26 hours, after which the IMHV was ablated bilaterally. Upon testing, the birds showed retention (Fig. 9.1*d*). There is thus evidence for storage in S′ when both the left and the right IMHV are intact, indicating that the storage can occur whether or not the left IMHV is present, and that integrity of the right IMHV is necessary for storage in S′.

THE TIME COURSE OF EVENTS FOLLOWING IMPRINTING

The effect of bilateral lesions to IMHV depends on the time relative to training at which the lesions are placed. It has been found that bilateral lesions placed in IMHV up to 6 hours after training produced amnesia, and that lesions placed after this time had no significant effect on retention (Davey *et al.* 1987; Davey 1988*a*). After this time therefore, S′ presumably is capable of supporting retention. These experiments have yielded an insight into the dynamics of left and right IMHV function following training; not only do the functions of the two sides of IMHV differ, but the nature of the difference appears to be time dependent.

Electrophysiological changes have been observed in the right IMHV 6 hours after training, i.e. at the time when S′ becomes capable of supporting retention. In the right IMHV both neuronal mean firing rate relative to that of the left, and frequency of multiple unit bursting activity, are significantly lower than the corresponding measures in dark-reared chicks (Davey 1988*a*,*b*). These results could reflect functional reorganization in IMHV following storage in S′.

THE EFFECTS OF UNILATERAL ABLATION OF IMHV BEFORE TRAINING

What would be the predictions of the new model if the left or the right IMHV were lesioned unilaterally *before* training? One would expect that early destruction of the right IMHV would preclude the storage of information in S′, and that therefore the left IMHV would subsequently become critical for retention. On the other hand, if the left IMHV were destroyed unilaterally before training, storage in S′ would be expected to proceed normally under the influence of the right IMHV and subsequent destruction of the right IMHV would not then be expected to impair retention. The experimental results were as follows:

Unilateral ablation of the right IMHV before training was found not to impair imprinting. Subsequent ablation of the remaining left IMHV resulted in amnesia (Fig. 9.3*a*). These results are consistent with the new model. If the left IMHV was lesioned before training, imprinting was

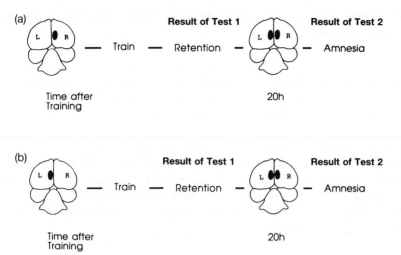

Fig. 9.3 (a) The effects of lesioning the right IMHV before training and the remaining left IMHV after training. Under these conditions the left IMHV is critical for retention and there is no evidence of storage in S'. (b) The effects of lesioning the left IMHV before training and the remaining right IMHV after training. This procedure also resulted in amnesia at the end of the experiment, suggesting that storage in S' did not occur when only the right IMHV was intact during training. The right IMHV was incapable of performing its normal function of establishing storage in S' if the left IMHV was absent during training.

unimpaired: this is also consistent with the new model which states that the right IMHV, being a buffer store, is capable of sustaining retention. However, when the remaining right IMHV was destroyed after training, the animals were, unexpectedly, amnesic: there was no evidence of storage in S' having occurred (Fig. 9.3b). It was concluded that, if the left IMHV is not present during training, the right IMHV becomes critical for retention in the same way as the left IMHV in the intact animal. It would appear that when the right IMHV is performing this modified function it can no longer exert its usual influence on storage in S'. There is thus a link between a putative mechanism for information storage and an enabling mechanism for storage in S', since there is evidence that either mechanism may occur in the right IMHV, depending on whether or not the left IMHV is intact. Furthermore, a constraint may operate on these mechanisms such that the same neural network cannot perform both functions simultaneously. These features may be important properties of the mechanism of information storage in the chick brain and other systems (see below).

It is possible that loss of the left IMHV before training results in the remaining right IMHV 'taking over' the role of the left IMHV; and that the assumption of this function by the right IMHV is incompatible with its normal function.

INTERACTION BETWEEN THE LEFT AND THE RIGHT IMHV AS A POSSIBLE EXPLANATION FOR THE EFFECTS OF SEQUENTIAL UNILATERAL LESIONS BEFORE TRAINING

The mechanism by which destruction of the left IMHV may prevent storage in S′ is not known. It is possible that the left IMHV is connected (perhaps multisynaptically) to the right IMHV and that this connection can trigger the right IMHV's function of establishing storage in S′. Removal of the left IMHV would then be expected indirectly to disable storage in S′ (see Horn 1985).

COMPARISON WITH HEMISPHERIC ASYMMETRIES IN OTHER SPECIES

Nottebohm and colleagues have suggested that, in the canary, destruction of the left side of the hyperstriatum ventrale pars caudale (HVc), a forebrain region which has a major role in the control of song (Nottebohm et al. 1976), results in a change in the function of the right HVc. After a left-sided lesion was made in adult birds, the characteristic song pattern initially disappeared. After seven months, however, there was substantial increase in the complexity of the song. The component syllables were predominantly new rather than similar to those acquired preoperatively, leading to the suggestion that memory of the song repertoire had been associated preoperatively with the left HVc. Subsequent section of the right hypoglossus (activated synaptically by the right HVc) led to a major reduction in song complexity, a result interpreted as the right HVc now being dominant for song control. Destruction of the right HVc in the previously intact bird gave no permanent impairment of song. Accordingly, in the intact bird the role of the right HVc in song control was assumed to be minor, but dominant in canaries which had lost the left HVc (Nottebohm 1977). There is a clear affinity between this suggestion and the effect of unilateral destruction of the left IMHV before imprinting, raising the possibility that there may be common neural mechanisms for the two types of learning.

In humans, the left cerebral hemisphere is usually dominant for language, and accordingly if the left parieto-temporal cortex is destroyed in adult life, aphasia results (Moscovitch 1977). If, however, such damage occurs in infancy, language can develop (Dennis and Kohn 1975; Hécaen

1976; Trevarthen 1983), presumably under the control of the right hemi-sphere. These clinical results are strongly reminiscent of those obtained in the experiments in which the left IMHV was lesioned before training, where there was evidence for the intact right IMHV assuming the function normally subserved by the left. If there are common features in the underlying mechanisms in the chick and human, the chick could provide a particularly useful neurological model.

WHY HEMISPHERIC ASYMMETRY?

The above results raise the possibility that when the right IMHV cell assembly takes on the putative storage function of the left IMHV it is unable to perform its normal function. If both functions are to be performed simultaneously during and/or after learning, this problem could be solved by the two functions being served separately by the left and right IMHV. A similar hypothesis has been advanced by Levy (1969), who compared dextral with sinistral human subjects with respect to their scores on the Wechsler Adult Intelligence Scale. She found that dextrals, in whom linguistic function was presumed to be strongly lateralized, had verbal scores which were virtually identical with those of sinistrals, in whom linguistic function was presumed to be more evenly distributed between hemispheres. In contrast, the 'performance' score, presumed to be principally under the control of the minor hemisphere, was significantly greater in dextrals than sinistrals. The results were interpreted as evidence that control of linguistic function in the minor hemisphere tended to preclude other types of processing in that hemisphere. Thus it was suggested that the language processing which engaged both hemispheres in sinistrals interfered with their minor hemisphere control of perform-ance. The results from the chick raise the interesting possibility that the neural basis of lateralization in humans and chicks may have underlying similarities which are amenable to study in the chick (see also Chapter 21).

HEMISPHERIC ASYMMETRY AND PAL

Passive avoidance training with an aversive (methylanthranilate-coated) bead is associated with a number of changes in IMHV (cf Chapters 10 and 11). The fact that IMHV is the locus of the changes is noteworthy because of the strong evidence implicating this region in the learning process of imprinting. Of further interest is the evidence that some of these effects are lateralized. The mean number of vesicles per synapse was significantly increased following training, in the left but not the right medial hyperstria-tum ventrale (Stewart *et al.* 1984). Significant interactions between training and hemisphere were found for numbers of vesicles per synapse, volume density of presynaptic boutons and the mean length of postsynaptic thickenings (Stewart *et al.* 1984). The numerical density and shape of dendritic spines on large, multipolar projection neurons were increased significantly in the left but not the right IMHV following PAL, and there was a significant training × hemisphere interaction (Patel and Stewart 1988). Subconvulsive transcranial electric shock rendered apparently amnesic a proportion of shocked, methylanthranilate-trained chicks; in such chicks, the increase in spine density in the left IMHV induced by training was abolished (Patel *et al.* 1988).

There are thus similarities between the effects of imprinting and the effects of passive avoidance training. In both cases there is evidence linking sequelae of training in IMHV with learning, and of lateralization. Moreover, the left side of IMHV in particular has repeatedly been implicated. Are the effects of lesions to IMHV similar for the two types of learning? Davies *et al.* (1988) placed lesions bilaterally in IMHV and found that this procedure, which prevents imprinting (see above), also blocked PAL. Patterson *et al.* (1990) made bilateral and unilateral lesions in IMHV before and after passive avoidance training. Bilateral and left IMHV lesions placed before training prevented acquisition of the passive avoidance behaviour, wherease right IMHV lesions had no effect. There is therefore evidence of functional lateralization in IMHV in relation to PAL. These results are reminiscent of those of Patterson *et al.* (1986), who injected L-glutamate into the right or the left cerebral hemisphere. Injection into the left hemisphere shortly before training significantly impaired PAL whereas injection into the right hemisphere was without effect.

DO THE LEFT AND THE RIGHT IMHV HAVE SIMILAR ROLES IN IMPRINTING AND IN PAL?

It is immediately apparent that there is a difference between the effects of lesions in IMHV on the two types of learning: unilateral destruction of the left IMHV does not affect imprinting (Horn *et al.* 1983) but a similar lesion does block PAL (Patterson *et al.* 1990). The disparity is unlikely to be due simply to PAL being associative and imprinting not, because at least two types of associative learning are unaffected by bilateral IMHV lesions (McCabe *et al.* 1982; Johnson and Horn 1986) and therefore do not depend critically on this brain region. Perhaps the right IMHV needs to be activated for at least several minutes before it can support acquisition—such prolonged activation may occur in imprinting but not PAL. This issue will fuel research for some time to come.

Barber (1990) found that intracerebral injection of 2-deoxygalactose (an inhibitor of glycoprotein synthesis—Rose and Jork 1987) into the right cerebral hemisphere within approximately 1 hour before or after training, impaired PAL or the retention of a passive avoidance response. Unilateral ablation of the right IMV does not block imprinting (Horn *et al.* 1983). These results are difficult to compare, but presumably the effect of the 2-deoxygalactose injection was not due to impairment of the right IMHV function because destruction of the right IMHV was found not to impair PAL (Patterson *et al.* 1990). It would appear that some region in the right hemisphere outside IMHV may be important for PAL.

LEARNING-RELATED LATERALIZATION STUDIED BY MONOCULAR OCCLUSION

There is evidence that the left and right eyes of the young chick have access to different brain systems, at least partly located in the right and left sides, respectively, of the brain (see Chapters 19, 20 and 21). The different roles of the two eye systems have been investigated by training and/or testing with one eye occluded. Evidence has accumulated of different roles for the left and right eye systems in the methylanthranilate bead-pecking and relating tasks, and also of interaction between the left and right eye systems at particular times after training. Whereas it is not known whether the IMHV is involved in such interaction, the possibility warrants serious consideration since one mechanism suggested to underlie the roles of the two sides of IMHV in imprinting proposes interaction between the left and right IMHV (Horn 1985). Andrew and Brennan (1985) trained and tested chicks monocularly on the methylanthranilate bead task. Both right- and left-eyed chicks showed retention, expressed as aversion to a clean bead identical to one previously covered with aversant. However, if, 25 minutes after training, a disruptive agent (sotalol) was injected into the right hemisphere of right-eyed chicks, retention was impaired. There was no effect on retention if the left hemisphere was injected at this time. Within a relatively short interval, it would seem that the left and right hemispheres interact. Evidence for an impairment was also found when left-eyed chicks received an injection in the left hemisphere 32.5 minutes after training (Andrew and Brennan 1985; Andrew and McKenzie, personal communication). Again there is evidence for interaction between the right and left hemispheres, but acting at particular times after training. At least some of the interactions between hemispheres are likely to be dynamic.

274   *B. J. McCabe*

VISUAL EXPERIENCE AND HEMISPHERIC ASYMMETRY

Many other cases of hemispheric asymmetry have been reported in the chick (see Chapters 19–21). Whether the asymmetries discussed previously in this chapter are associated with them is entirely a matter of speculation. There are, however, some clues. Some morphological and behavioural forebrain asymmetries have been shown to depend on unequal exposure of the two eyes to light during the perihatching period (Rogers 1982; Rogers and Sink 1988; Chapter 20). The chicks used for the above-mentioned experiments on imprinting hatched from eggs which had received no more than dim illumination for less than the minimum period of 1 hour necessary to establish the asymmetries described by Rogers (1982). There is therefore no reason to suppose that unequal stimulation of the two eyes, which produces lateralization of visual forebrain connections, visual discrimination learning and the control of copulation and attack behaviour (Chapter 20), is necessary for the hemispheric asymmetry associated with imprinting. See Chapter 21 for further discussion of this matter.

REFERENCES

Andrew, R. J. and Brennan, A. (1985). Sharply timed and lateralized events at time of establishment of long term memory. *Physiology and Behavior*, **34**, 547–56.
Barber, A. (1990). PhD dissertation, Open University.
Bradley, P., Horn, G., and Bateson P. P. G. (1979). Morphological correlates of imprinting in the chick brain. *Neuroscience Letters Supplement*, **3**, S84.
Bradley, P., Horn, G., and Bateson, P. (1981). Imprinting: an electron microscopic study of chick hyperstriatum ventrale. *Experimental Brain Research*, **41**, 115–20.
Cipolla-Neto, J., Horn, G., and McCabe, B. J. (1982). Hemispheric asymmetry and imprinting: the effect of sequential lesions to the hyperstriatum ventrale. *Experimental Brain Research*, **48**, 22–7.
Davey, J. E. (1988a). Time dependent changes in the neural systems underlying imprinting in the domestic chick. PhD dissertation, University of Cambridge.
Davey, J. E. (1988b). Imprinting and spontaneous activity in the hyperstriatum ventrale of the chick: a developing asymmetry. *Neuroscience Letters Supplement*, **32**, S46.
Davey, J. E., McCabe, B. J., and Horn, G. (1987). Mechanisms of information storage after imprinting in the domestic chick. *Behavioural Brain Research*, **26**, 209–10.
Davies, D. C., Taylor, D. A., and Johnson, M. H. (1988). The effects of hyperstriatal lesions on one-trial passive-avoidance learning in the chick. *Journal of Neuroscience*, **8**, 4662–6.

Dennis, M. and Kohn, B. (1975). Comprehension of syntax in infantile hemiplegics after cerebral hemidecortication: left-hemisphere superiority. *Brain and Language*, **2**, 472–82.

Errington, M. L., Lynch, M. A., and Bliss, T. V. P. (1987). Long-term potentiation in the dentate gyrus: induction and increased glutamate release are blocked by D(-)aminophosphonovalerate. *Neuroscience*, **20**, 279–84.

Hécaen, H. (1976). Acquired aphasia in children and the ontogenesis of hemispheric functional specialization. *Brain and Language*, **3**, 114–34.

Horn, G. (1985). *Memory, imprinting, and the brain*. Clarendon Press, Oxford.

Horn, G., Bradley, P., and McCabe, B. J. (1985). Changes in the structure of synapses associated with learning. *Journal of Neuroscience*, **5**, 3161–8.

Horn, G., McCabe, B. J., and Cipolla-Neto, J. (1983). Imprinting in the domestic chick: the role of each side of the hyperstriatum ventrale in acquisition and retention. *Experimental Brain Research*, **53**, 91–8.

Johnson, M. H. and Horn, G. (1986). Dissociation of recognition memory and associative learning by a restricted lesion of the chick forebrain. *Neuropsychologia*, **24**, 329–40.

Johnson, M. H. and Horn, G. (1987). The role of a restricted region of the chick forebrain in the recognition of individual conspecifics. *Behavioural Brain Research*, **23**, 269–75.

Levy, J. (1969). Possible basis for the evolution of lateral specialization of the human brain. *Nature*, **224**, 614–15.

McCabe, B. J., Cipolla-Neto, J., Horn, G., and Bateson, P. (1982). Amnesic effects of bilateral lesions in the hyperstriatum ventrale of the chick after imprinting. *Experimental Brain Research*, **48**, 13–21.

McCabe, B. J., Horn, G., and Bateson, P. P. G. (1981). Effects of restricted lesions of the chick forebrain on the acquisition of filial preferences during imprinting. *Brain Research*, **205**, 29–37.

McCabe, B. J. and Horn, G. (1988). Learning and memory: regional changes in N-methyl-D-aspartate receptors in the chick brain after imprinting. *Proceedings of the National Academy of Sciences of the USA*, **85**, 2849–53.

Moscovitch, M. (1972). The development of lateralization of language functions and its relation to cognitive and linguistic development: a review and some theoretical speculations. In *Language development and neurological theory* (ed. S. J. Segalowitz and F. A. Gruber), pp. 193–211. Academic Press, New York.

Nafstad, P. H. J. (1967). An electron microscope study of the termination of the perforant path fibers in the hippocampus and the fascia dentata. *Zeitschrift für Zellforschung und Mikroskopische Anatomie.*, **76**, 532–42.

Nottebohm, F. (1977). Asymmetries in neural control of vocalisation in the canary. In *Lateralization in the nervous system* (ed. S. Harnad, R. W. Doty, L. Goldstein, J. Jaynes, and G. Krauthamer), pp. 23–44. Academic Press, New York.

Nottebohm, F., Stokes, T. M. and Leonard, C. M. (1976). Central control of song in the canary, *Serinus canaria*. *Journal of Comparative Neurology*, **165**, 457–86.

Olverman, H. J., Jones, A. W., and Watkins, J. C. (1984). L-Glutamate has higher affinity than other amino acids for [³H]-D-AP5 binding sites in rat brain membranes. *Nature*, **307**, 460–2.

Patel, S. N., Rose, S. P. R., and Stewart, M. G. (1988). Training induced dendritic spine density changes are specifically related to memory formation processes in the chick, *Gallus domesticus*. *Brain Research*, **463**, 168–73.

Patel, S. N. and Stewart,M. G. (1988). Changes in the number and structure of dendritic spines 25 hours after passive avoidance training in the domestic chick, *Gallus domesticus*. *Brain Research*, **449**, 34–46.

Patterson, T.A., Alvarado, M. C., Warner, I. T., Bennett, E.L., and Rosenzweig, M.R. (1986). Memory stages and brain asymmetry in chick learning. *Behavioral Neuroscience*, **100**, 856–65.

Patterson, T. A., Gilbert, D. B., and Rose, S. P. R. (1990). Pre- and post-training lesions of the intermediate hyperstriatum ventrale and passive avoidance learning in the chick. *Experimental Brain Research*. (In press.)

Rogers, L. J. (1982). Light experience and asymmetry of brain function in chickens. *Nature*, **297**, 223–5.

Rogers, L. J. and Sink, H. S. (1988). Transient asymmetry in the projections of the rostral thalamus to the visual hyperstriatum of the chicken, and reversal of its direction by light exposure. *Experimental Brain Research*, **70**, 378–84.

Rose, S. P. R. and Jork, R. (1987). Long-term memory formation is blocked by 2-deoxygalactose, a fucose analog. *Behavioral and Neural Biology*, **48**, 24–58.

Snedecor, G. W. and Cochran, W. G. (1982). *Statistical methods*, 7th edn. Freeman, New York.

Stewart, M. G., Rose, S. P. R., King, T. S., Gabbott, P. L. A., and Bourne, R. (1984). Hemispheric asymmetry of synapses in chick medial hyperstriatum ventrale following passive avoidance training: a stereological investigation. *Developmental Brain Research*, **12**, 261–9.

Trevarthen, C. (1983). Development of the cerebral mechanisms for language. In *Neuropsychology of language, reading and spelling* (ed. U. Kirk), pp. 47–82. Academic Press, London.

10

Biochemical mechanisms involved in memory formation in the chick

S. P. R. Rose

INTRODUCTION

If memory formation requires, as we must assume, some lasting modification of cellular connectivity within the brain, a construction of new circuits or remodelling of old ones, then biochemical events that are directly associated with the novel construction or remodelling must occur. This is not an act of faith, or some reversion to the discarded views of the 1960s about memory molecules which in themselves, and independently of brain structure, encode for new information within the brain. Rather, it is a truism, which would be the case even if current connectionist models of memory storage were to be discarded in favour of more global phenomena of current flow and modulation of sinks and sources.*

The problem is of a different type; granted that such changes do occur, is it possible to measure them; and if one can measure biological changes during or consequent on some new experience which includes memory formation, how can one be sure that any such changes are indeed a direct aspect of the memory formation process? The two issues are of course related. The brain expresses a higher proportion of the genome than any other organ (some 30 000 different proteins in primates; the figure is not known in the chick), but only a few hundred of these are present in quantities sufficient to detect by conventional techniques; changes of a few per cent in the quantity of a rare protein confined to only a handful of cells would be beyond present methods of detection, and if the relevant changes were in conformation of membrane molecules rather than in their rate of synthesis or total quantity then detection would be even harder.

In fact it is the converse problem which is thrown up most regularly in studies of biochemical changes in memory—following experiences that include learning it has proved almost embarrassingly easy to detect changes

---

* I will not discuss theories of memory storage in general here: connectionist models are described in, e.g. Rumelhart and McClelland (1986), non-connectionist ones by Skarda and Freeman (1987): for a critique see Rose (1988).

in all sorts of measure—glucose utilization, enzyme activity, transmitter or receptor levels, or protein synthesis. The difficulty has been to show that these observed changes represent some direct aspect of the memory formation process.* This phrase masks two distinct categories of problem. First, it is not possible to induce memory formation in animals in a manner which is devoid of behavioural manifestation. For an experimenter to be sure that an animal is learning, it must be exposed to aversive conditions which it needs to avoid, or appetitive ones which require it to approach some goal to satisfy. To show that there is memory for what has been learned requires that the animal is placed in some type of test situation. In either case the experimental method involves the animal in motor, sensory, stress and arousal activities which may themselves result in biochemical change. As measurable memory formation cannot occur without the involvement of some or all of these other phenomena, it becomes necessary to devise a series of control experiments designed to show that motor, sensory, stress, arousal activity and so forth, in themselves, and in the absence of memory formation, do not result in the biochemical change. In relation to the chick, this was the purpose of a series of experiments run by Bateson, Horn, and myself during the early 1970s (reviewed in, e.g. Horn *et al.* 1973 and Rose 1977). A general discussion of the issues involved, and the criteria that must be met if any biochemical event is to be associated directly with (be a 'correspondent of') memory formation forms the substance of my 1981 paper (Rose 1981) and will not be discussed further here.

The second category of problem is, however, worth rehearsing. There may be a wide variety of biochemical processes that are triggered when an animal learns. For instance, there may be enhanced release of neuromodulator; increased cell firing will demand increases in glucose utilization and localized changes in cerebral blood flow. If synaptic connections are to be reconstructed then almost by definition there will be new protein synthesis, itself calling for changes in ATP turnover, whilst the membrane and genomic activation involved in any of these processes will need a cascade of other biochemical processes, from changes in second and third messengers to the expression of the products of 'early genes' like c-fos. To what extent may any of these necessary biochemical processes be defined as 'the' biochemical events subserving memory? This is a non-trivial question, for if immense research effort is required merely to reveal that during memory perfectly standard and well recognized biochemical processes occur that can more easily be studied in other contexts and simpler systems, then what is the whole exercise for? These phenomena are

---

* Once again a caveat. The discussion in this chapter is entirely concerned with mechanisms involved in the registration of learned events—memory formation—not with issues of the nature of representation or of recall processes.

sometimes called cellular housekeeping functions (often 'mere' housekeeping!), and the term itself is intended to sound somewhat derogatory—possibly reflecting the fact that it is coined by male biochemists who tend to under-rate the work involved in housekeeping. The point is not to minimize the importance of such functions but to define a different research task—the search for biochemical processes, localized in time and space, that *directly* subserve memory encoding events—those that in some sense can be regarded as aspects of the memorial code itself, or, as I describe them elsewhere (Rose 1981, 1988) the *necessary, sufficient* and *specific* biochemical correspondents of memory formation.

The distinction is perhaps worth expanding on. Neuromodulation may be a *necessary* part of the cellular processes subserving memoy formation, in the sense that whenever something is required to be learned, or fixed in long-term memory, then some type of burst of secretory activity is required. One could envisage that during the learning process a particular set of synapses were activated as a result of coupled pre- and postsynaptic changes in current flow, but that only in the presence of some extracellular signal—a particular concentration of a neuromodulator, or even a small glycoprotein molecule like an ependymin (Shashoua 1985)—did the synaptic activation become converted into lasting changes in synaptic structure. But what provides the specific learned information—say, about the actual quality of the conspecific on which imprinting is occurring, or the colour and shape of the bead to be avoided—is not the neuromodulator but the pattern of modified synapses. It is this pattern that must be determined to satisfy the criteria of *sufficiency* and *specificity*.

Because of the act of faith that memory involves such an altered pattern of synaptic connectivity, studies of long-term memory formation in vertebrates have placed much emphasis on altered synthesis of macromolecules, especially proteins and glycoproteins, which as membrane components might be presumed to be associated with changes in cellular form. By contrast, in the early years at least of the invertebrate studies by Kandel and Alkon and their collaborators with *Aplysia* and *Hermissenda*, studies on associative learning followed on from work on shorter term processes like habituation and sensitization (e.g. Horn and Hinde 1970). These transient phenomena seemed to require mechanistic explanation at the level of changed current flow and membrane channels. It is only within the last few years that Kandel and his colleagues have explicitly recognized that long-term processes are likely to require different types of cellular processes and have therefore turned their attention to the possible roles of protein synthesis and genomic activation (Goelet *et al.* 1986); in doing so they have run into many of the same methodological difficulties that have beset some of the vertebrate studies.

Nonetheless, one of the encouraging features of work in this area is the extent to which there has been a convergence amongst researchers working with the different current model systems for the study of the biochemistry of memory formation. The molluscan work is well known; it has seemed to offer the merit of apparently 'simple systems' with defined connections between small numbers of relatively large and identifiable neurons; its demerits have included the difficulty of convincing vertebrate neurobiologists that the processes being studied in *Aplysia* (and to a lesser extent *Hermissenda*) are really analogues of vertebrate associative learning, and that synaptic or molecular rules uncovered in invertebrates are generalizable to vertebrates. The discovery of hippocampal long-term potentiation by Bliss and Lømo (1973) was widely recognized as offering an alternative, vertebrate system demonstrating a form of neural plasticity which could be taken as a model for memory—and the fact that in mammals the hippocampus is known to be functionally involved in memory formation— has led to the wide assumption that hippocampal LTP is not merely a model but possibly even a mechanism for memory (Matthies 1989). The biochemical findings from *Aplysia* and from the hippocampal studies have at last begun to inform each other, and certain common biochemical features—especially concerning the role of Ca^{2+} and membrane phosphorylation processes—may even be emerging (Lynch and Baudry 1984; Byrne 1987). A further useful model, in which mechanisms of neural plasticity may follow rules that cast light on those involved in memory formation, are the various forms of developmental plasticity in sensory systems, and especially what Singer has called 'experience-dependent self-organization' (Singer 1987) in the visual system. This process of rewiring consequent upon constraints of visual experience during early postnatal development, may also be regarded as a form of memory.

THE CHICK AS A MODEL SYSTEM

Despite the array of model systems that has emerged in the last decades for the study of the cellular mechanisms of memory formation, the young chick retains considerable advantages, many of which have been rehearsed in earlier chapters; the well-organized behavioural repertoire which goes with a precocial animal, large and well developed brain and relatively high brain/body weight ratio. Of particular relevance to biochemical studies, though, is the additional feature that, in common with other very young animals the chick has a reduced blood–brain barrier, thus enabling rapid diffusion of injected precursors (or pharmacologically active substances) into the brain. Similarly, its thin skull makes localized intracerebral injections relatively easy. No other vertebrate model has lent itself to the range of studies which has been reported in the chick.

However, there are disadvantages. The fact that chick neuroanatomy is not well understood (but see Chapters 2, 3) may be of less importance in the context of biochemical studies than in many others, as (with the exception of autoradiographic or immunocytochemical procedures) one is generally analysing changes in fairly large tissue masses, or samples derived from homogenates, whose preparation in any case destroys morphological order. The problem of working with a rapidly developing organism is, however, a serious matter. Learning-induced changes are being superimposed upon a highly dynamic and plastic situation. Biochemical variability, even in control birds, is relatively large, both within and between hatches, by contrast with the inbred strains of rats with which biochemists are more familiar. Severalfold differences in the activity of enzymes or in metabolic measures can occur in apparently identical preparations. This is particularly problematic when one is searching for relatively small biochemical differences between 'trained' and 'control' birds. Average differences between conditions of no more than, in most cases, 15–30 per cent need to be detected against high control levels and a variability even amongst these controls which means that within-group standard error rarely falls below 10 per cent. Reliable detection of such small changes requires large experimental numbers, care in experimental design, the use of balanced replications, and interbatch standardization. The use of internal controls, for instance forebrain regions like ectostriatum, or cerebellum, assumed not to show learning-related changes in these paradigms, is often important, and now that many of the memory-related effects have been lateralized it also becomes possible to consider making interhemispheric comparisons and hence paired statistical procedures.

The reasons for this biological variability, which is seemingly more marked biochemically than it is behaviourally, are unknown, and can be troubling. It might for instance reflect subtle posthatch developmental differences which would be flattened out within a few days (Chapter 7). If so, the variability is simply a manifestation of the fact that in development there may be multiple pathways to a final common developmental endpoint, and is therefore of no great biological relevance. However, as well as methodological problems, such an explanation for the inter-bird variability raises the more interesting theoretical question of the implications of biochemical changes found consequent on training. Are they cases of 'speeded up development' or are they distinct processes? This is particularly at issue in the context of the frequently-observed hemispheric asymmetries, which occur as much in biochemical as in other measures. The conclusions from our own data on the asymmetric distribution of some synaptic markers, detected using monoclonal antibodies (p65 and SV2, vesicle markers, and 411B, a postsynaptic density marker), suggest that asymmetries present at day 1 between left and right IMHV, PA, and LPO in communally reared chicks persist until at least four weeks posthatch (Bullock *et al*, 1987).

Of the two forms of early learning which have been widely studied with the chick, imprinting and passive avoidance learning, I am now prepared, having worked with both, to make an unqualified argument in favour of the latter for biochemical studies, despite the fascination of the imprinting phenomenon and the flow of exciting results that has continued to pour from the Cambridge laboratories of Horn and Bateson. The reasons for my claim lie in the precision of timing that is possible with passive avoidance learning, a one-trial event in which the behavioural act which induces memory formation, the peck at a bitter-tasting bead, can be unequivocally observed and timed. This means that the events surrounding the training experience itself can be more readily dissociated from the biochemical processes occurring during memory formation phases when the training stimulus is no longer present. Biochemical studies are particularly suited to addressing the question of time-dependent processes subserving different phases of memory formation, and in passive avoidance learning these time courses, derived from pharmacological interventions, have been particularly well mapped (see Part V of this book).

In the older literature on the biochemistry of learning a distinction was often made between so-called correlative and interventive approaches (e.g. Agranoff et al. 1976). Measuring biochemical changes consequent on training is an example of the first approach; interfering with retention by injection of agents with relatively well-defined sites of biochemical actions exemplifies the second. Passive avoidance learning in the chick is the model, above all, in which it has been possible to synthesize insights from the two. There are of course methodological problems with both approaches; the issue of artefact in the correlative approach derives from the point made above concerning the difficulty of resolving genuinely underlying correspondents from effects which may be the merely passive consequence of changes in cerebral blood flow or other general metabolic process. Nor can one without hesitation infer that if a pharmacological treatment results in amnesia, then the cause of that amnesia is a chemical lesion in the system with which the pharmacological agent is believed to interfere. A clear case in point is the demonstration by Hambley and Rogers (1979) that inhibition of cerebral protein synthesis results in the accumulation of intracellular pools of amino acids, and that injection of certain of these amino acids, notably glutamate or taurine, can itself produce amnesia. Further, there may well be a delay between the injection of an agent and the onset of its effects, as it may require time to diffuse to an active site, and for an inhibitory effect to build up. Equally, unless it can be shown that following localized injection of an agent it does not diffuse far from the site of application, conclusions concerning localization may be hazardous. Such caveats mean that conclusions about the precise timing or mechanisms of memory phases based exclusively on interpreting the amnestic effects of pharmacological agents need to be viewed with caution.

BIOCHEMICAL STUDIES IN THE CHICK

In the remainder of this chapter I propose to review data on the biochemical sequelae of training in the chick, based largely but not entirely on the correlative approach using the passive avoidance model introduced in the previous chapter. In this context, the time-courses of the measured biochemical changes are important (Rose 1981) because if memory formation does involve a number of separable sequential or parallel behavioural processes, then we have to assume different biochemical processes, and perhaps even differently localized sites or cell-ensembles, underlying each phase. However, each successive phase of memory formation will also require distinct biochemical 'mobilization' steps. Hence biochemical and behavioural time-courses may not march mechanically in step, and it becomes difficult to assign precise relationships between the timecourses described here and the specific phases of memory dissected pharmacologically and described in Section 4 of this book. For instance, if new proteins have to be made this will require genomic activation and new or enhanced RNA synthesis which must precede in time the enhanced protein synthesis. If the protein synthesis is associated with long-term memory, it may well be that the enhanced RNA synthesis is observed at a time after training which is associated not with the long but with an intermediate phase of memory. The associated RNA synthesis, however, is not a 'correspondent' of the intermediate phase but is an 'enabling process' required for the long-term phase. It is because the issue of time dependency is important in unraveling biochemical mechanisms that, as mentioned above, the sharply-timed training experience of passive-avoidance learning may be preferable to the longer-drawn out processes of imprinting.

The evidence from which the biochemical model I present here is derived comes primarily from our own laboratory and the passive avoidance studies, but also including those by Bradley and by Davies, and will draw on some of the imprinting data from the Cambridge group. Other highly relevant work is of course represented in other chapters. The data drawn on below is structured in a logical rather than a historical manner. I want to argue that we can best understand the results in terms of a time-dependent sequence of biochemical events, as shown in Table 10.1. Implicit in this table is the assumption that the sequence is all taking place in the same ensemble of cells, and indeed this idea underlies most current connectionist modelling. However, it must be recognized that the lesioning data both in imprinting (see Chapters 8 and 9) and passive avoidance (Patterson *et al.* 1990) imply that this is at best an oversimplification. I do not propose to address these issues here in any detail as they are discussed in other chapters.

Table 10.1   Temporal processes in vertebrate memory storage, based mainly on chick studies.

Timescale		Processes	Region
Very short term	**s –> min**	Pre/post depolarizations?, Ca^{2+} flux? Transmitter release?	
		Increased glucose utilization	**IMHV + LPO, PA**
Short term	**min –> h**	Pre/post-antidromic signals (arachidonic acid?)	
		Translocation of PKC	**Left IMHV**
		C-fos and c-jun expression	**IMHV, LPO**
		Presynaptic phosphorylation of B50	**Left IMHV**
		Transient increases in receptor binding	**IMHV**
		Increased neuronal bursting	**IMHV, LPO**
Long term	**h –> days**	**Changed neuronal connectivity via:**	
		Protein synthesis, including tubulin	**'roof'**
		Pre and postsynaptic membrane glycoprotein synthesis	**IMHV, LPO + (PA?)**
		Presynaptic increases in synaptic vesicle numbers	**Left IMHV Left LPO**
		Postsynaptic increases in synaptic apposition zone length	**Left IMHV, + Left LPO**
		Increased dendritic spine density on IMHV projection neurons	**Left IMHV**
		Increased spine head diameter on IMHV projection neurons	**Left IMHV**

Bold face = results established in chick
Where no lateralization is mentioned, this has not yet been determined.

One further qualification is appropriate: because the biochemical data to be discussed are based on a decade of studies, conducted with varying methodologies, we do not know whether all of the changes observed are confined to, e.g. IMHV, or whether or to what extent they are lateralized. The sensitivity of our measures does not always permit one to look for changes in such small tissue blocks as IMHV, especially if we are attempting to make biochemical measures not in whole tissue samples but in subcellular fractions or separated proteins. Therefore the sequence in Table 10.1 should be regarded as primarily of heuristic value, summarizing the periods over which different biochemical processes predominate, without making any assumptions about the specific population of neurons involved in these responses.

SHORTER-TERM PROCESSES

If the immediate cerebral response to the experience of a novel set or combination of stimuli and experiences is an increased neuronal firing rate, then there will be changes in pre- and postsynaptic depolarization, the opening of membrane channels, modifications to ion fluxes and increased transmitter release. Such short-term processes have been studied in the molluscan and hippocampal systems, but not so far in the chick, where the methodology has hitherto been lacking. If it becomes possible, by analogy with the hippocampal slice, to develop an 'IMHV-learning-slice,' then the chick will also become open to such studies; failing this, the argument about the involvement of these processes is based on analogy with other learning systems and inference from the time-courses of amnesia-inducing agents.

However, an excellent marker of neuronal firing and synaptic activity is provided by the intracellular accumulation of radioactivity from systematically injected ^{14}C- or ^{3}H- labelled 2-deoxyglucose (2-DG). As is well known, 2-DG is taken up into neural tissue as if it were glucose; within the neurons it is converted into 2-deoxyglucose 6-phosphate but cannot be further metabolized. Serial autoradiography of brain sections following a pulse of 2-DG enables the sites of any change in accumulation of radioactivity from 2-DG to be determined. Comparing 2-DG labelling in brain sections from methylanthranilate-trained (Tr) and water-control (C) chicks during or following training can provide an index of where in the brain increases in metabolism or neuronal activity associated with training or memory formation may be occurring.

The first 2-DG experiments with the chick were made following an imprinting task by Kohsaka *et al.* (1979) shortly after Horn, McCabe, and Bateson had identified IMHV as the site of increased labelling from the RNA precursor uracil during imprinting (Horn *et al.* 1979). The Japanese group found increased accumulation of radioactivity from 2-DG in the IMHV. However, the design of their training situation meant that they were not looking at 2-DG metabolism during the period in which their birds were learning the imprinting, but subsequently, when they were being tested for their propensity to follow the object on which they had been imprinted. Nor was it possible to determine whether any increase in metabolism was associated with a 'pure' recall process or with the increased motor activity of the following activity in which the birds were engaged. The use of 2-DG measures in the context of acoustic imprinting is reviewed elsewhere by Scheich (1989).

In our own initial 2-DG experiments (Kossut and Rose 1984; see also Chapter 11) the labelled sugar was injected just prior to training, into C and Tr birds, which were tested, killed after half an hour and serial autoradiograms analysed for training-related differences. Increased accumulation of radioactivity was found in Tr compared to C birds in the posterior portion of the MHV, the PA and LPO. We had anticipated finding changes in HV because of the earlier observations of the Cambridge group with uracil accumulation after imprinting, and the fact that we had already found that passive avoidance produced changes in protein synthesis in the 'anterior roof' dissection, which includes HV. But the findings in LPO and PA, forebrain 'base' regions, were not predicted. It is still not known whether imprinting also results in changes in these regions, but it would be interesting to look.

Because in these first 2-DG experiments the sugar was injected prior to training, the study did not allow us to dissociate training effects from those occurring during the consolidation period; hence we repeated the study (Rose and Csillag 1985), this time injecting the sugar either 5 minutes before, or 10 or 30 minutes after training, and studying left and right IMHV, LPO and PA separately by micropunch rather than autoradiography. Enhanced radioactivity was found to persist in the left LPO in birds injected 10 minutes but not 30 minutes after training. In IMHV, even with injections of 2-DG 30 minutes after training, and hence accumulation of radioactivity in a time window 30–60 minutes following training, there was still a significant excess of activity in the left hemisphere, implying that in this region training produces a very persistent increase in metabolic, and hence presumably neuronal activity over a period which includes short and intermediate phases of memory formation. This was our first evidence for lateralization of a biochemical measure following training. Another indication that the increase in 2-DG uptake into these regions is associated with memory formation, rather than merely the concomitants of the bead pecking, comes from an unpublished negative experiment by Margaret Boxer and myself. In this, instead of pairing the beadpeck with a bitter taste, it was paired with footshock. The chicks are unable to learn this pairing, at least within a small number of trials, and continue to peck the bead despite the shock. Under these circumstances there are no differences in subsequent 2-DG uptake into the forebrain regions between birds which have experienced the paired beadpeck and shock, shock alone, or bead alone.

Another phenomenon which is associated in time with the intermediate phase of memory formation, and was incidentally the first biochemical measure we ever attempted in the passive avoidance model, is a transient increase in the maximal binding activity of the muscarinic cholinergic ligand QNB to forebrain roof homogenates. There is no difference in binding activity between Tr and C samples obtained 10 minutes or 3 hours after training, but a substantial (21 per cent) increase at 30 minutes(Rose et al. 1980). The significance of these changes in maximal binding activity is not clear, and we have not pursued these observations further, but it is presumably relevant that IMHV is exceptionally rich in muscarinic cholinergic receptors (Coulter 1988) and one could well envisage that a temporary increase (up-regulation) of these receptors could be part of the mechanism of transient modulation of synaptic connectivity pending more permanent structural modification.

Of more interest to us at present is that methylanthranilate training results in a transient, specifically presynaptic change in the phosphorylation of a particular membrane protein, with a molecular weight of 52 kDa. To explain the significance of this observation, it needs to be set within a broader biochemical context. It has been known for a long time that phosphorylated membrane proteins play key roles in a number of vital general cellular, and specifically neuronal functions. (For reviews, e.g. Heald 1960; Gispen and Routtenberg 1982, 1986). They serve as sites of interaction between cell surface signals (first messengers) and intracellular second messenger systems (cAMP, phosphoinositide, etc.). In addition, changing the phosphorylation state of synaptic membrane proteins serves to open or close ion channels across the membrane (especially Ca^{2+}). Subcellular fractionation procedures make it possible to isolate both synaptic plasma membrane (SPM) preparations, and, derived from these, fractions enriched in postsynaptic densities (PSDs) (Murakami *et al.* 1986). Brief (15 second) incubation of these membrane preparations with ^{32}P-labelled ATP results in labelling of a number of polypeptides which can then be separated by polyacrylamide gel electrophoresis. One of these polypeptides, with an apparent molecular weight of around 50 kDa, has been identified in a number of laboratories as showing changes in phosphorylation dependent on the past history of the tissue from which it has been isolated. Nelson and Routtenberg (1985) and others have shown that the phosphorylation state of this protein in rat hippocampus (which Routtenberg calls F1) alters after long-term potentiation; and it has been extensively characterized by Gispen's group (e.g. Oestreicher *et al.* 1981, 1983) who call it B50. The phosphorylation/dephosphorylation state of B50, which is regulated by the Ca^{2+}-dependent enzyme protein kinase C (PKC), is currently regarded as a key factor in the transition between the initiation phase and the maintenance phase of long term potentiation (Reymann *et al.* 1988). However, it must also be understood that there are problems of interpretation involved if one finds a difference in the *in vitro* phosphorylation of such a membrane protein. Thus an *in vitro* increase in phosphorylation could result from an increased availability of potentially phosphorylable sites, following a *decrease* in *in vivo* phosphorylation. An alternative would be that the phosphorylation is regulated by a redistribution of PKC between synaptosol and synaptic membrane (Akers *et al.* 1986).

When we came to examine the phosphorylated proteins, of SPM and PSD fractions derived from chick forebrain, we found that there was one protein in particular, with an apparent molecular weight of 52 kDa, which could be phosphorylated in SPMs, but not in PSDs; thus it appeared to be specifically presynaptic. Comparing phosphorylation patterns in SPMs and PSDs isolated from Tr and C chicks, the only difference appeared in this 52 kD protein, whose phosphorylation was reduced at 10 minutes and significantly lowered by 30 minutes after training in the M birds, but had reverted to control (W) levels in samples prepared from tissue taken 3 hours after training (Ali *et al.* 1988*a*). The reduction appears to be confined to the left hemisphere (we have not yet been able to measure specific regions like IMHV). Immunologically, Gispen and his colleagues have shown that our 52 kDa protein is identical to B50 (Bullock *et al.* 1990), and like B50, it is phosphorylated by protein kinase C. We have immunological evidence that training does indeed result in a redistribution of the PKC in left IMHV towards a membrane-bound form (Burchuladze *et al.* 1990), which could provide the mechanism for the change in phosphorylation and the 52 kDa protein.

The sensitivity of this particular membrane protein to training suggests parallels in mechanism in the biochemical responses to training in the chick and mammalian phenomena such as LTP (similar phosphorylation processes have also been claimed to show training-associated lability in *Aplysia* and *Hermissenda*). The fact that in the chick the effect is a purely presynaptic one is also potentially significant in developing a cellular theory of sequential processes in memory formation. Any model of memory formation that assumes that some type of Hebbian mechanism is involved—that is, that more-or-less continuous firing of pre- and postsynaptic cells strengthens the connections between them by growth or modulation of synaptic structures in both cells—must also postulate a signalling mechanism which relays information antidromically, from post- to presynaptic side. In the context of LTP, there is growing interest in the possibility that this retrograde signal may be carried by way of the postsynaptic release of one of the products of the phosphoinositide second messenger cascade, arachidonic acid, which then triggers a further presynaptic cascade via interaction with presynaptic membrane phosphorylated proteins. This idea, for which there is now some supportive evidence in the hippocampus (Lynch and Bliss 1986), points to the importance of unravelling further these second- and third-messenger processes within the chick system.

That the phosphorylation of the 52 kDa protein is dependent on protein kinase C opens a further interesting experimental possibility, for there exist a number of rather specific inhibitors of this enzyme. If the phosphorylation of the 52 kDa protein is necessary for memory formation, then inhibiting this phosphorylation should prevent memory being formed. We have recently shown that intracerebral injection of several such inhibitors, including mellitin, prior to training, does indeed result in amnesia (Ali, *et*

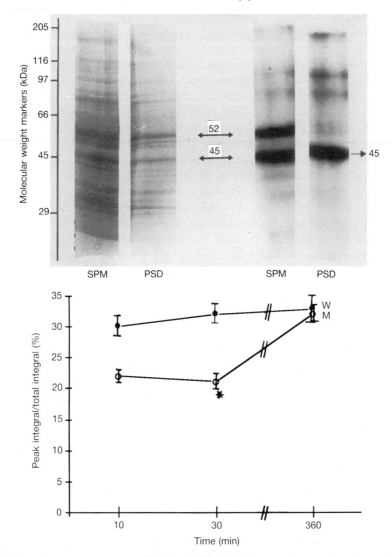

Fig. 10.1 Synaptic membrane phosphorylation following passive avoidance training. *Upper panel*: SDS polyacrylamide gel separation of proteins from chick brain synaptic plasma membranes (SPM) and postsynaptic densities (PSD). *Left-hand tracks*—proteins stained with Coomassie blue. *Right-hand tracks*—proteins phosphorylated from AT^{32}P during a 15-s incubation period in an *in vitro* phosphorylation system. Note the prominent bands at 45 and 52 kDa. Despite the fact that there is a protein band staining with Coomassie Blue at 52 kDa in the PSD as well as the SPM, this fraction is only phosphorylated in the SPM but not in the PSD. *Lower panel*: phosphorylation of the 52 kDa band in SPMs derived from Tr (*M*) and C (*W*) chick brain at varying times after training. There is a significant reduction in incorporation into the 52 kDa band 30 min after training on the passive avoidance task. (Data from Ali *et al.* 1988a).

al. 1988*b*). The amnestic effect of mellitin is confined to left hemisphere injections (Burchuladze *et al.* 1990). However, intriguingly, the amnesia does not occur at 30 minutes after training, when the change in phosphorylation can be measured biochemically, but only after 1.5–3 hours, when phosphorylation would have reverted to control levels. An equivalent observation concerning the effects of PKC inhibition on the maintenance of long-term potentiation has been made by the Magdeburg group (Reymann *et al.* 1988). The straightforward interpretation of this experiment is that phosphorylation of the 52 kDa protein is *not* an aspect of the biochemistry of early phases of memory formation, but is rather to be regarded as an *enabling* process involved in the transition to long-term memory, so that inhibition prevents the transition from occurring, just as is the case with inhibitors of protein synthesis. However, the kinetics of the inhibition requires more thorough investigation before this interpretation can be confirmed. It is of interest that similar delayed onset of amnesia is apparent with a number of other amnestic agents including certain amino acids and 5HT1 blockers (see Chapters 13, 16 and 19).

LONGER-TERM BIOCHEMICAL PROCESSES

The transition to long-term memory is clearly a behaviourally important event and not one which is by any means automatic. Presumably only those experiences which are judged by some type of adaptive criterion to be significant are carried over into long-term store. There are two examples of this from amongst our own experiments with the passive avoidance system. If the bitter-tasting methylanthranilate is replaced as an aversive stimulus by quinine (Q), which appears to be less unpleasant tasting, then Q-trained chicks will avoid a dry bead when presented within the first hours after training, but the amount of avoidance will rapidly decline, so that by 24 hours they are indistinguishable from water-trained birds. This type of observation is not novel (see Chapter 17); from the present point of view, however, what is interesting is that in the Q-birds, short-term memory has not been translated into long-term avoidance. One might therefore expect that only those biochemical events necessary for the early, but not the later, phases of memory will be occurring. Recently joint experiments by Michael Stewart and Rachel Bourne from our group and Ceri Davies in London (submitted) have tested this hypothesis using as biochemical marker the incorporation of radioactively-labelled fucose into glycoprotein (see below); the increased fucose incorporation over water controls which occurs during long-term memory formation for the methylanthranilate bead pairing does not occur when quinine is the aversive agent. However, it should be borne in mind that the act of pecking at a water-coated bead itself seems to be sufficient to result in some increase in protein and glycoprotein synthesis, compared with 'quiet control' birds which remain in their pens, as the experiments described in the following paragraphs suggest.

A recent experiment which casts some light, albeit slightly paradoxically, on this process derives from work by Barber, Gilbert, and myself (1989) on the conditioned taste aversion paradigm in the chick. It is well known (Chapters 1, 18) that chicks, like mammals, can associate tasting a novel food or drink (for instance, green-coloured saccharine solution) with subsequent sickness induced by injection of lithium chloride—a version of the classical Garcia effect (Gaston 1977). We have shown that if chicks peck at a dry bead—for instance a green LED—and half an hour later are made sick by lithium chloride injection they will avoid the bead on retest several hours later. What biochemical processes are required for retention of the memory of this apparently neutral stimulus in the period prior to its association with the LiCl injection? Retention seems to require the synthesis of glycoproteins, because the intracerebral injection of an inhibitor of glycoprotein synthesis (2-deoxygalactose; see below) at the time of the initial peck (but not later) will prevent the bird making the association of the bead with the subsequent sickness. Thus the chick must be (a) making representations of the bead in its brain even when not explicitly paired with an aversive taste, and (b) these representations involve the synthesis of macromolecules. This result has implications for memory models which demand contiguous firing of otherwise unpaired cells *à la* Hebb, in order to produce pre- and postsynaptic modifications; clearly if synaptic modification is taking place as result of pecking at the neutral stimulus, it cannot be occurring as a result of the associative pairing of hypothetical visual/peck neurons with taste neurons.

What biochemical processes are required for the transition from the earlier phases of memory to long-term storage? In the earliest of the imprinting studies (Bateson *et al.* 1972) we showed that exposure to an imprinting stimulus resulted in an increase in incorporation of labelled uracil into RNA, implying that training resulted in an increase in RNA synthesis. This increase seemed to begin relatively soon after the onset of exposure to the stimulus, but the nature both of the training procedure and of the biochemical measure made exact timing difficult. Incorporation studies are of their nature cumulative; they can only tell you what is going on over a period of time, generally at least 30 minutes. By contrast, studies on binding or enzyme acitivities provide a snapshot; they tell what is the state of this particular substance at time X (assumed to be the time of killing the animal). Enhanced synthesis of RNA implies an increase in the activity of the RNA-synthesizing enzyme RNA polymerase, and we showed that 30 minutes after the onset of the exposure to the imprinting stimulus, there was indeed an increase in RNA polymerase activity in the forebrain roof (Haywood *et al.* 1975). The events that might precede even this mobilization of RNA polymerase are not known, but there is at present widespread interest in the possibility that an apparently universal eukaryotic oncogene, which expresses a protein called c-fos, might play an important role in the conversion of synaptic membrane signals (such as those involving Ca^{2+} and phosphorylated proteins) to nuclear genomic activation (Sagar *et al.* 1988; Chiarugi *et al.* 1989). We have recently been able to test this possibility by measuring c-fos expression in IMHV and LPO of chicks 30 minutes after training on a methylanthranilate bead by comparison with water and quiet controls. There is a very substantial increase in the amount of c-fos message detectable by c-DNA hybridization in both IMHV and LPO in the trained group in these conditions (Anokhin *et al.*, in press).

As emphasized above, increased RNA synthesis is best regarded as an enabling process for increased synthesis of protein, and there is increased incorporation of radioactive lysine into protein in the anterior forebrain roof after imprinting (Bateson *et al.* 1972). So far as the passive avoidance paridigm is concerned, we already knew from the work of Gibbs (see Chapter 17) before we began working with the model that protein synthesis inhibitors like cycloheximide (or, later, anisomycin) prevented long- but not short-term memory for the avoidance. However, there are always ambiguities in the interpretation of such inhibitor experiments, as pointed out above [see, e.g. Hambley and Rogers 1979; or the contrasting recent papers of Bradley and Galal (1988), and Patterson *et al.* (1989); see Chapter 15]. Hence the merits of using the correlative as well as interventive approach. Again, for non-biochemists, it is important to point out that there is a very substantial distinction to be drawn between the transient modification of existing protein structures, for instance by phosphorylation, and the *de novo* synthesis of quite new molecules. It is this second which demands genomic activation, which in turn implies that signals from the synapse must be transmitted to the nucleus in order to trigger the process.

Using the passive avoidance model, we were able to show that training chicks on methylanthranilate beads resulted in a persistent increase in incorporation of labelled leucine into soluble protein in the forebrain roof, measured any time up to 24 hours after training. This seemed to imply that the single peck at the bead was resulting in a prolonged period of cellular reconstruction. What was of particular interest, though, was that the increase in incorporation (and total quantity) was not general but into specific proteins, and in particular, into the prominent 'housekeeping' protein tubulin (Mileusnic *et al.* 1980). Tubulin is the major constituent of microtubules which run down axons and dendrites and into pre- and postsynaptic apparatus, and are centrally involved in intracellular signalling and transport of key constituents by axonal or dendritic flow. In any cellular reconstruction, through sprouting, spine or synapse formation, increased tubulin production could be expected to occur. Later, we were also able to show that this increased protein synthesis could be mimicked *in vitro*, if tissues slices cut from the forebrain roof of Tr compared with C chicks, were incubated in oxygenated medium with labelled leucine, giving an opportunity to study in greater detail the exact nature of the protein species involved (Schliebs *et al.* 1985).

But of somewhat greater interest to us was the possible involvement of a major subclass of proteins, the glycoproteins. Glycoproteins are extensively present in the plasma membrane, where,because of the large variety of possible permutations of the glyco-moiety of their structure, which can protrude from the membrane surface into the intracellular matrix, they play an important role in intracellular recognition processes (Margolis and Margolis 1977). Glycoproteins such as N-CAMs (neuronal cell adhesion molecules) are closely involved in the molecular events of neuronal growth and differentiation. They may be synthesized on freshly-made proteins within the Golgi apparatus in the cell soma, or they may be modified *in situ* in the membrane rather like the protein phosphorylation phenomena discussed above. If long-term memory involves pre- and postsynaptic reorganization, we argued, it is likely to require synthesis of new or modification of existing glycoproteins. Indeed, there is evidence from other systems of the increased synthesis of glycoproteins during memory consolidation phases (Routtenberg *et al.* 1974; Popov *et al.* 1981), and antisera to specific glycoproteins can produce amnesia for avoidance tasks in rodents (Nolan *et al.* 1987). The ependymins, shown by Shashoua (1985) and Schmidt (1987) to play a role in consolidation processes, are a family of low molecular weight extracellular glycoproteins.

A favoured marker for glycoprotein synthesis is the sugar fucose, which, if injected systemically or intracerebrally is almost exclusively incorporated into glycoproteins rather than being metabolized by other routes. Early in our work with the passive avoidance model we were able to show that, following training, there was a prolonged enhancement of fucose incorporation into glycoproteins of the SPM (Burgoyne and Rose 1980; Sukumar *et al.*, 1980). As with leucine incorporation, the increase could be detected for up to 24 hours training, and could also be found in the tissue slice *in vitro* (McCabe and Rose 1985). Fucosylation depends on an initial activation of the fucose molecule by phosphorylation, dependent on the enzyme fucokinase, followed eventually by insertion into the growing glycoprotein chain, a process requiring the enzyme fucosyl transferase. Training increases the activity of the former, fucokinase, but not the latter enzyme (Losser and Rose 1983); the former is presumably the rate-limiting step. The training-induced fucosylation is a post-translational modification of existing proteins, as it is not prevented by the protein synthesis inhibitor cycloheximide, at least *in vitro* (McCabe and Rose 1987).

Although our earliest experiments with fucose incorporation pointed to an increase in the anterior forebrain roof region (i.e. presumed IMHV), the later experiments revealed repeatedly that effects were appearing in the base—and the right base at that (Lossner and Rose 1983; Rose and Harding 1984; McCabe and Rose 1985). At the time I was puzzled by this, as so much of the data, both from our laboratory and that of Horn was pointing to the importance of the IMHV. I now think, though, that the right base (LPO, PA) location may be telling us something important. Both in imprinting (Chapters 8, 9 and 12) and in passive avoidance (Patterson et al. 1990), pre-training lesions of IMHV prevent long-term memory formation, but post-training lesions do not, implying, as Horn has argued, transfer of memory to a second store outside the IMHV. Could this second store lie in the LPO/PA complex? By contrast with IMHV lesions, pretraining LPO lesions do not result in amnesia, but post-training lesions do (Patterson et al, 1990). The LPO, but not IMHV, thus seems necessary for long-term storage once memory has been formed. In this context the changes in synaptic and vesicle numbers found in the LPO 24 hours after training by Stewart (Chapter 11) may be particularly relevant.

If, as these correlative experiments indicate, there is a role for glycoprotein synthesis in long-term memory formation, then it becomes of interest to ask what interventive approaches might reveal of the necessity for such synthesis. Cycloheximide inhibition of protein synthesis does not immediately affect the conversion of existing proteins to glycoproteins, as mentioned above. But there does exist a more specific inhibitor of glycoprotein synthesis, the sugar 2-deoxygalactose (2-D-gal). This sugar competes with galactose for incorporation into glycoproteins; once incorporated the glycoprotein would normally be 'completed' by addition of a fucose moiety to the preterminal galactose. When 2-D-gal replaces galactose, however, its chemical structure means that it cannot accept the fucose addition. Behavioural studies using 2-D-gal were pioneered in Magdeburg by the Matthies group (Jork et al. 1986). In the chick, 2-D-gal injected at any time between 2 hours before and 2 hours after training on the passive avoidance task, (but not outside this time window) produces amnesia in birds tested 1 hour later; this amnesia can be prevented if excess galactose is injected together with the 2-D-gal, but not by excess fucose, a result in accord with the presumed biochemical mode of action of the inhibitor (Rose and Jork 1987). Thus prevention of glycoprotein synthesis prevents long-term memory formation.

An inverted form of this experiment is also possible; if memory formation results in enhanced glycoprotein synthesis, then preventing long-term memory should prevent this increase. The experimental trick required to achieve this, discussed also by Stewart (Chapter 11), is supplied by the observation due originally to Benowitz and Magnus (1972), that brief subconvulsive transcranial electric shock applied within 1 minute of training on the passive avoidance task produces amnesia (that is pecking rather than avoidance) in birds tested half an hour or more subsequently; by contrast, if the same shock is applied at 10 minutes after training the majority of birds show recall and avoid the bead. Thus it is possible to compare glycoprotein synthesis in the hours following training and testing in two groups of birds, each of which has pecked at and evinced the disgust response for the bitter tasting bead, and each of which has subsequently had a subconvulsive electric shock. The full experiment requires six groups of birds, three Tr, (a, unshocked, b, immediate shocked, and c, delayed shock); and a corresponding three C. If elevated glycoprotein synthesis only occurs when memory formation is taking place, then both the unshocked and delayed shocked Tr group will show increased fucosylation over the C birds, while the immediate shocked Tr group will not; if, conversely, the increased fucosylation is something to do with the taste of the methylanthranilate or some other feature of the training experience the immediate shock group will also show the effect. In fact, the immediate shocked, amnesic group shows a level of fucose incorporation indistin-guishable from that of its control, and, fortunately, shock itself is without effect on the rate of fucose incorporation at least at the time, several hours later, at which it is measured in this experiment (Rose and Harding 1984). Thus inhibiting glycoprotein synthesis prevents memory formation, and *vice versa*.

The fact that 2-D-gal produces amnesia, however, is potentially of more than just behavioural significance. So far I have referred to the synthesis of synaptic membrane glycoproteins as a generic group, rather than distiguish individual molecular species. However, the biochemical task at this stage is to identify which of this rather broadly defined group of proteins is specifically involved in the presumed synaptic reorganizations. It is relatively easy to separate the membrane glycoproteins, first by comparing SPM with PSD fractions, and then by submitting each mem-brane fraction to one- or two-dimensional gel electrophoresis. However, unless specific new glycoproteins are being made during memory forma-tion, which is improbable, it is likely only that some subset of the molecules is turning over faster or showing a net increase. Identifying this subset by fractioning fucose-labelled material from specific brain regions like IMHV is beyond the sensitivity of currently available techniques. However, 2-D-gal provides a novel dissecting tool, by enabling an easier, purely biochem-ical question to be asked. Which synaptic membrane glycoproteins are *not* synthesized in the presence of 2-D-gal? If we can identify these, then they must include amongst them at least some of those glycoproteins whose synthesis is required for memory formation to occur. We have conducted preliminary experiments along these lines, and found significant effects in a group of SPM glycoproteins of molecular weights in the region of 150–180 kD (Bullock *et al.* 1990). Probably, however, more precise identification is going to have to depend on raising specific antibodies to some amongst this group of glycoproteins (Bullock *et al*. 1988).

FROM BIOCHEMISTRY TO PHYSIOLOGY

If our working assumption is correct, that changes in synaptic membrane biochemistry during memory formation are associated with altered synaptic connectivity, then these connectivity changes should be reflected in altered physiological properties of the neurons. Such changes have now indeed been found (Mason and Rose 1987; 1988). In these experiments, chicks were trained as usual, tested after 30 minutes, and at various times therafter anaesthetized with equithesin and bilateral penetrations made with low impedance micropipettes filled with sodium acetate. Extracellular recordings of spontaneous multi-unit neuronal activity were made by moving the electrodes sequentially through HA, HD, IMHV and PA regions. Examination of the traces showed that they could be resolved into four general categories:

(1) bursting epochs containing high frequency (400–450 Hz) large amplitude (200–450 μV p–p) spikes, burst duration 15–40 ms;
(2) non-bursting (i.e tonically firing) spikes of amplitude to those similar to those occurring in bursts;
(3) non-bursting small amplitude spikes (100–175 μV p–p); and
(4) noise (36 μV p–p max).

Recordings made from animals anaesthatized between 2 and 12 hours after training showed a small but generalized bilateral increase in firing activity in all regions examined. However, when the bursting and non-bursting activity were considered separately, we found a substantial increase, of some fourfold, in bursting activity in right and left IMHV, but in no other region. To check whether this increased bursting activity was indeed associated with memory formation, we used the subconvulsive electroshock procedure described above, recording only from the IMHV. Trained, shocked but non-amnesic birds showed the increase in bursting, but in the shocked amnesic group the increase was abolished. By contrast, both groups showed an increase in non-bursting activity compared with shocked controls, suggesting that the generalized increased non-bursting activity found in both this and the first experiment is a consequence of the training experience—perhaps the taste of the methylanthranilate—rather than an aspect of memory formation *per se* (Fig. 10.2). This interpretation is strengthened by the observation that if small quantities of methylanthranilate are placed in the oral cavity of anaesthetized chicks there is a transient increase in non-bursting activity but no change in bursting.

Thus prolonged increases in phasic bursting, of high-frequency large amplitudes spikes in the IMHV, appears to be a neurophysiological correspondent of memory formation. While we do not yet understand its significance, analogous bursting activity has been found in mammals. Thus there are resemblances with the population firing in LTP, and with the phasic activity of theta rhythm, both believed to be associated with memory formation.

FROM BIOCHEMISTRY TO MORPHOLOGY

It is the thesis of this paper that in the long term, the brain represents experience—that is, stores memory—in the form of stable patterns of synaptic connections distributed across relatively small ensembles of neurons. The biochemical events that are catalogued above are therefore to be seen as aspects of the mobilization of processes of specific synaptic formation, growth or modulation, which, once achieved, are maintained in the same way as other stable synaptic connections are maintained within the brain. (This is, I am aware, a euphemism for saying that we don't at all understand how they are maintained, but that at least in this context the problem of memory reduces to a particular case of the general problem of the maintenance of neural specificity.) The merit of this formulation, however, is that it makes clear that we need not expect that the biochemical processes required for the induction of synaptic change are still required for its maintenance; in this sense we may expect that after the burst of activity involved in the remodelling (and other) processes, the biochemistry of the cell ensemble will revert to some hypothetical 'ground state' once more.

In the case of passive avoidance learning, we do not know quite how long the changed rates of protein and glycoprotein synthesis persist after training; they are still apparent after 24 hours, but no longer after 48 hours (Mileusnic *et al.* 1980; Sukumar *et al.* 1980). However, it was their persistence until 24 hours which led to the choice of this time point at which to search for the morphological changes which are described in Chapter 11. The increased synthesis of synaptic membrane glycoproteins is likely to be required for the production of the increased numbers of dendritic spines on projection neurons, and the increased length of the postsynaptic thickening of the left IMHV, amongst the other morphological phenomena discussed therein. It would be predicted from the morphology, however, that there should be other more lasting biochemical changes. Thus if the dendritic surface has been expanded by the appearance of more spines serving as synaptic contact zones, then one should expect changes in the total quantity (but no longer in the synthesis) of specific postsynaptic membrane glycoproteins. It is for the purpose of

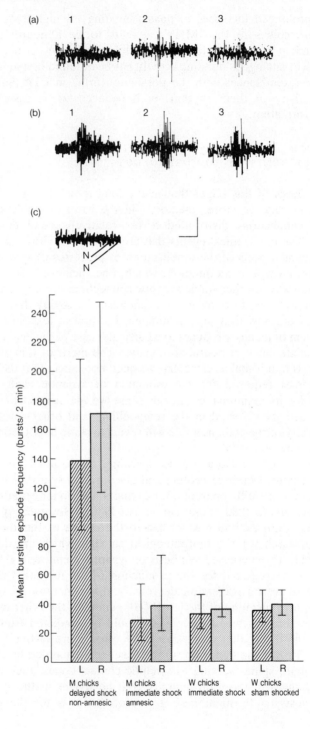

Fig. 10.2   Passive avoidance learning and bursting activity. *Upper panel*: patterns of multi-unit neuronal activity recorded from IMHV of anaesthetized chicks during the period 1–12 hours following training on the passive avoidance task. (a) 'Non-bursting' firing. (b) Bursting episodes. (c) Noise. For definitions of bursting and non-bursting, see text. *Lower panel*: bursting activity in left and right IMHV of Tr (*M*) and C (*W*) chicks in the electroshock amnesia paradigm. Bursting activity is increased only in those chicks which have pecked at the methylanthranilate bead but are not amnesic; all other groups show no differences in bursting activity. The experimental paradigm is described in the text. (Data from Mason and Rose 1987, 1988.)

identifying and quantifying any such membrane components that we are now attempting to raise antibodies to PSD proteins. Similarly, the increased numbers of synaptic vesicles found by Stewart *et al.* (1984) in left IMHV might be anticipated to have a biochemical reflection in terms of changed quantities of vesicle-specific components. The search for these led us to measure the binding of monoclonal antibodies for two specific vesicle constituents to material from IMHV, PA and LPO. The two antibodies we chose were SV2, which is a marker for cholinergic vesicles, and p65 which recognizes an apparently universal integral vesicle membrane protein (Matthew *et al.* 1981; Buckley and Kelly 1985). We were able to find left/right asymmetries in the titres of these antibodies which resembled those from the morphological data (Bullock *et al.* 1987) but although these were training-induced changes, they could not readily be mapped onto the morphological ones.

Perhaps, granted the very different methodologies involved [for instance a change in antibody titre can reflect a difference in the availability of an epitope (the form of a macromolecule recognized by a specific antibody), or differential masking, as well as changes in the quantity of the structure in which the antigen is embedded] this is not so surprising, but it points to some of the difficulties which still lie in the way of ready translation between biochemistry and morphology, let alone biochemistry and behaviour. Nonetheless, this must remain our goal, and we are committed to the view that passive avoidance learning in the chick is about as good a vertebrate model as we are likely to find in which to achieve it.

Acknowledgements

The research described in this chapter has been carried out under grants from the NIH, SERC, and MRC, and is presently supported by grants from the SERC and MRC, as well as a personal Wolfson Research Award. Support for visitors to the laboratory who been involved in this work has come from the British Council, Royal Society, and Wellcome Trust. Apart from visitors and students whose contribution is indicated amongst the references below, I would like particularly to acknowledge the continued collaboration of Sarah Bullock, Jenny Potter, and Mike Stewart in the experiments described here, and the work of our colleagues in the Animal House Dawn Sadler and Steve Walters. I thank Konstantin Anokhin, Alistair Barber, Margaret Boxer, Rachel Bourne, Dave Gilbert, Ceri Davies, Terry Patterson, and Mike Stewart for permission to quote unpublished work.

REFERENCES

Agranoff, B. W., Burrell, H. R., Dokas, L. R., and Springer A. D. (1976). Progress in biochemical approaches to learning and memory. In *Psychopharmacology* (ed. M. Lipton, A. De Mascio, and K. Killam), pp. 623–35. Raven Press, New York.

Akers, R. F., Lovinger, D. M., Colley, P. A., Linden, D. J., Routtenberg, A. (1986). Translocaton of protein kinase C activity may mediate hippocampal long-term potentiation. *Science*, **231**, 587–9.

Ali, S., Bullock, S., and Rose, S. P. R. (1988*a*). Phosphorylation of synaptic proteins in chick forebrain: changes with development and passive avoidance training. *Journal of Neurochemisty*, **50**, 1579–87.

Ali, S., Bullock, S., and Rose, S. P. R. (1988*b*). Protein kinase C inhibitors prevent long-term memory formation in the one-day-old chick. *Neuroscience Research Communicatons*, **3**, 133–9.

Anokhin, K. V., Mileusnic, R. M., Shumakina, I. Y., and Rose S. P. R. (1990). Effects of early experience on c-fos expression in the chick forebrain. (In press.)

Barber, A., Gilbert, D., and Rose, S. P. R. (1989). Glycoprotein synthesis is necessary for memory of sickness-induced learning in chicks. *European Journal of Neuroscience*, **1**, 673–7.

Bateson, P. P. G., Horn, G., and Rose, S. P. R. (1972). Effects of early experience on regional incorporation of precursors into RNA and protein in the chick brain. *Brain Research*, **39**, 449–65.

Benowitz, L. and Magnus, J. G. (1972). Memory storage processes following one-trial passive aversive conditioning in the chick. *Behavioral Biology*, **8**, 367–80.

Bliss, T. V. P. and Lømo T. (1973). Long lasting potentiation of synaptic transmission in the dentate area of the unanaesthetised rabbit following stimulation of the perforant path. *Journal of Physiology*, **232**, 331–56.

Bradley, P. M. and Galal, K. M. (1988). State dependent recall can be induced by protein synthesis inhibition: behavioural and morphological observations. *Developmental Brain Research*, **40**, 243–51.

Buckley, K. and Kelly, R. B. (1985). Identification of a transmembrane glycoprotein specific for secretory vesicles of neural and endocrine cells. *Journal of Cell Biology*, **100**, 1284–94.

Bullock, S., Csillag, A., and Rose, S. P. R. (1987). Synaptic vesicle proteins and acetylcholine levels in chick forebrain nuclei are altered by passive avoidance training. *Journal of Neurochemistry*, **49**, 812–20.

Bullock, S., Gordon Weeks, P. R., and Csillag, A. (1988). Preparation and characterisation of a monoclonal antibody to an antigen in chick brain postsynaptic densities. *Journal of Neurochemistry*, **51**, 442–50.

Bullock, S., de Grace, P. N. E., Oestreicher, A. B., Gispen, W. A., and Rose, S. P. R. (1990). Identification of c52 kD chick brain membrane protein showing changed phosphorylation after passive avoidance training *Neuroscience Research Communications*, **6**, 181–6.

Bullock, S., Potter, J., and Rose, S. P. R. (1990). Effects of the amnesic agent 2-deoxygalactose on incorporation of fucose into chick brain glycoproteins. *Journal of Neurochemistry*, **54**, 135–42.

Burchuladze, R., Potter, E., and Rose, S. P. R. (1990). Memory formation in the chick depends on membrane-bound protein kinase c. *Brain Research*. (In press.)

Burgoyne, R. and Rose, S. P. R. (1980). Subcellular localisation of increased incorporation of ^{3}H fucose following passive avoidance learning in the chick. *Neuroscience Letters*, **19**, 343–8.

Byrne, J. H. (1987). Cellular analysis of associative learning. *Physiological Reviews*, **67**, 329–439.

Chiarugi, V. P., Ruggiero, M., and Corradetti, R. (1989). Oncogenes, protein kinase C, neuronal differentiation and memory. *Neurochemistry International*, **14**, 1–9.

Coulter, J. C. (1988). Cholinergic receptors studied by antagonist labelling distribution; ontogeny and function. Thesis, Open University.

Gaston, K. (1977). An illness-induced conditioned aversion in domestic chicks: one-trial learning with a long delay of reinforcement. *Behavioral Biology*, **20**, 441–53.

Goelet, P., Castelucci, V. F., Schacher, S., and Kandel E. R. (1986). The long and the short of long-term memory—a molecular framework. *Nature*, **322**, 419–22.

Gispen, W.-H. and Routtenberg, A. (eds) (1982 and 1986). *Phosphoproteins in neuronal function. Progress in Brain Research*, Vols 58 and 69: Elsevier, Amsterdam.

Haywood, J., Rose, S. P. R., and Bateson, P. P. G. (1975). Changes in chick brain RNA polymerase associated with an imprinting procedure. *Brain Research*, **92**, 227–35.

Hambley, J. and Rogers L. J. (1979). Retarded learning induced by amino acids in the neonatal chick, *Neuroscience*, **4**, 677–84.

Heald, P. J. (1960) *Phosphorus metabolism of brain*. Pergamon, Oxford.

Horn, G. and Hinde, R. (ed.) (1970). *Short-term processes in neural activity and behaviour*. Cambridge University Press.

Horn, G., McCabe, B., and Bateson, P. P. G. (1979). An autoradiographic study of the chick brain after imprinting. *Brain Research*, **168**, 361–73.

Horn, G., Rose, S. P. R., and Bateson, P. P. G. (1973). Experience and plasticity in the nervous system. *Science*, **181**, 506–14.

Jork, R., Grecksh, G., and Matthies H.-J. (1986). Impairment of hippocampal glycoprotein fucosylation—consequences on memory formation, In *Learning and memory: mechanisms of information storage in the nervous system* (ed. H.-J. Matthies), pp. 223–8. Pergamon, Oxford.

Kohsaka, S., Takamatsu, K., Aoki, E., and Tsukada, Y. (1979). Metabolic mapping of chick brain after imprinting using ^{14}C 2-deoxyglucose technique. *Brain Research*, **172**, 539–44.

Kossut, M. and Rose, S. P. R. (1984). Differential 2-deoxyglucose uptake into chick brain structures during passive avoidance training. *Neuroscience*, **12**, 971–7.

Lossner, B. and Rose, S. P. R. (1983). Passive avoidance training increases fucokinase activity in right forebrain base of day old chicks. *Journal of Neurochemistry*, **41**, 1357–63.

Lynch, G. and Baudry, M, (1984). The biochemistry of memory—a new and specific hypothesis. *Science*, **224**, 1057–63.

Lynch, M. and Bliss, T. V. P. (1986). Long-term potentiation of synaptic transmission in the hippocampus of the rat; effect of calmodulin and oleoyl-acetyl-glycerol on release of $[^3\text{-H}]$ glutamate. *Neuroscience Letters*, **65**, 171–6.

McCabe, N. R. and Rose, S. P. R. (1985). Passive avoidance training increases fucose incorporation into glycoproteins in chick forebrain slices *in vitro*. *Neurochemical Research*, **10**, 1083–95.

McCabe, N. R. and Rose, S. P. R. (1987). Increased fucosylation of chick brain proteins following training: effects of cycloheximide. *Journal of Neurochemistry*, **48**, 538–42.

Margolis, R. H. and Margolis, R. K. (1977). Metabolism and function of glycoproteins and glycosaminoglycans in nervous tissue. *International Journal of Biochemistry*, **8**, 85–91.

Mason, R. J. and Rose, S. P. R. (1987). Lasting changes in spontaneous multi-unit activity in the chick brain following passive avoidance training. *Neuroscience*, **21**, 931–41.

Mason, R. J. and Rose, S. P. R. (1988). Passive avoidance learning produces focal elevation of bursting activity in the chick brain: amnesia abolishes the increase. *Behavioral and Neural Biology*, **49**, 280–92.

Matthew, W. D., Tsavaler, L., and Reichardt, L. F. (1981). Identification of a synaptic vesicle-specific membrane protein with a wide distribution in neuronal and neurosecretory tissue. *Journal of Cell Biology*, **91**, 257–69.

Matthies H.-J. (1989). Neurobiological aspects of learning and memory. *Annual Review of Psychology*, **40**, 381–404.

Mileusnic, R., Rose, S. P. R., and Tillson, P. (1980). Passive avoidance learning results in region-specific changes in concentration of and incorporation into colchicine-binding proteins in the chick forebrain. *Journal of Neurochemistry*, **34**, 1007–15.

Murakami, K., Gordon Weeks, P. R., and Rose, S. P. R. (1986). Isolation of postsynaptic densities from day-old chicken brain. *Journal of Neurochemistry*, **46**, 340–7.

Nelson, R. B. and Routtenberg, A. (1985). Characterisation of the 47 kDa protein F1 (pI 4.5), a kinase C substrate dirctly related to neural plasticity. *Experimental Neurology*, **89**, 213–24.

Nolan, P. M., Bell, R., and Rega, C. M. (1987). Acquisition of a brief behavioural experience in the presence of neuron-specific and D2-CAM/N-CAM-specific antisera. *Neurochemical Research*, **12**, 619–24.

Oestreicher, A. B., Zwiers, H., Schotman, P., and Gispen, W.-H. (1981). Immunohistochemical localisation of phosphoprotein (B-50) isolated from rat brain synaptosomal plasma membranes. *Brain Research Bulletin*, **6**, 145.

Oestreicher, A. B., Van Drougen, C. J., Zwiers, H., and Gispen W.-H. (1983).

Affinity-purified anti-B-50 antibody: interference with the function of the phosphoprotein B-50 in synaptic plasma membrane. *Journal of Neurochemistry*, **41**, 331–40.

Patterson, T. A., Gilbert, D., and Rose, S. P. R. (1990). Pre- and post-training lesions of the IMHV and passive avoidance learning in the chick. *Experimental Brain Research*, **80**, 189–95.

Patterson, T. A., Rose, S. P. R., and Bradley, P. (1989). Anisomycin and amnesia in the chick; state-dependent effects are not present with intracranial injections. *Developmental Brain Research*, **49**, 173–8.

Popov, N., Schulzeck, S., Pohle, W., and Matthies, H.-J. (1981). Changes in the incorporation of ^{3}H-fucose into rat hippocampus after acquisition of a brightness discrimination reaction: an electrophoretic study. *Neuroscience*, **5**, 161–7.

Reymann, K. G., Schulzeck, K., Kase, H., and Matthies, H.-J. (1988). Phorbol ester-induced long-term potentiation is counteracted by inhibitors of protein kinase C. *Experimental Brain Research*, **71**, 227–30.

Rose, S. P. R. (1977). Early visual experience, learning and neurochemical plasticity in the rat and the chick. *Philosophical Transactions of the Royal Society of London*, **278**, 307–18.

Rose, S. P. R. (1981). What should a biochemistry of learning and memory be about? *Neuroscience*, **6**, 811–21.

Rose, S. P. R. (1988). Mind and memory between molecule and metaphor. In *Systems with learning and memory abilities* (ed. J. Delacour and J. C. S. Levy), pp. 177–97. Elsevier, Amsterdam.

Rose, S. P. R. and Csillag, A. (1985). Passive avoidance training results in lasting changes in deoxyglucose metabolism in left hemisphere regions of chick brain. *Behavioral and Neural Biology*, **44**, 315–24.

Rose, S. P. R., Gibbs, M., and Hambley, J. (1980). Transient increase in forebrain muscarinic cholinergic receptors following passive avoidance learning in young chicks. *Neuroscience*, **5**, 169–72.

Rose, S. P. R. and Harding, S. (1984). Training increases ^{3}H fucose incorporation in chick brain only if followed by memory storage. *Neuroscience*, **12**, 663–7.

Rose, S. P. R. and Jork, R. (1987). Long-term memory formation in chicks is blocked by 2-deoxygalactose, a fucose analogue. *Behavioral and Neural Biology*, **48**, 246–58.

Routtenberg, A., George, D. A., Davis, L. G., and Brunngraber, E. G. (1974). Memory consolidation and fucosylation of crude synaptosomal glycoproteins resolved by gel electrophoresis. *Behavioural Biology*, **12**, 461–75.

Rumelhart, D. E., McClelland, J. L., and the PDP Research Group (1986). *Parallel distributed processing* (2 vols.). MIT Press, Cambridge, Mass.

Sagar, S. M., Sharp, F. P., and Curran, T. (1988). Expression of c-fos protein in brain: metabolic mapping at the cellular level. *Science*, **240**, 1328–31.

Schliebs, R., Rose, S. P. R., and Stewart, M.G. (1985). Effects of passive avoidance learning on protein synthesis in forebrain slices of day old chicks. *Journal of Neurochemistry*, **44**, 1014–28.

Scheich, H. (1989). *Physiological Reviews*. (In press.)

Schmidt, R. (1987). Changes in subcellular distribution of ependymins in goldfish brain induced by learning. *Journal of Neurochemistry*, **48**, 1870–8.

Shashoua, V. E. (1985). The role of brain extracellular proteins in neuroplasticity and learning. *Cellular and Molecular Neurobiology*, **5**, 183–207.

Singer, W. (1987). Developmental plasticity—self-organisation or learning? In *Imprinting and cortical plasticity* (ed. J. P. Rauscheker and P. Marler), pp. 171–6. Wiley, New York.

Skarda, C. and Freeman, W. (1987). How brains make chaos in order to make sense of the world. *Behavioural and Brain Sciences*, **10**, 161–73.

Stewart, M. G., Rose, S. P. R., King, T. S., Gabbott, P. L. A., and Bourne R. (1984). Hemispheric asymmetry of synapses in chick medial hyperstriatum ventrale following passive avoidance training: a stereological investigation. *Developmental Brain Research*, **12**, 261–9.

Sukumar, R., Rose, S. P. R., and Burgoyne, R. (1980). Increased incorporation of ^{3}H fucose into chick brain glycoprotein following training on a passive avoidance task. *Journal of Neurochemistry*, **34**, 1000–7.

11

Changes in dendritic and synaptic structure in chick forebrain consequent on passive avoidance learning

M. G. Stewart

PASSIVE AVOIDANCE LEARNING—INTRODUCTION

Newly hatched domestic chicks peck indiscriminately at small objects in their field of view but quickly learn to distinguish between food and non-food objects; this is clearly most important in selection of food in the natural environment. Knowledge of this discrimination ability has allowed development of an experimental learning task centred on avoidance by the chick of pecking at unpleasant tasting substances (Chapter 1). This paradigm, which involves one-trial passive avoidance learning, was first introduced by Cherkin (1969), and was subsequently developed further by Gibbs and Ng (1977). It has been extensively studied for some time in our laboratories as a model for the cellular correlates of memory formation. In this chapter I will consider the avoidance learning paradigm as used at the Open University and review some of the data relating both to the discovery of the loci of memory formation for the avoidance task within the forebrain, and its structural basis at the neuronal and synaptic level. The changes that I will describe occur some 24 hours post-training and are therefore presumed to represent long-term memory store. We do not yet know the time course of these morphological changes though some, at least, must have correlates in the biochemical changes which are known to occur at particular times during the 24 hours post-training (Rose 1981). Where possible, comparisons will be made with known morphological changes in chick brain resulting from other types of learning, notably filial imprinting. The preceding Chapter (10), which forms a pair with this, considers molecular mechanisms of learning in the chick.

BEHAVIOURAL PROCEDURES

The training procedure for passive avoidance learning used in our laboratory has been described in detail elsewhere (Stewart *et al.* 1984) and will only be briefly considered here. Chicks (at 24–30 hours post-hatch) are placed in pairs in a small pen (pairing of chicks reduces the distress often observed in chicks housed singly). Chicks are pre-trained with three presentations of a small white bead 2–3 cm in front of the beak. Ten minutes after the third pre-training trial birds are presented in the training trial with a chrome bead (4 mm diameter) either dipped in water (W: *control chicks*), or in a bitter tasting substance, methylanthranilate (M: *trained chicks*). At training, behaviour is scored as peck, or peck and shake head, with beak wiping on the floor of the pen (the disgust response to methylanthranilate), or avoid (about 10 per cent of chicks, which are not used for further analysis). The chicks are tested 30 minutes later by a single presentation of a dry but otherwise identical chrome bead and scored for peck or avoidance, and then re-tested at a selected experimental time up to 25 hours later. Birds are used for subsequent anatomical work only if they give the correct response on this final test (approximately 80 per cent), i.e. by pecking if water controls (W- chicks) or avoiding if methylanthranilate trained (M- chicks). Birds are coded, all subsequent procedures being performed blind, with the codes broken only when all experimental work is completed.

STATISTICAL METHODS

Following experimental work the data are analysed using rigorous statistical procedures: in the case of studies of altered synaptic or dendritic structure this involves taking means of measurements for individual parameters from each hemisphere of each chick, and then using these mean values in an appropriate analysis of variance (ANOVA)—a split plot ANOVA for data from synaptic measurements—with control versus training as one factor and hemisphere (left versus right) as another. For data from studies involving dendritic measurements a nested, repeated-measures analysis of variance (training by order within hemisphere) is adopted. Differences are considered to be significant where F values correspond to a value of $p < 0.05$.

LOCATION OF FOREBRAIN REGIONS INVOLVED IN PASSIVE
AVOIDANCE TRAINING

The initial biochemical studies from our group on the avoidance paradigm
involved measures made on relatively large regions of the forebrain
dissected into roof (anterior and posterior) and base. Many of the
alterations following training, such as a rise in quinuclidinyl benzilate
(QNB) binding to putative muscarinic receptors (Rose *et al.* 1980) and of
(^{14}C)-leucine incorporation into tubulin (Mileusnic *et al.* 1980) were
localized to the anterior forebrain roof, whereas others such as enhanced
(^{14}C)-fucose incorporation into glycoproteins were found in the forebrain
base regions. To investigate the localization of the metabolic changes
more precisely, the 2-deoxyglucose (2DG) autoradiographic technique of
Sokoloff *et al.* (1977) was used, 2DG being taken as a general marker of
metabolic activity (presumably in this case, mainly due to increased
electrical activity). In these studies chicks were pre-trained as described
above and then immediately before the actual training trial, using either
water (W) or methylanthranilate (M), were injected with 10 μmCi (^{14}C)
2DG. The birds were tested 30 minutes later and were then killed by
decapitation, and the brains frozen and prepared for apposition autoradiography (Kossut and Rose 1984). The overall labelling patterns of the
autoradiograms of coronal serial sections of M and W birds were qualitatively similar throughout the forebrains. However, a quantitative study
(Table 11.1), in which measurements were made of the optical densities of
13 regions of the autoradiograms of coronal serial sections of M and W
birds, showed that there was altered 2DG labelling in three main regions
of M-chicks, the hyperstriatum ventrale posterior region (HVp), and in
two parts of the palaeostriatal complex, the paleostriatum augmentatum
(PA) and the lobus parolfactorius (LPO). In subsequent experiments these
data were replicated when 2DG metabolism following passive avoidance
learning was measured (via scintillation counting methods) in small regions
of the chick forebrain removed from fresh tissue using a microdissection
technique (Rose and Csillag 1985). However, in this case the regions of
change identified were the medial hyperstriatum ventrale (MHV) and the
LPO, with no elevations in incorporation of 2DG being found in the PA.
The differences in the data from the two experiments were taken to reflect
the large areas sampled in the autoradiographic study. The palaeostriatal
regions, the PA and LPO, had not previously been identified as loci of
memory formation in the chick, but the involvement of the hyperstriatum
ventrale in learning was not surprising given its supposed role as a
polysensory processing centre (Benowitz 1980; Horn 1985), analogous to
association cortex in mammals. Indeed lesions in the hyperstriatum
ventrale have been shown to affect both avoidance learning (Davies *et al.*

Table 11.1   Optical densities of 2-deoxyglucose autoradiograms of forebrain structures of trained (methylanthranilate) and control (water) chicks. (From Kossut and Rose 1984.)

Structure	(a) Methylanthranilate	(b) Water	(a)/(b) × 100
Ectostriatum	3.13±0.27	3.20±0.23	98
Archistriatum ventrale	2.26±0.20	2.27±0.32	104
Neostriatum	2.36±0.20	2.19±0.25	108
Area L4	2.24±0.13	2.17±0.09	103
Palaeostriatum augmentatum	2.40±0.11	2.13±0.08	113*
Area parahippocampalis	2.14±0.27	2.05±0.25	104
Lobus parolfactorius	2.14±0.06	1.92±0.08	111*
Hyperstriatum accessorium	1.85±0.10	1.90±0.13	97
Hyperstriatum dorsale/intercalatus	1.91±0.14	1.89±0.13	101
Neostriatum mediale	1.93±0.13	1.88±0.14	103
Nucleus septalis lateralis	1.87±0.14	1.76±0.10	106
Hyperstriatum ventrale (post)	1.90±0.14	1.72±0.13	110*
Hyperstriatum ventrale (medial)	1.72±0.17	1.65±0.13	104

Data are based on mean optical density, expressed in each case as ratio to reference structure ± SD; $n = 7$ in each case except for lobus parolfactorius, neostriatum mediale and nucleus septalis lateralis where $n = 4$.
* Differences are significant in paleostriatum augmentatum, lobus parolfactorius and hyperstriatum ventrale posterior.

1988; Chapters 10, 12) and imprinting of chicks (Horn 1985; Chapter 8). Moreover, the hyperstriatum ventrale was also identified as a key region in memory formation in imprinting studies by Horn *et al.* 1979 (Chapter 8), on the basis of studies which showed an increased incorporation of uracil into RNA in response to overtraining of chicks on a red flashing light. The part of the hyperstriatum ventrale involved in imprinting was termed by Horn (1985) the intermediate and medial hyperstriatum ventrale (IMHV), and is the same as that identified in the study of Rose and Csillag (1985). The hyperstriatum ventrale also includes part of the region MNH (medial neostriatum and hyperstriatum ventrale), which was identified by Scheich and his colleagues (following 2DG studies), as playing a key role in auditory imprinting in the guinea fowl (Scheich 1987).

MORPHOLOGICAL STUDIES OF CORRELATES OF AVOIDANCE
LEARNING IN THE CHICK

Synaptic changes

The changes in 2DG metabolism following training (reflected by the elevations in 2DG labelling) occur within 1 hour of training of chicks and must presumably represent a phase connected with short term memory formation. If this is to be translated into a lasting change (i.e. into long term memory) it seems reasonable to expect that there will be alterations in connectivity between nerve cells, which on most current models of learning means modifications in efficacy at the synaptic level (Thompson *et al.* 1983). Such changes are likely to result in remodelling of existing circuitry with the loss of under-specified pathways and strengthening of other synaptic connections, but formation of new pathways may also occur.

Therefore in a series of experiments we investigated the nature of changes in synaptic morphology in the HV (both the IMHV and the HVp), PA, and LPO, as a consequence of training. In all these experiments the possibility of lateralization of changes was examined because of the considerable evidence of hemispheric asymmetry of avian brain function (Andrew 1983; Horn 1985; Mench and Andrew 1986; Rogers 1986: Chapters 20, 21).

One important point to note is that any possible morphological changes in the forebrain at either the neuronal or synaptic level will undoubtedly take place against a background of continuing developmental maturation. Regions so far investigated are the IMHV and LPO (Bradley 1985; Curtis and Stewart 1989; Hunter and Stewart 1989). In the IMHV we have shown that in the first week post-hatching, there is a marked increase in total synapse numerical density ($N_{v.syn}$), from 30 synapses per 100 μm^3 at 1 day post-hatch to 50 synapses per 100 μm^3 at 9 days post-hatch, and there are differences between the development profiles for synapses with asymmetric as compared to symmetrical synaptic junctions (Curtis and Stewart 1989). Similar changes are observed in the LPO (Hunter and Stewart 1989). In contrast to synaptic development, in the IMHV the number of neurons per unit volume, ($N_{v.neu}$), decreased by approximately 50 per cent from the value at 16 days *in ovo* to that at day 0 (hatching), then remained stable to 3 days post-hatch, before declining to almost a quarter of the original population size in 9-day-old birds. When the synapse to neuron ratio was examined in the IMHV, a trend was observed of a gradual increase with age. No hemispheric differences existed in the synaptic or neuronal measures in the IMHV during the period of development that we investigated but in the LPO there is a hemispheric asymmetry of

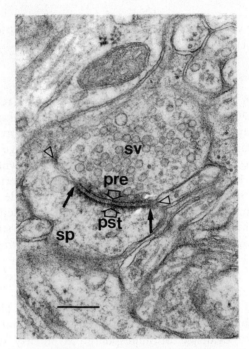

Fig. 11.1 Electron micrograph from chick IMHV synapse showing a synapse containing spheroid shaped vesicles (sv) and making a synaptic contact on a spine head (sp). The total synaptic apposition zone is between the open arrowheads. The limits of the postsynaptic thickening (pst) are indicated by the solid arrows; measurement of the length of the postsynaptic thickening (pst) is made between these; pre = presynaptic thickening. Scale bar = 0.2 μm.

synaptic number at 9 days post-hatch, with the left hemisphere containing 1.6 times more synapses than the right hemisphere.

In the passive avoidance learning studies the chicks were trained at 24 hours post-hatch, as described above, but were left for 24–25 hours before being killed in order to allow time for any possible morphological alterations to occur. The chicks were then intracardially perfused with a glutaraldehyde/formaldehyde mixture and the brains exposed. Tissue samples from the left and right forebrain hemispheres of the IMHV, PA and LPO of up to eight W-and eight M-chicks were removed either stereotaxically, or via a microdissection technique (Rose and Csillag 1985), and the tissue was processed for electron microscopy. In all experiments chicks were coded and the codes were only broken when all the experiments and measurements were complete. Electron micrographs (25 micrographs from each hemisphere of each animal) of neuropil only were taken on either Philips 301 or JEOL 100S electron microscopes using rigorous

Table 11.2 Summary of changes in synaptic structure in three regions of the chick forebrain, 24 h following passive avoidance training.

Hyperstriatum ventrale. HVp (hyperstriatum ventrale posterior) no synaptic changes; *IMHV* (intermediate and medial hyperstriatum ventrale) synaptic changes are lateralized: there is a hemispheric asymmetry in *postsynaptic thickening* (PST) length in W-chicks; that of the right hemisphere is greater than the left by 12 per cent and this difference is abolished on training. There is an increase in *presynaptic bouton volume* and a large increase in *synaptic vesicle number*, in the left hemisphere of M-chicks.

Lobus parolfactorius. Synaptic changes (some lateralized, some not). There is a hemispheric asymmetry in *PST* length in control chicks: that of the right hemisphere is 10 per cent greater than the left and this difference is reversed on training. There is a large increase in number of *synaptic vesicles* in the left hemisphere following training. In contrast to the IMHV there is an increase in *synaptic number*, in both hemispheres after training.

Paleostriatum augmentatum. Synaptic changes: there is a *hemispheric asymmetry* in *vesicle number*; that of the right is greater than the left in control chicks and this disappears on training. Bouton volume is greater in left hemisphere than right following training.

---

stereological techniques (Stewart *et al.* 1984; 1987). Photomicrographs were printed to a magnification of approximately 45 000 and synaptic measurements were made using a semi-automatic measuring device (digitizing tablet with mouse, attached to a microcomputer running with appropriate morphometric software). The following synaptic parameters were measured (Fig. 11.1): numerical density of synapses ($N_{v.syn}$); length of postsynaptic thickening (PST, sometimes also expressed as mean diameter, D); volume density of the presynaptic bouton (V_v): i.e. volume per unit volume; numerical density of synaptic vesicles ($N_{v.ves}$), and number of vesicles per presynaptic bouton (*ves/syn*). In addition in the paleostriatal regions synaptic contact curvature, which is considered to be an index of structural efficacy or maturity (Dyson and Jones 1980; Wesa *et al* 1982), was also measured.

A summary of the synaptic morphometric changes in the HV, LPO and PA is given in Table 11.2. These data demonstrate clearly that passive avoidance training causes alteration in synaptic morphology in one part of the hyperstriatum ventrale, the IMHV (but not the HVp) and in both of the paleostriatal regions, the PA and LPO. However, as is discussed below, the synaptic changes are not all similar in each region, and synaptic contact curvature (measured only in the paleostriatal regions) showed no significant changes following training. What is perhaps most striking is the lateralization of some of the synaptic parameters in all three regions.

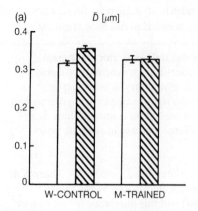 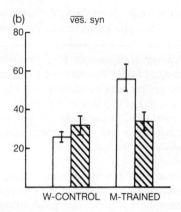

Fig. 11.2 (a) Length ($\bar{D}$) of postsynaptic thickening in left (open bar) and right (cross-hatched bar) hemispheres of the IMHV of control (W)- and trained (M)-chicks 24 h after initial training on a one-trial passive avoidance task. There is a significant interaction of hemisphere and training; each bar is the mean of eight replicate determinations ± SE (from Stewart *et al.* 1984). (b) Synaptic vesicle number expressed as the mean vesicle number per presynaptic bouton (*ves. syn*): the large increase in vesicle number in the left hemisphere of trained (M-) chicks, produces an interaction (Training × Hemisphere) which is statistically highly significant (from Stewart *et al.* 1984).

These may exist before training and be abolished after training: for example, PST length (D) in the IMHV of W-chicks in the right hemisphere is greater than in the left by 12 per cent and this difference is abolished in M-chicks (Fig. 11.2*a*). However, in the LPO where PST length is 10 per cent greater in the right than the left hemisphere in W-control chicks, training does not merely abolish the asymmetry but reverses it. A similar although not identical increase in PST length of left IMHV synapses has been observed by Bradley *et al.* (1981) and Horn *et al.* (1985) following overtraining of chicks on an imprinting stimulus. More recently Bradley (Bradley and Galal 1987) turned his attention to the passive avoidance learning paradigm and has shown that there is a significant increase in the length of the PST in the left IMHV of methylanthranilate trained chicks compared to water trained controls such that the small hemispheric asymmetry, in which PST length in the right hemisphere is greater than the left, is reversed post-training. In contrast to our findings, no other changes in synaptic morphology were observed by Bradley and Galal (1987), although their morphological investigations were carried out 12 hours after initial training in contrast to the 24 hour time point we have used. In our studies the greatest changes in synaptic morphology (number of vesicles per synapse: *ves.syn.*) in the IMHV, LPO, and PA are also lateralized. In the IMHV (Fig. 11.2*b*) the increase in number of vesicles per presynaptic bouton reaches about 60 per cent following training, a figure similar to that observed in the LPO. The synaptic changes in the LPO following avoidance training exhibit differences from those in the IMHV. Whereas synaptic alterations in the IMHV are largely restricted to the left hemisphere, the increase in synaptic numerical density ($N_{v.syn}$) following training (which is not observed in the IMHV) is present in both hemispheres of the LPO. Moreover, the PA synaptic changes are largely different than those in either the LPO or IMHV, involving only a loss of the hemispheric asymmetry in synaptic vesicles in W-chicks and an increase in presynaptic bouton volume in the left hemisphere of M-chicks.

Dendritic changes

The changes in synaptic morphometry in the IMHV and paleostriatal regions together with the demonstration of altered metabolism (from the 2DG studies) are evidence of altered neural function following avoidance learning but are not in themselves proof of memory storage in these regions. For this to be so we would need additional evidence of, e.g. impairment of memory recall following lesions in the region. Such evidence is, as we discuss below, available in the IMHV; consequently, in further morphological studies, in which the nature of postsynaptic changes following passive avoidance learning was to be examined (Patel and Stewart 1988; Patel *et al.* 1988), we concentrated upon the IMHV. The rationale for examination of postsynaptic changes was that alterations in synaptic efficacy brought about by the changes in presynaptic morphology would be likely to be reflected also in changes in dendritic parameters such as spine shape, spine number or pattern of dendritic branching. This approach was additionally attractive to us because of the possibility of using the Golgi technique selectively to examine dendritic parameters of a particular class, or subclass, of morphologically identified neurons, a selectivity denied in our synaptic studies in which all synapses within a hemisphere were, by necessity of the stereological techniques used, measured as a single class without regard to their postsynaptic location.

Chicks were trained and tested approximately 24 hours after initial training as described above, at a similar time to that at which changes in synaptic morphology were recorded. Slabs of IMHV tissue were dissected from perfused brains of M- and W-chicks, Golgi-impregnated using the rapid Golgi technique of Valverde (1970), and then cut into sections of 90–120 μm thickness. Cells in the chick hyperstriatum are all multipolar in nature (based on the number and form of dendrites emanating from the cell body) and these may be divided into two major classes (Tombol *et al.* 1988*a*): putative projection neurons (PNs) (with long axon projecting away some distance from the cell body), and putative local circuit neurons (LCNs, with axon ramifying within the vicinity of the cell body). There are several subclasses of these two main types as detailed in Tombol *et al.* (1988*a*). In preliminary studies only large multipolar projection neurons (LMPNs) (Fig. 11.3*a,b*) showed qualitative changes in spine density 24 hours after passive avoidance training and hence further studies on dendritic parameters were restricted to this neuronal subclass.

A total of 52 LMPNs from 9M-, and 50 LMPNs from 8 W- chicks (~1779 dendrite branches) were analysed. Dendrites were ordered centrifugally, i.e. starting from the cell body, according to the method of Coleman and Riesen (1968); up to 6 orders were present on each dendrite. Dendrite length (DL), dendrite diameter (DD), overall spine length (SL), spine head diameter (SHD), and spine stem length (STL: calculated from SL − SHD; Fig. 11.3*c*) of all the spines visible along each dendrite length, were measured using an ocular graticule at ×2000 in a Zeiss photomicroscope III. The true spine density (calculated using the correction formula of Feldman and Peters 1979), was expressed per μm of dendrite length for each branch order of dendrite. Any protrusions from the dendrite shaft less than 0.7 μm in length which could not be unequivocally identified as a spine were not included in the analysis (approximately 4 per cent of the true spine number). Any dendrites which were truncated or obscured in any way were not included in the measurements. The most striking results are shown in Fig. 11.4*a–d*. There is a highly significant hemispheric asymmetry in spine density in W-control chicks (Fig. 11.4*a*): the right hemisphere has more spines than the left in dendritic orders 2–5. This asymmetry disappears upon training in M-chicks (Fig. 11.4*d*). However, this loss of asymmetry is not simply due to an increase in spine density in the left hemisphere because, as Figs 11.4*a* and *b* show, there are highly significant increases in spine density in both hemispheres of M- compared with W-chicks (up to 113 per cent in the left and 69 per cent in the right hemisphere).

The other important alteration in spine measures following training was that of the spine head diameter and spine stem length (Fig. 11.5*a–d*). Although overall spine length did not increase in the left hemisphere of trained chicks spine head diameter increased (average 9 per cent: Fig. 11.5*a,b*) and spine stem length showed a significant decrease (average 17 per cent: Fig. 11.5*c,d*). There were no significant differences in mean dendrite lengths between M- and W-chicks, nor were there any differences in mean dendrite diameter.

SPECIFICITY OF MORPHOLOGICAL CHANGES TO MEMORY FORMATION

These dendritic changes were quite large; indeed, their size at first surprised us. The possibility existed that such effects might have been due

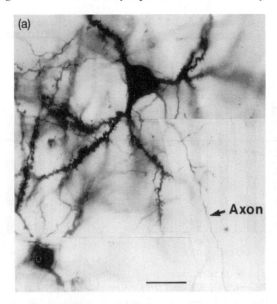

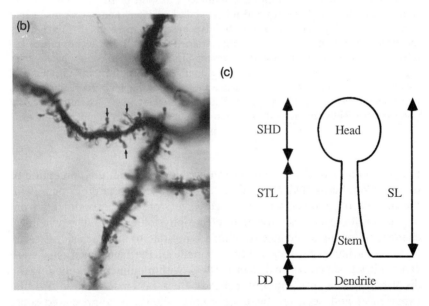

Fig. 11.3 (a) Photomicrograph of large spiny multipolar projection neuron with an axon (arrowed) stretching out into the tissue (scale bar = 20 μm). (b) Higher power photomicrograph of dendrite segment from a showing dendritic spines (arrowed) (scale bar = 10 μm). (c) Schematic representation of a dendritic spine showing the shape parameters measured: SHD = spine head diameter, SL = length of spine, STL = spine stem length (= SL − SHD), DD = dendrite diameter. [(a) and (b) from Patel and Stewart 1988).]

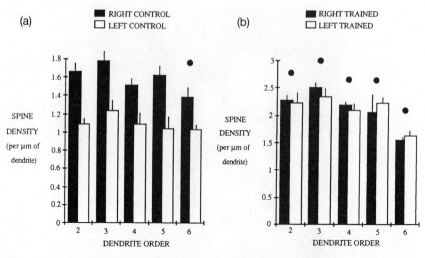

Fig. 11.4 (a) Spine density measures in multipolar projection neurons of the IMHV in water control chicks, and (b) in methylanthranilate-trained chicks, 25 h after training. There is a hemispheric asymmetry in spine density in control chicks (right hemisphere > left—(a) and this is abolished after training (b). Note that spine density in both hemispheres of trained chicks also increases (b). Each bar is the mean spine density value from nine trained (52 cells) and eight control (50 cells) chicks and the vertical bars represent SEs. All the left hemisphere versus right differences for control chicks (a) are significant except for that indicated by a solid circle; the solid circles in (b) indicate that none of the hemispheric differences in trained chicks are significant (from Patel and Stewart 1988). The differences in spine density between trained and control chicks are highly significant for each hemisphere.

to concomitants of the training procedure, for example, the perception of the taste of the methylanthranilate, and are not associated directly with the process of memory formation. However, previous experiments from our laboratory have shown that electrophysiological and biochemical changes following avoidance training are not due to any such side-effects. In these earlier experiments, use was made of the fact that if chicks are given a brief, subconvulsive electric shock within moments of eliciting the disgust response for the bitter bead, they become amnesic for the experience, and peck the bead vigorously when it is re-presented some time later. However, if the shock is delayed to 10 minutes after training, the chicks show recall and avoid the bead on test. By altering the time of administration of the shock relative to the training experience, it is possible to alter the proportion of birds showing recall in relation to those which are amnesic. If a population of trained birds is shocked 5 minutes after training, approximately one half will show recall whereas the other half

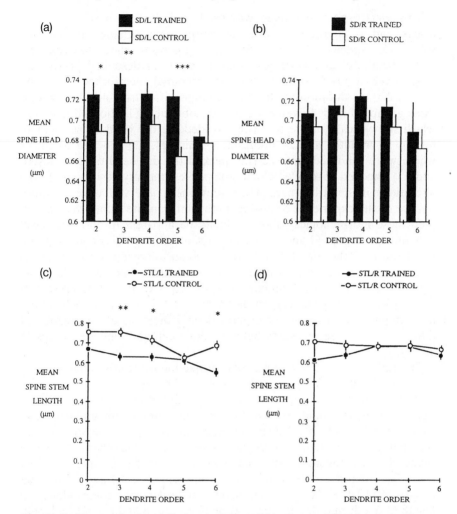

Fig. 11.5 Mean spine head diameter changes 25 h after training. (a) Only the left hemisphere shows significant increases in spine head diameter in orders 2(*), 3(**), and 5(***); (b) the small differences in spine head diameter in the right hemisphere are not significant (L = left, R = right hemisphere); (c) mean spine stem length changes 25 h after training; a significant effect of training is shown only in the left hemisphere in orders 3, 4, and 6; (d) no significant differences are found in the right hemisphere between trained and control chicks (from Patel and Stewart 1988)

are amnesic on test. Chicks trained on a water-coated bead and sub-sequently shocked in a similar way do not show any changes either in pecking behaviour, or in the biochemical and physiological measures so far studied.

This electroshock paradigm was used to induce amnesia in trained chicks, and to determine whether the morphological changes in dendritic spines were specific to memory formation processes related to avoidance of the bead. M- and W-chicks, trained exactly as described previously, were given a brief, subconvulsive, transcranial electroshock (12 mA, 110 V, 220 ms duration at 50 Hz), 5 minutes after training. As a result, three groups of birds (seven in each) were obtained: (1) shocked M-chicks which show recall for the task (i.e. avoided the dry bead on subsequent testing 30 minutes and 24 hours after training), (2) shocked M-chicks where were rendered amnesic (i.e. pecked the dry bead on both tests), and (3) shocked W-chicks which still pecked the dry test bead. If the alterations in dendritic parameters previously observed were a consequence of the experience of tasting methylanthranilate rather than water, then these morphological changes should be apparent in both the recall and amnesic groups (1 and 2) by comparison with the water control group (3). If on the other hand, the dendritic modifications are associated with storage of memory for avoidance of the bead rather than the taste experience of methylanthranilate, then the changes should be present in the shocked recall group (1), but not in the amnesic group (2), when both are compared with the water group (3), and there should be significant differences in these measures between the recall and amnesic groups (1 and 2).

The cells examined were multipolar projection neurons but the analyses were restricted to the third order branches because our previous study (detailed above) demonstrated that only third order branches showed significant changes in all three of the following parameters: an increase in spine density, spine head diameter enlargement, and spine stem length shortening. Other branch orders showed only one or the other of the spine shape changes, together with a concomitant spine density increase. The spine head diameters (SHD), overall spine lengths (SL) and spine stem lengths (STL) (i.e. SL − SHD), of the visible dendritic spines along the length of the third order dendrites were measured, and the dendrite length (DL) and dendrite diameter (DD) were also noted. Measurements and analytical methods were exactly as described above.

Spine density significantly increased in chicks showing recall of the training task, compared to those either rendered amnesic or to the shocked water controls (Fig. 11.6), with the changes showing a significant hemispheric asymmetry. There was a 28 per cent increase in the recall group in the left hemisphere compared to the amnesic group and the water group. The 15 per cent increase in the right hemisphere was not significant compared to the amnesic or water group. These results support the argument that the increase in spine density after passive avoidance training is specifically related to memory processes, because the chicks that were rendered amnesic did not show any change in spine density

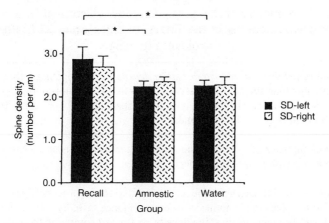

Fig. 11.6 Spine density changes in third order dendrites of multipolar projection neurons from electroshocked chicks. Chicks which recalled the task showed an increase in spine density compared to those which were rendered amnesic and to the water controls. Significant changes were observed only in the left hemisphere. Each bar is the mean of estimations from cells from seven chicks ± SE (from Patel *et al.* 1988). (* = *p* < 0.02.)

compared to the shocked water controls. There were no significant changes in dendrite length or dendrite diameter between chicks in the three groups. The significant spine shape changes (increases in spine head diameter and spine stem length shortening) found between unshocked M- and W-birds in our first study 25 hours after passive avoidance training (Patel and Stewart 1988), were not observed in the electroshock experiments. There were no significant differences in spine shape in trained chicks that were shocked, but still showed recall of the task, compared to chicks rendered amnesic by the electroshock. This suggests that changes in spine shape may not be connected with engram formation *per se*, but might possibly result from physiological factors relating to the training experience itself. Electroshock may also possibly have had a disruptive effect on the structure of the spines, over and above those changes due to memory formation processes, because dendritic spines are very plastic structures, whose shape can change rapidly (within 4 minutes) upon intense electrical stimulation (Van Harreveld and Fifkova 1975). A summary of the dendritic spine changes which occur in the IMHV following passive avoidance learning is shown in Table 11.3.

Table 11.3   Summary of changes in dendritic structure of large multipolar projection type neurons in the IMHV of chick brain 25 h after passive avoidance training.

There is a *hemispheric asymmetry of spine density* in control chicks: that of the right is greater than the left. This asymmetry is abolished on training due to an increase in spine density in both hemispheres, reaching 113 per cent in the left, and 69 per cent in the right hemisphere.

Spine head diameter in left hemisphere also increases after training (by 9 per cent) but with a decrease in *spine stem length* (by 17 per cent).

The *spine density* increases are specifically related to the process of memory formation; in chicks made amnesic for the avoidance task, by subconvulsive electroshock, the increase in spine density, in trained compared to control chicks, is abolished.

THE SIGNIFICANCE OF MORPHOLOGICAL CHANGES ASSOCIATED WITH PASSIVE AVOIDANCE LEARNING

A complex set of morphological changes occur in the chick forebrain following avoidance learning. At the synaptic level these changes are not restricted to a single brain region, the IMHV, but are present in at least two other regions, the PA and LPO, both of which are part of the paleostriatal complex. However, dendritic changes have so far been investigated only in the IMHV. The lesioning experiments of Horn (1985), Davies *et al.* (1988) and Patterson *et al.* (1990), and our neurophysiological data (Mason and Rose 1987; 1988), suggest that the IMHV is at least one of the sites of engram storage both for imprinting, and passive avoidance learning. This information, together with the evidence from the electroshock experiments which shows that the increase in spines is memory related, means that we can be confident that changes in morphology within the IMHV are related to an aspect of the formation of long term memory rather than being connected with stress or some general effect associated with administration of methylanthranilate. In addition, the changes in synapses (at least in postsynaptic thickening length) parallel those shown by Bradley *et al.* (1981) in the IMHV of chicks following imprinting, where the effects are also lateralized to the left hemisphere.

What is much more difficult to determine, in the absence of similar electrophysiological or lesioning data, is whether the changes in the paleostriatal complex are connected directly with long-term memory formation, and if so the functional relationship between the PA, LPO, and the IMHV. The fact that the synaptic changes in the LPO and PA are not all similar to those in the IMHV makes such comparisons more difficult and, whereas synaptic alterations in the IMHV are largely restricted to the left hemisphere, the increase in synaptic numerical density ($Nv._{syn}$) following training (which is not observed in the IMHV) is present in both hemispheres of the LPO. We have previously suggested (Stewart *et al.* 1987) that alterations in synaptic structure in the LPO and PA could represent an additional aspect of the memory trace observed in the IMHV, perhaps a second memory store as has been argued to exist outside the IMHV following imprinting of chicks (Horn 1985). But it may also be that the changes in the palaeostriatal regions (homologues of the mammalian caudate–putamen and nucleus accumbens: Karten and Dubbledam 1973; Chapter 2), represent another aspect of the memory processes involved in learning to avoid the aversive substance, or are even connected with altered motor function. Passive avoidance learning involves not only processing of visual information but also suppression of innate pecking behaviour. The IMHV plays a major role in visual information processing (Horn 1985) and it is interesting that there is a hemispheric asymmetry of morphometric changes in this region following avoidance learning with changes restricted to the left hemisphere. This would appear to be in agreement with the studies of Rogers (1986) which indicate the importance of the left hemisphere in visual discrimination tasks relating to food selection (see Chapters 19, 20, 21). The absence of similar hemispheric asymmetries following training in some of the modifications in synapses in the LPO (e.g. bouton volume) and the finding of increases in synapse number in both hemispheres may indicate differences in the function of this region compared with the IMHV, though what this means in functional terms is difficult to explain at present. However, given the differences in the cytoarchitectonic nature of the IMHV, the PA and LPO (Tombol *et al.* 1988*a,b*), and in their connections with other forebrain regions (Chapters 2, 8; specifically, MHV projects directly to PA but not LPO, Horn 1985), the dissimilar morphological responses of these two paleostriatal regions to passive avoidance training are not perhaps surprising.

One of the key questions arising from this work is how to interpret the relationship between the alterations in synaptic and spine morphology, spine density, and the process of memory formation. Because of the unavailability of data on dendritic changes in the palaeostriatal regions, such considerations must at present be restricted to the IMHV. One fact which might appear to run contrary to the observed increases in spine density is that no significant changes in the numbers of synapses in the IMHV have been found. An essential difference between the dendritic and synaptic studies is that the latter did not differentiate between the neuronal classes to which the synapses belonged, and thus measured total synapse numbers after passive avoidance training, whereas in the dendritic study differences in spine number were analysed only in one specific class of neuron. Also, an increase in spine number does not necessarily indicate an increase in synapse number: the latter would remain unchanged if shaft synapses become spine synapses after training (Chang and Greenough 1984). Therefore, the results of the two studies are not necessarily incompatible. One other important consideration is whether the increases in spine number which are present at 25 hours post-training, a period considered to represent the phase within which long term memory formation occurs (Gibbs and Ng 1977), really last for more than a few days. A loss of spines has been found by Wallhauser and Scheich (1987), who imprinted chicks (on auditory stimuli) in the first 2 days post-hatch, and then measured spine densities in large multipolar neurons (similar to those analysed in our work) in the NMH (medial neostriatum and hyperstriatum) when the chicks were 7 days old. Spine density fell from ~2.3 spines per μm to ~1.8, 5 days after auditory imprinting. In our studies chicks were trained when they were 1 day old, and the spine density of projection neurons analysed 25 hours later increased from ~1.8 spines per μm to ~2.5 spines per μm. Whether there is a selective stabilization of dendritic (and synaptic) contacts which have been initially over produced in response to the training paradigm has yet to be determined for passive avoidance learning. Such a process, which leads long term to a decrease in spines, may be peculiar to acoustic imprinting. However, the possibility of a loss of unwanted spines, some time after the sensitive period, is supported by the finding that large multipolar type neurons in the hyperstriatum ventrale, pars caudale, of 1-year old mynah birds have 50 per cent of the spine complement of that class of neurons in 10-day-old birds. In addition, in mammals, developmental decreases in spine density are also observed in rats (Rothblat and Schwartz 1979), and in monkeys (Boothe *et al.* 1979) after the first 2 months from birth. It would be important to know the nature (if any) of dendritic spine changes in the chick IMHV following filial imprinting (as investigated by Horn's group), especially since there are similarities in the nature of the synaptic morphological changes with those found following avoidance training. Whilst this is of course a matter for speculation (I am not aware that spine density changes have been measured following imprinting by Horn) it is most interesting that the changes in PST length in the IMHV of chicks following overtraining on the imprinting stimulus occur on spine rather than shaft synapses.

A consistent and most interesting finding is that postsynaptic changes in the IMHV following avoidance training appear to be lateralized, with spine density and shape changes being significantly altered only in the left hemisphere (as are the presynaptic changes). These changes appear to be imposed upon a pre-existing asymmetry in the 'control' group; some of the possible reasons for lateralization of function and structure in the avian brain are discussed elsewhere (Chapters 9, 20, 21). The alterations in postsynaptic thickening length in the IMHV together with the increased vesicle number in the left hemisphere of M-, compared with W-chicks are likely to indicate an enhancement in the transmissive capability of synapses. Whether such changes are also connected with presynaptic zone modification in the chick is unknown at present but in amphibian motor nerve terminals, Herrera *et al.* (1985) have provided evidence to support the view that changes in presynaptic zone size may be the structural basis of long-term changes in transmitter release and alterations in synaptic efficacy. Altered synaptic vesicle number in the left IMHV (and LPO) of M-chicks may directly affect synaptic efficacy.

Jack *et al.* (1975) have suggested that a high density of synaptic vesicles would enhance the electrical field potential in the vicinity of the synaptic membrane. Marked changes in synaptic vesicle density following various training paradigms in other animals are also known. In the robustus archistrialis (RA) of canaries there is an increase in synaptic vesicle number associated with acquisition of a new behaviour (DeVoogd 1976; DeVoogd *et al.* 1985), which has been suggested to be related to enhancement of synaptic transmission, and similar suggestions have been made for the increase in synaptic vesicle number following a simple form of non-associative learning (sensitization) in the nudibranch mollusc *Aplysia* (Bailey and Chen 1983). Another (possibly related) correlate of this altered synaptic efficacy is the increase in presynaptic bouton volume in the left IMHV following training, a feature which is also observed in *Aplysia* synapses following long-term sensitization (Bailey and Chen 1988).

If the formation of a memory trace in the chick IMHV involves Hebbian-type circuitry (Hebb 1949), where the efficacy of certain critical synapses (either newly formed or already existing) is increased and strengthened to retain the engram in a neuronal network, then the importance of dendritic spines becomes clear too, in view of their ability to enlarge the surface area of a neuron's receptive field and facilitate impulse transmission to the cell body (Miller *et al.* 1985; Perkel and Perkel 1985; Pongracz 1985; Shepherd *et al.* 1985). We do not have definitive evidence for the chick IMHV, but synaptic inputs onto spines are generally believed to be excitatory (Chapter 8). If this is the case for the chick, greater impulse transmission could therefore also occur due to the shortening of the spine stem, which is believed to result in a lowering of the spine stem resistance and so increase current flow into and along the dendrite. The 'weight' of a synapse onto a spine can, in effect, be changed by alteration in neck length, such as occurs in chick spines. If in addition, the spine heads possess excitable properties, rather than simply possessing passive properties, then the synaptic response is theoretically amplified relative to the passive case (Rall and Sergev 1987). Should this be so in the chick, the potential functional importance of the increase in spine number we have observed becomes even greater.

NECESSARY FURTHER WORK TO HELP UNDERSTAND
MORPHOLOGICAL CHANGES THAT OCCUR FOLLOWING LEARNING

The data discussed above tell us that morphological changes occur at the dendritic and synaptic level following learning but say little about how these events fit into the overall process of altered brain function in the chick that results from storage of the engram. A fundamental problem experienced when working with the chick is that much basic information on the structure and function of the avian brain is lacking. The situation is perhaps analogous to that existing for workers on the mammalian CNS 15 years ago. Yet there are very considerable advantages to working with avian species where behavioural paradigms such as learning tasks can be better controlled than in most mammals. There are several key areas in which further research is needed to provide a better understanding of the synaptic and dendritic changes that occur in the chick forebrain following a learning experience such as one-trial passive avoidance learning.

We need to:

1. Fully identify inputs and outputs of morphologically identified cells within regions of known change, of which the IMHV and LPO appear to be most central to avoidance training studies.
2. Ask whether, and how, inputs and outputs are modified following learning; in other words, we need to determine the neural circuitry involved by use of Golgi, HRP, and tracing studies.
3. Determine the electrophysiological characteristics of the representatives of the class (or classes) of cells in IMHV and LPO which are involved in events associated with learning.
4. Determine the transmitters involved in the identified cells, responsible for modifying their physiological characteristics.

Acknowledgements

Thanks are due to the many colleagues at the Open University, and visitors to the Brain and Behaviour Research Group, who have contributed to the work described here, in particular Dr Sanjay Patel, Professor Steven Rose, Professor Terez Tombol, Ms Rachel Bourne, Dr Andras Csillag, Dr Liz Curtis, Dr Paul Gabbott, Mr Alistar Hunter, Mr Tony King, Mr Mike Lowdnes, Mr David Stanford, and Mr Steve Walters.

REFERENCES

Andrew, R. J. (1983). Lateralization of emotional and cognitive function in higher vertebrates with special reference to the domestic chick. In *Advances in vertebrate neuroethology* (ed J. P. Ewert and D. J. Ingle), pp. 477–509. Plenum, New York.

Bailey, C. H. and Chen, M. (1983). Morphological basis of long-term habituation and sensitization in *Aplysia, Science*, **220**, 91–3.

Bailey, C. H. and Chen, M. (1988). Long-term sensitization in *Aplysia* increases the number of pre-synaptic contacts onto the identified gill motor neuron L7. *Proceedings of the National Academy of Sciences (USA)*, **85**, 9356–9.

Benowitz, L. (1980). Functional organization of the avian telencephalon. In *Comparative neurology of the telencephalon* (ed. S. O. E. Ebbesson), pp. 389–421. Plenum Press, New York.

Boothe, R. G., Greenough, W. T., Lund, J. S., and Wrege, K. (1979). Quantitative investigation of spine and dendrite development of neurons in the visual cortex (area 17) of *Macaca nemestrina* monkeys. *Journal of Comparative Neurology*, **186**, 473–90.

Bradley, P. (1985). Development of two regions of the chick telencephalon. *Developmental Brain Research*, **20**, 83–8.

Bradley, P. G., Horn, G., and Bateson, P. (1981). Imprinting: an electronmicroscope study of chick hyperstriatum ventrale. *Experimental Brain Research*, **41**, 115–20.

Bradley, P. M. and Galal, K. M. (1987). The effect of protein synthesis inhibition on structural changes associated with learning in the chick. *Developmental Brain Research*, **37**, 267–76.

Chang, F.-L., F., and Greenough, W. T. (1984). Transient and enduring morphological correlates of synaptic activity and efficacy change in the rat hippocampal slice. *Brain Research*, **309**, 35–46.

Cherkin, A, (1969). Kinetics of memory consolidation: role of amnestic treatment parameters. *Proceedings of the National Academy of Sciences (USA)*, **63**, 1094–101.

Coleman, P. D. and Riesen, A. H. (1968). Environmental effects on cortical dendritic fields 1. Rearing in the dark, *Journal of Anatomy*, **102**, 35–46.

Curtis, E. M., Stewart, M. G., and King, T. S. (1989). Quantitation of synaptic, neuronal and glial development in the intermediate and medial hyperstriatum ventrale (IMHV) of the chick, *Gallus domesticus*, pre- and post-hatch, *Developmental Brain Research*, **48**, 105–18.

Davies, D. C., Taylor D. C., and Johnson, M. H. (1988). The effects of hyperstriatal lesions on one-trial passive learning in the chick, *Journal of Neuroscience*, **8 (12)**, 4662–6.

DeVoogd, T. J. (1976). Steroid interactions with structure and function of avian song control regions, *Journal of Neurobiology*, **17(3)**, 177–201.

DeVoogd, T. J., Nixdorf, B., and Nottebohm, F. (1985). Synaptogenesis and changes in synaptic morphology related to acquisition of new behaviour, *Brain Research*, **329**, 304–8.

Dyson, S. E. and Jones, D. G. (1980). Quantitation of terminal parameters and their inter-relationships in maturing central synapses, a perspective for experimental studies. *Brain Research*, **183**, 43–59

Feldman, M. L. and Peters, A. (1979). A technique for estimating total spine number on Golgi impregnated dendrites. *Journal of Comparative Neurology*, **188**, 527–42.

Gibbs, M. E. and Ng, K. T. (1977). Psychobiology of memory, towards a model of memory formation, *Biobehavioural Reviews*, **1**, 113–36.

Greenough, W. T. and Chang, F., F. (1985). Synaptic structural correlates of information storage in mammalian nervous systems. In *Synaptic plasticity* (ed. C. W. Cotman), pp. 335–72. Guilford Press, New York.

Hebb, D. O. (1949). *The organization of behaviour: a neuropsychological theory*. John Wiley, New York.

Herrera, A. A., Grinnell, A. D., and Wolowske, B. (1985). Ultrastructural correlates of experimentally altered transmitter release efficacy in frog motor nerve terminals. *Neuroscience*, **16 (3)**, 491–500.

Horn, G. (1985). *Memory, imprinting and the brain, an inquiry into mechanisms*. Clarendon Press, Oxford.

Horn. G., McCabe, B. J., and Bateson, P. (1979). An autoradiographic study of the chick brain after imprinting. *Brain Research*, **168**, 361–73.

Horn, G., Bradley, P., and McCabe, B. J. (1985). Changes in the structure of synapses associated with learning. *Journal of Neuroscience*, **5(12)**, 3161–8.

Hunter, A. and Stewart, A. (1989). The synaptic development of the lobus parolfactorius of the chick, *Gallus domesticus*. *Experimental Brain Research*, **78**, 425–34.

Jack, J. J. B., Noble, D., and Tsien, R. W. (1975). *Electric current flow in excitable cells*. Clarendon Press, Oxford.

Karten, H. J. and Dubbledam, J. L. (1973). The organization and projections of the paleostriatal complex in the pigeon (*Columba livia*). *Journal of Comparative Neurology*, **148**, 61–91.

Kossut, M. and Rose, S. P. R. (1984). Differential 2-deoxyglucose uptake into chick brain structures during passive avoidance training. *Neuroscience*, **12(3)**, 971–7.

Mason, R. J. and Rose, S. P. R. (1987). Lasting changes in spontaneous multi-unit activity in the chick brain following passive avoidance training. *Neuroscience*, **21 (3)**, 931–41.

Mason, R. J. and Rose, S. P. R. (1988). Passive avoidance learning produces focal elevation of bursting activity in the chick brain: amnesia abolishes the increase. *Behavioural and Neural Biology*, **49**, 280–92.

Mench, J. A. and Andrew, R. J. (1986). Lateralisation of food search task in the domestic chick. *Behavioural and Neural Biology*, **46**(2) 107–14.

Mileusnic, R., Rose, S. P. R., and Tilson, P. (1980). Passive avoidance learning results in region specific changes in concentration and incorporation into colchicine-binding proteins in the chick forebrain. *Journal of Neurochemistry*, **34**, 1007–15.

Miller, J. P., Rall, W., and Rinzel, J. (1985). Synaptic amplification by active membrane in dendritic spines. *Brain Research*, **325**, 325–30.

Nottebohm, F. (1977). Asymmetries in neural control of vocalization in the canary.In *Lateralization in the nervous system* (ed. S. Harnad, D. W. Doty, L. Goldstein, J. Jaynes, and G. Krauthamer), pp. 23–4. Academic Press, New York.

Patel, S. N. and Stewart, M. G. (1988). Changes in the number and structure of dendritic spines, 25 h after passive avoidance training in the domestic chick, *Gallus domesticus. Brain Research*, **449**, 34–46.

Patel, S. N., Rose, S. P. R., and Stewart, M. G. (1988). Training induced spine density changes are specifically related to memory formation processes in the chick, *Gallus domesticus. Brain Research*, **463**, 168–173.

Patterson, T., Gilbert, D., and Rose, S. P. R. (1990). *Experimental Brain Research*. (In press.)

Perkel, D. H. and Perkel D. J. (1985). Dendritic spines: role of active membrane in modulating synaptic efficacy. *Brain Research*, **325**, 331–5.

Pongracz, F. (1985). The function of dendritic spines: A theoretical study. *Neuroscience*, **15, (4)**, 933–46.

Rall, W. and Sergev, I. (1987). Functional possibilities for synapses on dendrites and dendritic spines, In *Synaptic function* (ed. G. M. Edelman, W. E. Gall, and W. M. Cowan). John Wiley, New York.

Rogers, L. J. (1986). Lateralization of learning in chicks. *Advances in Studies in Behaviour*, **16**, 147–89.

Rose, S. P. R. (1981). What should a biochemistry of learning and memory be about? *Neuroscience*, **6**, 811–21.

Rose, S. P. R., Gibbs, M. E., and Hambley, J. (1980). Transient increase in forebrain muscarinic cholinergic receptor binding following passive avoidance learning in the young chick. *Neuroscience*, **5**, 169–72.

Rose, S. P. R. and Harding, S. (1984). Training increases (^{3}H) fucose incorporation in chick brain only if followed by memory storage. *Neuroscience*, **12(2)**, 663–7.

Rose, S. P. R. and Csillag, A. (1985). Passive avoidance training results in lasting changes in deoxyglucose metabolism in left hemisphere regions of chick brain. *Behavioural and Neural Biology*, **44**, 315–24.

Rothblat, L. A. and Schwartz, M. L. (1979). The effect of monocular deprivation on spines in visual cortex of young and adult albino rats: evidence for a sensitive period. *Brain Research*, **161**, 156–61.

Scheich, H. (1987). Neural correlates of auditory imprinting. *Journal of Comparative Physiology*, **A 161**, 605–19.

Shepherd, G. M. and Brayton, R. K. (1987). Logic operations are properties of computer simulated interactions between excitable dendritic spines. *Neuroscience*, **21 (1)**, 151-65.

Shepherd, G. M., Brayton, R. K., Miller, J. P., Segev, I., Rinzel, J., and Rall, W. (1985). Signal enhancement in distal cortical dendrites by means of interactions between active dendritic spines. *Proceedings of the National Academy of Sciences (USA)*, **82**, 2192–5.

Sokoloff, L. (1977). Relation between physiological function and energy metabolism in the central nervous system. *Journal of Neurochemistry*, **29**, 13–26.

Stewart, M. G., Rose, S. P. R., King, T. S., Gabbott, P. L. A., and Bourne, R. (1984). Hemispheric asymmetry of synapses in chick medial hyperstriatum ventrale following passive avoidance training: a stereological investigation, *Developmental Brain Research*, **12**, 261–9.

Stewart, M. G., Csillag, A., and Rose, S. P. R. (1987). Alterations in synaptic structure in the paleostriatal complex of the domestic chick, *Gallus domesticus*, following passive avoidance training. *Brain Research*, **426**, 69–81.

Thompson, R. F., Berger, T. W., and Madden, J. (1983). Cellular processes of learning and memory in the mammalian CNS. *Annual Review of Neuroscience*, **6**, 447–91.

Tombol, T., Csillag, A., and Stewart, M. G. (1988a). Cell types of the hyperstriatum ventrale of the domestic chicken, *Gallus domesticus*: a Golgi study. *Journal fur Hirnfornschung*, **3**, 319–34.

Tombol, T., Csillag, A., and Stewart, M. G. (1988b). Cell types of the paleostriatal complex of the domestic chicken, *Gallus domesticus*: a Golgi study. *Journal fur Hirnfornschung*, **5**, 493–507.

Valverde, F. (1970). The Golgi method: a tool for comparative structural analyses. In *Contemporary research methods in neuroanatomy* (ed. W. J. Nauta and S. O. E. Ebbesson), pp. 12–31. Springer Verlag, London.

Van Harreveld, A. and Fifkova, E. (1975). Swelling of dendritic spines in the fascia denta after stimulation of the perforant fibres as a mechanism of post-tetanic stimulation. *Experimental Neurology*, **49**, 736–49.

Wallhauser, E. and Scheich, H. (1987). Auditory imprinting leads to differential 2-deoxyglucose uptake and dendritic spine loss in the chick rostral forebrain. *Developmental Brain Research*, **31**, 29–44.

Wesa, J. H., Chang, F. F., Greenough, W. J., and West, R. W. (1982). Synaptic contact curvature: effects of differential rearing on rat occipital cortex. *Developmental Brain Research*, **4**, 253–7.

12

Lesion studies and the role of IMHV in early learning

D. C. Davies

INTRODUCTION

The results of experiments designed to investigate the effects of brain lesions on behaviour can be particularly difficult to interpret since they do not necessarily provide unambiguous information about the localization of function within the brain. Ablation of a particular brain region may indeed cause a behavioural deficit because the neural basis of that behaviour is truly localized in the ablated region. Alternatively, a similar behavioural deficit could result if the lesioned area was not directly related to the behaviour, but was part of a system of interrelated neuronal networks which might become functionally disconnected by the lesion. Such a disconnection could also endow the system as a whole with quite different properties to normal. Furthermore, a lesion might not reveal the true function of a brain region if that function is only expressed under particular circumstances, or if that function can be taken over by other brain regions. Nevertheless, when designed and interpreted carefully in the light of other experimental data, lesion studies have proven exceptionally useful in extending our knowledge of brain function, since they have allowed theoretical models of brain function to be tested and have facilitated the formulation of new hypotheses. Thus, bearing in mind the caveats outlined above, lesion studies have contributed greatly to our knowledge of the neural basis of learning in the chick. In this chapter I will compare the effects of lesions to a single region of the chick brain, the intermediate part of the medial hyperstriatum ventrale (IMHV), on a number of behavioural tasks and discuss their implications for the function of IMHV.

FILIAL IMPRINTING

Filial imprinting is the process by which a chick learns to recognize and form a preference for the first visually conspicuous object to which it is exposed (Bateson 1966; Sluckin 1972). In nature, the first such object to which a chick is normally exposed is its mother. The chick will then approach the fowl, learn its characteristics and form a social attachment to it (see Chapter 5 for a fuller description). However, the object need not be an adult fowl and a wide range of artifical objects can be employed as imprinting stimuli, with varying degrees of success. In the laboratory, imprinting can be used to narrow the range of objects that the chick will approach. Thus, if a chick is imprinted onto an object (the training object) and has consequently learnt its characteristics, when the chick is subsequently given a choice between the training object and a novel object, it will prefer the training object. The chick's preference for the training object can therefore be used as an index of learning.

A series of early biochemical experiments (Bateson *et al.* 1973; Horn *et al.* 1973; Bateson *et al.* 1975) which investigated the incorporation of radioactive uracil into the chick brain following imprinting, implicated the dorsal forebrain as being specifically involved in this process. Subsequent studies using autoradiographic techniques (Horn *et al.* 1979) localized this biochemical change resulting from imprinting to the IMHV. No other brain regions were implicated in this process. The finding of Kohsaka and colleagues (1979) that the metabolic marker ^{14}C-2-deoxyglucose was also accumulated in IMHV following imprinting, supported the view that this region of the forebrain was specifically involved in the process of imprinting. Furthermore, electrophysiological evidence has also supported the idea that IMHV is involved in filial imprinting (Payne and Horn 1982, 1984). These experiments are reviewed in more detail in Chapter 8.

Although the above studies strongly suggested the involvement of IMHV in filial imprinting, it was essential to directly test the hypothesis that an intact IMHV is necessary for the learning process of imprinting by a series of lesion experiments. In the first study (McCabe *et al.* 1981), bilateral radiofrequency coagulation of IMHV was found to prevent chicks from acquiring a preference for their training object on the following day, in contrast to sham-operated controls which strongly preferred the training object. This lesion-induced deficit could have been due to a non-specific sensory or motor deficit. Such an interpretation is unlikely, because lesioned chicks performed a visuomotor co-ordination task equally as well as sham-operated controls. Although the above experiment strongly suggested that IMHV was critically involved in the acquisition of an imprinted preference, it could not shed any light on the role of IMHV in the retention of the preference. Consequently, in a second study (McCabe *et al.* 1982) bilateral lesions were placed in IMHV 3 hours after imprinting and the chicks' preference for the training object tested 15–20 hours later. In addition to sham-operated controls, the design of this experiment included two other groups of chicks, with bilateral lesions to either the hyperstriatum accessorium (HA) or the lateral cerebral area (LCA). On testing, the sham-operated chicks and those which received lesions in HA or LCA exhibited a strong preference for the training object, but the

IMHV-lesioned chicks did not. Thus, bilateral lesions placed in the IMHV after training prevented the retention of an imprinted preference. Once again this deficit was unlikely to be a consequence of impaired sensory processing or motor performance, since all four groups of chicks performed equally well in tests of visuomotor co-ordination. Furthermore, since HA and LCA-lesioned chicks showed retention, the amnestic effect of similar sized IMHV lesions is unlikely to be due to brain damage *per se*.

Although bilateral lesions to IMHV have been shown to prevent acquisition of a preference through imprinting, it was not known if a single IMHV would be sufficient to support this process. In order to investigate this question, Horn *et al.* (1983) lesioned the left or the right IMHV prior to training and subsequently tested the chicks' preference for the training object compared to a novel stimulus. Both groups of chicks showed a similar, significant preference for the training stimulus. Thus, a single IMHV is sufficient for the acquisition of a preference by imprinting and the left or right IMHV appeared to be equally effective. In order to test whether the IMHV that was intact during training was necessary for retention of the preference, the remaining IMHV was then ablated. When the preferences of the chicks were tested again, neither of the groups showed any significant retention. This result led Horn *et al.* (1983) to conclude that if only one IMHV is present during training, then it must also be present for the expression of the preference.

Although it would appear that either the right or left IMHV alone is equally effective in mediating imprinting, there is some information to suggest that the two IMHVs do not have an identical role in imprinting. It has long been suggested that learning involves the formation and strengthening of synaptic connections (Cajal 1911; Hebb 1949). Since an increase in protein synthesis has been observed in IMHV as a result of imprinting (Horn *et al.* 1979), Bradley *et al.* (1981) investigated the effect of training on an imprinting stimulus on synaptic morphology in IMHV. In under-trained chicks there was a hemispheric asymmetry in the mean length of the postsynaptic density, with that in the right IMHV being greater than that in the left. This asymmetry was not present in overtrained chicks. The principal effect of training appeared to be to increase the length of the postsynaptic density in the left IMHV, suggesting that there may be an asymmetry in the roles of the right and left IMHV in imprinting.

The results of a further lesion study helped to clarify the roles of the right and left IMHVs in imprinting. In a two stage operation Cipolla-Neto *et al.* (1982) placed lesions in either the right or left IMHV approximately 3 hours after the end of training. The chick's preference for their training object was then tested 15–20 hours later. In this test, all chicks strongly preferred the training stimulus. A second lesion was subsequently placed in the IMHV contralateral to the first lesion and the chick's preferences tested 15–20 hours later. Chicks which received their initial lesion in the right IMHV did not show a preference for the training object. However, chicks which received an initial lesion in the left IMHV continued to show a preference for their training object in the second test.

The results of the studies involving unilateral/sequential lesions to IMHV are not easy to interpret and are considered in detail by McCabe in Chapter 9. However, in brief, Horn and co-workers have interpreted the results to mean that there are two distinct memory systems that can operate in imprinting. One system requires the presence of the left IMHV and the other is formed under the influence of the right IMHV, which possibly acts as a buffer store. The exact time-course of formation of this second memory store, which has been termed S' (Cipolla-Neto *et al.* 1982), is unknown, but it appears to be fully functional by 6 hours after training, since bilateral lesions placed in the IMHV after this time have no significant effect on retention (Davey *et al.* 1987). The location of S' is also unknown; however, it may be interesting to note that Salzen *et al.* (1975) reported that lateral forebrain lesions in newly hatched chicks prevent imprinting when tested 3–10 days later. In addition, if chicks are imprinted and similar lesions given on the sixth day post-hatch, Salzen *et al.* (1978) found retention to be impaired on testing on the 9th, 12th, or 14th day after hatching. The region lesioned includes the dorso-lateral corticoid area which Bradley *et al.* (1985) have shown to receive efferent projections from IMHV.

ONE-TRIAL PASSIVE AVOIDANCE LEARNING

Young chicks will spontaneously peck at small visually conspicuous objects in their field of view and they can learn to discriminate between unpleasant and neutral tasting objects. This behaviour underlies the one-trial passive avoidance (PAL) paradigm first developed by Cherkin (1969). Chicks which are presented with a small bright bead will peck at it. If the bead has been coated with a distasteful substance such as methylanthranilate (MeA), the chicks can learn in a single trial not to peck at a similar bead on a subsequent presentation.

A number of biochemical changes have been found in the chick forebrain following one-trial PAL. In initial experiments, an increased incorporation of radioactive leucine into protein was found in the forebrain roof of trained chicks both *in vivo* (Mileusnic *et al.* 1980) and later *in vitro* (Schliebs *et al.* 1985). Moreover, increased incorporation of the radiolabelled glycoprotein precursor ^{14}C-fucose has been shown in the forebrain roof after one-trial PAL and this elevated incorporation was demonstrated to be associated with synaptic membranes (Burgoyne and Rose 1980). Biochemical changes have also been indicated in the forebrain base, since *in vitro* studies have shown enhanced glycoprotein in this region following training (McCabe and Rose 1987).

More precise localization of the biochemical changes in the chick forebrain associated with one-trial PAL was obtained by autoradiography studies using the metabolic marker ^{14}C-2-deoxyglucose (Kossut and Rose 1984; Rose and Csillag 1985). Incorporation of ^{14}C-2-deoxyglucose was found to be enhanced in three regions of the chick forebrain following training: IMHV, lobus parolfactorius (LPO) and palaeostriatum augmentatum (PA). Electron microscopy has also revealed synaptic changes in these three brain regions following one-trial PAL (Stewart *et al.* 1984, 1987; Patel and Stewart 1988; Chapter 11).

Electrophysiological correlates of PAL have been demonstrated in IMHV by Mason and Rose (1987), who reported long-lasting changes in spontaneous bursting activity in IMHV neurons. These changes were prevented when trained chicks were made amnesic by subconvulsive electroshock (Mason and Rose 1988). Similar electroshock treatment has also been shown to prevent the training-related increase in dendritic spine number in IMHV (Patel *et al.* 1988).

Thus, three regions of the chick forebrain have been implicated in one-trial PAL, with the greatest weight of evidence supporting the involvement of IMHV, the brain region critically involved in filial imprinting. In an early attempt to use lesions to investigate the role of the chick hyperstriatum in one-trial PAL, Benowitz (1972) found that 'limited' hyperstriatal suction lesions (including the 'hyperstriatum accessorium, -dorsalis, intercalatus and overlying paleocortical tissue') impaired acquisition of a one-trial PAL task while 'extensive' lesions (which in addition 'more frequently included hyperstriatum ventrale, parts of adjacent neostriatum and medial portions of the hippocampal complex') impaired both acquisition and retention of the task. Although this study implicated the dorsal forebrain in one-trial PAL, it was not possible to associate any particular part of it with the learning process. More recently, Patterson *et al.* (1986) showed that bilateral injection of any one of a number of substances which disrupt neuronal function (L-glutamate, ouabain, cycloheximide, anisomycin or emetine) into the region of the chick's medial hyperstriatum ventrale prevents them from learning a one-trial PAL task. In an attempt to determine whether the same part of the hyperstriatum ventrale is critically involved in the process of filial imprinting and one-trial PAL, Davies *et al.* (1988) placed bilateral radiofrequency lesions in the IMHV of 12–18-hour-old chicks. Fifteen to twenty hours later, the chicks were trained in a one-trial PAL task and tested 3 hours later. Two other groups of chicks were subjected to the same training and testing procedure, sham-operated and LCA-lesioned chicks. Bilateral lesions of IMHV prevented the acquisition of the one-trial PAL task; however, neither bilateral lesions of a similar volume of tissue of the LCA, nor sham operation affected learning. Thus, the role of IMHV in learning is not restricted to filial imprinting, but it is also critically involved in one-trial PAL.

The findings of Davies et al. (1988) that, bilateral pre-training radio-frequency lesions of IMHV prevent learning of a one-trial PAL task have been replicated by Patterson et al. (1990). These authors then investigated the effect of unilateral pre-training lesions on acquisition and bilateral post-training lesions on retention of the one-trial PAL task. Lesions of the left IMHV combined with sham lesions of the right IMHV placed before training impaired the chicks' ability to learn the task. However, lesions of the right IMHV and sham lesions of the left IMHV did not impair the chicks' ability to learn the task. Thus, it would appear that only the left IMHV is involved in the formation of a memory for the one-trial PAL task. This finding is consistent with the results of studies of brain ultrastructure which have indicated the importance of the left IMHV in passive avoidance learning (Stewart et al. 1984; Rose and Csillag 1985; Patel and Stewart 1988; Chapter 11). Although similar hemispheric asymmetries have been reported for filial imprinting (Bradley et al. 1981; Chapter 9), unilateral IMHV lesions given before training appear to affect imprinting and one-trial PAL differently. In one-trial PAL, only the left IMHV appears to be involved in the learning process (Patterson et al. 1990) whereas in imprinting, the results indicate that either IMHV alone is capable of mediating the acquisition of a preference (Horn et al. 1983).

Bilateral post-training lesions to IMHV placed 1 or 6 hours after one-trial PAL did not produce any impairment of learning (Patterson et al. 1990), thus indicating that the IMHV is not necessary for the retention of the avoidance response once it has been learnt. In contrast, bilateral lesions placed in IMHV 3 hours after imprinting did impair the retention of a learned preference (McCabe et al. 1982). This difference may, however, be more apparent than real, since it is known that S′ is formed by 6 hours after training and bilateral lesions to IMHV given after this time do not impair retention of an imprinted preference (Davey et al. 1987), and one-trial PAL is a much faster process than imprinting. It is therefore possible that lesions given earlier than 1 hour after one-trial PAL might impair retention. In filial imprinting, it appears that the left IMHV acts as a permanent memory store, whereas the right IMHV functions as a 'buffer' store which transfers information to a permanent store, the location of which is as yet unknown (see Horn 1985). The failure of post-training bilateral IMHV lesions to impair one-trial PAL may therefore be due to the relatively rapid transfer of the learned information to other brain areas for permanent storage. Candidate brain regions for this permanent store may be the LPO and PA for the reasons outlined above. However, it should be borne in mind that there is as yet no firm evidence for the critical involvement of either of these areas in one-trial PAL or imprinting and that the changes reported in these areas might simply reflect some aspect of the training process such as olfaction in the case of LPO (Rieke and Wenzel 1978) or motor activity in the case of PA (Karten and Dubbeldam 1973) and not learning *per se*. The true nature of the involvement of the LPO and PA in learning as yet awaits elucidation by lesion and other studies.

ASSOCIATIVE LEARNING

In their study of the effect of post-training bilateral IMHV lesions on imprinting, McCabe *et al.* (1982) also investigated the effect of these lesions on an associative learning task. Chicks were imprinted on a training object and then the lesions were placed. After recovery, the chicks were given a preference test. The IMHV-lesioned chicks did not show a preference for the training object. However, sham-operated, Wulst-lesioned and LCA-lesioned chicks did show a preference for their training object. All four groups of chicks were then trained on a simultaneous visual discrimination task using heat reinforcement (Zolman 1968, 1976). Half of each group of chicks was required to approach one visual pattern (vertical black bars on a yellow background) and the other half required to approach another (black spots on a blue background). The experiment was performed in a room maintained at 12 °C and correct responses were reinforced by a current of warm air. All four groups of chicks were equally successful in learning this task. Thus, in the same chicks, bilateral IMHV lesions impaired retention of a preference for an imprinting stimulus but did not affect the chicks' ability to selectively approach a visual pattern that was associated with a heat reward. However, Johnson and Horn (1986) did not consider that this experiment provided conclusive evidence that IMHV is not essential for associative learning for three reasons:

1. Simultaneous discrimination may be easier than successive discrimination tasks; the stimuli were presented simultaneously in the visual discrimination task, whereas in the imprinting task chicks were trained on a single stimulus and their preferences were measured in a test comprising sequential presentation of the training and a novel object.
2. The chicks were trained on the heat reinforcement task after they had been imprinted and therefore age differences could prejudice the results.
3. The stimuli used in the imprinting and heat reinforcement tasks were not identical.

Johnson and Horn (1986) therefore designed an experiment to control for these possible confounding variables. Young chicks quickly learn to press a pedal in order to be presented with a rotating red or blue illuminated box (Bateson and Reese 1969). When the chick learns to associate the pressing of the pedal with the presentation of the reinforcer, it also learns the visual characteristics of the object which will elicit filial behaviour. Thus the two processes, filial imprinting and associative learning, can take place at the same time, leading Johnson and Horn (1986) to inquire whether these two learning processes could be dissociated by means of IMHV lesions.

Chicks were given bilateral IMHV lesions 12 hours after hatching and the operant training commenced 8–12 hours later. Sham-operated chicks served as controls. The reinforcing object was either a red box or a stuffed jungle fowl. The IMHV-lesioned chicks were not impaired in the operant task or in measures of general activity, compared to sham-operated controls. However, 2 hours after the end of the operant training when each chick was given a simultaneous choice test (Bateson and Wainwright 1972) between the reinforcing object in the operant task and a novel object, IMHV-lesioned chicks apparently failed to recognise the reinforcing object and did not show a preference for it. In contrast, sham-operated chicks showed a strong preference for their reinforcing object. Thus, bilateral IMHV lesions impaired imprinting, but were without effect on the operant task. These findings are in accord with those of McCabe et al. (1982) and strengthen the view that there is a dissociation between the learning process of imprinting and associative learning and that IMHV is critically involved in the former but not in the latter.

RECOGNITION OF INDIVIDUAL CONSPECIFICS

There is considerable evidence to suggest that there are two distinct neural systems involved in filial preference behaviour in the chick. One entails the predisposition of a newly-hatched chick to approach objects resembling adult conspecifics and the other is a 'learning system' which can be focused on a variety of visually conspicuous objects (Horn and McCabe 1984; Bolhuis et al. 1985; Johnson et al. 1985; Johnson and Horn 1986; Chapters 5 and 8). It seems likely that in natural filial imprinting, the predisposition serves to direct the chick towards adult fowl in general and the 'learning system' allows it to learn the characteristics of an individual conspecific, normally the chick's own mother. Lesions to IMHV impair the acquisition and retention of the learned component of a filial preference (see above) but they do not affect the development of the predisposition (Horn and McCabe 1984; Johnson and Horn 1986). It could therefore be predicted that following ablation of IMHV, the brain region critically involved in the 'learning system', chicks should not be able to recognize the characteristics of individual adult conspecifics. Johnson and Horn (1987) tested this prediction by placing bilateral radiofrequency lesions in IMHV in chicks 6–10 hours after hatching. Twenty to twenty eight hours after surgery each chick was trained on one of two stuffed jungle fowl and 2 hours after the end of training each chick was given a simultaneous choice preference test (Bateson and Wainwright 1972) employing the two stuffed jungle fowl. IMHV-lesioned chicks did not show a preference for either of the stuffed jungle fowl. However, sham-operated controls and Wulst-lesioned chicks showed a significant preference for the particular stuffed fowl that they had been exposed to during training. There was no difference in activity in the test between the three groups of chicks. Thus, sham-operated and Wulst-lesioned chicks were capable of learning to recognize a particular individual adult fowl, but bilateral IMHV lesions prevented the recognition of individual adult conspecifics during imprinting.

Sexual imprinting is also likely to involve the recognition of individuals (Bateson 1979) and there is evidence to suggest that lesions to IMHV also impair sexual imprinting by preventing chickens from learning the characteristics of individual conspecifics. Bolhuis *et al.* (1989) placed bilateral lesions in the IMHV of female chicks 6–10 hours after hatching. These chicks and sham-operated female controls were allowed to recover and were reared in small social groups with males from the same hatch. At 12 weeks of age the sexual preferences of the females were measured. On the first day of testing the females were given a choice between a male with which they had been reared (familiar white) and a novel male of the same strain (novel white). On the second day of testing the chickens were given a choice between a novel white male and a novel brown (Rhode Island Red) male. On the third day of testing the chickens were given a choice between a novel white male and a rotating red box. Sham-operated females significantly preferred novel white males. This finding is in accord with that first reported for female Japanese quail, which prefer individuals that differ slightly from those they have been raised with (Bateson 1978, 1980, 1982). Female chicks given IMHV lesions shortly after hatching subsequently showed no preferences for any of the males. However, given a choice between a male and a red box, both groups of females showed a preference for the male. Thus, IMHV lesions impair sexual imprinting. This impairment is unlikely to be due to the general impairment of the lesioned birds' performance in the test, since given a choice between a male and an artificial stimulus (red box), they showed a strong preference for the male. However, the lesioned chicks could not distinguish between the individual males, suggesting that the lesion had disrupted the birds' ability to learn the characteristics of individuals. The processes underlying filial imprinting and sexual imprinting therefore show similarities in that they both appear to involve the recognition of individuals and the IMHV is critically involved in this recognition process.

CONCLUSION

Bilateral lesions to the chick IMHV prevent filial imprinting, sexual imprinting, learning the characteristics of individual adult conspecifics and one-trial passive avoidance learning. However, such lesions are without effect on a visual discrimination task associated with a heat reward or a pedal-pressing operant task associated with the presentation of a reinforcer. IMHV must therefore play a critical role which is common to the first four learning processes but is not shared by the associative learning tasks. A common feature uniting filial imprinting, sexual imprinting and learning the characteristics of individual adult conspecifics is the ability to recognize objects. However, it is not immediately clear how one-trial PAL fits into this category. In the one-trial passive avoidance task, chicks may associate pecking the bead with the unpleasant taste of MeA and subsequently avoid the bead. This task is therefore, at least in part, an associative learning task. However, there are features of the one-trial PAL task employed by Davies *et al.* (1988) that might explain the effect of IMHV lesions in preventing learning. When sham-operated and LCA-lesioned chicks were trained on a red MeA-coated bead, they avoided a similar coloured bead in the test. However, when the chicks were subsequently presented with a blue bead of similar size in the test, a significant number of chicks pecked this bead. Thus, the chicks had not simply associated the act of pecking with the aversive taste, but had also learned information about the visual characteristics of the training bead which subsequently allowed the chicks to discriminate between a red and a blue bead. IMHV lesions may therefore prevent one-trial PAL by impairing the chicks' ability to recognize a particular bead. This inability to recognize the red training bead may then prevent the formation of an association between the unpleasant taste and the particular training bead, resulting in the amnesia observed. The view that there is indeed a recognition element in the one-trial PAL bead pecking task is supported by the work of Roper and Redston (1987). These authors demonstrated that after a single trial chicks show stronger and longer lasting avoidance if the MeA-coated training bead is conspicuous (red bead on white background or *vice versa*) rather than cryptic (red bead on a red background or white bead on a white background). Thus, chicks can recognize individual exemplars of the same class of objects and form a learned association between bead colour and noxious taste which is stronger when the stimulus is conspicuous than when it is cryptic.

A second feature common to filial imprinting, one-trial PAL, recognition of adult conspecifics, and sexual imprinting is the inhibition of an inborn tendency. In filial imprinting, when a chick is presented with an appropriately-sized and visually conspicuous object, it will approach that object and gradually restrict its filial behaviour to that object and avoid other, novel objects. Thus, filial imprinting may involve the selective inhibition of an inborn tendency to approach, especially if the object resembles an adult conspecific. Young chicks spontaneously peck at small visually conspicuous objects (e.g. coloured beads) in their field of view. If the bead is coated in an aversive substance (MeA) in the one-trial PAL task, this tendency to peck is inhibited on subsequent presentation of the bead. In the recognition of individual adult conspecifics, young chicks exhibit a predisposition to approach any object resembling an adult fowl, but once they have learnt the characteristics of an individual, they restrict their approach behaviour to this individual. A similar situation may also apply in the case of sexual imprinting, where a female chicken restricts her sexual behaviour to an individual male. Thus, IMHV lesions may affect all of these behaviours by preventing the inhibition of an inborn response. In contrast, in neither the heat-reinforced visual discrimination task nor in the acquisition of the pedal-pressing task, is the inhibition of an inborn response required and IMHV lesions do not affect the acquisition of these tasks. However, it would be interesting to investigate whether reversals of these associative learning tasks are affected by IMHV lesions.

Although it is argued here that the role of IMHV in learning is in general concerned with object recognition and possibly response inhibition, the precise role of IMHV in each of the tasks in which it is involved may vary and requires further investigation. In particular, the hemispheric asymmetries revealed by lesion studies may be important for our understanding of these differences, which imply that both IMHVs are involved, and there are two types of memory store in filial imprinting, but only the left IMHV appears to play a role in one-trial PAL. Furthermore, in filial imprinting IMHV is involved in both acquisition and retention but in one-trial PAL it may only be involved in acquisition. Unfortunately there is currently no information available concerning the role of IMHV in the retention of information about the characteristics of individual adult conspecifics or about the retention of a preference in sexual imprinting. Neither is there any information about the role of the individual right or left IMHV in these processes.

The key to understanding the differences in the function of IMHV in the tasks in which it is involved is likely to lie in the interaction of IMHV with other brain regions. It is known that in filial imprinting, the right IMHV passes information to another brain region (S') of unknown location for storage and the LPO and PA have been implicated in one-trial PAL. Thus, although IMHV may have a general function in learning, the particular nature of the individual learning tasks in which it is involved may determine the exact involvement of IMHV by its interaction with other brain structures. Investigation of the cerebral networks with which

IMHV is involved is therefore of fundamental importance for a full understanding of the role of IMHV in learning.

Acknowledgements

I wish to thank Grant McLennan and Jane Davey for constructive criticism of this manuscript.

REFERENCES

Bateson, P. P. G. (1966). The characteristics and context of imprinting. *Biological Reviews*, **41**, 177–220.

Bateson, P. (1978). Sexual imprinting and optimal outbreeding. *Nature*, **273**, 659–60.

Bateson, P. (1979). How do sensitive periods arise and what are they for? *Animal Behaviour*, **27**, 470–86.

Bateson, P. (1980). Optimal outbreeding and the development of sexual preferences in Japanese quail. *Zeitschrift fur Tierpsychologie*, **53**, 231–44.

Bateson, P. (1982). Preferences for cousins in Japanese quail. *Nature*, **295**, 236–7.

Bateson, P. P. G. and Reese, E. P. (1969). The reinforcing properties of conspicuous stimuli in the imprinting situation. *Animal Behaviour*, **17**, 692–9.

Bateson, P. P. G. and Wainwright, A. A. P. (1972). The effects of prior exposure to light on the imprinting process in domestic chicks. *Behaviour*, **42**, 279–90.

Bateson, P. P. G., Horn, G., and Rose, S. P. R. (1975). Imprinting: correlation between behaviour and incorporation of [^{14}C] uracil into chick brain. *Brain Research*, **84**, 207–20.

Bateson, P. P. G., Rose, S. P. R., and Horn, G. (1973). Imprinting: lasting effects on uracil incorporation into chick brain. *Science*, **181**, 576–8.

Benowitz, L. (1972). Effects of forebrain ablations on avoidance learning in chicks. *Physiology and Behavior*, **9**, 601–8.

Bolhuis, J. J., Johnson, M. H., and Horn, G. (1985). Effects of early experience on the development of filial preferences in the domestic chick. *Developmental Psychobiology*, **18**, 299–308.

Bolhuis, J. J., Johnson, M. H., Horn, G., and Bateson, P. (1989). Long-lasting effects of IMHV lesions on social preferences in domestic fowl. *Behavioral Neuroscience*, **103**, 438–41.

Bradley, P., Davies, D. C., and Horn, G. (1985). Connections of the hyperstriatum ventrale of the domestic chick (*Gallus domesticus*). *Journal of Anatomy*, **140**, 577–89.

Bradley, P., Horn, G., and Bateson, P. (1981). Imprinting: an electron microscopic study of chick hyperstriatum ventrale. *Experimental Brain Research*, **41**, 115–20.

Burgoyne, R. D. and Rose, S. P. R. (1980). Subcellular localisation of increased incorporation of [^{3}H] fucose following passive avoidance learning in the chick. *Neuroscience Letters*, **19**, 343–8.

Cajal, S. R. (1911). *Histologie du système nerveux de l'homme et des vertébrés*, Vol. 2, pp. 886–90. Maloine, Paris. (Republished 1952, Instituto Ramón y Cajal, Madrid.)

Cherkin, A. (1969). Kinetics of memory consolidation. Role of amnesic treatment parameters. *Proceedings of the National Academy of Science, USA*, **63**, 1094–101.

Cipolla-Neto, J., Horn, G., and McCabe, B. J. (1982). Hemispheric asymmetry and imprinting: the effect of sequential lesions to the hyperstriatum ventrale. *Experimental Brain Research*, **48**, 22–7.

Davey, J. E., McCabe, B. J., and Horn, G. (1987). Mechanisms of information storage in the domestic chick. *Behavioural Brain Research*, **26**, 209–10.

Davies, D. C., Taylor, D. A., and Johnson, M. H. (1988). The effects of hyperstriatal lesions on one-trial passive-avoidance learning in the chick. *Journal of Neuroscience*, **8**, 4662–6.

Hebb, D. O. (1949). *The organization of behaviour*. John Wiley, New York.

Horn, G. (1985). *Memory, imprinting and the brain. An inquiry into mechanisms*. Clarendon Press. Oxford.

Horn, G., Bradley, P., and McCabe, B. J. (1985). Changes in the structure of synapses associated with learning. *Journal of Neuroscience*, **5**, 3161–8.

Horn, G. and McCabe, B. J. (1984). Predispositions and preferences. Effects on imprinting of lesions to the chick brain. *Animal Behaviour*, **32**, 288–92.

Horn, G., McCabe, B. J., and Bateson, P. P. G. (1979). An autoradiographic study of the chick brain after imprinting. *Brain Research*, **168**, 361–73.

Horn, G., McCabe, B. J., and Cipolla-Neto, J. (1983). Imprinting in the domestic chick: the role of each side of the hyperstriatum ventrale in acquisition and retention. *Experimental Brain Research*, **53**, 91–8.

Horn, G., Rose, S. P. R., and Bateson, P. P. G. (1973). Experience and plasticity in the central nervous system. *Science*, **181**, 506–14.

Johnson, M. H., Bolhuis, J. J., and Horn, G. (1985). Interaction between acquired preferences and developing predispositions during imprinting. *Animal Behaviour*, **33**, 1000–6.

Johnson, M. H. and Horn, G. (1986). Dissociation of recognition memory and associative learning by a restricted lesion of the chick forebrain. *Neuropsychologia*, **24**, 329–40.

Johnson, M. H. and Horn, G. (1986). An analysis of predisposition in the domestic chick. *Behavioural Brain Research*, **20**, 108–9.

Johnson, M. H. and Horn, G. (1987). The role of a restricted region of the chick forebrain in the recognition of individual conspecifics. *Behavioural Brain Research*, **23**, 269–75.

Karten, H. J. and Dubbeldam, J. L. (1973). The organisation and projections of the paleostriatal complex in the pigeon (*Columba livia*). *Journal of Comparative Neurology*, **148**, 61–9.

Kohsaka, S., Takamatsu, K., Aoki, E., and Tsukada, Y. (1979). Metabolic mapping of chick brain after imprinting using [^{14}C]2-deoxyglucose. *Brain Research*, **172**, 539–44.

Kossut, M. and Rose, S. P. R. (1984). Differential 2-deoxyglucose uptake into chick brain structures during passive avoidance training. *Neuroscience*, **12**, 971–7.

Mason, R. J and Rose, S. P. R. (1987). Lasting changes in spontaneous multi-unit activity in the chick brain following passive avoidance learning. *Neuroscience*, **21**, 931–42.

Mason R. J. and Rose, S. P. R. (1988). Passive avoidance learning produces focal elevation of bursting activity in chick brain: amnesia abolishes the increase. *Behavioral and Neural Biology*, **49**, 280–92.

McCabe, B. J., Horn, G., and Bateson, P. P. G. (1981). Effects of restricted lesions of the chick forebrain on the acquisition of filial preferences during imprinting. *Brain Research*, **205**, 29–37.

McCabe, B. J., Cipolla-Neto, J., Horn, G., and Bateson, P. (1982). Amnesic effects of bilateral lesions placed in the hyperstriatum ventrale of the chick after imprinting. *Experimental Brain Research*, **48**, 13–21.

McCabe, N. R. and Rose, S. P. R (1987). Increased fucosylation of chick proteins following training: effects of cycloheximide. *Journal of Neurochemistry*, **48**, 538–42.

Mileusnic, R., Rose, S. P. R., and Tillson, P. (1980). Passive avoidance learning results in region-specific changes in concentration of and incorporation into colchicine binding proteins in the chick forebrain. *Journal of Neurochemistry*, **34**, 1007–15.

Patel, S. N. and Stewart, M. G. (1988). Changes in the number and structure of dendritic spines 25 h after passive avoidance training in the domestic chick. *Gallus domesticus*. *Brain Research*, **449**, 34–46.

Patel, S. N., Rose, S. P. R., and Stewart, M. G. (1988). Training induced dendritic spine density changes are specifically related to memory formation processes in the chick, *Gallus domesticus*. *Brain Research*, **463**, 168–73.

Patterson, T. A., Alvarado, M. C., Warren, I. T., Bennett, E. L., and Rosenzweig, M. R. (1986). Memory stages and brain asymmetry in chick learning. *Behavioral Neuroscience*, **100**, 856–65.

Patterson, T. A., Gilbert, D. B., and Rose, S. P. R. (1990). Pre- and post-training lesions of the intermediate medial hyperstriatum ventrale and passive avoidance learning in the chick. *Experimental Brain Research*, **80**, 189–95.

Payne, J. K. and Horn, G. (1982). Differential effects of exposure to an imprinting stimulus on 'spontaneous' neuronal activity in two regions of the chick brain. *Brain Research*, **232**, 191–3.

Payne, J. K. and Horn, G. (1984). Long-term consequences of exposure to an imprinting stimulus on 'spontaneous' impulse activity in the chick brain. *Behavioural Brain Research*, **13**, 163–72.

Rieke, G. K. and Wenzel, B. M. (1978). Forebrain projections of the pigeon olfactory bulb. *Journal of Morphology*, **158**, 41–56.

Roper, T. J. and Redston, S. (1987). Conspicuousness of distasteful prey affects the strength and durability of one-trial avoidance learning. *Animal Behaviour*, **35**, 739–47.

Rose, S. P. R. and Csillag, A. (1985). Passive avoidance training results in lasting changes in deoxyglucose metabolism in left hemisphere regions of chick brain. *Behavioral and Neural Biology*, **44**, 315–24.

Salzen, E. A., Parker, D. M., and Williamson, A. J. (1975). A forebrain lesion preventing imprinting in domestic chicks. *Experimental Brain Research*, **24**, 145–57.

Salzen, E. A., Parker, D. M., and Williamson, A. J. (1978) Forebrain lesions and retention of imprinting in domestic chicks. *Experimental Brain Research*, **31**, 107–16.

Schliebs, R., Rose, S. P. R., and Stewart, M. G. (1985). Effect of passive avoidance learning on *in vitro* protein synthesis in forebrain slices of day old chicks. *Journal of Neurochemistry*, **44**, 1014–28.

Sluckin, W. (1972). *Imprinting and early learning*. Methuen, London.

Stewart, M. G., Csillag, A., and Rose, S. P. R. (1987). Alterations in synaptic structure in the paleostriatal complex in the domestic chick, *Gallus domesticus*, following passive avoidance training. *Brain Research*, **426**, 69–81.

Stewart, M. G., Rose, S. P. R., King, T. S., Gabbott, P. L. A., and Bourne, R. (1984). Hemispheric asymmetry of synapses in chick medial hyperstriatum ventrale following passive avoidance training: a stereological investigation. *Developmental Brain Research*, **12**, 261–9.

Sukumar, R., Rose, S. P. R., and Burgoyne, R. D. (1980). Increased incorporation of [³H] fucose into chick brain glycoproteins following training on a passive avoidance task. *Journal of Neurochemistry*, **34**, 343–8.

Zolman, J. F. (1968). Discrimination learning in young chicks with heat reinforcement. *Psychological Record*, **18**, 303–9.

Zolman, J. F. (1972). Developmental constraints on conditioning. In *Knowing, thinking and believing* (ed. L. Petrinovitch and J. L. McGaugh), pp. 85–114. Plenum Press, New York.

PART V

Memory formation

Introduction

R. J. Andrew

The hypothesis that memory formation is organized into phases, each of which is sensitive to a different group of amnestic agents, is well established (Chapters 14, 15) for both mammals and birds. Work on phases of memory in the chick by Gibbs and Ng (1977; Chapters 13, 17) has demonstrated a series of remarkable phenomena, including the following.

1. Sensitivity ends sharply at a time which is different for each group of amnestic agents, and (like other timings of processes in chick memory formation) is remarkably consistent across populations of chicks.
2. Both delayed loss of memory and temporary amnesia (Chapter 14) can be produced, depending upon which amnestic agent is employed. Loss, and return of memory occur with the same timing in the two cases.
3. Some classes of events in memory formation, although constant in timing when experimental conditions are held constant, shift predictably when hormonal status is changed.

It has commonly been assumed that, during the course of memory formation, the availability of information for retrieval shifts between a series of different bases of memory, the 'phases'. Three are usually recognized : short term, intermediate term and long-term memory. Very short-term memory is sometimes added (Chapter 15), and ITM is now divided into two phases. A phase is assumed to form before it becomes available to retrieval, and to be sensitive to disruption whilst forming, so that the deletion of a phase becomes evident only some time after administration of the amnestic agent, at the time when the deleted phase would normally become available for retrieval.

The physical bases of successive phases might be (to take one extreme theoretical position) successive stages in the consolidation of the trace within a single population of neurons. The neurons holding the trace would have to be labelled in some way to allow access to retrieval mechanisms, and the type of labelling would change with the transition to a new phase. Each type of labelling would have a period of preparation before it came into use, and during this period, disruption by amnestic agents might occur.

Such an explanation for memory phases is attractive in its economy. However, it is not easily reconciled with evidence for temporary amnesias lasting only for the duration of ITM (Chapter 14); it might perhaps be argued that such amnesias resulted from interference with the form of labelling necessary for retrieval during this period.

Even more serious problems for the hypothesis are raised by the extensive evidence that both hemispheres, and within them, at least three structures (Chapters 8–12, 15, 16, 19) are involved in memory formation. This suggests the existence of more than one version of the trace, held in different sites In fact, there would probably be little dispute that memory formation proceeds to some extent independently in the two hemispheres. Rosenzweig *et al.* (Chapter 15), using the aversive bead task, have shown, in addition, that at least two separate areas of the forebrain go through the same sequence of sensitivity to different agents, but do so independently. Horn (Chapter 8), using the imprinting task, summarizes extensive evidence for two sites of storage in at least the right hemisphere.

It remains true that amnestic agents which act on STM or ITM often cause the loss in addition of all subsequent phases. One way of reconciling this with more than one site of storage is to suppose that some agents reach and disturb corresponding processes in all sites of storage.

If indeed there is more than one version of the trace, then it is necessary to ask what sorts of role do different versions play during memory formation. One possibility is that, from the start, permanent memory is one independent version. There is general agreement that the first steps in its formation occur very soon after learning. These are the 'enabling' changes discussed by Rose (Chapter 10); they include amino acid uptake (Chapter 13), the expression of particular genes, increased RNA synthesis and then synthesis of at least two classes of protein (tubulin, glycoproteins: Chapter 10), which may occur in two separate bursts (Chapter 14). Disturbance in any one of these processes has been shown to result in permanent amnesia; in some cases, amnesia is known to occur only after delay, appearing at the time when retrieval has been held to shift to LTM. It could therefore be argued that one version is formed soon after learning, but becomes available for retrieval only at the end of memory formation. Other versions are available to retrieval before this time, perhaps so as to protect the route to permanent memory during consolidation.

However, it is at least equally possible that permanent memory takes on its final form during memory formation. In the case of imprinting, it is thought that permanent memory is formed by transfer of information from a buffer store to a final site of storage. Evidence for interaction between the hemispheres, which may involve the transfer of information is considered in Chapter 19. Once it is supposed that a series of stores may be involved in memory formation, then a wide range of processes have to be considered as open to disturbance by amnestic agents, in addition to primary processes of consolidation. These might include systems which are not concerned directly with storage but which provide 'hold' or 'clear' signals, or timing inputs of a more general character; and systems which are responsible for the transfer of information.

The reinstatement of sensitivity to amnestic agents at times of processing thus becomes a real possibility. Lewis (1979) argued that all amnestic action which does not occur in a brief period after learning is associated with re-activation of the trace due to reminiscence (which results when the animal is reminded of circumstances associated with training, but without any opportunity for re-training). Sensitivity associated with episodes of processing may provide a second source of delayed sensitivity. The processes open to disturbance at such times are potentially diverse. Changes in a version of the trace (as a result of information transfer, for example) would presumably require changes in neuronal state like those which occur at learning, and so might reinstate sensitivity in the neurons holding the memory. It is also possible that disturbance of inputs (e.g. an incorrect 'clear' signal) might occur. The most interesting possibility is that disturbance of transfer of information might result in the incorporation into the trace of degraded information, and thereby produce a final version which is distorted and inadequate to support normal response.

Noradrenergic systems are obvious candidates for systems which might provide inputs to the trace(s). They are clearly important in a number of amnestic effects. Opposition of amnestic effects by noradrenaline is common (Chapters 13, 14); certain protein synthesis inhibitors such as cycloheximide may act on memory formation, at least in part, by interfering with catecholamine synthesis (Chapter 13). Stephenson (Chapter 16) shows that beta-2-antagonists are potent amnestic agents, and that they fall into two groups. One appears to act on a system which helps to maintain the trace(s) until at least 40 minutes after learning; the other group acts specifically in brief windows of time associated with a series of events (below) which occur during memory formation (Chapter 19; see also Allweis, Chapter 14: role of noradrenaline in formation of memory phases).

Much remains to be done in studying the role of other neuromodulators and neurotransmitters in memory formation of the chick. Rosenzweig *et al.* (Chapter 15) demonstrate a role for opiates immediately after learning; up-regulation of cholinergic and NMDA receptors is considered in the previous section.

A new explanation for many of these features of chick memory formation is provided by the evidence which is given in Chapter 19 for cyclically recurring episodes of good retrieval. The cycle period differs between right and left hemispheres; the first four retrieval events occur at crucial timings which are already well established by earlier work. The last of these timings, at 50 minutes, has the special property that it involves, for the first time, coincidence of retrieval episodes in both hemispheres. Differing specialization of the two hemispheres for different types of analysis of perceptual information (Chapter 21) may result in the initial elaboration of somewhat different versions of the training experience. Coincidence of retrieval episodes at 50 minutes may allow exchanges of information between these two versions; disturbance of such exchange, following the administration of an amnestic agent may explain both delayed loss of memory, and the return of memory at this time. Which will occur depends (according to the hypothesis) on which hemisphere was predominantly affected by the amnestic agent. Asymmetry of action is known to occur for some agents, with the hemisphere which is predominantly sensitive changing with time of application (Chapters 15, 19). The hypothesis also assumes that one hemisphere (the left: Chapter 21) is predominantly responsible for the control of pecking after the aversive bead task. Disturbance of the left hemisphere trace(s) is thus likely to lead to immediate amnesia, whereas a corresponding effect on the right hemisphere might affect overt behaviour only after interaction between the hemispheres at 50 minutes.

Gibbs (Chapter 17) discusses the postponement of certain features of memory formation by hormonal action. The standard timings of these features hold only for chicks which are not stressed by isolation, and therefore are not exposed to elevated ACTH and glucocorticoid levels. Two types of feature may be postponed: endings of sensitivity to particular amnestic agents, and spontaneous points of poor retrieval ('dips'). Such dips are interpreted as being caused by the shift of retrieval from one phase to the next. Both peptide and steroid hormones are effective in producing postponement. It is possible that effects of this sort partly explain the much more protracted course of memory formation following imprinting (Chapter 8).

Clifton (Chapter 18) describes a different set of effects on memory formation, in which hormones enhance the ability of one experience to compete with the effects of a second comparable but discrepant experience. The effectiveness of such competition changes sharply as the interval between the two experiences is progressively changed; strikingly, but perhaps by now not unexpectedly, the sharpest changes occur at timings already familiar from studies of memory phases.

These effects have many points of resemblance with the stabilization of attention by the same hormones. Indeed, when intervals between the two experiences are very short, it is likely that stabilization of information derived from the first experience, and used to control attention (i.e. to control the selection and appraisal of stimuli) is responsible for hormonally enhanced competition.

REFERENCES

Lewis, D. J. (1979). Psychobiology of active and inactive memory. *Psychological Bulletin,* **86**, 1054–83.

13

Stages in memory formation: a review

K. T. Ng and M. E. Gibbs

INTRODUCTION

With notable exceptions (Craik and Lockhart 1972; Gold and McGaugh 1975), the idea that memory formation (conceptualized as those brain states and activities associated with the consolidation of a learning experience into a more or less permanent neural representation) occurs in behaviourally distinct stages, has been widely accepted (Hebb 1949; Halstead and Rucker 1968; Booth 1970; Gibbs and Ng 1977, 1979). Disagreements persist, however, on the number of stages involved (Hebb 1949; Gibbs and Ng 1977; Frieder and Allweiss 1978; Patterson *et al.* 1986), the sequential dependence or otherwise of the stages (Gibbs and Ng 1977; Frieder and Allweiss 1978), the temporal parameters associated with each stage (Booth 1970) and the neuronal mechanisms and processes underlying each stage (Gibbs and Ng 1977; Dunn 1980; McGaugh 1983; Ng and Gibbs 1988). To a large extent, the absence of consensus regarding the number of stages and the temporal characteristics of these may be attributed to the use of a wide range of species and learning tasks (Booth 1970). The resolution of these two issues is crucial to any attempt to identify the neuronal substrates underlying the various memory stages and the relationships between these stages.

Cherkin (1971) introduced a single trial passive avoidance learning task for day-old chicks which has proved particularly useful in attempts to isolate possible stages in memory formation. In essence, the task involves training day-old chicks to avoid a small chrome bead previously coated with a chemical aversant, methylanthranilate, and presented to the chick for 10 seconds. Chicks pecking at this stimulus exhibit typical disgust reactions and have been shown to avoid the bead in subsequent retention tests carried out several days later. In this paper, we summarize the findings from a range of pharmacological–behavioural studies carried out in our laboratories using a modified version of Cherkin's paradigm.

EXPERIMENTAL PARADIGM

Day-old chicks, normally black Australorp-white Leghorn cockerels, are obtained from a local hatchery on the morning of each experiment. The chicks are delivered in cardboard boxes housing approximately 100 chicks in each box, with each box divided by cardboard dividers into four compartments. A number of holes in the lid and sides of the boxes allow light to filter into the boxes. On arrival at the laboratory, the chicks are kept in the delivery boxes for approximately 30 minutes prior to being placed in pairs in wooden experimental boxes (Chapter 1) with chick mash *ad libitum*. The experimental boxes are arranged in blocks of five boxes. Typically, 20 different chicks are used for each data point, with the 20 chicks housed in two blocks of five boxes each, placed on two shelves. Each laboratory normally houses no more than 12 blocks of boxes (i.e. 120 chicks). The temperature in each laboratory is maintained at 22–26 °C by red 60 W light globes suspended above the experimental boxes.

The experimental protocol is outlined in Table 13.1. Briefly, 30 minutes after placement in the experimental boxes, chicks are exposed to a pre-training trial with a small chrome bead (2 mm diameter), attached to a straight wire, and coated with water. The attention of each pair of chicks is attracted by tapping lightly on the front of the box and the bead is introduced into the box for up to 20 seconds. This pre-training trial is followed by a second similar pre-training trial. Following the second chrome bead trial, a red glass bead (4 mm diameter), dipped in water, is presented to each pair of chicks for 10 seconds. The number of pecks and the latency to first peck at this bead are recorded for each chick using a manually operated handset connected to a computer. All chicks in each group of 20 are given this pre-training trial before being presented with a blue glass bead (4mm diameter), dipped in water, for 10 seconds. The number of pecks and the latency to the first peck for each chick on this trial are also recorded.

The training trial is started 30 minutes after the last pre-training trial. Each pair of chicks is presented with a red glass bead, identical to that used in the pre-training trial, but coated with the chemical aversant methylanthranilate, for 10 seconds. The number of pecks and the latency to first peck for each chick are recorded. Chicks which fail to peck at the training bead on this trial or which fail to show the typical disgust reactions of beak-wiping and distress calls are eliminated from data analyses at the end of the experiment. In general, no more than 10 per cent of chicks are eliminated for this reason.

Retention tests are carried out at various times after the training trial. These consist of a 10 second presentation of a dry red bead, identical to that used in the training trial, to each pair of chicks in a block of 20, followed by a 10 second presentation of a dry blue bead, also identical to that used in the pre-training trial. The number of pecks and the latency to first peck for each chick are recorded for each of the retention trials.

In earlier papers, the measure of retention used was the proportion of chicks in any group which avoided the training (typically red) bead, while avoidance of the never-aversive blue bead was taken either as generalized learning or a performance deficit. Recently, we have introduced two more indices of retention which more clearly reflect discrimination memory (Ng and Gibbs 1988):

1. Per cent discrimination, defined as the proportion of chicks which avoid the red bead and peck the blue bead, among those chicks that peck the blue bead. Thus, chicks that avoid the blue bead on the retention test are excluded from the definition of the index. This is a more or less arbitrary criterion adopted to make this index more comparable with the next one.

2. Discrimination ratio, defined as the ratio of the number of pecks at the red bead to the total number of pecks at the blue and the red bead for a given chick, excluding any chick which avoids the blue bead on the retention test. This is thus a continuous measure of retention, unlike the others.

DRUGS

All drugs, unless otherwise stated, are prepared in 154 mM NaCl and administered in 100 μl volumes subcutaneously or 10 μl volumes intracranially. Subcutaneous injections are administered into a fold of skin on the ventral side of the rib cage. Intracranial injections are given freehand into the centre of each forebrain to a depth of 3 mm, using a Hamilton repeating dispenser syringe.

PHARMACOLOGICAL EVIDENCE FOR MEMORY STAGES

Pharmacological evidence for various stages in memory formation arises from the use of drugs which inhibit, interfere with, or attenuate neuronal processes which are suspected to be involved in memory formation, and observing the consequent effects on behavioural evidence of memory. In addition, agents which are known to counteract the actions of the above drugs on the relevant neuronal processes are used to challenge the behavioural effects of these drugs.

The effective times of administration of an amnestic agent after learning provide an indication of when a stage of memory processing involving the

Table 13.1   Effects of amnestic agents on long-term memory

Agents	Effective post-training times of injection (min)	Earliest appearance of amnesia (post-training) (min)	Postulated common pharmacological action
Antibiotics			
1. Cycloheximide	0–20	60	Direct protein
2. Anisomycin	0–20	60	synthesis inhibition
Amino acids			
Most non-essential amino acids	0–5	60	Indirect synthesis inhibition— imbalance of amino acids— possibly involving sodium-pump transport
Antibodies			
Anti-chick-THY-1 Antibodies:	0–10 (latest time tested)		
1. Polyclonal ascites		60	Possible blocking
2. Monoclonal ascites			of THY-1
3. Purified IgG			molecules
4. Fab			

neuronal process affected by that agent may be taking place. To the extent that the degree of memory loss decreases with increasing interval between learning and drug administration, the drug may be said to affect the development phase of that stage of memory, provided allowance is made for the latency of action of the drug. This latency can be estimated to some extent from the effective pre-training times of administration. The earliest time of onset and the progression of amnesia are taken to indicate the decay phase of the memory stage immediately preceding the stage inhibited by the amnestic agent. Thus, the time of administration function of an amnestic agent and the consequent retention function together provide the temporal boundaries of a stage of memory.

Evidence for long-term memory stage

One of the most enduring hypotheses regarding memory processing is that protein synthesis underlies permanent memory encoding (Dunn 1980).

Support for this proposition comes in part from consistent reports that protein synthesis inhibitors, including a range of antibiotics, inhibit consolidation of memory, although the basis of antibiotic inhibition of memory consolidation remains a point of contention (Dunn 1980; McGaugh 1983). Whatever the basis of action of the antibiotics, the findings from the use of these agents point to multiple stages in memory formation.

As shown in Table 13.1, post-learning intracranial administration of the antiobiotics cycloheximide or anisomycin results in amnesia appearing some 60 minutes after the training trial, with no evidence of recovery by 180 minutes post-learning (Fig. 13.1). Furthermore, these drugs are non-effective if administered later than 20 minutes post-learning (Fig. 13.2). These results suggest an antibiotic-sensitive stage of memory, fully developed some time after 20 minutes post-learning and available for recall after 60 minutes post-learning.

Consistent with the view that antibiotics induce amnesia through inhibition of protein synthesis is the finding that the non-metabolizable amino acid α-amino isobutyrate produces amnesia at 60 minutes following learning, provided it is administered intracranially by 5 minutes post-learning (Robertson *et al.* 1978). A similar effect is observed with a number of non-essential amino acids (Table 13.1; Gibbs *et al.* 1987). The difference in effective times of administration between the antibiotics and the amino acids will be dealt with later.

Finally, it is of interest to note that anti-chick anti-Thy-1 antibodies administered intracranially also yield amnesia beginning 60 minutes post-learning (Table 13.1; Lapukke *et al.* 1987; Bernard *et al.* 1983). Recent evidence from our laboratories suggests that effect is obtained with the Fab but not the Fc fragment (Fig. 13.3, Feng, H., unpublished data). While it is not suggested that this glycoprotein is a substrate for long-term memory, the findings are consistent with the notion that protein synthesis may play a significant role in memory consolidation.

Evidence for an intermediate memory stage

The fact that normal retention levels are observed up to 60 minutes post-learning in the presence of protein synthesis inhibitors suggests that there is a stage of memory preceding the antibiotic-sensitive long-term memory (LTM) stage. More direct evidence for this comes from experiments showing that the sodium pump inhibitors ouabain and ethacrynic acid, given intracranially up to 5 minutes post-learning, induce amnesia after 10 minutes post-learning (Table 13.2; Fig. 13.4; Gibbs and Ng 1977). Neither ouabain nor ethacrynic acid is effective when administered 10 minutes later following learning (Fig. 13.5). These results suggest that there is a stage of memory processing preceding the long-term memory stage which is susceptible to blockade by sodium pump inhibitors, which is formed

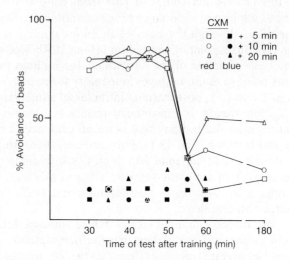

Fig. 13.1 Retention function for CXM administered intracranially at various times after training. Retention levels are high until after 50 minutes post-learning. (Taken from Gibbs and Ng 1984.)

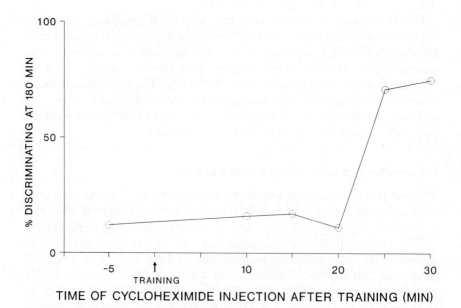

Fig. 13.2 Effect of varying time of administration of CXM for retention tested at 180 minutes post-learning. Retention is measured as per cent of chicks avoiding the red and pecking the blue bead.

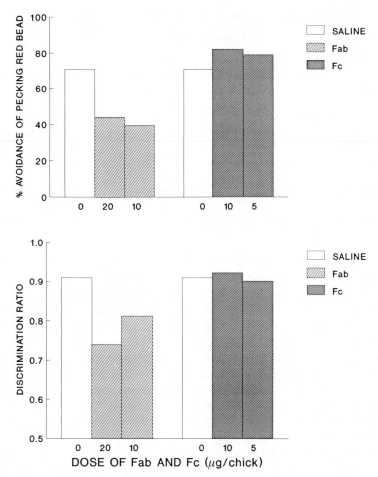

Fig. 13.3 Effects of intracranially administered Fab and Fc fragments of anti-chick Thy-1 IgG on one-trial passive avoidance learning task.

some time between learning and 10 minutes post-learning, and which is available for recall after 10 minutes post-learning, and lasts up to 60 minutes post-learning. We have now called this stage intermediate memory (ITM). It corresponds to the 'labile memory' stage reported in early papers (Watts and Mark 1971; Gibbs and Ng 1977).

We have tentatively suggested that development of ITM may be dependent upon the action of an electrogenic sodium pump (Gibbs and Ng 1977) and may involve a phase of neuronal hyperpolarization associated with the pump (Jansen and Nicholls 1973; Gibbs *et al.* 1978). Support for this hypothesis comes from the observation that the amnestic effect of ouabain may be prevented by subcutaneous injections of the anticonvulsant

Table 13.2   Effects of amnestic agents on intermediate memory

Agents	Effective post-training times of injection (min)	Earliest appearance of amnesia (post-training) (min)	Postulated common pharmacological action
Ouabain (digitalis)	0–5	20	Inhibition of sodium pump activity (Na^+/K^+ ATPase)
Ethacrynic acid	0–5	20	
2,4-Dinitrophenol	5–25	5 min after injection	Inhibition of ATP synthesis

diphenylhydantoin, which has been shown to stimulate Na^+/K^+ ATPase activity at the anti-amnestic dose of 0.1 M (Gibbs and Ng 1977). This conclusion is also consistent with the finding that ouabain-induced amnesia can be counteracted by noradrenalin and amphetamine, drugs which share with diphenylhydantoin the action of stimulating sodium pump activity (Gibbs and Ng 1979).

In this context, the earlier reported observation that α-amino isobutryate and some non-essential amino acids are effective only if given by 5 minutes post-learning suggests that, in inducing amnesia, transport of these amino acids may be sodium pump mediated. This being the case, sodium pump inhibitors may in fact interfere with transport and balance of amino acids necessary for long-term memory consolidation.

If sodium pump activity is critical to the development of ITM, it may be expected that the metabolic inhibitor 2, 4-dinitrophenol (DNP) would also inhibit development of this stage. This is indeed the case, with 0.2 mM of DNP administered intracranially 5 minutes after learning resulting in evidence of amnesia after 10 minutes following learning (Fig. 13.6). However, unlike ouabain and ethacrynic acid, DNP is effective in inducing amnesia when given after 5 minutes and up to 25 minutes post-learning, with amnesia being evident 5 minutes after the administration of the drug. Injection of DNP 30 minutes or later after learning does not produce amnesia (Fig. 13.6). These findings suggest that:

1. The development of ITM may involve a state of neuronal hyperpolarization associated with Na^+/K^+ ATPase activity;

2. When fully developed, intermediate memory may be maintained in two distinct phases: phase A, lasting from about 20 to about 30 minutes post-learning, susceptible to inhibition by DNP, and phase B, lasting from

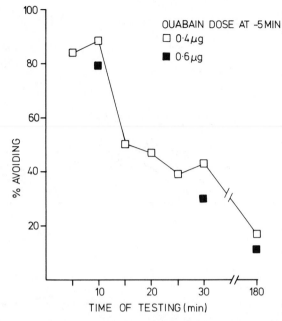

Fig. 13.4   Retention function for 0.4 μg ouabain given intracranially 5 minutes before learning, compared with retention levels at selected TTI for chicks treated with 0.6 μg ouabain. Percentage avoidance of the aversive training bead is shown. (Taken from Ng and Gibbs 1988.)

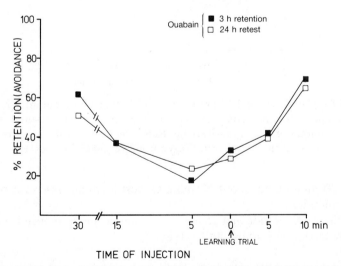

Fig. 13.5   The effects of varying the time of intracranial injection of 0.4 μg ouabain, with retention tested at 180 minutes or 24 hours post-learning. Only training (aversive) bead results are shown. (Taken from Ng and Gibbs 1988.)

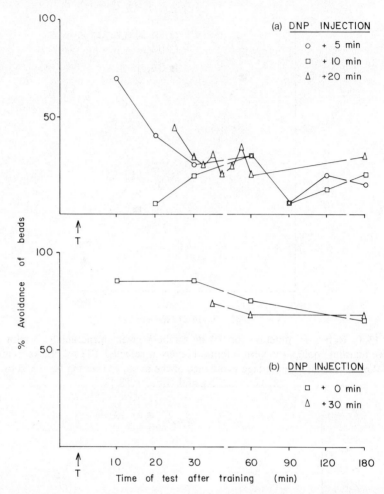

Fig. 13.6 The effects of 2, 4-dinitrophenol (DNP) administered intracranially at various times before and after training (T) on retention levels measured at various times (5 minutes or later) post-learning. Retention levels for the aversive training bead only are shown. (Taken from Ng and Gibbs 1984.)

about 30 minutes to about 50 minutes post-learning, not susceptible to DNP inhibition;

3. Phase A is not maintained by sodium pump-induced neuronal hyperpolarization (Gibbs and Ng 1984).

We are at present unable to state with certainty just what neuronal mechanisms underpin phases A and B of intermediate memory. However, it is useful to note that cycloheximide, administered intracranially 2.5

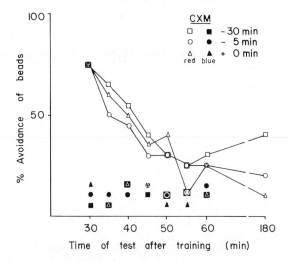

Fig. 13.7 The effects of CXM given intracranially immediately after or before learning. Unlike the case with CXM administered 5 minutes or later after learning (cf. Fig. 13.1), retention levels decline after 30 minutes post-learning. (Taken from Ng and Gibbs 1984.)

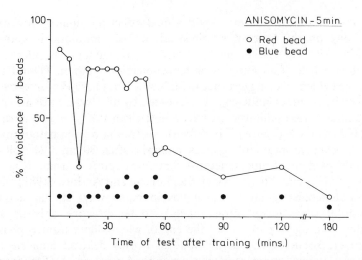

Fig. 13.8 Retention function for ANI given intracranially 5 minutes before learning. Retention levels are high until after 50 minutes following learning. Note the low retention level at 15 minutes post-learning. (Taken from Bernard *et al.* 1983.)

minutes after learning or earlier, yields amnesia after 30 minutes following learning (Fig. 13.7). This contrasts markedly with the effect of cyclohex-imide given 5 minutes later after learning and with that of anisomycin given 5 minutes before learning (Fig. 13.8; Gibbs and Ng 1984). It seems

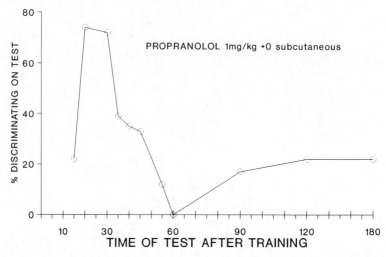

Fig. 13.9 Retention function resulting from the subcutaneous administration of propranolol (1 mg/kg) immediately after learning. Retention is measured as the percentage of chicks avoiding the red bead and pecking the blue bead.

clear that cycloheximide may exert a dual effect on memory processing, depending on the time of administration. This antibiotic is known to interfere with catecholamine synthesis, in a manner dissimilar to the inhibitory effect of anisomycin on catecholamine synthesis (Dunn 1980). We have evidence to suggest that the inhibition of phase B of intermediate memory by cycloheximide can be prevented by dibutryl-cAMP and by the phosphodiesterase inhibitor theophylline (Brown 1987), and by noradrenalin (Gibbs and Ng, unpublished data). Furthermore, the beta-noradrenergic blocker propranolol induces amnesia after 30 minutes following learning when given subcutaneously 5 minutes before learning (Fig. 13.9; Gibbs and Ng, unpublished data). Stephenson and Andrew (1981) showed a beta-antagonist, sotalol (which has in many ways similar action to propanolol when given intracranially), to be effective only up to 25 minutes, thus again picking out the end of what is here termed phase A. Moreover, sotalol given at 25 minutes causes delayed amnesia at 60 minutes, thus suggesting interference with the formation of LTM (Stephenson and Andrew, *loc. cit*). The action of beta-antagonists is discussed further in Chapter 16. Routtenberg (1979) has provided evidence to suggest that glycoproteins may be implicated in long-term memory consolidation, while phosphoproteins may be involved in shorter-term memory processing. Since DNP is a known uncoupler of oxidative phosphorylation (Lehninger 1965), it is possible to speculate that phase A of intermediate memory may be associated with a state of neuronal hyperpolarization

Table 13.3   Effects of amnestic agents on short-term memory

Agents	Effective post-training times of injection (min)	Earliest appearance of amnesia (post-training) (min)	Postulated common pharmacological action
1. 1–2 mM KCl 2. 154 mM KCl 3. Monosodium glutamate	0–2.5	5	Depolarization of neurons through interference with K^+ conductance
Lanthanum chloride	0–2.5	5	Depolarization of neurons by blocking calcium channels

involving cAMP-mediated phosphorylation of proteins (Despopoulos and Silbernagl 1986). We are presently exploring this possibility.

Evidence for a short-term memory stage

The presence of a normal level of retention up to 10 minutes following learning when the chicks are treated with ouabain or ethacrynic acid suggests the existence of an early stage of memory not sensitive to the effects of sodium pump inhibition. This stage appears to have a decay function beginning after 10 minutes following learning. We have shown that this short-term stage is susceptible to blocking by depolarizing agents such as 4 mM glutamate, a low dose (1–2 mM) of potassium chloride and isotonic potassium chloride, given intracranially up to 2.5 minutes post-learning. Later administrations of these drugs have no effect (Table 13.3). With these drugs, amnesia is evident by 5 minutes after learning. It would appear, therefore, that a short-term memory (STM) stage is formed by 5 minutes post-learning and survives for a further 5 minutes before decaying.

There is evidence to suggest that this stage of memory may be associated with a phase of neuronal hyperpolarization arising from changes in K^+ conductance across neuronal membranes following neural input. Such an initial phase of hyperpolarization has been isolated in small diameter unmyelinated fibres in the leech (Jansen and Nicholls 1973). These authors have shown that this phase of hyperpolarization may be enhanced by increased extracellular calcium. If the proposed short-term memory stage is associated with such a phase of hyperpolarization, it may be expected that the characteristics of this stage will be altered by changing Ca^{2+} levels. This is in fact the case. Calcium chloride, given intracranially immediately

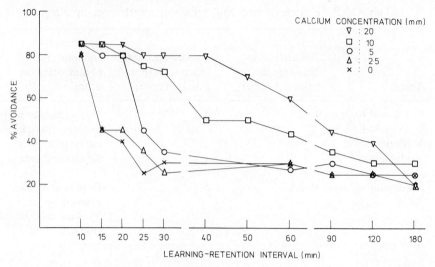

Fig. 13.10   Effect of increasing concentrations of calcium on the retention function in the presence of ouabain. Retention is measured as the percentage of chicks avoiding the red bead. (Taken from Gibbs *et al.* 1979.)

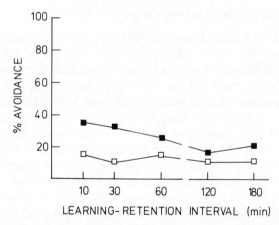

Fig. 13.11   Blocking of calcium channels by lanthanum chloride and subsequent amnesia. Retention is measured as the percentage of chicks avoiding the red bead. (Taken from Gibbs *et al.* 1979.)

after learning to chicks pretreated with ouabain 5 minutes before learning to prevent formation of intermediate memory, produces an extension of the duration of the postulated short-term stage in a dose-dependent manner (Fig. 13.10). Moreover, the calcium channel blocker lanthanum chloride prevents formation of this stage of memory (Fig. 13.11).

BEHAVIOURAL EVIDENCE FOR STAGES IN MEMORY PROCESSING

If, as the pharmacological evidence would appear to suggest, there are clearly defined stages in memory formation, it is of interest to determine whether there are behavioural markers of such stages. We have presented data suggesting that chicks trained on the single trial discriminated passive avoidance task and tested for retention at various times after training show normal retention levels at all training-test intervals except at 15 and 55 minutes after learning. At these times there is a clear transient retention deficit (Gibbs and Ng 1979). We interpreted these 'dips' in retention levels as indicating the cross-over of succeeding stages of memory, since the times of these dips correspond to the times of first appearance of amnesia resulting from the use of pharmacological inhibiting agents, such as ouabain and cycloheximide. Since these purely behavioural findings were not carried out in completely 'blind' experiments, we have repeated the experiments using double blind procedures. The results, which are set out in Chapter 17 (Fig. 17.1), clearly confirm earlier behavioural evidence for at least three stages in memory processing with temporal parameters commensurate with those suggested by the pharmacological studies.

CONCLUSION

The pharmacological evidence, taken together, argues for a model of memory processing involving at least three distinct stages, with distinct neuronal processes underlying them, and with reasonably well-defined temporal characteristics: a short-term stage (STM) formed by 5 minutes after learning and decaying after 10 minutes following learning, susceptible to inhibition by a range of neuronal depolarizing agents; an intermediate stage (ITM) formed by 20 minutes following learning and decaying after 50 minutes post-learning, consisting of an energy-dependent phase A and an energy-independent phase B, susceptible to inhibition by sodium pump blockers and the metabolic inhibitor dinitrophenol during development, and by dinitrophenol during phase A; a long-term memory stage formed by 60 minutes post-learning and inhibited by protein synthesis inhibitors, some amino acids, and specific antibodies to certain glycoproteins (Fig. 13.12). Furthermore, the temporal parameters established in these pharmacological studies are consistent with results from purely behavioural observations which show that the retention function consists of three distinct stages of high levels of retention separated by two points of transient retention deficit, one at 15 minutes and the other at 55 minutes post-learning.

We have reason to believe that the existence of phase B of ITM is

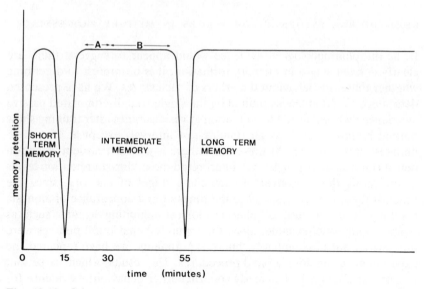

Fig. 13.12   Schematic representation of three-stage model of memory. (Taken from Gibbs and Ng 1984.)

essential for the ultimate consolidation of the learning experience into long-term memory (see also Andrew and Brennan 1985), and that a triggering mechanism for this consolidation is initiated in the transition from phase A to phase B. This possibility is canvassed in detail by Marie Gibbs in Chapter 17. In brief, chicks trained on a weakly-reinforced version of the single trial passive avoidance task, obtained by diluting methylanthranilate in alcohol, yield evidence of STM and ITM (A), but not ITM (B) or LTM. Retraining with this task or post-training administration of a range of pituitary adrenal hormones yield LTM only when the number of retraining trials or the dose of hormones leads to the occurrence of phase B. Furthermore, in chicks trained on the normal task, the administration of these doses of hormones (1) extends the duration of phase A of ITM, (2) delays the appearance of phase B of ITM, and (3) delays the post-training period of sensitivity of LTM to inhibition by CXM. The evidence suggests that those neuronal processes underlying the development of LTM which are susceptible to antibiotic inhibition are initiated at the time of transition from phase A to phase B of ITM. Furthermore, the presence of phase B is necessary, although not sufficient, for LTM development.

While the mechanisms underlying these proposed stages of memory remain speculative, the evidence for the existence of these stages, at least in the limited case of a single trial discriminated passive avoidance learning in the day-old chick, is overwhelming. Our findings and conclusions have been substantially confirmed in a recent report from Patterson *et al.*

(1986). Differences between our findings and those of Patterson *et al.* with respect to the temporal parameters defining the various stages may be attributed to procedural differences, particularly the pairing of chicks in our experiments and the use of isolated chicks in theirs. The effect of isolating chicks may be to induce hormonal release associated with stress and hence alter the timing of the stages. This issue is taken up in detail by Marie Gibbs in Chapter 17.

It is also encouraging that a similar multi-stage model, with comparable temporal parameters and possible underlying mechanisms, has been postulated for a learning task in rats (Frieder and Allweis 1978), although these authors suggest an additional very short-term stage. The chick paradigm does not permit investigation of such a very short-term stage because of the persistence of the taste of methylanthranilate for a couple of minutes after the training trial. Frieder and Allweis have also suggested that the long-term memory stage is dependent only on the short-term stage and not on the intermediate stage, in view of the finding that a period of temporary amnesia occurs during the ITM stage in both the chick and the rat following hypoxia treatment (Frieder and Allweis 1978; Allweis *et al.* 1984). While the explanation for this effect of hypoxia remains conjectural, this and other results from Frieder and Allweis (1978) provide striking confirmation that the underlying neuronal processes are similar in memory formation across the two species.

The evidence presented in this paper, as well as reports in the literature from our and other laboratories, is persuasive with respect to the existence of stages in memory processing. Just how many stages there are, the relationships between them, the temporal parameters governing them, and the neuronal mechanisms underlying them are matters which require further investigation before unequivocal conclusions can be drawn, and may depend upon the species of animals, the learning task, and the particulars of the experimental protocol used. In the case of the single trial discriminated passive avoidance task with day-old chicks trained and tested in pairs, we are satisfied that the schematic model outlined in Fig. 13.12 is appropriate.

REFERENCES

Allweis, C., Gibbs, M. E., Ng, K. T., and Hodge, R. J. (1984). Effects of hypoxia on memory consolidation: Implications for a multistage model of memory. *Behavioural Brain Research*, **11**, 117–21.

Andrew, R. J. and Brannan, A. (1985). Sharply timed and lateralised events at time of establishment of long term memory. *Physiology and Behavior*, **34**, 547–56.

Bernard, C. C. A., Gibbs, M. E., Hodge, R. J. and Ng, K. T. (1983). Inhibition of long-term memory formation in the chicken by anti chick Thy-1 antibody. *Brain Research Bulletin*, **11**, 111–36.

Booth, D. A. (1970). Neurochemical changes correlated with learning and memory retention. In *Molecular mechanisms in memory and learning* (ed. G. Ungar), pp. 1–57. Plenum Press, New York.

Brown, D. F. (1987). The role of adenosine 3′, 5′-cyclic monophosphate (cAMP) in memory formation: a behavioural, pharmacological, and biochemical study. PhD Dissertation, LaTrobe University, Melbourne.

Cherkin, A. (1971). Biphasic time course of performance after one-trial avoidance training in the chick. *Communications in Behavioral Biology*, **5**, 379–81.

Craik, F. I. M. and Lockhart, R. S. (1972). Levels of processing: A framework for memory research. *Journal of Verbal Learning and Verbal Behavior*, **11**, 671–84.

Despopoulos, A. and Silbernagl, S. (1986). *Color atlas of physiology*. George Thieme, Stuttgart.

Dunn, A. J. (1980). Neurochemistry of learning and memory: an evaluation of recent data. *Annual Review of Psychology*, **31**, 343–90.

Frieder, B. and Allweis, C. (1978). Transient hypoxic-amnesia: evidence for a triphasic memory-consolidating mechanism with parallel-processing. *Behavioral Biology*, **22**, 178–89.

Gibbs, M. E. and Ng, K. T. (1977). Psychobiology of memory: towards a model of memory formation. *Biobehavioral Review*, **1**, 113–36.

Gibbs, M. E. and Ng, K. T. (1979). Behavioral stages in memory formation. *Neuroscience Letters*, **13**, 279–83.

Gibbs, M. E. and Ng, K. T. (1984). Dual action of cycloheximide on memory formation in day-old chicks. *Behavioural Brain Research*, **12**, 21–7.

Gibbs, M. E., Gibbs, C. L., and Ng, K. T. (1978). A possible physiological mechanism for short-term memory. *Physiological Behavior*, **20**, 619–27.

Gibbs, M. E., Gibbs, C. L., and Ng, K. T. (1979). The influence of calcium on short-term memory. *Neuroscience Letters*, **14**, 355–60.

Gibbs, M. E., Richdale, A. L., and Ng, K. T. (1987). Effects of excess intracranial amino acids in memory: a behavioural review. *Neuroscience and Biobehavioral Reviews*, **11**, 331.

Gold, P.E. and McGaugh, J. L. (1975). A single-trace two-process view of memory storage processes. In *Short term memory* (ed. D. Deutsch and J. A. Deutsch), pp. 355–78. Academic Press, New York.

Halstead, W. C. and Rucker, W. B. (1968). Memory: a molecular maze. *Psychology Today*, **2**, 38–41 and 66–7.

Hebb, D. O. (1949). *The organization of behavior: a neuropsychological theory*. John Wiley, New York.

Jansen, J. K. S. and Nicholls, J. G. (1973). Conductance changes, an electrogenic pump and the hyperpolarization of leech neurons following impulses. *Journal of Physiology*, **229**, 635–55.

Lappuke, R., Bernard, C. C. A., Gibbs, M. E., Ng, K. T., and Bartlett, P. F. (1987). Inhibition of memory in the chick using a monoclonal anti-Thy-1 antibody. *Journal of Neuroimmunology*, **14**, 317–24.

Lehninger, A. L. (1965). *Bioenergetics*. Benjamin, New York.

McGaugh, J. L. (1983). Hormonal influences on memory. *Annual Review of Psychology*, **34**, 297–323.

Ng, K. T. and Gibbs, M. E. (1988). A biological model for memory formation. In *Information processing by the brain* (ed. H. Markowitsch). Hans Huber, Toronto.

Patterson, T. A., Alvarado, M. C., Warner, I. T., Bennett, E. L., and Rosenzweig, M. R. (1986). Memory stages and brain asymmetry in chick learning. *Behavioral Neuroscience*, **100**, 856–65.

Robertson, S., Gibbs, M. E., and Ng, K. T. (1978). Sodium pump activity, amino acid transport and long-term memory. *Brain Research Bulletin*, **3**, 53–8.

Routtenberg, A. (1979). Anatomical localization of phosphoprotein and glycoprotein substrates of memory. *Progress in Neurobiology*, **12**, 85–113.

Stephenson, R. M. and Andrew, R. J. (1981). Amnesia due to β-antagonists in a passive avoidance task in the chick. *Pharmacology, Biochemistry and Behavior*, **15**, 597–604.

Watts, M. E. and Mark, R. F. (1971). Drug inhibition of memory formation in chickens. II. Short-term memory. *Proceedings of the Royal Society of London B*, **178**, 455–64.

14

The congruity of rat and chick multiphasic memory-consolidation models

C. Allweis

INTRODUCTION

The first experimental evidence for a progressive increase in the stability of the memory trace or engram following training was presented some 40 years ago by Duncan (1949), who made use of electroconvulsive shock (applied after each daily trial) to test the stability of the engram. His conclusions are well worth quoting today.

When the shock is interpolated sooner after each trial, less time is allowed for consolidation and there is a greater interference with retention. When the shock is applied after consolidation has ceased, no retention loss is found.

Duncan's pioneering experiment has been repeated with numerous variations hundreds of times. It also inspired many hundreds of experiments using a variety of chemical agents, the most popular of which were cycloheximide and later anisomycin, which were used in attempts to establish a role for protein synthesis in LTM formation.

The purpose of this paper is to summarize the key facts which led Kobiler and Allweis (1973) to extend Duncan's hypothesis and propose their three-phase model of memory consolidation following active avoidance training in the rat, and to compare it with the three-phase model of memory consolidation in the chick which was proposed independently by Gibbs and Ng (1976). The key results of these studies are summarized in Figs. 14.2, 14.9, and 14.12 and Table 14.1, which may be consulted for orientation. The fact that the necessity for similar three-phase models of memory consolidation to encompass a great deal of experimental data was perceived independently by two groups using different species, tasks, and interfering agents lends greater weight to both models.

A subsequent collaborative study using hypoxia in the chick carried out by Allweis et al. (1984) which is described later is crucial in that it is indicative of a very close correspondence between these models and hence between the neurochemical processes which are responsible for the various phases of memory in these two very different species and tasks.

Taken as a whole, the results of these investigations, which have been reviewed by Andrew (1985), seem to establish the viability of the multiphase consolidation hypothesis as the basis of a valuable heuristic programme for memory research.

EXPERIMENTAL PROCEDURES

The shock avoidance apparatus (Kobiler and Allweis 1974) consisted of a wooden box $91 \times 25 \times 46$ cm high, divided into two equal compartments, one of which was black, and one white, by a vertical sliding door. In the bottom of the box was a grid floor which could be electrified with 50 cps current which was limited to 330 μA_{RMS} by a series resistor.

At the start of training, the rat was placed in the white side with the door closed. After a 1 minute delay, the door opened automatically and the rat was transferred to the black side by hand. If the rat remained in the black side for 7 seconds it received an electric shock and the trial was scored as a failure. (If the rat did not run to the safe side after the first shock further brief shocks were given at 1 second intervals until it did so). Running to the safe side (white) within 7 seconds of being transferred to the black side, and thus avoiding electrical shock, was scored as a successful response. Training was continued until the rat achieved a series of five successful responses out of five trials (5/5 criterion). With naïve rats an average of 5.0 ± 1.3 (standard deviation) trials to criterion (TTC) were needed, excluding the five successive successful trials ($n = 294$). Rats which during training had less than three or greater than seven TTCs (about 22 per cent of the animals trained) were excluded from the experiment.

At test (which followed training at various intervals) the number of trials to criterion was again measured. TTCs of treated animals and controls were compared using the Mann–Whitney one-tailed test to determine if memory was impaired by the treatment or not.

Rats were subjected to hypoxia by thrusting them individually into a 10 l transparent plastic bag which had been freshly filled with 2 per cent O_2 in N_2 (Frieder and Allweis 1978). This gas mixture was used to produce hypoxia, since it usually produced severe hypoxia rapidly without the convulsive activity which results when pure N_2 is used. As soon as the rat appeared to have lost consciousness, which took 30–40 seconds, it was returned to room air. About 10 per cent of the rats showed signs of convulsive activity or respiratory irregularity and these were eliminated from the experiments.

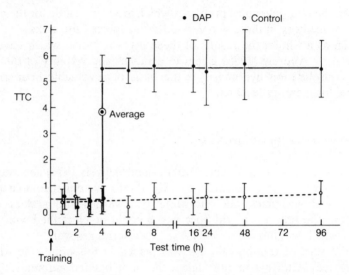

Fig. 14.1 The effect of DAP on the consolidation of memory. Retention was measured as the number of trials to criterion (TTC). The lower this measure the better was retention. Training was completed at zero time. The rats which had received DAP became amnesic about 4 hours after training. Memory did not reappear up to 96 hours after training. Note the break in the abscissa.

THE EFFECT OF DAP ON LTM FORMATION

We chose to work initially with 2,6-diaminopurine (DAP) an inhibitor of RNA synthesis, because its effects are competitive and can be reversed by the injection of adenosine. All drugs were injected intracisternally under very light ether anaesthesia to limit their actions to the CNS as far as possible. Control experiments with fluorescein solution (40 mg per ml) showed that within 15 minutes of injection fluorescence was seen over the entire brain surface.

The timecourse of the inhibitory effect of DAP on RNA synthesis was followed with the aid of uridine-5-^{3}H, which was also injected intracisternally. Incorporation was measured 30 minutes after injection on RNA isolated from brain (Kobiler and Allweis 1974).

Figure 14.1 summarizes behavioural data from some 90 rats. Experimental animals received DAP intracisternally and controls received the same volume of 0.15 M sodium bicarbonate.

The results show that DAP does not affect learning or the formation of memory and its recall; however, 4 hours after training, memory disappeared in the experimental group and was absent for at least 96 hours after training. The control group retained memory for at least 96 hours.

By varying the dose and timing of the DAP injection in relation to training we were able to show that DAP produced retrograde amnesia, provided that the dose and its timing resulted in a more than 60 per cent decrease in the rate of incorporation of labelled uridine into brain RNA over the period from 30 to 200 minutes after training.

THE PREVENTION OF THE AMNESIA-INDUCING EFFECT OF DAP BY ADENOSINE ADMINISTRATION

By injecting 150 μg of adenosine, which is known to reverse the effect of DAP on RNA synthesis, we were able to restore the rate of incorporation of radioactive uridine to 95–100 per cent of its control value within 15 minutes of the injection.

The injection of adenosine (following a 120 μg dose of DAP) also prevented the amnestic action of DAP, providing it was made before or within 3 hours after training. This indicates that it is the RNA synthesis-inhibiting activity of DAP specifically rather than some side-effect on brain metabolism which is responsible for its amnestic effect.

The inability of adenosine injection to re-enable LTM formation after the earlier holding phase has decayed may indicate that the neurobiological processes underlying that earlier phase determine the nature of the RNA subsequently synthesized and this RNA in turn codes for a protein which is essential for LTM formation.

These results, which were presented as a series of 3-dimensional graphs (Kobiler and Allweis 1974), showed that RNA synthesis must occur in the brain over some period between 30 and 200 minutes after training in order for memory to be consolidated for the long term.

THE DISCOVERY OF MEDIUM-TERM MEMORY

In our attempts to augment the extent and duration of RNA synthesis inhibition, we increased the volume of solution injected intracisternally from 10 to 20 μl and were amazed to find that control animals which received saline alone became amnesic provided the injection was given within 1 hour after training. We lost no time exploiting this serendipitous finding by combining it with DAP treatment. We found that, although the 20 μl injection alone is effective in causing amnesia only if given within 60 minutes after training, in the presence of DAP it was effective up to over 200 minutes after training (Kobiler and Allweis 1977).

We interpreted this finding to indicate the existence of a hitherto unrecognized memory-holding mechanism having the following three characteristics.

1. Its formation is not affected by the inhibition of RNA synthesis and is therefore unlikely to be dependent on training-specific protein synthesis.
2. It is susceptible to disruption by a 20 μl intracisternal injection of saline up to 1 hour after training.
3. The effective duration of this postulated memory-holding mechanism is up to about 200 minutes but this can only be demonstrated if LTM formation is prevented by DAP. In the normal course of events LTM is formed about 60 minutes after training, so that beyond that time, the disruption of MTM if it occurred would not be detectable because it would be masked by the presence of LTM. We termed this postulated memory-holding mechanism 'medium-term memory'.

The concept of the masking of one memory holding mechanism by the presence of another became part of our thinking from this point on. It follows that memory-based behaviour is not 'stronger' when two or more different holding mechanisms are active at the same time.

These experiments, together with numerous other experiments combining the procedures mentioned above in various ways, led us to propose a more detailed model of memory consolidation. (Fig. 14.2)

Medium-term memory (so designated on the basis of the criteria discussed previously) is present from about 15 minutes to 200 minutes after training. However, in the normal course of events MTM is masked from about 75 minutes onwards by LTM, which appears to be formed independently by a parallel process necessitating RNA synthesis (and presumably subsequent protein synthesis based on the newly synthesized RNA).

The division of the RNA synthesis period into two distinct phases is based on the following experimental observations. In a normal rat, it takes about 75 minutes until LTM, which is resistant to a 20 μl intracisternal injection of saline, is formed. However, when adenosine is injected intracisternally and competitively reverses the inhibition of RNA synthesis brought about by an earlier injection of DAP, it takes only about 45 minutes for 20 μl-resistant memory (LTM) to be formed. We suggested that the 30 minute discrepancy represented the time required for pre-RNA synthetic processes to occur, and that these processes were not affected by the presence of DAP. This 30 minute period might thus be required for an extracellular signal $\rightarrow$ intracellular signal $\rightarrow$ regulatory gene activation sequence.

As already noted, if RNA synthesis was 60 per cent inhibited over the period from 30 to 200 minutes after training, LTM was not formed. This result poses a problem. For, as is very well known, protein synthesis inhibitors must act during or at least immediately after learning in order for them to produce amnesia. Yet, as we see here, if synthesis of RNA,

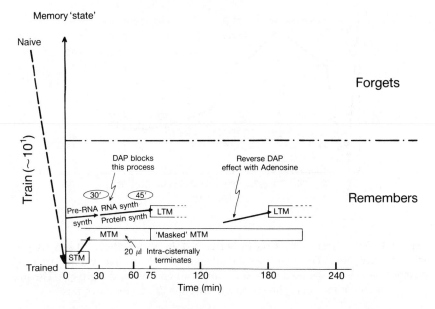

Fig. 14.2 Our first schematic three-phase model of memory consolidation in the rat. The ordinate serves only to differentiate between two ungraded memory states, 'remembers or forgets', which are separated by the horizontal broken line. The abscissa shows time of testing. Illustrative times of injection are shown by the bent arrows: thus DAP (2,6-diaminopurine) injected at about 40 minutes blocks LTM formation, saline ('20 μl') at about 50 minutes disrupts MTM, and adenosine at about 150 minutes reverses the effects of an earlier injection of DAP, and allows the development of LTM. Note that the transcription of STM to MTM depicted here was subsequently shown to be incorrect (cf. Fig. 14.12).

which presumably codes for a burst of protein synthesis which is essential for LTM formation, is inhibited some 30 minutes after training, it nevertheless results in amnesia. Furthermore, if RNA synthesis is reinstated as late as 150 minutes after training by the injection of adenosine, LTM is formed. It appears then that if the commonly used protein synthesis inhibitors prevent LTM formation by preventing protein synthesis soon after training, as most investigators appear to believe, a second and later protein synthesis phase is also required for the formation of LTM. This second phase, unlike the first, requires *de novo* synthesis of mRNA. We have recently presented confirmatory evidence, in that this latter protein synthesis phase is inhibited by chloramphenicol and probably therefore occurs on mitochondria (Fride *et al.* 1989).

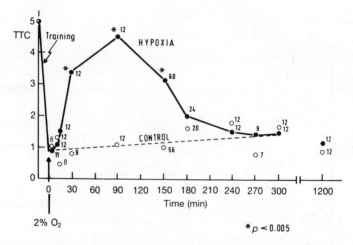

Fig. 14.3 The effect of hypoxia (2 per cent O_2 in N_2 for about 30 seconds) on memory retention. The hypoxia was administered immediately after training. Numbers alongside the points are the number of animals in the groups. The first point of the curve shows trials to criterion (TTC) for naïve rats.

HYPOXIA AS A TOOL IN THE ELUCIDATION OF MULTIPHASIC CONSOLIDATION PROCESSES

At this point in our programme we decided to look into the '20 μl effect' more closely. It transpired that the volume injected and the rate of injection were the critical factors which determined whether or not amnesia was caused. We deduced that the rise in CSF pressure brought about by the rapid injection must produce a transient fall in cerebral blood flow and that the resulting brain anoxia interferes with some stage in the consolidation of memory.

In order to test this hypothesis, we subjected rats to brief hypoxia by placing them in pure 2 per cent O_2 in N_2 immediately after training, as described by Frieder and Allweis (1978). The time-course of the amnesia produced by 30-second exposure to this gas mixture, and its implications for the theory of memory consolidation in the context of other experiments, will now be described.

The basic phenomenon is shown in Fig. 14.3. If rats are subjected to acute hypoxia immediately after training, memory persists for about 15 minutes, disappears over the next 75 minutes and then reappears spontaneously, so that rats tested 240 minutes after the hypoxia are indistinguishable from trained rats which were subjected to the same procedure with air in the plastic bag.

Before the effect of hypoxia on test performance can be interpreted as a true retrograde amnesia, one must show that it is not due to delayed interference with recall mechanisms or a non-specific behavioural deficit in the test situation. We did this by delaying equally the times of hypoxia treatment and testing following training to obtain hypoxia-test intervals of 30, 90 and 150 minutes. All of these hypoxia-test intervals resulted in amnesia, when 2 per cent O_2 was given immediately after training (Fig. 14.3). If hypoxia interfered with memory recall, then it would be expected that the same hypoxia-test intervals would produce amnesia even if hypoxia occurred some time after training. However, as may be seen in Fig. 14.4, amnesia was not obtained in those cases where both hypoxia and testing were delayed.

These findings strongly suggest that we are dealing with a true retrograde amnesia. We called it 'delayed post-hypoxic transient amnesia' (DPHTA). The next question which arose is whether this phenomenon is related to the consolidation of memory.

As may be seen from Fig. 14.5, the results we obtained using hypoxia to test the stability of the engram show that, as the interval between training and hypoxia is increased, the amnesia-inducing effect of the hypoxia decreases.

If hypoxia is administered 30 minutes after training no effect on retention is discernible.

These experiments show that delayed post-hypoxic transient amnesia may be interpreted within the framework of consolidation theory. Before dealing with the important contribution of this phenomenon to consolidation theory, I would like to consider briefly the mechanism involved.

Although we took great pains to eliminate from our experiments uncertainties of interpretation which might arise as a result of the presence of convulsions which accompany hypoxia induced with pure N_2, we could not be sure that covert electrical seizure activity was not responsible for the amnesia observed (Cohen and Barondes 1967). We therefore carried out an investigation in which we compared the effects of N_2 and 2 per cent O_2 in N_2 on the electrical activity of the brain (Frieder and Allweis 1982).

In order to compare the effects of N_2 and 2 per cent O_2 in N_2 on the ECoG we selected five major features of the ECoGs (normal, high frequency, flattening, high amplitude slow waves, and separate slow waves) and plotted the percentage of animals whose ECoGs contained each of these features against time after exposure to the gas.

These graphs (Fig. 14.6) show clearly that, although overt convulsions accompanied by typical electrical seizure activity (i.e. high frequency, followed by flattening, or high amplitude slow waves) was prevalent in the N_2-treated group, convulsions were absent in the 2 per cent O_2-treated group and covert brief electrical seizure type activity was seen only in very few of the 2 per cent O_2 in N_2-treated animals.

These facts, when taken together with the important observation that 2

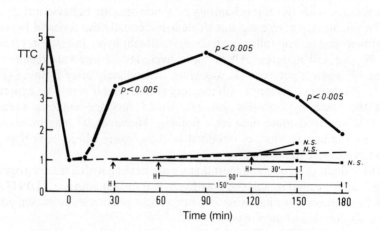

Fig. 14.4 The effect of delaying equally both hypoxia administration and testing on memory retention. All rats were trained at zero time. H indicates the time at which hypoxia was administered, and T the time of test. The curves show the results of testing at the time shown on the abscissa. Transient amnesia occurred only when hypoxia was administered immediately after training (*heavy line*). In all other cases (lower timing bars; N.S. = not significant) in which training and hypoxia were equally delayed, no amnesia was found. This is so even though the three intervals between hypoxia and testing (30, 90 and 150 minutes) *did* result in transient amnesia, if hypoxia followed the end of training closely. The first point shows trials to criterion for naïve rats.

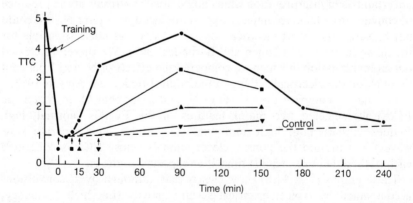

Fig. 14.5 The effect of change in the interval between training and hypoxia on memory retention. Hypoxia was administered immediately after training, or 10 minutes, 15 minutes, or 30 minutes after training. As the interval was increased, the effect diminished. The first point shows trials to criterion for naïve rats; the abscissa otherwise shows time of testing.

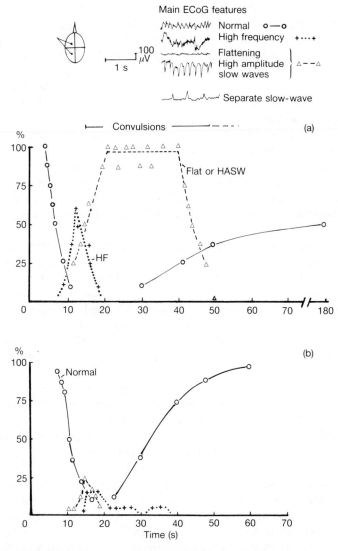

Fig. 14.6 Times of occurrence of prominent abnormal features in rat ECoGs following brief exposure to either N_2 (a) or 2 per cent O_2 in N_2 (b). The features selected are high frequency (HF) and high amplitude slow waves (HASW). Percentage of animals whose ECoGs contained a given feature or group of features is plotted against time after exposure to the gas. The duration of this exposure was about 30 seconds with 2 per cent O_2 in N_2 but only about 15 seconds in pure N_2. With N_2, the occurrence of ECoG features associated with electrical seizures was prevalent over the period from 10 to 40 seconds. In the case of 2 per cent O_2 in N_2, such features were observed only in a very small proportion of the animals and were of very short duration.

per cent O_2 (which did not cause convulsions) was just as effective an amnestic agent as pure N_2 (which did), both with respect to the degree of amnesia produced and the percentage of animals rendered amnesic, indicate that the mechanism whereby DPHTA is induced is not linked to ECoG changes of the type seen during electrical brain seizures.

Having shown that DPHTA is caused by hypoxia *per se*, that it is not due to a recall deficit, and that it is critically dependent on the interval between training and hypoxia (and not on the interval between training and testing) we next tried to determine which of the phases of memory consolidation is affected by hypoxia.

We had already shown in earlier experiments that 2,6-diaminopurine, an RNA synthesis inhibitor, produced a permanent amnesia beginning about 200 minutes after training. This observation was taken to indicate that long-term memory starts about 200 minutes after training and that RNA synthesis is essential for its formation.

Since hypoxia did not abolish memory or interfere with its recall, we proposed that hypoxia prevents the formation of an hypoxia-resistant memory-holding mechanism that is normally established by about 20 minutes after training and which persists at least until LTM becomes effective about 200 minutes after training. We further suggested that this hypoxia-resistant memory-holding mechanism whose formation is prevented is identical with medium-term memory (MTM). This medium-term memory-holding mechanism was operationally defined previously on the basis of its susceptibility to disruption by a rapid intracisternal injection of 20 μl of saline (Kobiler and Allweis 1977). The time after training at which MTM becomes effective could not be determined in that series of experiments, but the course of its decay about 200 minutes after training was unmasked by preventing the development of LTM with DAP. On the basis of these results we proposed that hypoxia prevents the occurrence of the processes responsible for the transcription of memory from STM (or some briefer memory-holding mechanism) to MTM (Frieder and Allweis 1978).

The delayed spontaneous appearance of DAP-resistant LTM about 180 minutes after training followed by hypoxia, and so in the absence of MTM, suggests that the learning process initiates a sequence of neurochemical reactions capable of transcribing the engram directly from STM (or some briefer memory-holding mechanism) to LTM. It seems reasonable to assume that in the absence of experimental interference, memory is transcribed to MTM and to LTM in parallel. Parallel processing of memory has been discussed by Kesner and Conner (1972) and Daniels (1971). This interpretation of our data was supported by the results of subsequent experiments using two other inhibitors which will be described briefly.

Diethyldithiocarbamate (DDC), a dopamine hydroxylase inhibitor which interferes with noradrenalin (NA) synthesis, was found (following intracisternal injection) to produce a delayed transient amnesia identical

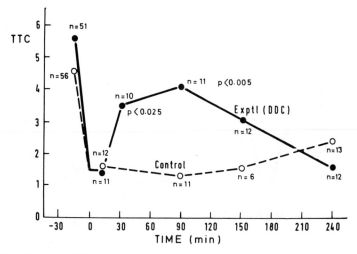

Fig. 14.7   Effect of DDC on active avoidance learning and memory formation in rats. DDC 3 mg was injected intracisternally 30 minutes before training. DDC-treated animals have a delayed transient amnesia, the time-course of which is identical to that produced by hypoxia. Controls which received saline show full retention. The abscissa shows time of testing.

in its time-course with that produced by acute hypoxia (Frieder and Allweis 1982; Fig. 14.7)

Our use of the next agent, ethacrynic acid (EA), which inhibits Na^+/K^+ ATPase and thereby interferes with the transport of Na^+ and K^+ across cell membranes, was prompted by a report by Rogers *et al.* (1977). Using a visual discrimination task in chicks they found that EA, if injected 10 minutes before training, prevents STM formation, so that learning appears to be absent. Nevertheless, memory (presumably intermediate memory) did emerge spontaneously about 20–30 minutes after training. In our rat experiments, EA produced a delayed transient amnesia with a much more rapid onset and much briefer time-course than DPHTA, just as would be expected if it prevented the formation of short-term memory specifically (Frieder and Allweis 1982; Fig. 14.8).

The subsequent appearance of MTM and later LTM in this experiment seems to indicate that STM is not necessary for the formation of these later phases. This in turn suggests that both MTM and LTM are transcribed from some yet briefer trace, VSTM, whose decay is represented by the increase in TTC between 0 and 10 minutes after training in Fig. 14.8. In order to integrate all of the above data into a coherent picture, it is helpful to normalize them. The result is shown in Fig. 14.9.

It is only when the pattern of the data points is given an interpretation in terms of the consolidation hypothesis that a four-phase model of

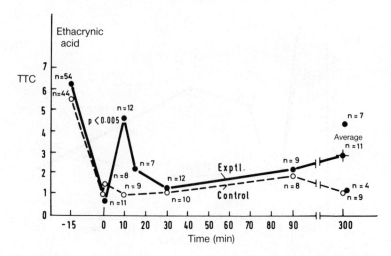

Fig. 14.8 Ethacrynic acid (4 μg in 10 μl of water injected intracisternally 30 minutes before training) does not affect learning. However, it produces a brief delayed transient amnesia which is maximal 10 minutes after the end of training. From 30 to 300 minutes after training retention does not differ from that observed with saline-injected animals. We interpreted the initial decline of memory (0–10 minutes) as the unmasking of the decay of very short-term memory whose existence was earlier inferred from hypoxia-hyperoxia experiments (Frieder and Allweis 1982). The abscissa shows time of testing.

memory consolidation emerges. The relationships between the various phases and the experimental procedures which revealed their existence are summarized in Table 14.1, which also includes corresponding information with respect to the Gibbs and Ng three-phase memory consolidation model to be described next.

EVIDENCE FOR THREE-PHASE CONSOLIDATION FROM PASSIVE-AVOIDANCE EXPERIMENTS ON CHICKS

Independent evidence favouring the concept of multiphasic memory consolidation was obtained by Gibbs and Ng (1976; see also Chapters 13 and 17). Their experimentally-derived three-phase model of consolidation based on the peck inhibition test in 1-day-old chicks (Gibbs 1982) is described in the preceding chapter (Fig. 13.13).

They have presented evidence for the existence of: (1) STM (with a time-course similar to our STM) based on post-neural activity hyperpolarization due to a K^+ permeability change; (2) 'Labile Phase' or 'Intermediate Memory' (IM) (with a time-course considerably briefer than that of

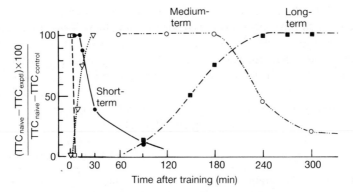

Fig. 14.9 Graphic representation of our three-phase model of memory consolidation for an active avoidance task in the rat. All of the points are experimental data. The agents used to unmask the segments of the various phases are given in Table 14.1. The measure used (% memory effectiveness: % ME) is derived from number of trials to criterion (TTC) by the expression

$$\%ME = 100 \, \frac{(TTC_{naive} - TTC_{experimental})}{TTC_{naive} - TTC_{control}}, \text{ where } TTC_{naive} \text{ is the average training}$$

TTC for untreated animals (7.6 ± 3.1, $n = 202$). $TTC_{control}$ is the average TTC for saline-treated animals during re-training at test, and $TTC_{experimental}$ is the average TTC for drug-treated animals during re-training at test. The decay is shown of a postulated fourth very early phase of memory consolidation, which we have referred to as very short term memory, VSTM. There is only a limited amount of evidence for the existence of this phase, based on the experiments with EA, and on experiments in which the effect of hypoxia on consolidation was reversed by the administration of 100 per cent O_2, provided this was done within 2.5 minutes of the hypoxia (Frieder and Allweis 1982). This phase will not be discussed further here, but it is noteworthy that the existence of a pre-STM phase in the chick has also been postulated by Gibbs and by Rosenweig (Chapter 15).
$\nabla \cdots \nabla$ The time-course of formation of MTM as deduced from delayed hypoxia exeriments. $\bullet\!\!-\!\!-\!\!\bullet$ The time-course of the decay of STM deduced from experiments using hypoxia or DDC. $\circ\!\!-\!\!\cdot\!\!-\!\!\circ$ The plateau and decay of MTM deduced from experiments with DAP. $\blacksquare\!\!-\!\!\cdot\!\!-\!\!\blacksquare$ The time-course of the formation and plateau of LTM deduced from experiments with hypoxia and DDC.

our MTM) based on post-neural activity hyperpolarization due to Na^+/K^+ pump activity; (3) Long-term memory dependent on protein synthesis. An important feature of their model is that the stages are sequential (see Fig. 14.12).

They have also shown two dips in the control retention curve which coincide with the times at which successive phases of memory are supplanting each other (Gibbs and Ng 1979, and Fig. 14.10).

Their introduction of the use of an additional non-aversive discriminatory blue bead to control for possible non-specific effects of various agents

Table 14.1 A comparison of the multiphase memory consolidation models which have been proposed for rat and chick. Two complementary aspects of the experimental strategy which underlies these research programmes are distinguished in this table: firstly, the prevention of the formation of one or more phases of consolidation by a specific treatment and secondly, the consequent unmasking of the time-course of formation and/or decay of other phases of consolidation (see also Fig. 17.1 in Rosenzweig and Bennett 1984).

Rat active avoidance			Chick passive avoidance	
Formation-preventing agent	Duration: unmasking agents	Phase and sub-phases	Duration: unmasking agents	Formation-preventing agents
	Up to 10min — EA	**VSTM** Development plateau and decay		EA
EA	Up to 90 min — Hypoxia, DDC	**STM** Development plateau and decay	Up to 10 min Ouabain, EA	LiCl, KCl
Hypoxia, DDC	20–200 min Delayed-hypoxia DAP	**MTM/IM** Development Plateau and decay	20–50 min CXM & ANI	OU, EA, hypoxia
	200 min onwards Hypoxia, DDC —	**LTM** Development	60 min onwards Hypoxia	ANI, CXM, AIB

AIB = α-amino isobutyrate; ANI = anisomycin; CXM = cycloheximide; DAP = 2,6-diaminopurine; DDC = diethyldithiocarbamate; EA = ethacrynic acid; OU = ouabain.

on the peck-response latency was an important advance in technique which lends considerable weight to the validity of their peck-inhibition data.

The agents which they used to prevent the formation of various memory phases in the chick are detailed in Table 14.1.

In view of the similarities between these two models, it was clearly of great interest to find out if post-training hypoxia in the chick would induce

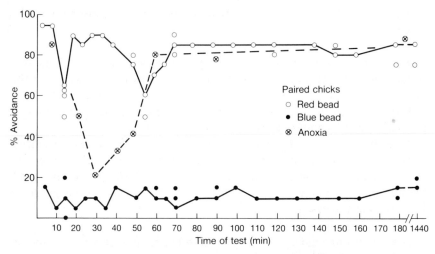

Fig. 14.10 Discriminative memory of an aversive-tasting bead followed over time after learning. The red bead was dipped in methylanthranilate for the learning trial; both red and blue beads were dry on the test trial. Separate groups of 20 chicks were tested at each time interval. The dips in avoidance at 15, and around 55 minutes are held, in the Gibbs–Ng model, to represent transition from STM to MTM, and from MTM to LTM. The delayed post-hypoxic transient amnesia found in the chick in a separate series of experiments is superimposed on this control data. Modified from Gibbs (1976), with superimposition of data resulting from anoxia.

DPHTA. On the basis of the results obtained with rats and the interpretation of those results within the framework of consolidation theory, we predicted that post-training hypoxia in the chick would also prevent MTM (IM) formation and thereby unmask both the declining phase of STM and the ascending phase of LTM. This of course is a very strong prediction in that it calls not only for a shorter DPHTA in the chick but also predicts that its timing should fit that of all three of the experimentally-derived curves for the three successive phases in the Gibbs and Ng model. Note that these were obtained by using quite different agents to interfere with the formation of the various phases of memory.

In a collaborative investigation it was found that hypoxia administered 5 minutes after training produced DPHTA (for response to red bead) but had no effect on blue bead pecking. In this crucial experiment the temporal course of DPHTA showed a remarkable fit to our prediction (Allweis *et al.* 1984; and Fig. 14.10). Hypoxia neatly eliminated the memory-holding mechanism which lay between the two dips on the control retention curve, whilst leaving the memory-holding mechanisms on either side of it quite unaffected.

It may therefore be concluded that the models are consonant to the extent that

- DPHTA can be induced in both species under similar experimental conditions, with respect to the reduced partial pressure of oxygen in the inspired gas and the duration of exposure to the gas mixture;
- the delay in the onset of amnesia following the return of the chick to room air is similar to the delay observed in the rat;
- the time-course of the DPHTA (which was found to be much shorter in the chick than in the rat) is just the time-course which one would expect, if the hypoxia prevented the formation of IM in the chick and thereby unmasked the declining phase of STM and the rising phase of LTM (as was the case in the rat).

There is strong evidence that hypoxia in the rat prevents the formation of MTM specifically. Hence, and in the light of the strong evidence for three-phase consolidation in the chick, it is reasonable to conclude that it has a similar action in the chick.

These results fully accord with the strong predictions referred to above and conversely constitute very strong evidence for the validity of the models on which the predictions were based. This result also marks the confluence of two independent research programmes. In view of the use of different species, different tasks and different agents to interfere selectively with the formation of the different memory phases, this outcome is most remarkable. It also demonstrates the heuristic value of the consolidation hypothesis.

From the result of this experiment it may be further inferred that the neurochemical processes underlying MTM formation in both rat and chick are similar in nature. This is a striking inference which needs confirmation by further experiments with different agents in both species.

The validity of the above inferences is strongly supported by a comparison of the periods of susceptibility of MTM/IM formation to hypoxia in rat and chick in relation to the time of training. Hypoxia in the rat has a maximal amnestic effect if it administered immediately after training, but if it is administered to the chick immediately after training it has no discernible effect on memory (Fig. 14.11). Its effect on MTM formation in the chick is maximal if it is administered 5 minutes after training.

This seemingly discrepant aspect of the data was, however, entirely resolved *post hoc* with the realization that, in the active avoidance test, each rat is obliged to perform five trials to criterion, each lasting about 1 minute, after it has learned to make the escape response. Hence, in effect, the administration of hypoxia to a rat immediately after training is temporally equivalent to the administration of hypoxia to a chick 5 minutes

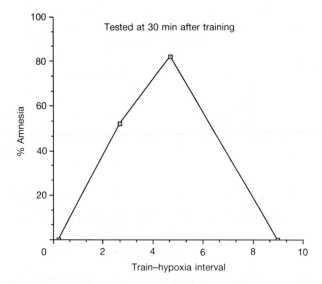

Fig. 14.11 The effect of change in the interval between training and hypoxia on the degree of amnesia measured 30 minutes after training in chicks. Per cent amnesia is calculated as (100 − per cent memory effectiveness); see legend to Fig. 14.9 for definition of memory effectiveness.

after single-trial training, with respect to the dynamics of the consolidating mechanisms.

Figure 14.12 is a schematic depiction of the temporal relationship between the various phases of memory in rat and chick. Their sequential dependencies, as inferred from many experiments (see Table 14.1) are indicated by arrows.

DPHTA in the chick has been ascribed (Allweis *et al.* 1984) to a retrieval deficit. The basis for this interpretation of the data was the previously observed necessity of the presence of IM for LTM formation in experiments with ouabain-like compounds in the chick. These compounds were shown to prevent both IM and LTM formation in the chick and this fact served as one of the arguments for the serial model proposed by Gibbs and Ng. However, the interpretation of DPHTA as a retrieval deficit now appears to me to be untenable for the following reasons.

- Rogers *et al.* (1977) showed that EA can eliminate STM in the chick whilst leaving LTM intact. This implies that there exists a parallel pathway from training or some subsequent brief trace to LTM, and that this pathway does not require the presence of STM.
- It has been clearly demonstrated by means of extensive control

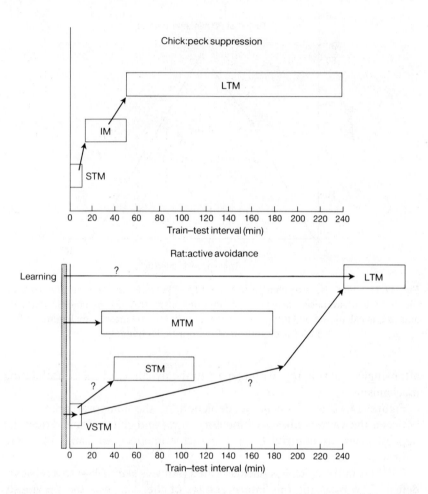

Fig. 14.12 A schematic comparison of the relationships between the various phases of memory consolidation in rat and chick. The ordinate has no significance in these figures other than indicating zero time. The arrows represent the dependence of the formation of a later phase (arrow-head) on the prior existence of an earlier phase. In the case of the chick, the pattern of dependence, which was deduced from the experiments depicted in Table 14.1, is strictly serial: i.e. the formation of each phase is dependent on the integrity of the antecedent phase. The evidence from hypoxia, as set out in the text, is more consistent with the parallel processes of memory formation, found in the rat. Memory consolidation of active avoidance in the rat, apart from taking much longer, appears to be more complex in that parallel dependence seems to be a major feature of consolidation; and the formation of all phases except STM may be initiated by the learning process itself which occurs about 5 minutes prior to the end of training as explained in the text.

experiments in the rat (involving some 150 rats) that DPHTA is not an MTM retrieval deficit (Frieder and Allweis 1978).

• If hypoxia is administered to a chick immediately after training and memory assessed 30 minutes later when IM is the only form in which it exists, no deficit is seen. In order to maintain the IM retrieval-deficit explanation, it would be necessary to explain why a 5 minute delay between training and hypoxia was essential for the prevention of retrieval 30 minutes later.

The fact that the two multiphasic consolidation models proposed to encompass a large body of experimental data so obtained are consonant with respect to DPHTA strengthens the argument for the existence of at least three operationally distinguishable neurochemical processes and memory holding mechanisms in the consolidation of memory in both species. Both models provide valuable clues with respect to the timing and nature of the neurochemical changes which are responsible for the observed experience-induced changes in behaviour, changes which are still ascribed by many to an elusive abstraction termed memory.

Long-term potentiation in hippocampal slices is also maintained by a multiphasic mechanism (Reyman *et al*. 1988). These authors describe three distinct phases whose significance in relation to the multiphasic consolidation hypothesis remains to be clarified.

Turning now to the mechanism whereby DPHTA is produced brings us face to face with a mystery.

Recovery from hypoxic collapse is very rapid in the absence of convulsions if the animal is returned to room air immediately, as was done here.

As shown in Fig. 14.13, the animal's cortical P_{O_2} (Cross and Silver 1962), its extracellular potassium concentration (Morris 1974), and its cortical NADH concentration (Mayevsky and Chance 1975) all return to normal values within about 1 minute. At that time its EEG appears to be normal and the animal appears to recover completely and regain its normal adenylate energy charge shortly thereafter (Ridge 1972). STM is also present. What consequence of hypoxia is then responsible for the failure to form MTM?

Although the hypoxic episode in our experiments is rapid in onset and severe, it is very brief in duration. It is therefore very unlikely that it brings brain cells to the state in which membrane failure and rapid Ca^{++} entry lead to long-lasting or irreversible changes. It appears rather that some specific and more moderate effect of hypoxia is involved.

The following evidence suggests that if this is so, the locus coeruleus (A6) might be involved. This group of cells is the origin of the dorsal noradrenergic pathway which innervates mainly the hippocampus and the cerebral cortex (Ungerstedt 1971).

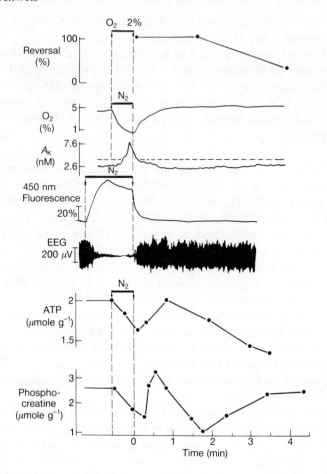

1. DPHTA can be prevented by the prior intracisternal injection of 10 μg of NA.
2. Rats which received an intracisternal injection of DDC showed a delayed transient amnesia identical to DPHTA.
3. The induction of DPHTA by DDC could be prevented by injecting 10 μg of NE intracisternally with the DDC.

   The remarkable coincidence of the timecourses of DPHTA and the DDC-induced delayed transient amnesia, when viewed in the light of the multiphasic consolidation theory and the other experimental results described here, suggests the following interpretation.

a. The DDC-induced amnesia is a specific consequence of its NA-depleting effect, since it is preventable by NA injection.

Fig. 14.13 The effect of brief hypoxia on several CNS variables. In the uppermost graph, the ability of post-hypoxic hyperoxia to reverse the effect of post-training hypoxia, is plotted as a function of the interval between hypoxia and hyperoxia (Frieder and Allweis 1982). The measure Reversal (%) is calculated as $100 \frac{(x - y)}{(x - z)}$, where x = TTC with hypoxia followed by air, y = TTC with hypoxia followed by hyperoxia, and z = TTC for controls receiving no treatment. The other curves have all been replotted from various sources (text) on the same time-scale for ease of comparison. A_k is the extracellular concentration (activity) of potassium. The 450 nm fluorescence curve is a relative (not absolute) measure of the state of oxidation of pyridine nucleotides and therefore indicative of the balance between energy-consuming and energy-accumulating reactions. Note how rapidly the pre-hypoxic level of these variables is re-established when the inspired gas is changed back to air. The EEG, which was virtually flat after 1 minute of anoxia, regains its pre-hypoxic amplitude about 30 seconds after returning the animal to air. The decrease in the concentrations of the high-energy phosphates, adenosine triphosphate and phosphocreatine is also rapidly reversed (within 1 minute), though the phosphocreatine concentrations appears to undergo a second transient decrease. References are given in the text.

b. NA is necessary for MTM formation but not for the formation of STM or LTM.
c. Since hypoxia also prevents MTM formation and its effect may also be prevented by NA injection, it probably acts by depleting cortical NA as does DDC.

These experimental results also imply that cortical NA is not required for acquisition but is essential for MTM formation specifically.

It seems possible that the activation of the locus coeruleus by hypoxia (Elam *et al.* 1981) depletes the terminals of the projection system of NA so that insufficient is available at the time when it is necessary for MTM formation. NA may facilitate the modification of functional connections in the cortex (Kasematsu *et al.* 1979), possibly exerting its action by increasing cortical cyclic AMP concentration (Korf *et al.* 1979).

Acknowledgements

The support of the Israel Centre of Psychobiology, Charles E. Smith Foundation during the early part of this investigation is gratefully acknowledged.

REFERENCES

Allweis, C., Gibbs, M. E., Ng, K. T., and Hodge, R. J. (1984). Effects of hypoxia on memory consolidation: implications for a multistage model of memory. *Behavioural Brain Research*, **11**, 117–21.

Andrew, R. J. (1985). The temporal structure of memory formation. In *Perspectives in Ethology*. (ed. P. P. G. Bateson and P. H. Klopfer), vol. 6, Ch. 7, pp. 219–55. Plenum Press. London.

Cohen, H. H. and Barondes, S. H. (1967). Puromycin effect on memory may be due to occult seizures. *Science*, **157**, 333–4.

Cross, B. A. and Silver, L. A. (1962). Some factors affecting oxygen tension in the brain and other organs. *Proceedings of the Royal Society*, **156**, 483–99.

Daniels, D. (1971). Acquisition, storage and recall of memory for brightness discrimination by rats following intracerebral infusion of acetoxycycloheximide. *Journal of Comparative Physiology and Psychology*, **76**, 110–18.

Davis, H. P., Rosenzweig, M. R., Jones, O. W., and Bennett, E. L. (1981). Inibition of cerebral protein synthesis does not prolong short-term memory. *Journal of Comparative Physiology and Psychology*, **95**, 556–64.

Duncan, C. P. (1949). The retroactive effect of ECS on learning. *Journal of Comparative Physiology and Psychology*, **42**, 32–3.

Elam, M., Yao, T., Thoren, P., and Svensson, T. H. (1981). Hypercapnia and hypoxia: chemoreceptor-mediated control of locus coeruleus neurons and splanchnic sympathetic nerves. *Brain Research*, **222**, 373–81.

Fride, E., Ben-Or, S., and Allweis, C. (1989). Mitochondrial protein-synthesis may be involved in long-term memory formation. *Pharmacology Biochemistry and Behaviour* (in press).

Frieder, B. and Allweis, C. (1978). Transient hypoxic-amnesia: evidence for a triphasic memory-consolidating mechanism with parallel processing. *Behavioural Biology*, **22**, 178–89.

Frieder, B. and Allweis, C. (1982). Delayed post hypoxic transient amnesia is not associated with brain seizures. *Physiology and Behaviour*, **29**, 1059–64.

Frieder, B. and Allweis, C. (1982). Memory consolidation: further evidence for the four-phase model from the time-course of diethyldithiocarbamate and ethacrynic acid amnesias. *Physiology and Behaviour*, **29**, 1071–5.

Frieder, B. and Allweis, C. (1982). Prevention of hypoxia-induced transient amnesia by post-hyperoxia. *Physiology and Behaviour*, **29**, 1065–9.

Gibbs, M. E. (1976). Behavioural stages in memory formation. *Neuroscience Letters*, **13**, 279–83.

Gibbs, M. E. (1979). The molecular mechanism of memory. *New Scientist*, 25 Jan, 261–3.

Gibbs, M. E. (1982). Memory and behaviour: birds and their memories. *Bird Behaviour*, **4**, 93–107.

Gibbs, M. E. and Ng, K. T. (1976). Memory formation: a new three-phase model. *Neuroscience Letters*, **2**, 165–9.

Gibbs, M. E. and Ng, K. T. (1979). Behavioral stages in memory formation. *Neuroscience Letters*, **13**, 279–83.

Kasamatsu, T., Pettigrew, J. D., and Ary, M. (1979). Restoration of visual cortical plasticity by local microperfusion of norepinephrine. *Journal of Comparative Neurology*, **185**, 163–81.

Kesner, R. P. and Conner, H. S. (1972). Independence of short and long term memory: A neural system analysis. *Science*, **176**, 432–4.

Kobiler, D. and Allweis, C. (1973). The prevention of long-term memory from formation by the intracisternal administration of 2, 6 diaminopurine, a reversible inhibitor of RNA synthesis. Joint Meeting of the European Brain and Behaviour Society and the Israel Centre for Psychobiology, April 1972. *Israel Journal of Medical Sciences*, **Vol. 9**, (supplement).

Kobiler, D. and Allweis, C. (1974). The prevention of long-term memory formation by 2, 6 diaminopurine. *Pharmacology Biochemistry and Behaviour*, **2**, 9–17.

Kobiler, D. and Allweis, C. (1977). Retrograde amnesia production by the intracisternal injection of 20 μl of saline in rats. *Pharmacology Biochemistry and Behaviour*, **6**, 255–8.

Korf, J. and Sebens, J. B. (1979). Cyclic AMP in the rat cerebral cortex after activation of noradrenaline neurons of the locus coeruleus. *Journal of Neurochemistry*, **32**, 463–8.

Mayevsky, A. and Chance, B. (1975). Metabolic responses of the awake cerebral cortex to anoxia, hypoxia, spreading depression and epileptiform activity. *Brain Research*, **98**, 149–65.

Morris, M. E. (1974). Hypoxia and extracellular potassium activity in the guinea-pig cortex. *Canadian Journal of Physiology*, **52**, 872–82.

Reyman, K., Frey, U., and Matthies, H. (1988). A multiphase model of synaptic long-term potentiation in hippocampal CA1 neurons: protein kinase C activation and protein synthesis are required for the maintenance of the trace. In *Synaptic plasticity in the hippocampus* (ed. H. L. Haas and G. Buzsaki). Springer, Berlin.

Ridge, J. W. (1972). Hypoxia and the energy charge of the cerebral adenylate pool. *Biochemical Journal*, **127**, 351–5.

Rogers, L. J., Oettinger, R., Szer, J., and Mark. F. (1977). Separate chemical inhibitors of long-term and short-term memory: contrasting effects of cyclohex-imide, ouabain and ethacrynic acid on various tasks in chickens. *Proceedings of the Royal Society*, **196**, 171–95.

Rosenzweig, M. R. and Bennett, E. L. (1984). Basic processes and modulatory influences in the stages of memory formulation. In *The neurobiology of learning and memory* (ed. G. Lynch *et al.*), pp. 263–88. Guilford Press, New York.

Ungerstedt, U. (1971). Stereotaxic mapping of the monoamine pathways in the rat brain. *Acta Physiological Scandinavia*, Supplement 367, 1–49.

15

Stages of memory formation in the chick: findings and problems

M. R. Rosenzweig, E. L. Bennett, J. L. Martinez, Jr, D. Beniston,
P. J. Colombo, D. W. Lee, T. A. Patterson, G. Schulteis, and P. A. Serrano

The meeting of many investigators who work on neural plasticity and learning in the chick provides an opportunity not only to learn recent findings but also to examine and discuss methodological issues that affect the discovery and understanding of these findings. Our paper therefore presents some results of our recent research and also takes up several methodological issues.

This paper consists of five main parts:

(1) Evidence for multiple stages in memory formation in the chick;
(2) State dependency as an alternative to amnesic effects;
(3) Participation of different regions of the chick brain in stages of memory formation;
(4) Effects of opioid agonists and antagonists on learning and memory in the chick; and
(5) Some problems encountered in research with chicks.

EVIDENCE FOR MULTIPLE STAGES IN MEMORY FORMATION

A review of research and hypotheses on multiple stages in memory formation

Evidence of many sorts has been offered since the work of Ebbinghaus for the existence of at least two stages of memory, now usually called short-term (STM) and long-term memory (LTM), and research with chicks is contributing to this topic. Parametric differences between short-term and long-term memory in human verbal learning convinced many that these are two quite different stages. A basis for this work had been provided by Mueller and Pilzecker (1900) in their perseveration-consolidation hypothesis of the formation of memory. References to the term 'short-term memory (STM)' began to appear in the 1950s and they continued at a high rate through the 1970s, then falling off in the 1980s. Neuropsychological

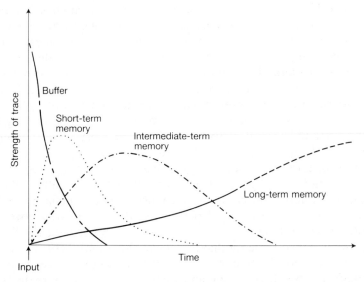

Fig. 15.1 Diagram of a multiple-trace hypothesis of memory storage (from McGaugh 1968). Separate traces begin to form immediately after training for short-term, intermediate-term and long-term memories, and these traces have successively later peaks. (Reprinted by permission of Academia Nazionale dei Lincei, Rome.)

studies also support a dissociation between STM and LTM. Deficits of memory often affect formation of LTM but leave STM intact, as in the well-known case of H.M. (Corkin 1984). On the other hand, there are reports of impairment of STM with LTM intact (Baddeley and Warrington 1970; Warrington 1982). Thus the effects of certain brain lesions may dissociate the two stages. Some believe that the concept of a separate short-term memory has outlived its usefulness (e.g. Crowder 1982), but others continue to view the distinction between STM and LTM as fundamental or at least highly useful (e.g. Horton and Mills 1984; Simon 1986).

Studies with animal subjects on consolidation of memory began with the work of Duncan in 1949, and in the same year Hebb (1949) and Gerard (1949) independently set forth dual-trace hypotheses of memory. In 1968 McGaugh published a schematic graph (Fig 15.1) suggesting that perform-ance after a learning trial is held very briefly by a sensory buffer and then by three overlapping stages: short-, intermediate-, and long-term memor-ies; this figure has been adapted and reprinted by many authors, often without acknowledgement of the original.

In 1972 McGaugh and Herz edited an important volume that reviewed animal research on consolidation of memory. By that time, the concept of consolidation had almost disappeared from research on human memory.

Since then there has been some revival of research on consolidation in normal human subjects and there has also been interesting research on consolidation in patients with impaired memory (e.g. Weingartner and Parker 1984). In animal research, Bennett *et al.* (1972) introduced the use of the protein synthesis inhibitor anisomycin for work on formation of LTM. [It is true that in the previous year Schwartz *et al.* (1971) had shown that anisomycin does not prevent short-term sensitization in *Aplysia*, but they did not show that anisomycin can prevent formation of long-term memory, nor did they deal with associative memory.] The findings of Bennett *et al.* appeared to demonstrate that anisomycin can prevent formation of LTM for associative learning in mammals. Anisomycin, a relatively non-toxic agent, overcame several of the difficulties that had complicated interpretation of research using other inhibitors such as puromycin and cycloheximide. Papers by Flood, Bennett, Rosenzweig and collaborators (e.g. Flood *et al.* 1972, 1973, 1975; Rosenzweig and Bennett 1984*a* and *b*) added evidence that protein synthesis must occur in a narrow time window following training if LTM is to be formed. They suggested (Rosenzweig 1984; Rosenzweig and Bennett 1984*a*) that proteins might be required, in part at least, for the changes seen in synaptic number and structure as a result of differential experience (Diamond *et al.* 1975) or of formal training (Chang and Greenough 1982). Control experiments were performed to test whether the protein synthesis inhibitors (PSIs) affected formation of LTM as such, or whether the effects could be attributed to influences on factors such as perception, motivation, learning, or motor performance. For example, administration of PSIs an hour or more before training did not affect learning in mice even though it affected other aspects of behaviour. A large dose of anisomycin 5 hours pre-training reduced locomotor activity and caused signs of illness (including watery eyes, diarrhoea, piloerection and low arousal after handling) but did not interfere with retention, whereas a small dose that blocked protein synthesis in the immediate post-training period prevented formation of LTM but caused only minor motivational effects (Davis *et al.* 1980).

Meanwhile, the neurochemical bases of formation of the earlier stages as well as of LTM were investigated by Mark and Watts (1971; Watts and Mark 1971) and then by Gibbs (formerly Watts) and collaborators (e.g. Gibbs and Ng 1979, 1984). This research employed the one-trial peck-aversion training of chicks introduced by Cherkin (1969; Cherkin and Lee-Teng 1965). In this training, a chick pecks spontaneously at a small bright lure. If the lure is coated with an aversive substance, the chick will tend to avoid pecking when a similar lure is presented, whether the test occurs seconds, minutes, hours, or days later. Using this technique, Gibbs and Ng (1977) set forth a comprehensive model of memory formation, including three sequentially dependent stages, each depending upon different

Table 15.1 Some amnestic agents classified by the memory stages they affect

STM	ITM	LTM
Glutamate[1,2]	Ouabain[1,2]	Anisomycin[1,2]
LaCl$_3$[1,2]	Ethacrynic acid[1]	Cycloheximide[1,2]
KCl[1]	Scopolamine[2]	Aminoisobutyrate[1]
	Trifluoperazine[2]	Emetine[2]

[1] Reported in papers by Gibbs and Ng
[2] Reported in papers from our laboratory

neurochemical mechanisms. Formation of LTM in chicks requires synthesis of proteins in the brain shortly after training, as Flood, Bennett, and Rosenzweig and others had shown with rodents. An early stage (STM), lasting about 10 minutes, appeared to depend upon hyperpolarization due to potassium conductance; a later stage (called the labile stage but in later articles intermediate-term memory), lasting about 30 minutes, was hypothesized to depend upon hyperpolarization associated with sodium pump activity. Research in our laboratory with chicks has confirmed and extended many of the observations of Gibbs and Ng (e.g. Patterson *et al.* 1986) but has also indicated the importance for the early stages of memory formation of both calcium influx (see also Gibbs *et al.* 1979, and Ng, Chapter 13) and calmodulin (Patterson 1987).

Preliminary work of Bennett *et al.* (1988) has also yielded indications that β-endorphin leads to decline of memory by 10 seconds after training. If confirmed, this may reveal a stage of memory formation in the chick that resembles STM of human learners in its temporal parameters. For the present, however, we will continue to use the term STM to designate a stage that lasts about 10 minutes in research with chicks.

The existence of three main stages in memory formation is indicated by the fact that use of a variety of amnestic agents yields only three curves of appearance of amnesia and not a different curve for each agent. Table 15.1 shows some of the agents that produce each of the three time curves. It might be asked whether these curves, instead of suggesting different stages of memory formation, simply reflect the time required for various agents to diffuse or to act. That the latter alternative is not correct is demonstrated by the fact that an amnestic agent causes the same temporal curve of decline of memory whether it is given early or late within its time window of amnestic effectiveness. See, for example, Fig. 5 in Gibbs and Ng (1977), where the memory decline after administration of ouabain follows the same curve whether the drug is given 15 or 5 minutes pretraining or 5 minutes post-training. See also Figs 2.5 and 2.6 in Patterson (1987); Patterson (1987) compared time-courses of level of amnesia when amnestic agents were given either 10 or 5 minutes pre-training. The curves of memory decline for glutamate and anisomycin showed no differences related to time of administration; the results for ouabain seemed to indicate a shift, but this was probably due to deficiency in performance of the saline control groups rather than to performance of the ouabain groups. Serrano *et al.* (1989) showed that amnesia appeared at the same time whether emetine was injected 20 minutes or 5 minutes pre-training in the region of the IMHV of the chick. Thus the results support the hypothesis of three stages of formation of memory.

Evidence from animal behaviour for the existence of stages of memory

Even if there are biochemical stages in formation of memory, they may not necessarily coincide with separate behavioural stages of memory. Could direct behavioural evidence be found for the existence of stages of memory that might coincide with the biochemical stages? Behavioural studies by Kamin (1957, 1963) and others indicated that the course of memory strength following training may not be monotonic but may include one or more dips (see the review by Gisquet-Verrier 1983, and Andrew, Chapter 19). In general, however, the complex time course was interpreted as indicating motivational factors rather than stages of memory formation. Furthermore, studies of the Kamin effect did not investigate in detail the changes in the strength of memory within the first hour after training. Gibbs and Ng (1977, 1984), however, reported that memory of chicks for peck-aversion training shows dips or 'fissures' at about 12 and 55 minutes post-training, and they interpreted the earlier dip as marking the transition from STM to ITM and the second dip as marking the transition from ITM to LTM (Chapter 17). They also reported that the timing of these dips could be shifted by various pharmacological agents. The existence of two sharp dips has not yet been confirmed by publications from other laboratories, so far as we know, and doubts have been raised about them (Roberts 1987; see also the rejoinder by Ng and Gibbs 1987)

We have recently obtained evidence that bears upon this question. In order to conduct research on enhancing memory formation by pharmacological agents (including opioid agonists and antagonists), Lee in our laboratory has been giving chicks weaker training by using dilute solutions of methylanthranilate (MeA) as the aversive substance, rather than the 100 per cent MeA used in most of our experiments and those of other laboratories. The MeA was diluted in ethyl alcohol. In these experiments, as in most of our work, the chicks are trained with single presentation of a bead rather than with successive presentations of beads as described in other chapters of this volume. More complete descriptions of our methods can be found in Patterson *et al.* (1986, 1989).

Earlier work using dilute MeA was reported by Cherkin (1971) and

Gibbs (1983). Cherkin (1971) tested the course of memory when chicks were trained with a bead coated with 0.25 per cent MeA dissolved in distilled water. He used latency to peck as the measure of retention and tested recall times from 10 seconds post-training to 24 hours. Gibbs (1983) also tested memory after training with 0.25 per cent MeA and recorded the percentage of chicks that avoided the target, using recall times from 10 minutes to 24 hours post-training. Both Cherkin and Gibbs reported no evidence of recall 24 hours after the weak training. Cherkin reported good recall at 10 and 20 seconds post-training, with a dip at 2–5 minutes; his graph shows a sizeable decline in latency by 40 and 80 seconds. Cherkin did not test at or near 15 minutes or 60 minutes and wrote of a biphasic time course of performance. In spite of Cherkin's emphasis on the early dip, Gibbs did not test at any time under 10 minutes; she reported a dip at 15 minutes and decline of memory by 60 minutes (see Chapter 17 for more recent findings).

With 5 per cent or 10 per cent MeA producing somewhat stronger training in our experiments than the 0.25 per cent MeA used by the earlier workers, our chicks showed retention at 24 hours although significantly weaker than the 24 hour retention after training with 100 per cent MeA. We then wondered whether testing their memory at different times following training might reveal successive drops in performance, like the hypothetical curves of McGaugh (1968), and thus indicate stages in memory formation. This research is in progress (Rosenzweig *et al.* 1989); the results to date (based on 20–25 animals per point) are shown in Fig. 15.2. They do suggest successive stages in memory formation, but the strengths of the presumed stages do not drop off monotonically as do McGaugh's curves. Note that we have indications of cusps around 1 minute, 15 minutes and 60 minutes, the last two being close to the times of the dips reported by Gibbs and Ng (1984). We are doing further studies to define these time regions more clearly. It seems quite possible that weaker training allows the transitions between stages to appear rather clearly, whereas stronger training pushes behaviour toward the ceiling at all time points. In fact, for the weakest training (5 per cent MeA) the initial dip at 30 seconds is significantly lower than the 10 second value ($p < 0.004$) and also than the succeeding peak at 10 minutes ($p < 0.03$); the second dip at 20 minutes does not differ significantly from the 10 minute peak but does differ significantly from the succeeding peak, whether this is measured at 45 minutes ($p < 0.04$), 60 minutes ($p < 0.06$), or 90 minutes ($p < 0.005$). We will also be testing the effects of various amnestic agents on performance after weaker training in an attempt to define more completely the shapes of each of the component curves. The first component is seen more clearly in a graph that expands the time scale (Fig. 15.3); this is a limb that descends steeply to 60 seconds. It appears like the component labelled 'sensory buffer' in McGaugh's presentation,

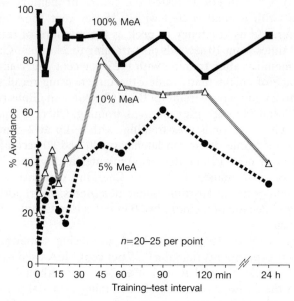

Fig. 15.2   Effect of training strength on retention of the peck-aversion response. Training strength was varied by diluting the concentration of the aversive substance on the training bead (MeA 100%, 10%, 5%). Training-to-test intervals were the following: 10, 30 s; 1, 5, 10, 15, 20, 30, 45, 60, 90, 120 min; 24 h. % Avoidance is the percentage of chicks that refrained from pecking in the 10-second test period. Separate groups of chicks were tested for each time point. The results are cumulative data from three successive experiments in which 8–10 chicks were tested at each time point.

but note that it has approximately the duration of short-term memory in studies of human verbal learning. Perhaps this should be labelled STM, and two intermediate-term stages follow before protein-synthesis-dependent LTM appears. It has been suggested that this short downward component is caused by the taste of MeA remaining briefly on the chick's bill (Andrew, personal communication). We know of no attempt to test between this hypothesis and STM; perhaps this could be done by using a nonchemical aversive stimulus such as electric shock.

Thus our data are consistent with a four-stage hypothesis, with approximate durations of the stages as follows, under the conditions of our experiment: (1) a sensory buffer or very short-term memory, lasting up to 1 minute; (2) STM, becoming apparent after 1 minute and lasting until about 15 minutes post-training; (3) ITM, becoming apparent about 15 minutes post-training and lasting until about 60 minutes post-training, and (4) LTM, becoming apparent at about 60 minutes post-training, and still present at 24 hours. Clearly, there is much more research to do along

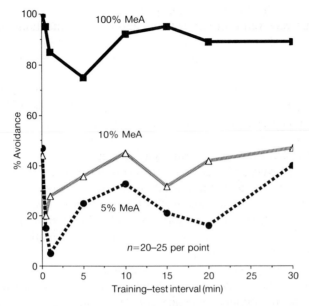

Fig. 15.3   The data of Fig. 15.2 are replotted here for the first 8 time points. This shows a very brief initial limb that may reflect activity of a sensory buffer or perhaps a true short-term stage of memory.

these lines. The appearance of distinct successive stages in the behav-ioural curves opens up new possibilities for research and for understand-ing of memory, and we have begun to pursue them in research with chicks.

CAN SOME OF THE APPARENT AMNESIC EFFECTS BE ATTRIBUTED TO STATE DEPENDENCY?

Before presenting some of the main results of our research, let us deal briefly with the question of state dependency. In experiments of the kind we have been considering, there exists the possibility that information acquired under a particular drug state is stored but can be retrieved best or only if the subject is placed at the time of test under the same drug state as during acquisition. State-dependent learning (SDL) for some drugs is well documented in both animals and humans (Overton 1984; Järbe 1986). To test whether drugs that we have used with chicks might cause SDL rather than amnesia, we have conducted experiments with glutamate, ouabain, and anisomycin in which chicks were given intracerebral injec-tions of the agent both 5 minutes before peck-aversion training and 5 minutes before testing. The experiments with glutamate or ouabain did not give any indications of state dependency; amnesia was as complete in groups that received both pre-training and pre-test injections of the agent as in groups that received only pre-training injections. However, the experiments with anisomycin indicated recall when the drug was given pre-test.

After we had undertaken these experiments on the possibility of SDL, we saw the preliminary report of Bradley and Galal (1987) claiming that anisomycin causes state-dependent recall in the chick and that long-term memories can be formed even when protein synthesis is inhibited in the brain. The claim that long-term memories can be formed when protein synthesis is prevented in the brain runs counter to a multitude of studies, including many conducted in our laboratory (e.g. Flood *et al.* 1973, 1975; Gibbs and Ng 1977; Patterson *et al.* 1986). Moreover, we had introduced the use of anisomycin for the study of LTM (Bennett *et al.* 1972; Flood *et al.* 1973), so the claim that it does not prevent formation of LTM was particularly challenging to us.

Bradley, along with Patterson and Rose at the Open University, undertook further work on this problem, and we continued to gather evidence and to conduct necessary control studies. All of the papers are now published (Bradley and Galal 1988; Lee *et al.* 1989; Patterson *et al.* 1989), so detailed exposition here would be redundant. We found that even chicks trained with a non-aversive water-coated bead showed avoidance at test if they were given anisomycin pre-test, regardless of whether the pre-training injection was anisomycin or physiological saline. We conclude that a generalized avoidance induced by pre-test anisomycin accounts for the appearance of SDL for peck-aversion training.

ROLES OF DIFFERENT BRAIN REGIONS IN MEMORY FORMATION IN THE CHICK

Different sites in chick brain do not all have the same significance for formation of memory. Our research on this topic was made possible by the finding that certain amnestic agents, administered in rather low doses, affect only a small volume of tissue around the site of injection (Patterson *et al.* 1986). Among such agents are glutamate, which impairs formation of STM, ouabain, which impairs formation of ITM, and emetine, which impairs formation of LTM. (These designations of memory stages are used here as we and others have used them in previous publications, although for the reason suggested earlier we are not convinced that they are really correct.) Our first studies on this topic were made by Patterson, using injections into or close to two regions of the chick forebrain that are analogous to cerebral cortex in mammals: the intermediate and medial hyperstriatum ventrale (IMHV) and the lateral neostriatum (LNS). Injections are made into regions of the brain of the unanaesthetized chick with a hypodermic needle. The head is held by hand in a Plexiglass headholder, and the direction of the needle is guided by a hole in the top plate of the headholder. The depth is determined by a stop fitted around the upper part of the needle and made from plastic tubing. This technique follows that devised by Davis *et al.* (1982). Examination of needle tracks indicates that the ventral end of the needle track in three-quarters of the cases falls within 1 mm of the target structure; therefore we speak of our injections as being made 'within the region of' a particular anatomical target. The effects reported below indicate that we do, in fact, influence different brain sites.

The importance of the IMHV for memory formation was first reported by Horn *et al.* (1979), and work at this site is reported by Horn and Rose in Chapters 8 and 10. With bilateral injections, IMHV and LNS show rather similar dose-response functions for amnesic effects (Table 15.2). Some problems of interpretations of the dose–response functions will be discussed on pp. 411–14. Unless otherwise noted, all injections were made 5 minutes before training, and testing was done 24 hours later. To show some of the main data without making the tables too full, the dose-response functions in the table have been abbreviated.

The fact that IMHV and LNS yield similar results with bilateral injections does not allow us to conclude that these two sites play identical roles in memory formation. *Unilateral* injections produce mirror-image effects at these two loci (Fig. 15.4): injections in the region of the left IMHV cause amnesia, whereas injections into the region of the right IMHV produce no significant effect. At the LNS the situation is reversed; injections into the region of the left LNS are without effect, but injections into the region of the right LNS cause amnesia. At each site, each amnestic agent causes amnesia to appear according to the temporal characteristic of that agent—STM, ITM, or LTM. A small qualification should be added: although the decline of memory after training showed similar time functions for injections in the region of the left IMHV and right LNS for glutamate (inhibition of STM) and emetine (inhibition of LTM), for ouabain (inhibition of ITM) amnesia occurred slightly but significantly later with injection into LNS compared with injection into IMHV (Patterson *et al.* 1988). The effects at each site showed sequential dependence; that is, preventing formation of one stage of memory also prevented the appearance of the later stages.

Serrano in our laboratory has been exploring further brain sites. One of these is the cerebellum. Recent research (e.g. Thompson 1986) has shown that mechanical or chemical lesions of the deep cerebellar nuclei prevent formation of conditioning of somatic responses. Serrano therefore tested the same three amnestic agents with injections into the centre of the

Table 15.2   Abridged dose-response curves for three amnestic agents in two regions of chick brain (% chicks showing avoidance at 24-h test)

		IMHV[a]						LNS[b]		
Glutamate	(mM) Sal	25	37	50				Sal	50	
TP[c]	n	25	25	25	25			58	57	
	%	85	70	55*	38*			76	49*	
PS[d]	n	66		58						
	%	86		42*						
Ouabain	(mM) Sal	0.007	0.014	0.027				Sal	0.027	
TP	n	25	25	25	25			58	55	
	%	85	87	49*	25*			76	28*	
PS	n	50		44						
	%	84		34*						
Emetine	(mM) Sal	0.08	1.5	3.0	4.0	4.5		Sal	1.5	2.25
TP	n	25	25	25	25		25	58	52	32
	%	82	70	24*	40*		40*	76	45*	40*
PS	n	52		50		44	42			
	%	81		55*		50*	45**			

[a] Intermediate and medial hyperstriatum ventrale
[b] Lateral neostriatum
[c] TP, T. A. Patterson
[d] PS, P. Serrano
* $p < 0.01$

cerebellum 0.5 mm dorsal to the ventral cerebellar commissure, between the lateral cerebellar nuclei (Table 15.3). The results showed a lack of amnesic effect for doses that are amnestic in the regions of the IMHV or the LNS; even tripling effective doses for the other sites did not cause amnesia when the agents were injected into the centre of the cerebellum. It is, of course, possible that injections into other cerebellar sites would be amnestic, but the central region appears not to be involved in memory formation.

Thus far it appeared that a brain site was either involved in memory formation for the peck aversion response in the chick (as in the case for IMHV and LNS) or that it was not involved (as is the case for the central cerebellum). Exploration at a further site revealed another possibility (Table 15.4): this is the lobus parolfactorius (LPO), first studied in relation to learning and memory by Rose and Csillag (1985). We tested this region with the same agents producing local effects as were used in

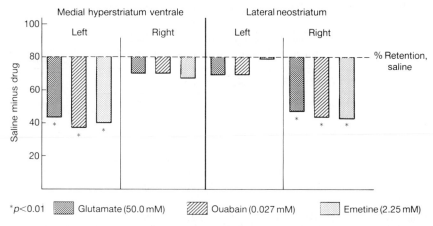

Fig. 15.4 Comparison of effects of unilateral injection of amnestic agents into the regions of the left or right intermediate and medial hyperstriatum ventrale (*IMHV*) or into the regions of the left or right lateral neostriatum (*LNS*). Injections were made 5 min pre-training, and memory was tested at 24 hours. Saline control groups were run with each of the 12 drug groups. Since the per cent retention of the saline control groups varied from 74 to 86 per cent, each of these control values has been normalized to 80, for clarity of presentation, but the magnitude of the difference between each drug groups and its control group was kept unchanged. The numbers ranged from 39 to 58 per group. Each of the three agents caused significant amnesia when injected into the region of the left but not the right IMHV; each caused significant amnesia when injected into the region of the right but not the left LNS. (Data from Patterson 1987.)

the IMHV and the cerebellum (Serrano *et al.* 1988). Bilateral injections of glutamate into the LPO did not cause amnesia within or even beyond the dose range that was amnestic in IMHV or LNS. Injections of emetine into LPO were largely without effect, although at a high dose a small amnesic effect was observed. However, ouabain produced amnesia when injected into LPO, and at the same dose that we used for most of the experiments with IMHV and LNS. The time curve of amnesia produced by ouabain in LPO was similar to the curves found with injections into IMHV and LNS. Moreover, another agent found to prevent formation of ITM in IMHV— scopolamine—was also found to be effective in LPO. Thus we have presumptive evidence that LPO plays a role in formation of ITM but not in the formation of STM or LTM. It should be noted that although LPO does not appear to be involved directly in formation of LTM, the same sequential dependence is seen here as at IMHV and LNS; that is, prevention of formation of ITM by intervention at LPO causes failure of LTM, since the test was made at 24 hours.

LPO also appears to show an asymmetric hemispheric involvement in

Table 15.3   Abridged dose–response data for three amnestic agents in cerebellum

% Chicks showing avoidance at 24-h test				
Glutamate	(mM)	Sal	45	60	90
	n	65	58	53	47
	%	81	68	65	68
Ouabain	(mM)	Sal	0.025	0.035	0.05
	n	71	63	50	53
	%	94	77	89	92
Emetine	(mM)	Sal	1.0	2.0	8.0
	n	73	67	62	60
	%	81	71	94	88

Table 15.4   Abridged dose-response data for three amnestic agents in lobus paraolfactorius

(% Chicks showing avoidance at 24-h test)					
Glutamate	(mM)	Sal	35	50	70	
	n	46	24	48	22	
	%	89	78	77	83	
Ouabain	(mM)	Sal	0.02	0.03	0.04	0.05
	n	48	49	44	50	40
	%	87	65	43**	38**	40**
Emetine	(mM)	Sal	2.25	3.0	6.0	
	n	82	82	75	23	
	%	82	79	72	61*	

*$p < 0.05$; **$p < 0.01$

formation of ITM, although this is not as strong as the asymmetry found in IMHV or LNS. Injection of ouabain into either the left or the right LPO causes amnesia, but the effect is significantly stronger in the left hemisphere.

Exploration is continuing at other brain sites. Possibly some will be found that appear to have special significance for formation of STM or

LTM, as LPO appears to for ITM. Even among the sites already identified, it will be necessary to trace their connections and interactions and to try to find how each fits into an overall picture of formation of the stages of memory.

The evidence we present about hemispheric asymmetry for learning/ memory in the chick should be related to findings of several other participants in the Sussex Conference, namely Andrew, Horn, Rogers, and Rose (see Chapters 8, 9, 10, 20, 21). More broadly, attempts should be made to integrate the chick findings with the growing work on hemispheric asymmetry in both humans and animals (for reviews, see Geschwind and Galaburda 1984, 1987; Hellige 1987, 1990). Within the field of interhemispheric interaction, Hellige (1990) reviews several specific topics: co-operative collaboration in performing various subprocesses that one or the other hemisphere handles best, cross-hemispheric integration, and metacontrol—determination of which hemisphere controls a cognitive operation (and this is not necessarily the hemisphere with greater ability to perform the task). Can the chick model be used to obtain information on these questions?

EFFECTS OF OPIOID AGONISTS AND ANTAGONISTS ON LEARNING AND MEMORY IN THE CHICK

Because we were finding many similarities between chicks and laboratory rodents in their responses to amnestic agents, we decided to determine whether chick learning and memory formation might provide a useful model system for the study of effects of opioid agonists and antagonists. A paper reporting our initial findings has appeared (Patterson *et al.* 1989*b*), and other findings have been reported at the Society for Neuroscience (Bennett *et al.* 1988; Colombo *et al.* 1989; Lee *et al.* 1989); some of the results will be reported briefly here.

β-Endorphin (β-END) injected bilaterally 5 minutes before peck-aversion training into the region of the IMHV made the chicks amnesic at tests conducted 24 hours later. Three doses of β-endorphin (0.01, 0.10., 1.0 nmole/hemisphere) produced significant amnesia, compared to retention of control animals that received injections of physiological saline solution.

To test whether the effect of β-END was an opioid effect and not due to some other type of action of the drug, we tested whether it could be reversed by naloxone. β-END given alone or in combination with a low dose of naloxone (16.0 nmole/hemisphere) produced significant amnesia compared to saline controls. A higher dose of naloxone (50.0 nmol/ hemisphere) reversed the amnesia caused by β-END. Flood *et al.* (1987) have reported that naloxone administered immediately post-training enhanced memory formation in both chicks and mice. In their experiments naloxone was approximately 1000-fold more potent when administered

408   M. R. Rosenzweig et al.

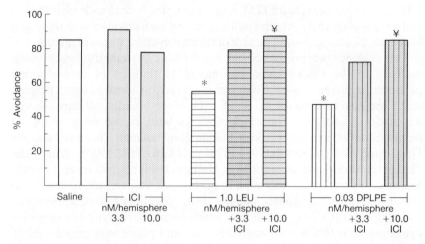

Fig. 15.5 Reversal of amnesia produced by [D-pen², L-pen⁵] enkephalin (*DPLPE*) or [leu⁵] enkephalin (*LEU*) by the delta selective antagonist ICI 174,864 (*ICI*). ICI administered alone did not produce either enhancement of memory or amnesia. LEU or DPLPE given alone produced significant amnesia compared to saline controls (LEU vs saline $\chi_i^2[1, n = 41] = 6.7$; DPLPE vs saline $\chi_i^2[1, n = 43] = 8.9$; *, $p < 0.01$). Administration of ICI, along with the amnestic drug, reversed amnesia produced by either LEU or DPLPE in a dose-dependent manner ($\chi_i^2[1, n= 45] = 6.2$, mixture or LEU and ICI compared to LEU alone; $\chi_i^2[1, n=41] = 6.4$, mixture of DPLPE and ICI compared to DPLPE alone; Y, $p < 0.05$). All injections (10 µl/hemisphere) were made bilaterally into the region of the intermediate medial hyperstriatum ventrale, 5 minutes before training, and chicks were tested 24 hours after training. (From Patterson *et al.* 1989. Reproduced with permission of the American Psychological Association.)

intracerebroventricularly than subcutaneously, so it appears to exert its effect within the central nervous system.

[Leu⁵]enkephalin (LEU), employed in similar experiments, was amnestic at a dose of 1.0 nmole/hemisphere. Since LEU works mainly on delta receptors, we tested the effects of an agonist that is highly selective for delta receptors, [D-Pen², L-Pen⁵]enkephalin (DPLPE). Injections of 0.03 nmole/hemisphere of DPLPE produced significant amnesia, so DPLPE is about 30 times more potent than LEU.

We then attempted to reverse amnesia produced by either LEU or DPLPE by the use of an antagonist, ICI 174,864, that is selective for the delta receptor. Figure 15.5 shows that LEU and DPLPE again produced significant amnesia compared with saline-injected controls. ICI 174,864 reversed these amnesias in a dose-dependent manner.

In recent experiments, Lee *et al.* (1989) have found that for weak training (10 per cent MeA) naloxone, administered 5 minutes pre-training,

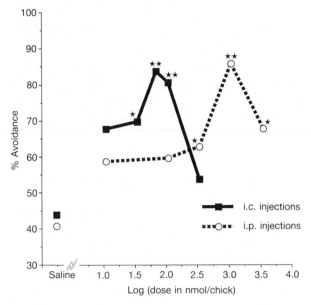

Fig. 15.6 Effect of naloxone dose and route of injection on mean per cent avoidance at 24 hour test. Half of the groups received intracerebral (i.c.) injections of saline or 10, 30, 60, 96, or 300 nmol/chick naloxone. The remaining groups were given intraperitoneal (i.p.) injections of saline or 10, 100, 300, 1000, or 3000 nmol/chick naloxone. Numbers per point ranged from 15 to 44 (*$p < 0.05$, **$p < 0.01$).

improves memory performance at 24 hours (Fig. 15.6). Enhancement was found with either intracerebral or intraperitoneal administration of naloxone, with intracerebral requiring about one-tenth the dosage of intraperitoneal for the largest effect. Both curves had an inverted U shape.

Colombo *et al.* (1989) have found that when LEU is injected in the region of the IMHV 5 minutes pre-training, memory remains strong for at least 180 minutes post-training. This is at least twice as long as occurs when the amnestic agent is an inhibitor of protein synthesis. We noted earlier that β-endorphin appears to cause an earlier decline of memory than agents that impair STM. Thus, opioids may affect memory formation through mechanisms other than those previously studied, and this is a focus of our ongoing research.

These indications of clear effects of opioid agonists and antagonists on learning/memory formation in chicks have encouraged us to develop further a chick model to investigate effects and mechanisms of drugs of abuse. Several lines of research are being followed. We are investigating whether the effects are on learning or on memory formation; in the latter case, we will test effects on different stages of memory formation. These experiments are studying enhancement as well as impairment of learning and memory. Different kinds of learning and different tests of memory are being investigated for their effectiveness with chicks. We are mapping concentrations of endogenous opioids and of their hydrolyzing enzymes in the chick brain. Among other things, this mapping will suggest further sites to investigate for their roles in learning and memory formation. We are also investigating effects of peripheral administration of opioid agonists and antagonists in the chick, following findings of effects of peripheral injections in rodents.

SOME PROBLEMS ENCOUNTERED IN RESEARCH WITH CHICKS

Although research with chicks on the neural bases of learning and memory is productive, problems encountered in this research cannot be over-looked. Among these problems are the following:

(a) A variety of methods is used for housing chicks, and a variety of protocols is used for training and testing; these appear to yield somewhat different results from one laboratory to another. Our discussion of this topic has been placed in Chapter 1.

(b) Different lines of chicks are used by different laboratories, and the lines differ somewhat in their behavioural characteristics. These differences may interact with the housing and training methods mentioned just above.

(c) When material is injected into the chick brain with a hypodermic needle, much of it often leaks out rapidly through the needle track, so it is difficult to determine accurately the effective dose.

We discuss each of these points.

Indications of strain differences

Our experience with two strains of chicks has made us aware of the potential influence of strain differences in studies of brain mechanisms of learning and memory in chicks. The two varieties we have used are egg layers available in California—DEKALB-Warren Sex-linked Browns (*DEKALB–Warren Sex-Sal-Link*, 1987) and DEKALB XL White Leghorns (*DEKALB XL-Link*, 1987).

We began our research using DEKALB-Warren Sex-linked Browns. They are a four-way genetic cross of females of two strains with white feather colouration and males of two strains of Rhode Island Reds which are responsible for the sex-linked red/brown feather colouration of the females. Exact information about the genetics of this and other commercial varieties is difficult to obtain, since this is proprietary information. The Browns are a quiet chicken with a relatively slow metabolism and low energy maintenance requirment (personal communication, J. J. Warren, Jr). We found chicks of this line to be calm, easy to work with, and good learners, but unfortunately their availability is limited, so since November 1987 we have used mainly DEKALB XL White Leghorns.

The DEKALB XL White Leghorns are also the product of a four-way cross in which all parental lines are derived from White Leghorns. Compared with the Browns, the Leghorns are smaller, more aggressive, with a quicker and stronger reaction to stress, higher activity levels, and higher metabolic rate (personal communication, J. J. Warren, Jr). The energy maintenance requirement for the Leghorns is about 20 per cent greater than that for the Browns. The Leghorns are slightly more nervous and therefore chicks of this line require greater care to train, but they are available in the quantities that our research requires.

Recently we compared activity of the two lines by counting in several batches of 30 chicks the number of times a chick jumped to the top of its container. Immediately after being placed in its cardboard cylinder, a White XL chick averages 2.1 jumps/minute. Two hours later the rate has fallen to 1.4. In contrast, the Brown XL chick averages 0.6 jumps/minutes at the start and 0.2 2 hours later. Thus the White chick after 2 hours of acclimatization is more active than the Brown chick at the start.

Chicks do not differ from rodents or other laboratory animals in showing strain differences. It is possible that the strain differences in chicks interact with the variables mentioned in the part of our material that has been placed in Chapter 1 (pp. 32–4). It is also possible that the varieties of chick differ in seasonal variations in behavioural responsiveness and in susceptibility to various drugs. We are attempting to take such factors into account in our research, and we encourage other investigators to do so.

Problems with retention of material injected intracranially into the chick

A note of caution must be added here. The dosages stated in the sections above are based upon amounts injected into the chick brain, but we have found recently that half or more of the injected material often leaks rapidly out of the brain through the track of the hypodermic needle.

In early 1988 we began a series of experiments to determine the distribution and retention of several of the drugs we were then using—ouabain, glutamate, and [leu⁵]enkephalin (LEU). We had already obtained considerable data concerning protein synthesis inhibition which showed that after unilateral administration of anisomycin or cycloheximide into chick brain inhibition of protein synthesis occurred rapidly throughout the brain. On the other hand, inhibition of protein synthesis by emetine was localized and longer lasting.

Table 15.5   Recovery and distribution of drugs injected into chick brain

Drug[a]	Time after injection (min)	Number of chicks	Total recovered in brain [b] %	Total recovered in right hemisphere[c] %	Total recovered in right medial and posterior brain[d] %
[^{14}C]-glutamate	0.5–5	11	40 ± 18	84 ± 7	77 ± 6
	10–15	5	44 ± 21	78 ± 21	82 ± 4
	30–60	6	29 ± 12	78 ± 15	83 ± 6
	Overall	22	38 ± 17	81 ± 13	80 ± 6
[^{3}H]-[leu^5]-	5	3	22 ± 12	95 ± 3	90 ± 5
enkephalin	15	2	21 ± 8	96 ± 1	90 ± 4
	30–60	3	24 ± 8	87 ± 9	82 ± 10
	Overall	8	22 ± 9	92 ± 7	87 ± 7
[^{3}H]-ouabain	0.5–5	36	42 ± 20	90 ± 5	83 ± 7
	15	3	30 ± 12	93 ± 4	92 ± 4
	30–60	6	29 ± 12	89 ± 8	89 ± 7
	Overall	45	40 ± 19	90 ± 6	84 ± 8

[a] 10 μl of each labelled drug was injected unilaterally into the region of the right IMHV together with 10 μl of non-radioactive drug into the left hemisphere. The drugs injected were 50 mM [^{14}C]-glutamate, 0.1 mM [^{3}H]-[leu^5]-enkephalin, and 0.027 mM [^{3}H]-ouabain. All solutions contained approximately 100 000 dpm per 10 μl
[b] Expressed as a percentage of injected radioactivity
[c] Expressed as a percentage of total radioactivity found in the brain
[d] Expressed as a percentage of total radioactivity found in the right hemisphere

To our surprise and dismay, our first experiments using [^{14}C] glutamate yielded extremely erratic data for the retention of glutamate in chick brain as measured by the radioactivity remaining in brain areas. The results have led to a series of experiments on the retention and distribution of glutamate, ouabain, and LEU in the chick brain. A major focus has been to determine the effects of varying several aspects of administration: the volume of drug solution administered, the rate of administration, and the depth of administration.

In the first series of experiments in which the drugs were injected in a volume of 10 μl unilaterally into the region of the IMHV of the chick brain, we found high variability in the amount retained in the brain. In individual chicks the amount ranged from as low as 5 per cent to as high as 80 per cent shortly after injection. In preparing Table 15.5, in order to consider the time course and distribution of the material retained, we excluded animals with less than 10 per cent retention. Due to the variable initial retention, we were unable to determine a reliable 'half-life' of the drug measured by the radioactivity in the chick brain in time points up to

Table 15.6 Effect of injection volume on amount of radioactivity retained in brain. Labelled drug was injected unilaterally into the region of the right IMHV, and 10 μl of non-radioactive drug into the region of the left IMHV. Data were drawn from 12 experiments using [³H]-ouabain. Solution concentration and activity were adjusted so that total amount of drug and total dpm injected remained constant among volumes. Data for 1 μl were obtained from three animals sacrificed at each of the following time points: 5 min, 15 min, 30 min, and 60 min; data for 2 μl, from three animals at each of the following time points: 5 min, 10–15 min, 15–30 min; data for 5 μl, from 5 animals sacrificed at 1 min and 11 animals at 5 min; data for 10 μl, from 41 animals sacrificed at 5 min

Injection volume (μl)	Number of subjects	Percentage retained
1	12	0.4 ± 0.7
2	9	3.7 ± 5.4
5	16	27.6 ± 22.3
10	41	37.7 ± 22.2

1 hour. It is clear, however, that most of the radioactivity is retained over 1 hour. This does not address the rate of conversion of the injected drugs into other compounds. We believe that ouabain is still present primarily as ouabain, while LEU is hydrolyzed within minutes after administration.

On the positive side, these experiments showed that most of the radioactivity in the brain remained near the site of injection. An average of 81 per cent of the radioactivity in the brain after glutamate administration was found in the right hemisphere, and 92 per cent or 90 per cent of the radioactivity from LEU and ouabain, respectively, were found in the right hemisphere. More than 80 per cent of the radioactivity in brain was present in the medial and posterior brain near the site of injection after glutamate administration. These percentages were somewhat larger with LEU and ouabain, 86 per cent and 84 per cent, respectively, suggesting less diffusion than with glutamate (Table 15.5). Typically, less than 2 per cent of the injected radioactivity was found in the brainstem.

A further series of experiments investigated the influence of the amount of injection volume on the amount of drug retained in the brain using [³H]ouabain. We were disappointed to see that reducing the volume of material injected did not improve retention when the Hamilton repeating syringe was used (Table 15.6); in fact, per cent retention was positively related to the injection volume. However, when a syringe pump was used for relatively slow injection (13 seconds), better retention was obtained for a 1 μl volume than for 5 μl.

In another series of experiments, injections were made at 3 mm depth instead of the standard 4 mm. Slightly less ouabain was retained in the brain after injections at 3 mm compared with 4 mm. However, even less radioactivity was found in brain when the injections were made into the LPO, at a depth of 5 mm.

A third series of experiments investigated the suggestion that retention of drug would be improved by layering light mineral oil above the drug. This was achieved by filling the Hamilton syringe first with 5 or 10 μl of drug followed by 5 or 10 μl of light oil (Johnson baby oil). The oil was then injected first at a depth of approximately 3 mm, and then the syringe was lowered an additional 1 mm and the drug was injected. These experiments showed that the combination of 10 μl of drug together with 10 μl of oil was superior to the other combinations tested (10 μl drug, 5 μl oil; 5 μl drug, 10 μl oil, and 5 μl drug, 5 μl oil). The amount retained in brain was not clearly superior to that with the standard method of administration. In view of the additional problems of both carrying out the behavioural experiments as well as possible side effects of the oil and questions of interpretation, we have not pursued this method further.

Thus, using the present methods, dosages must be considered relative rather than absolute. Loss of material injected introduces variability into the data and makes it necessary to use relatively large numbers of subjects in order to obtain statistically reliable results.

CONCLUSIONS

On the basis of our research to date and of comparisons among reports of research groups that are using chicks and rodents for similar studies, we conclude that chicks are useful for studies of brain mechanisms of learning and memory. Stages of memory formation are seen more clearly in chicks than in rodents. The availability of chicks and the relatively low costs of acquiring and maintaining them make it feasible to design experiments in which several conditions are tested within the same batch. On the other hand, certain problems and drawbacks need to be faced and overcome in order to realize all of the potential benefits of this preparation: these include effects of strain differences and the variable retention of material injected into the chick brain.

Acknowledgments

The research was supported by NIDA grant DA04795 and NSF grants BNS-86-06938 and BNS-88-10528.

REFERENCES

Baddeley, A. D. and Warrington, E. K. (1970). Amnesia and the distinction between long and short-term memory. *Journal of Learning and Verbal Behaviour*, **9**, 176–89.

Bennett, E. L., Orme, A. and Hebert, M. (1972). Cerebral protein synthesis inhibition and amnesia produced by scopolamine, cycloheximide, streptovitacin A, anisomysin and emetine in rat. *Federation Proceedings*, **31**, 838.

Bennett, E. L., Patterson, T. A., Schulteis, G., Martinez, J. L. and Rosenzweig, M. R. (1988). Beta-endorphin administration impairs acquisition in the chick. *Society for Neuroscience Abstracts*, **14**, 1029.

Bradley, P. M. and Galal, K. M. (1987). Structural changes at the synapse associated with state dependent recall of a passive avoidance task. Poster presented at the *Third Conference on the Neurobiology of Learning and Memory*, University of California, Irvine, Calif.

Bradley, P. M. and Galal, K. M. (1988). State-dependent recall can be induced by protein synthesis inhibition: behavioural and morphological observations. *Developmental Brain Research*, **40**, 243–51.

Chang, F.-L. F. and Greenough, W. T. (1982). Lateralized effects of monocular training on dendritic branching in adult split-brain rats. *Brain Research*, **232**, 282–92.

Cherkin, A. (1969). Kinetics of memory consolidation: role of amnesic treatment parameters. *Proceedings of the National Academy of Science, USA*, **63**, 1094–101.

Cherkin, A. (1971). Biphasic time course of performance after one-trial avoidance training in the chick. *Communications in Behavioral Biology*, **5**, 379–81.

Cherkin, A. and Lee-Teng, E. (1965). Interruption by halothane of memory consolidation in chicks. *Federation Proceedings*, **24**, 328.

Colombo, P. J., Tsai, J., Bennett, E. L., Rosenzweig, M. R. and Martinez, J. L., Jr (1989). Delayed development of amnesia following intracranial injection of [leu]enkephalin in two-day-old chicks. *Society for Neuroscience Abstracts*, **15**, 1169.

Corkin, S. (1984). Lasting consequences of bilateral medial temporal lobectomy: clinical course and experimental findings in H. M. *Seminars in Neurology*, **4**, 249–59.

Crowder, R. G. (1982). The demise of short-term memory. *Acta Psychologica*, **50**, 291–323.

Davis, H. P., Rosenzweig, M. R., Bennett, E. L. and Squire, L. R. (1980). Inhibition of cerebral protein synthesis: dissociation of nonspecific effects and amnesic effects. *Behavioral and Neural Biology*, **28**, 99–104.

Davis, J. L., Pico, R. M. and Cherkin, A. (1982). Memory enhancement induced in chicks by L-prolyl-L-leucyl-glycineamide. *Pharmacology Biochemistry and Behavior*, **17**, 893–96.

DEKALB-Warren Sex-Sal-Link: *Pullet & layer management guide* (3rd edn) (1987). DEKALB Corporation, DeKalb, Ill.

DEKALB XL-Link: *Pullet & layer management guide* (3rd edn) (1987). DEKALB Corporation, DeKalb, Ill.

416   *M. R. Rosenzweig et al.* `

Duncan, C. P. (1949). The retroactive effect of electroshock on learning. *Journal of Comparative and Physiological Psychology*. **42**, 32–44.

Diamond, M. C., Lindner, B., Johnson, R., Bennett, E. L. and Rosenzweig, M. R. (1975). Differences in occipital cortical synapses from environmentally enriched, impoverished, and standard colony rats. *Journal of Neuroscience Research*, **1**, 109–19.

Flood, J. F., Bennett, E. L., Rosenzweig, M. R. and Orme, A. E. (1972). Influence of training strength on amnesia induced by pretraining injections of cycloheximide. *Physiology and Behavior*, **9**, 589–600.

Flood, J. F., Bennett, E. L., Rosenzweig, M. R. and Orme, A. E. (1973). The influence of duration of protein synthesis inhibition on memory. *Physiology and Behavior*, **10**, 555–62.

Flood, J. F., Bennett, E. L., Orme, A. E. and Rosenzweig, M. R. (1975). Relation of memory formation to controlled amounts of brain protein synthesis. *Physiology and Behavior*, **15**, 97–102.

Flood, J. F., Cherkin, A. and Morley, J. E. (1987). Antagonism of endogenous opioids modulates memory processing. *Brain Research*, **422**, 218–34.

Gerard, R. W. (1949). Physiology and psychiatry. *American Journal of Psychiatry*, **106**, 161–73.

Geschwind, N. and Galaburda, A. M. (eds) (1984). *Cerebral dominance: the biological foundations*. Cambridge: Harvard University Press.

Geschwind, N. and Galaburda, A. M. (1987). *Cerebral lateralization: biological mechanisms, associations, and pathology*. MIT Press, Cambridge, Mass.

Gibbs, M. E. (1983). Memory and behaviour: birds and their memories. *Bird Behaviour*, **4**, 93–107.

Gibbs, M. E., Gibbs, C. L. and Ng, K. T. (1979). The influence of calcium on short-term memory. *Neuroscience Letters*, **14**, 355–60.

Gibbs, M. E. and Ng, K. T. (1977). Psychobiology of memory formation. *Biobehavioral Reviews*, **1**, 113–36.

Gibbs, M. E. and Ng, K. T. (1979). Neuronal depolarization and the inhibition of short-term memory formation. *Physiology and Behavior*, **23**, 369–75.

Gibbs, M. E. and Ng, K. T. (1984). Hormonal influence on the duration of short-term and intermediate stages of memory. *Behavioral Brain Research*, **11**, 109–16.

Gisquet-Verrier, P. (1983). L'effet Kamin: description, analyse et interpretations. Revue critique. *Cahiers de Psychologie Cognitive*, **3**, 3–34.

Hebb, D. O. (1949). *The organization of behavior*. John Wiley, New York.

Hellige, J. B. (1987). Interhemispheric interaction: models, paradigms and recent findings. In *Duality and unity of the brain: Vol. 47. Wenner-Gren international symposium series* (ed. D. Ottoson), pp. 454–65. Plenum, New York.

Hellige, J. B. (1990). Hemispheric asymmetry. *Annual Review of Psychology*, **41**, 55–80.

Horn, G., McCabe, B. J. and Bateson, P. P. G. (1979). An autoradiographic study of the chick brain after imprinting. *Brain Research*, **168**, 361–73.

Horton, D. L. and Mills, C. B. (1984). Human learning and memory. *Annual Review of Psychology*, **35**, 361–94.

Järbe, T. U. C. (1986). State-dependent learning and drug discriminative control of behaviour: an overview. *Acta Neurologica Scandinavica*, **S109**, 37–60.

Kamin, L. J. (1957). The retention of an incompletely learned avoidance response. *Journal of Comparative and Physiological Psychology*, **50**, 457–60.

Kamin, L. J. (1963) The retention of an imcompletely learned avoidance response: some further analyses. *Journal of Comparative Physiological Psychology*, **56**, 713–18.

Lee, D. W., Means, M. K., Afinowicz, D. J., Bennett, E. L., Martinez, J. L., Jr, and Rosenzweig, M. R. (1989). Enhancement of memory for a one-trial passive avoidance task in chicks given peripheral and central injections of naloxone. *Society for Neuroscience Abstracts*, **15**, 1169.

Lee, D. W., Perlmutter, A. M., Beniston, D. S., Bennett, E. L., and Rosenzweig, M. R. (1989). Is anisomycin-induced amnesia for a passive avoidance task in chicks the result of state dependent learning? *Developmental Brain Research*, **49**, 179–84.

Mark, R. F. and Watts, M. E. (1971). Drug inhibition of memory formation in chickens. I. Long-term memory. *Proceedings of the Royal Society of London B*, **178**, 439–54.

McGaugh, J. L. (1968). A multi-trace view of memory storage processes. In *Attuali orentamenti della ricerca sull'apprendimento e la memoria* (ed. R. Bovet), pp. 13–24. N. 109 Academia Nazionale dei Lincei, Quaderno, Rome.

McGaugh,J. L. and Herz, M. J. (ed.) (1972). *Memory consolidation*. Albion, San Francisco.

Mueller, G. E. and Pilzecker, A. (1900). Experimentelle Beiträge zur Lehre vom Gedächtniss. *Zeitschrift für Psychologie*, Suppl. 1, 1–288.

Ng, K. T. and Gibbs, M. E. (1987). Less-than-expected variability in evidence for three stages in memory formation: a response. *Behavioral Neuroscience*, **101**, 126–30.

Overton, D. A. (1984). State dependent learning and drug discriminations. In *Handbook of psychopharmacology, Vol. 18* (ed. L. L. Iverson, S. D. Iverson, and S. H. Snyder), pp. 59–127. Plenum, New York.

Patterson, T. A., Alvarado, M. C., Rosenzweig, M. R. and Bennett, E. L. (1988). Time courses of amnesia, development in two areas of the chick forebrain. *Neurochemical Research*, **13**, 643–7.

Patterson, T. A. (1987). Neurochemical processes in memory formation in the chick. Unpublished doctoral dissertation, University of California at Berkeley.

Patterson, T. A., Alvarado, M. O., Warner, I. T., Bennett, E. L., and Rosenzweig, M. R. (1986). Memory stages and brain asymmetry in chick learning. *Behavioral Neuroscience*, **100**, 850–9.

Patterson, T. A., Rosenzweig, M. R., and Bennett, E. L. (1987) Amnesia produced by anisomycin in an appetitive task is not due to conditioned aversion. *Behavioral and Neural Biology*, **47**, 17–26.

Patterson, T. A., Schulteis, G., Alvarado, M. C., Martinez, J. L., Jr, Bennett, E. L., Rosenzweig, M. R., and Hruby, V. J. (1989). Influence of opioid peptides on memory formation in the chick. *Behavioral Neuroscience*, **103**, 429–37.

Patterson, T. A., Rose, S. P. R., and Bradley, P. M. (1989). Anisomycin and amnesia in the chick: not a state-dependent effect. *Developmental Brain Research*. (In press.)

Roberts, S. (1987). Less-than-expected variability in evidence for three stages in memory formation. *Behavioral Neuroscience*, **101**, 120–5.

Rose, S. P. R. and Csillag, A. (1985). Passive avoidance training results in lasting changes in deoxyglucose metabolism in left hemisphere regions of chick brain. *Behavioral and Neural Biology*, **44**, 315–24.

Rosenzweig, M. R. (1984). Experience, memory, and the brain. *American Psychologist*, **39**, 365–76.

Rosenzweig, M. R. and Bennett, E. L. (1984*a*). Direct processes and modulatory influences in the stages of memory formation. In *Neurobiology of learning and memory* (ed. G. Lynch, J. L. McGaugh, and N. M. Weinberger), pp. 264–88. Guilford Press, New York.

Rosenzweig, M. R. and Bennett, E. L. (1984*b*). Studying stages of memory formation with chicks and rodents. In *The neuropsychology of memory* (ed. N. Butters and L. R. Squire), pp. 555–65. Guilford Press, New York.

Rosenzweig, M. R. Lee, D. W., Means, M. K., Bennett, E. L., and Martinez, J. L. Jr (1989). Effects of varying training strength on short-, intermediate-, and long-term formation of memory (STM, ITM, LTM) for a one-trial passive avoidance task in chicks. *Society for Neuroscience Abstracts*, **15**, 1171.

Schwartz, J. H. Castellucci, V. F., and Kandel, E. R. (1971). Functioning of identified neurons and synapses in abdominal ganglion of *Aplysia* in absence of protein synthesis. *Journal of Neurophysiology*, **34**, 939–63.

Serrano, P. A., Ramus, S. J., Bennett, E. L. and Rosenzweig, M. R. (1988). A comparative study of the LPO and MHV in memory formation in the chick brain. *Society for Neuroscience Abstracts*, **14**, 250.

Serrano, P. A., Ramus, S. J., Bennett, E. L. and Rosenzweig, M. R. (1989). No evidence for time-locked effects of emetine injected into the MHV of the chick brain. *Society of Neuroscience Abstracts*, **15**, 1171.

Simon, H. (1986). The parameters of human memory. In *Human memory and cognitive capabilities; Symposium in memoriam Hermann Ebbinghaus* (ed. F. Klix and H. Hagendorf), Vol. A, pp. 299–309. Elsevier Science Publishers, Amsterdam.

Thompson, R. F. (1986) The neurobiology of learning and memory. *Science*, **233**, 941–47.

Warrington, E. K. (1982). The double dissociation of short- and long-term memory. In *Human memory and amnesia* (ed. L. S. Cermak). Lawrence Erlbaum, Hillsdale, NJ.

Watts, M. E. and Mark, R. F. (1971). Drug inhibition of memory formation in chickens. II. Short-term memory. *Proceedings of the Royal Society of London B*, **178**, 455–64.

Weingarter, H. and Parker, E. S. (ed.) (1984). *Memory consolidation: psychobiology of cognition*. Lawrence Erlbaum, Hillsdale, NJ.

16

Monoamine systems and memory formation

R. M. Stephenson

During the past decade, a large body of evidence has accumulated implicating monoamine function in memory processing. This has been interpreted in a variety of ways, ranging from direct effects upon learning and memory (Kety 1970; Crow and Arbuthnott 1972) to non-specific effects upon attentional processes (Mason 1984). I wish to argue here and have argued elsewhere (Stephenson 1981), that these views are not incompatible and that much confusion has ensued from ignoring the mechanisms by which retrieval may operate.

Recently central beta-adrenergic involvement in chick memory processing has become well established (Stephenson and Andrew 1981; Davies and Payne 1989). This is supported by clear evidence from the rat of changes in central noradrenalin turnover immediately after the acquisition of a one-trial (inhibitory) passive avoidance task (Gold and Walsh 1987). Other work in the chick has indicated that changes in central noradrenergic activity are equally likely to affect passive avoidance learning and imprinting (Davies *et al*. 1985).

BETA-ADRENERGIC SYSTEMS AND MEMORY FORMATION IN THE CHICK

Here I describe a number of experiments performed by myself and others, which indicate that beta-adrenergic systems play a crucial and specific role in memory formation. The experimental details of much of this work are described elsewhere (Stephenson and Andrew 1981; Davies and Payne 1989) and I shall only briefly refer to them here.

Much early work on the relationship between catecholamine systems and memory formation was hindered by the fact that many of the agents used to deplete central levels of these amines lacked specificity. For example, it was unclear whether the amnestic effects of powerful copper chelating agents such as diethyldithiocarbamate resulted from inhibition of dopamine hydroxylase activity or one of a number of non-specific side effects (Haycock *et al*. 1977). Later it became possible to attack the

Table 16.1   Effect of alpha and beta antagonists on retention

Treatment	Time of administration			
	5 min before training % not pecking		10 min after training % not pecking	
	Red	Blue	Red	Blue
Vehicle	79	15	70	16
Sotalol	18***	5	23**	6
Timolol	37**	16	29**	16
Atenolol	80	0	74	5
Piperoxane	53	5	75	30
Vehicle	79	21	75	18
Nadolol	29***	5	16***	16
Phenoxybenzamine	74	21	78	11

The percentage of birds not pecking the red and blue beads at test are shown. Statistical comparisons (χ^2) were between drug-treated groups (systemic route) and their appropriate controls (vehicle alone). Note that two series of experiments, each with a control group, are shown.
*** $p < 0.001$, ** $p < 0.01$

problem at the level of the receptor using antagonists which appeared to have a high degree of specificity and also a lack of complicating side-effects such as membrane stabilization and sympathomimetic effects (Clark 1976; Frishman 1979; Cruickshank and Prichard 1988; Wikberg 1979).

SUB-CUTANEOUS INJECTION OF ALPHA AND BETA ANTAGONISTS: BEFORE AND AFTER TRAINING.

The passive avoidance task used at Sussex (Table 1.3) was used in all the work described in this chapter, unless indicated otherwise. Briefly, it begins with pre-training (small white, and then larger red and blue beads); training (ill-tasting red bead) follows after 120 minutes. The retention test (a red, and then a blue bead) was administered 180 minutes after training. The measure shown here (% retention) is the percentage of birds which did not peck at test. All treatment groups were initially 20 birds; birds failing to peck at training were excluded, reducing group sizes to a minimum of 16.

From Table 16.1 it can be seen that the three beta-antagonists (sotalol, nadolol, and timolol) which are effective in mammals at both beta$_1$ and beta$_2$ receptor sites, markedly and significantly reduce retention, whether given 5 minutes before or 10 minutes after training. The beta$_1$ antagonist (atenolol), an alpha$_1$ antagonist (phenoxybenzamine) and an alpha$_2$ antagonist (piperoxane) had no effects on retention, whether given before or after training. The neutral blue bead which had been seen in pre-training but had not been used in training was pecked freely by all groups (Table 16.1). This suggests that none of the drugs effective in opposing retention at 180 minutes after training did so by a general depressive effect on performance.

STATE DEPENDENCY

The above experiments suggest that beta-mediated systems might have a role to play in memory consolidation in the chick. The absence of effect following injection of the antagonist after training can be taken as evidence that these antagonists do not interfere with acquisition. However, it was not possible to exclude direct effects of these antagonists upon performance at test. The plasma half-life of all these antagonists is well beyond the 3 hour injection-testing interval and may be as long as 18 hours in the case of nadolol (Lee 1977). It is also possible that state dependency (Overton 1973) might be involved; that is, learning (here, formation of the trace after the learning event) in a special physiological state induced by a drug might result in memory being accessible only when the same physiological state is again produced.

Experiments were performed to test the hypothesis that the injection of beta antagonists before training would not produce amnesia if an identical dose of the antagonist were injected 5 minutes before testing. Another group of animals was treated with appropriate vehicle before training and antagonist only before test. This investigated the possibility that the effects of the beta antagonists are upon performance at test. In another set of experiments groups were injected with an antagonist, at a time when this was fully effective, and were tested 24 hours later to examine further the possibility of drug effects at test and to see how permanent was the induced amnesia.

The results indicated (Stephenson and Andrew 1981) that the groups receiving a beta antagonist at both training and test showed a degree of disruption of retention, which would have been expected if the antagonist had been given only before training. The groups receiving a beta antagonist only at test showed no disruption of retention and differed significantly from the drug-drug groups. All groups pecked the neutral bead freely. The amnesia is still present 24 hours after injection and so well beyond a point at which the drug is presumed to be effective. It seems clear that the effects of beta antagonists are not a result of state dependency.

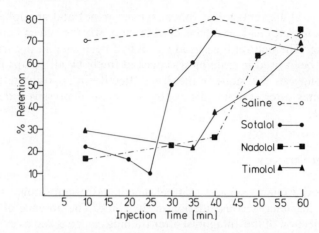

Fig. 16.1 The percentage retention (% of animals not pecking the red bead at test) is shown for groups of animals injected with beta antagonists (4 mg/kg) or saline (154 mM NaCl). The time of injection is shown for points between 5 and 60 minutes after training, with tests being made 3 hours after training in each case.

BETA ANTAGONISTS INJECTED AT DIFFERENT TIMES AFTER TRAINING

If the effects of beta antagonists are specifically upon memory formation, it might be expected that the antagonists would be effective in disrupting subsequent retention for only a limited period after training.

It can be seen (Fig. 16.1) that all three beta antagonists affected retention when given within a limited period after training. Unexpectedly, the duration of this period differed between antagonists; there appeared to be a relatively sharp loss of sensitivity to sotalol between 25 minutes after training (when it was maximally effective) and 35–40 minutes after training, with most of the change occurring between 25 and 30 minutes; sensitivity to both nadolol and timolol began to fall away later at around 35–40 minutes after training, and was not fully lost until 60 minutes. When injection was at 10 minutes after training the groups receiving sotalol, nadolol, and timolol all differed significantly from the matched control groups ($p < 0.02$, $p < 0.01$, and $p < 0.02$, respectively, χ_1^2). When injection was at 40 minutes after training the nadolol and timolol groups still differed significantly from the control groups ($p < 0.001$ and $p < 0.01$ respectively, χ_1^2). These data suggest that at the doses used, loss of sensitivity to sotalol follows a time course significantly different from that shown by the other two agents.

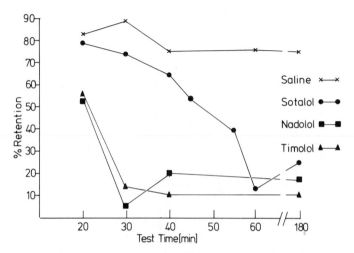

Fig. 16.2   The percentage retention (percentage not pecking the read bead at test) is shown for groups of animals injected with beta antagonists (1 mg/kg) or saline (154 mM NaCl) 15 minutes after training, and tested at the times shown.

TIME COURSE OF LOSS OF RETENTION AFTER THE
ADMINISTRATION OF BETA ANTAGONISTS

There did not appear to be any simple pharmacodynamic (mechanism of action) or pharmacokinetic (absorption, distribution, metabolism, excretion) explanation for the differences observed in the sensitivity time course; for example, they are effective in the same dosage range. This in itself is a strange result given that sotalol is 100-fold less effective than either nadolol or timolol in competition with isoprenaline (a specific beta agonist), *in vivo*. Indeed evidence indicated that sotalol would produce amnesia in the chick at lower doses than either nadalol or timolol.

After injection 5 minutes before training all three beta antagonists produced a similar rapid loss of retention (Stephenson and Andrew 1981). At 5 minutes after training retention was almost or quite complete, whilst at 10 minutes there was little retention. Retention levels did not fall further between 10 and 180 minutes. At all times the neutral bead was pecked freely.

Injection at 15 minutes after training, however, once again revealed a marked difference between sotalol and the other two beta antagonists (Fig. 16.2). Loss of retention was considerably delayed in groups receiving sotalol: the retention curve did not begin to diverge significantly from saline-injected controls until 45 minutes after training and did not show full loss until 60 minutes after training. The groups receiving nadolol and

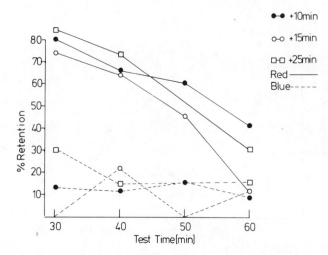

Fig. 16.3 The percentage retention (percentage of animals not pecking the red bead at test) and response to the neutral bead are shown. Animals were injected with sotalol at one of the indicated times (10 minutes, 15 minutes, 25 minutes, after training), and tests were performed between 30 and 60 minutes after training, (Test Time).

timolol already showed some signs of loss at 20 minutes after training. Loss was complete at 30 minutes, when nadolol and timolol groups differed significantly from the matched control groups ($p < 0.001$ and $p < 0.01$, χ_1^2). At 180 minutes after training, as expected from earlier experiments, sotalol, nadolol and timolol groups all differed significantly from controls ($p < 0.03$, $p < 0.01$, and $p < 0.001$ χ_1^2, respectively). Thus the time course of loss of retention in relation to the time of injection did not differ markedly in the case of nadolol and timolol between injection at 5 minutes before training and at 15 minutes after training; in both cases loss was largely complete 10–15 minutes afer injection. This was not true of sotalol.

It was possible that these differences in time course reflected a pharma-cokinetic difference between the drugs. To test this possibility the effects of variation of injection time were studied on the retention curve obtained. Injection at 10, 15 and 25 minutes after training (the latter being the latest time at which sotalol was expected to act at all) produced curves similar to each other (Fig. 16.3), and to that obtained in the previous experiment. It thus seems unlikely that the delay in loss of retention following sotalol reflects a substantially slower onset of action at a cellular level than occurs with nadolol or timolol. If this were so, then the curve for the 25 minute injection would be expected to be shifted to the right in comparison with the 10 minute injection curve, and it is not.

INTRACRANIAL ADMINISTRATION

Subcutaneous adminstration of beta antagonists is likely to induce beta blockade centrally as well as peripherally. Disturbance of noradrenergic (or adrenergic) function by beta antagonists might therefore affect memory by a central or peripheral route. Although it is not known how freely beta antagonists pass the blood–brain barrier in the young chick, its ineffectiveness as a barrier to other classes of agent (Spooner and Winters 1966) suggests that beta antagonists also might enter. However, it is possible that the permeability of the partially formed blood-brain barrier may be differentially selective to sotalol on the one hand and nadolol and timolol on the other. This may be related to differences in the intrinsic lipid solubility of the various agents used. To test this hypothesis, acute administration of beta antagonists was made to chick brain centrally, and sensitivity and retention time courses were produced.

All birds were pre-trained in the normal way and trained 2 hours later. Injections were made at a range of times between 10 and 40 minutes after training inclusive. Each bird received 25 μg/10 μl of beta antagonist in each hemisphere by free hand injection, to a depth of 2 mm in the centre of each hemisphere. Propranolol was included in this analysis as a comparison to the other beta antagonists and also because it had proved relatively ineffective when injected systemically. Although propranolol had been rejected as a first choice beta antagonist, because of its membrane stabilizing properties, its lack of effect when given peripherally in comparable doses to sotalol was interesting given its relatively high affinity for beta receptors. Propranolol's high binding affinity for serum albumin (Zaagsma and Meems 1976) was a possible explanation: this was excluded by central administration.

It can be seen (Fig. 16.4) that all the drug-injected groups show significant differences from saline-injected controls in the proportion of birds not pecking the red bead at test, when they were injected 10 minutes after training and tested 3 hours later (sotalol $p < 0.001$, timolol $p < 0.001$, propranolol $p < 0.01$ χ_1^2). However, if the injection of beta antagonist was delayed until 40 minutes after training only the timolol-treated group differed significantly from saline controls ($p < 0.001$ χ_1^2). This suggested that not only were the sensitivity time-courses very similar to those found with peripheral injection of sotalol and timolol but also that propranolol acted in a similar way to sotalol.

A retention time-course for intracranial injection also revealed similarity between the results obtained with peripheral injection (Fig. 16.5). When birds were injected 15 minutes after training and tested at either 30 or 60 minutes, only those treated with timolol showed a significant retention deficit at 30 minutes, when compared to the saline controls ($p < 0.005$

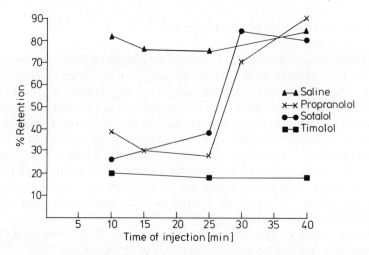

Fig. 16.4 The percentage retention is shown (percentage animals not pecking the red bead at test) for groups of animals injected intracranially with beta antagonists (25 μg/hemisphere) or saline (154 mM NaCl). The time of injection is given and all the points represent tests made 3 hours after training.

χ_1^2). At 60 minutes after training all three drug-treated groups differed significantly from vehicle-treated control groups in the proportion of birds not pecking the red bead at test ($p < 0.05$ propranolol, $p < 0.05$ timolol, $p < 0.001$ sotalol χ_1^2).

It is thus clear that propranolol and sotalol, on the one hand, and timolol and nadolol, on the other, form two groups of agents with strikingly different effects on memory formation.

LOCALIZATION OF ACTION OF BETA-ANTAGONISTS AT CENTRAL SITES

The above experiments do not entirely exclude the possibility that peripheral sites of action are involved in one or both of the defined types of amnesia. In those experiments leakage to the periphery was very likely with the large injection volume used, although the propranolol result suggests central sites of action to be more likely. In the following experiments birds were injected with a much smaller volume/hemisphere and the point of entry to the forebrain was recorded, in an attempt to localize any potential central site of action. The experiments here were conducted double blind, with both the experimenter and the person mapping the points of entry, being unaware of the behavioural results for each animal when mapping, the drug being injected or the point of entry

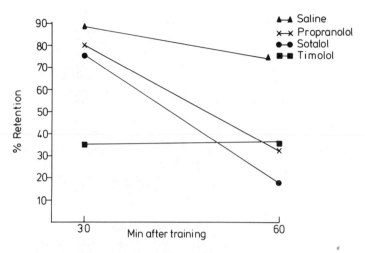

Fig. 16.5 The percentage retention (percentage not pecking the red bead at test) is shown for groups of animals injected intracranially with beta antagonists (25 μg/ hemisphere) or saline (154 mM NaCl). The injections were made 15 minutes after training and tests given at the points shown.

when recording the behaviour at test. Each animal was pre-trained in the usual way and trained 2 hours later. Injections of sotalol, timolol (both 12.5 μg/hemisphere), or saline were administered as 1 μl injections at a depth of 2 mm, 25 minutes after training. Each pair of birds was injected in approximately the same area but injections between each pair were positioned randomly. All birds were tested 3 hours after training and the proportion of birds pecking and the number of pecks made were recorded, for both the red and the blue presentations. The birds were then sacrificed and the position of entry of each injection was recorded, using a transparent cast of the skull roof. This could be placed in a standard position on the skull of the sacrificed chick and the points of entry to the brain were visible through it (p. 34). These points were plotted on a horizontal reconstruction of the chick brain for a depth of 2 mm below the surface of the brain. These plots revealed that the points of bilateral injection were largely symmetrical. Points that differed by more than 2 mm in any direction from the point of entry on the contralateral side were excluded. As there is no obvious bilateral asymmetry between the two sides, plots are presented in Fig. 16.6 for the left hemisphere (the side injected first in all cases) for saline-, sotalol-, and timolol-injected birds.

The proportion of birds pecking the red bead at test changes significantly when points are sampled posteriorly-anteriorly in equal 2 mm segments ($p < 0.01$, χ_{10}^2 timolol, $p < 0.01$, χ_{10}^2 sotalol) in the drug-treated groups. It is clear from Fig 16.6 that the points of injection that induce amnesia

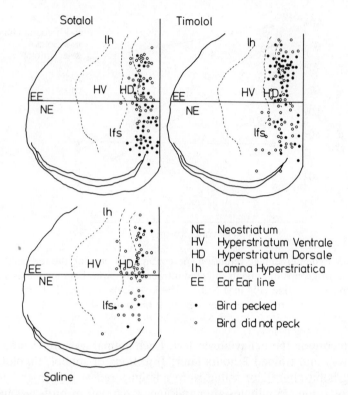

Fig. 16.6 Points of entry to the skull are shown for injection in the left hemisphere. Birds were injected to a depth of 2mm below scalp surface, with sotalol, timolol (both at 12.5 μg) or saline (154 mM NaCl) via 1 μl injection.

with timolol are different from those that produce amnesia with sotalol. If the proportion of birds not pecking the red bead at test for sotalol is compared with those for timolol for points lying between the ear/ear line (chosen as an arbitrary dividing line) and a line 6 mm posterior to it, timolol-treated birds differ significantly from sotalol-treated ($p < 0.001$ χ_1^2).

If such a comparison is made for the points lying in front of the ear/ear line (up to 6 mm anterior), timolol-treated birds differ significantly from sotalol-treated birds ($p < 0.001$ χ_1^2). The posterior sample for sotalol-injected birds differs significantly from vehicle injected controls ($p < 0.001$ χ_1^2); this is not so at the anterior site. Conversely, the timolol-treated sample does not differ significantly from vehicle-injected controls in the posterior segment but it does in the anterior segment ($p < 0.001$ χ_1^2).

BETA-ADRENERGIC SYSTEMS AND MEMORY FORMATION

The evidence presented here suggests that beta-mediated systems are important in memory consolidation. Three beta antagonists which are effective (sotalol, nadolol, timolol) all show broad opposition to $beta_1$ and $beta_2$ receptors and do not have sympathomimetic or membrane stabilizing effects. At similar doses $alpha_1$, $alpha_2$, and $beta_1$ antagonists were ineffective, suggesting specific action at $beta_2$ receptor sites. This is consistent (given a central site of action) with the finding that beta receptors in the chick brain are predominantly or entirely $beta_2$ in type (Nahorski 1978). More recently, the role of $beta_2$ sites has been confirmed by others using the specific $beta_2$ antagonist ICI 118.551 (Davies and Payne 1989). Their results show that birds injected with this compound 10 minutes after passive avoidance training with a methylanthranilate-coated red bead peck the red bead at test significantly more than vehicle-injected control groups. Noradrenalin has also been shown to be crucial for imprinting (Davies *et al.* 1985). In this study the noradrenergic neurotoxin DSP4 was used to reduce forebrain noradrenalin levels by about 65 per cent. This profoundly impaired imprinting for a rotating red box but not for a stuffed jungle fowl.

Clearly, the role of brain noradrenalin in modulating memory storage is as yet unclear. However, it is clear that noradrenergic systems accomplish diffuse innervation and that each noradrenergic neuron must branch thousands of times. One estimate for the rat brain (Descarries *et al.* 1977) estimates that the rat cortex contains 330,000 noradrenalin varicosities per mm^3. Thus every cell in the cortex may lie within 30 μm of a nonsynaptic bouton. This would suggest that large areas of cortex would be affected by NA activity and that NA may direct information storage in many brain regions at once. Pharmacologically, the neuromodulatory effects of noradrenaline (Rogawski and Aghajanian 1980; Waterhouse and Woodward 1980) and direct effects upon neural plasticity (Kasamatsu *et al.* 1983; Loeb 1987) make it a likely candidate for the mediation of a consolidatory process. However, we are a long way from discerning many of the cellular details.

At this stage it is important to consider the relationship between the effects of beta antagonists on memory formation and the phases of the Gibbs/Ng model (Gibbs and Ng 1977*a*).

If sotalol is injected after training both its sensitivity and retention time courses appear similar to those found with intracranial administration of the protein synthesis inhibitors cycloheximide and anisomycin. For example, if it is injected after 30 minutes following training, it has no effect upon retention at test. The retention time courses for these agents with injection 15 minutes after training are also similar: normal levels of retention being observed if birds are tested at 30 minutes after training but not at 60 minutes. It seems likely therefore that injection of sotalol after training affects a late stage of memory formation, most probably the hypothesized long-term memory (Gibbs and Ng 1977a). Nevertheless, the effects of protein synthesis inhibitors (such as anisomycin) and sotalol are certainly not identical: protein synthesis inhibitors injected before training still only affect the late stage already defined (Gibbs and Ng 1984). Sotalol on the other hand also affects an earlier processing stage, which, when prevented from operating normally, induces marked and significant retention deficits within 10 minutes of training. It thus appears that sotalol affects two processes in memory formation, one at or close to training and another about 30 minutes after training. Completely independent evidence for an important processing event between 25 and 30 minutes after learning comes from a procedure in which chicks are given two contradictory experiences with beads of identical type: at the first a red bead is without ill-taste, whereas at the second it is coated with methylanthranilate. If consolidation of the first experience is affected by the introduction of testosterone, it is able to interfere with subsequent avoidance training with the same type of bead (Andrew et al. 1981). If the interval between the two experiences is varied, interference which is marked when the interval is 30 minutes or greater largely disappears as it is shortened to 25 minutes or less (Clifton et al. 1982; see also Chapters 17, 18, 19). The processing event or events responsible for this change clearly coincides in time with the postulated transition between phases A and B of ITM (Chapter 13).

Timolol and nadolol given before or after training appear to affect memory formation in a way not previously described. Sotalol has two distinct time courses of action when given either before or after training. This is reminiscent of, but not identical with the dual action of cyclohex-imide (Gibbs and Ng 1984). Timolol and nadolol, on the other hand, induce retention deficits within 10 minutes of injection, when injected between 5 minutes before and 15 minutes after training and continue to produce amnesia when injected as late as 40 minutes after training.

These results suggest that timolol and nadolol affect a process which is necessary for retrieval for at least 40 minutes after training and one which relies on continued activity of a beta-adrenergic system throughout that period. It is possible, therefore, that the evidence which indicates that noradrenergic mimetics and agonists will attenuate the effects of both Na^+/K^+ ATPase inhibitors and protein synthesis inhibitors (Gibbs 1976; Gibbs and Ng 1977b) may reflect an amplification of a crucial process in memory formation quite independently of any effects upon a sodium pump intermediate stage. The fact that the estimated duration of an intermediate phase of memory, ITM (or 'labile memory', Gibbs and Ng 1977a) lasts for about as long as sensitivity to nadolol and timolol poses a new set of issues.

If nadolol and timolol do affect ITM they must affect not only its establishment but also its maintenance. This is quite distinct from the action of ouabain, which is not effective if given after the formation of ITM, i.e. later than 10 minutes after training. Further, whether nadolol and timolol act on ITM or not, it is striking that they still interfere with retention when given later than 30 minutes after training, a point in time when long-term memory is deemed to be fully established, although not yet retrievable (Gibbs and Ng 1977a). This suggests that long-term memory is not fully established until much later than 30 minutes after training, in the sense that it is still open to interference in a way which does not hold later. Such interference could be additional to the sequential dependence of LTM on ITM or could lead to re-interpretation of evidence for such dependence. In view of the implication of adrenergic systems in attentional mechanisms (Mason and Iverson 1979), it is possible that the system sensitive to nadolol and timolol is involved in functions of this type. If so, then it might act during memory formation on processes involving selection of material and rehearsal, so protecting temporarily held material against disruption (Robbins 1984). Evidence for brief events recurring during memory formation, which might involve such processes, is considered in Chapter 19.

The pharmacodynamic differences between the two groups of beta antagonists remain to be discussed. Clearly a number of hypotheses are possible. They may differ because:

(a) There are two types of $beta_2$ receptor in the chick brain, differently responsive to two types of beta antagonist. The classification of beta receptors is based on mammalian receptors and may not be complete even for these (Szabadi *et al.* 1978). Chick erythrocyte beta receptors have been shown to be divisible into subtypes which do not entirely correspond to the $beta_1$/$beta_2$ subdivision in mammals (Dickinson and Nahorski 1980).

(b) The beta antagonists may compete differently with different transmitters at the same type of beta receptor; adrenalin as well as noradrenalin appears to be important in the avian brain (Dickinson and Nahorski 1980). For example, it has been found that (^{3}H) antagonist/agonist competition curves tend to be shallow, with slope factors (on 'pseudo' Hill slopes) of less than one (Magurie *et al.* 1977), suggesting an apparent heterogeneity of the receptor population not found with (^{3}H) antagonist/antagonist competition curves. These observed differences between agonist and antagonist binding properties have led to the development of a model (Lefkowitz and Williams 1978) that proposes beta-adrenergic receptors can exist in either a high or a low affinity state. Non-mammalian beta adrenoceptors may have accessory binding sites which are different from those present in the beta receptor of the rat tissue; if so, they cannot be classified as $beta_1$ or $beta_2$ adrenoceptors.

It is possible, therefore, that these receptors may show differential selectivity to sotalol on the one hand and nadolol and timolol on the other.

(c) The third possibility is that one (or both) of the groups of beta anatagonist have effects at other receptor sites. It is now clear that many beta antagonists have effects at 5HT sites and it is this possibility and the role of 5HT systems in memory formation I now wish to discuss.

5-HT AND MEMORY FORMATION IN THE CHICK

Serotonin (5HT) autoreceptors, mediating negative feedback regulation of release of 5-HT, are located on 5-HT axon terminals in the CNS (Cerrito and Raiteri 1979). The autoreceptors present in cerebral cortex, cerebellum and hippocampus of the rat have been characterized pharmacologically and appear to belong to the $5-HT_{1b}$ subtype of 5-HT receptor (Bonanno et al. 1986; Middlemiss 1984). It was found that in slices of cortex from the rat brain (-)-propranolol has antagonistic properties at the 5-HT autoreceptor (Middlemiss 1984). This has been demonstrated for other nonselective beta antagonists (Nahorski and Willcocks 1983; Middlemiss 1986). It is a possibility therefore that antagonism by one or both groups of beta antagonists at this autoreceptor site might impair memory formation through the release of 5-HT. Work in the rat has indicated that elevated 5-HT levels centrally can induce specific memory deficits in both active and passive avoidance tasks (Ogren 1985).

The following experiments test the hypothesis that blockade of presynaptic $5-HT_{1b}$ autoreceptors may be responsible for some of the memory deficits induced by beta antagonists in the previous work.

THE EFFECTS OF SELECTIVE BLOCKADE OF CENTRAL $5-HT_{1b}$ RECEPTORS ON MEMORY FORMATION IN THE CHICK

Chicks were pre-trained and trained in the way previously described and tested and injected at a range of times. All experiments were performed blind with treatment groups randomized between cages containing two birds. In the first series of experiments the selective $5-HT_{1b}$ antagonist 21-009 (Sandoz) or saline were injected intracranially at a range of times from 60 minutes before, to 25 minutes after training at a dose of 15 μg/hemisphere in a 10 μl injection. Placement was not thought to be crucial at this stage (given the high volume) but the anterior site was consistently used.

From Fig. 16.7 it can be seen that if 21-009 is given 60 minutes before training it causes a marked and highly significant decrease in the number of birds avoiding the red bead at test when compared with the saline

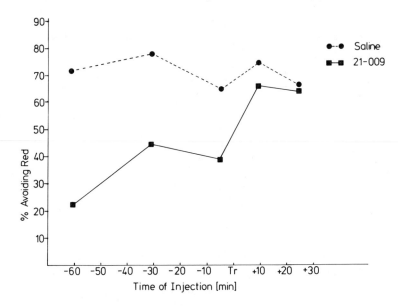

Fig. 16.7   The percentage retention (percentage not pecking the red bead at test) is shown for groups of birds injected intracranially with a 5-HT$_{1b}$ antagonist (15 μg/ hemisphere) or saline (154 mM NaCl) at the times shown. All tests were performed 3 hours after training.

controls ($p < 0.01$ χ_1^2). Injections given after training do not affect retention. These results are discussed in more detail elsewhere (Stephenson and Andrew, in preparation) but the sensitivity to 21-009 is evidently quite distinct from any sensitivity profile reported for the beta antagonists. Clearly any agent which acts only when given before training may be having nonspecific effects which may interfere with the learning of the task. It was therefore important to establish whether the animals showed any evidence of learning the task, and if so for how long. In order to test this, birds were injected with either 21-009 or saline 60 minutes before training and tested at one of four times (10, 30, 60 and 180 minutes) after training.

It can be seen from the results presented in Fig 16.8 that retention is good up to 60 minutes, and there is no significant difference between 21-009 and saline-injected control groups until 180 minutes after training ($p < 0.01$ χ_1^2). This, taken with other evidence showing normal pecking responses towards the blue neutral bead and no effect of injection of 21-009 just prior to test, suggests that the effects of 5-HT$_{1b}$ antagonism on memory formation are quite specific and do not affect learning, intermediate memory stages, or retrieval at test.

I have already suggested that the effects of 5-HT$_{1b}$ blockade would be

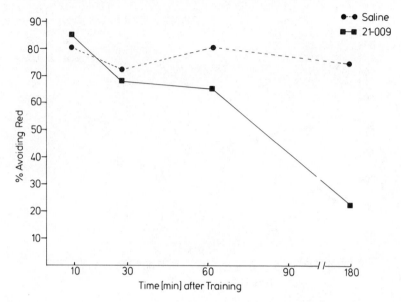

Fig. 16.8   The percentage retention (percentage not pecking the red bead at test) is shown for birds injected intracranially with 5-HT$_{1b}$ antagonist (15 μg/hemisphere) or saline (154 mM NaCl). Injections were made 60 minutes before training and retention was tested at 10, 30, 60, 90, and 180 minutes after training.

to elevate central 5-HT levels. If such elevation is necessary to produce amnesia, blockade of postsynaptic 5-HT receptors (5-HT$_2$ receptors in rats) should have little effect on memory formation. This hypothesis was tested by comparing the effects of ketanserin (selective 5-HT$_2$ antagonist), 21-009 (selective 5-HT$_{1b}$ antagonist) and ICS 204-930 (selective 5-HT$_3$ antagonist), when all three were injected 30 minutes before training.

It can be seen from the results presented in Fig. 16.9 that antagonism of 5-HT$_2$ or 5-HT$_3$ receptors does not result in any significant retention deficit when birds are tested at 180 minutes.

Ketanserin and ICS 205–930 are equally without effect when injected at other times before or after training.

DISCUSSION

The results presented above indicate that both catecholamine and indolamine systems are specifically involved in memory processing in the chick. While there may be a great deal of interaction between the two systems, two pieces of evidence indicate that the effects on 5-HT and noradrenergic systems are distinct.

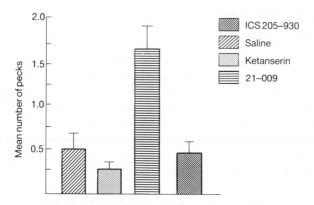

Fig. 16.9 The percentage retention is shown (percentage of birds failing to peck the red bead at test). Groups of birds were injected intracranially with a 5-HT$_2$ (ketanserin 15 μg/hemisphere), 5-HT$_3$ (ICS 205–930 15 μg/hemisphere) antagonist, or saline (154 mM NaCl) via a 10 μl injection, 30 minutes before training. Tests were performed 3 hours after training.

1. The sensitivity and retention profiles obtained with 21-009 do not repeat those found for any of the beta antagonists, suggesting a different site of action.

2. The specific beta$_2$ antagonist ICI 118.551 will induce specific retention deficits in the chick (Davies and Payne 1989) but does not bind to 5-HT$_{1b}$ receptor sites (Middlemiss 1986 and S. R. Nahorski, personal communication).

However, this does not rule out a close interaction between the two systems and their effects upon memory formation. It is now well established that enhanced serotonergic activity induced by subacute administration of selective serotonin uptake inhibitors like sertraline (Koe *et al.* 1987) induces down-regulation of the beta adrenoceptor subpopulation. Under conditions of impaired serotonergic activity, beta-adrenoceptors display a profound decrease in agonist but not antagonist affinity. While beta adrenoceptors are coupled to adenylate cyclase in a stimulatory fashion, 5-HT receptors are linked to phosphatidylinositol hydrolysis (Conn and Saunders-Bush 1985; Kendall and Nahorski 1985). The inositol triphosphate (IP$_3$) derived from this hydrolysis serves to mobilize calcium ions from the endoplasmic reticulum and calcium ions serve as a 'third messenger' by activating calcium/calmodulin-dependent protein kinases. Diacylglycerol activates protein kinase C. Both protein kinase C and calcium-dependent protein kinases are known to cause beta receptor desensitization in cell-free systems of turkey erythrocytes (Nambi *et al.* 1985). This elevated 5-HT activity, caused in this case by blockade of the autoreceptors, may impair normal consolidation as a result of impaired beta-adrenergic activity.

In conclusion, it seems likely that $beta_2$ mediated noradrenergic activity is crucial for a number of stages of memory formation in the domestic chick. It should be stressed that whatever combination of actions may underlie the differing pharmacodynamic effects of the two groups of $beta_2$ antagonists, three different sets of action on processes of memory formation have had to be postulated here. Sotalol affects processes at a crucial point 25–30 minutes after training; timolol and nadolol have an unusually extensive period of sensitivity, which may be additional to the mechanisms involved in phases of memory. 5-HT_{1b} antagonism at or just after training causes amnesia but with a very delayed loss. The beta receptor population is modulated by 5-HT systems (in mammals at least) and this modulation may play an important role in memory formation. Parallel routes of memory formation, discussed further in Chapters 14 and 19 also offer various possible ways by which very early disruption might only be revealed much later in memory formation.

Clearly, elevation of central 5-HT activity in the chick causes severe disruption of memory processing. It is not clear at this stage whether the groups of beta antagonists described above have differential activity at 5-HT_{1b} receptor sites or whether they have differential effects on high and low affinity beta receptor sites; either might explain their different actions.

REFERENCES

Andrew, R. J. Clifton, P. G., and Gibbs. M. E. (1981). Enhancement of effectiveness of learning by testosterone in the domestic chick. *Journal of Comparative Physiological Psychology*, **95**, 406–17.

Bonanno, G., Maura, G., and Raiteri. M. (1986). Pharmacological characterization of release regulating serotonin autoreceptors in rat cerebellum. *European Journal of Pharmacology*, **126**, 317–21.

Cerrito, F. and Raiteri, M. (1979). Serotonin release is modulated by presynaptic autoreception. *European Journal of Pharmacology*, **57**, 427–30.

Clark, B. J. (1976). Pharmacology of beta-adrenoceptor blocking agents. In *Beta-adrenoceptor blocking agents* (ed. P. R. Saxena and R. P. Forsyth), pp. 45–76. North-Holland, Amsterdam.

Clifton, P. G. Andrew, R. J., and Gibbs. M. E. (1982). Limited period of action of testosterone on memory formation in the chick. *Journal of Comparative Physiological Psychology*, **96**, 212–22.

Conn, P. J. and Saunders-Bush, E. (1985). Serotonin stimulated phosophoinositide turnover. Mediation by the S_2 binding site in rat cerebral cortex but not in subcortical regions. *Journal of Pharmacology and Experimental Therapeutics*, **234**, 195–208.

Crow, T. G. and Arbuthnott, G. W. (1972). Function of catecholamine-containing neurones in mammalian central nervous system. *Nature (New Biology)*, **238**, 245–6.

Cruickshank, J. M. and Prichard, B. N. C. (1988). *Beta-blockers in clinical practice*. Churchill Livingstone, Edinburgh.

Davies, D. C. Horn, G., and McCabe. B. J. (1985). Noradrenaline and learning: effects of the noradrenergic neurotoxin DSP4 on imprinting in the domestic chick. *Behavioural Neuroscience*, **99**, 652–60.

Davies, D. C. and Payne, J. M. (1989). Amnesia of a passive avoidance task due to the beta$_2$-adrenoceptor antagonist ICI 118.551. *Pharmacology Biochemistry and Behaviour*, **32**, 187–90.

Descarries, L., Watkins, K. C., and Bapherri, Y. (1977). Noradrenergic axon terminals in the cerebral cortex of rat. Topometric ultrastructural analysis *Brain Research*, **133**, 197–222.

Dickinson, K. E. J. and Nahorski, S. R. (1980). Atypical beta-adrenoceptors on frog and chick erythrocytes. *British Journal of Pharmacology*, **70**, 57–8.

Frishman, W. (1979). Clinical pharmacology of the new beta-adrenergic blocking drugs. Part 1. Pharmacodynamic and pharmacokinetic properties. *American Heart Journal*, **97**, 663–70.

Gibbs, M. E. (1976). Modulation of CXM-resistant memory by sympathomimetic agents. *Pharmacology Biochemistry and Behaviour*, **4**, 703–7.

Gibbs, M. E. and Ng, K. T. (1977a). Psychobiology of memory: towards a model of memory formation. *Behavioural Biology*, **1**, 113–36.

Gibbs, M. E. and Ng, K. T. (1977b). Counteractive effects of norepinephrine and amphetamine on ouabain induced amnesia. *Pharmacology Biochemistry and Behaviour*, **6**, 533–7.

Gibbs, M. E. and Ng, K. T. (1984). Dual action of cycloheximide on memory formation in day old chicks. *Behaviour and Brain Research*, **12**, 21–7.

Gibbs, M. E. Richards, A. L., and Ng K. T. (1987). Effect of excess intracranial amino acids on memory: a behavioural survey. *Neuroscience and Biobehavioral Reviews*, **11**, 331–9.

Gold, P. E. and Walsh, K. A. (1987). Regional brain catecholamines and memory: effects of footshock, amygdala implantation, and stimulation. *Behavioural and Neural Biology*, **47**, 116–29.

Haycock, J. W., Van Buskirk, R., and McGaugh, J. L. (1977). Effects of catecholaminergic drugs upon memory storage in mice. *Behavioural Biology*, **20**, 281–310.

Kasamatsu, T. (1983). Neuronal plasticity maintained by the central norepinephrine system in the cat visual cortex. In *Progress in psychobiology and physiological psychology* (ed. J. M. Sprague and A. N. Epstein), Vol. 10, pp. 1-112. Academic Press, New York.

Kendall, D. A. and Nahorski, S. R. (1985). 5-Hydroxytryptamine-stimulated inositol phospholipid hydrolysis in rat cerebral cortex slices: pharmacological characterization and effects of antidepressants. *Journal of Pharmacology and Experimental Therapeutics*, **233**, 473–9.

Kety, S. S. (1970). The biogenic amines in the central nervous system: their possible role in arousal, emotion and learning. In *The neurosciences second study program* (ed. F. O. Schmitt), pp. 324–36. Rockefeller University Press, New York.

Koe, B. K., Koch, S. W., Lebel, L. A., Minor, K. W., and Page, M. G. (1987). Sertraline, a selective inhibitor of serotonin uptake, induces subsensitivity of beta-adrenoceptor system of rat brain. *European Journal of Pharmacology*, **141**, 187–94.

Lee, R. J. (1977). Modification of developing infarct size by beta-adrenergic blockade. In *Pathophysiology and therapeutics of myocardial ischemia* (ed. A. M. Lefer and G. J. Kelliher), pp. 481–92. Spectrum Publications, New York.

Lefkowitz, R. J. and Williams, L. T. (1978). Molecular mechanisms of activation and desensitization of adenylate cyclase coupled beta-adrenergic receptors. In *Advances in cyclic nucleotide research* (ed. W. J. George and L. J. Iñarro), Vol. 9, pp. 1–17. Raven Press, New York.

Loeb, E. P., Chang, F. F., and Grennough, W. T. (1987). Effects of neonatal 6-hydroxydopamine treatment upon morphological organization of the poster medial barrel subfield in mouse somatosensory cortex. *Brain Research*, **403**, 113–20.

Magurie, M. E., Ross, E. M. and Gilman, A. G. (1977). Beta-adrenergic receptors: Ligand binding properties and the interaction with adenylate cyclase. In *Advances in cyclic nucleotide research* (ed. P. Greengard and G. A. Robinson), Vol. 8, pp. 1–83. Raven Press, New York.

Mason, S. T. (1984). *Catecholamines and behaviour*. Cambridge University Press.

Mason, S. T. and Iverson, S. D. (1979). Theories of the dorsal bundle extinction effect. *Brain Research Review*, **1**, 107–37.

Middlemiss, D. N. (1984). Stereoselective blockade at [^{3}H]5-HT binding sites and at the 5-HT autoreceptor by propranolol. *European Journal of Pharmacology*, **101**, 289–93.

Middlemiss, D. N. (1986). Blockade of the central 5-HT autoreceptor by beta adrenoceptor antagonists. *European Journal of Pharmacology*, **120**, 51–6.

Nahorski, S. R. (1978). Heterogeneity of central beta-adrenoceptor binding sites in various vertebrate species. *European Journal of Pharmacology*, **51**, 199–209.

Nahorski, S. R. and Willcocks, A. L. (1983). Interactions of beta-adrenoceptor antagonists with 5-hydroxytryptamine receptor subtypes in rat cerebral cortex. *British Journal of Pharmacology*, **78**, 107.

Nambi, P., Peters, J. R. and Sibly, D. R. (1985). Desensitization of the turkey erythrocyte beta-adrenergic receptor in a cell-free system. *Journal of Biological Chemistry*, **260**, 2165–77.

Ogren, S. O. (1985). Evidence for a role of brain serotonergic neurotransmission in avoidance learning. *Acta Physiologica Scandinavica*, **125**, Supplementum 544.

Overton, D. A. (1973). State dependent or dissociative learning. *Science*, **180**, 878–80.

Robbins, T. W. (1984). Cortical noradrenaline, attention and arousal. *Psychological Medicine*, **14**, 13–21.

Rogawski, M. A. and Aghajanian, C. K. (1980). Modulation of lateral geniculate neurone excitability by noradrenaline microiontophoresis or locus coeruleus stimulation. *Nature*, **287**, 731–4.

Spooner, C. E. and Winters, W. D. (1966). Neuropharmacological profile of the young chick. *International Journal of Neuropharmacology*, **5**, 215–36.

Stephenson, R. M. (1981). Memory processing in the domestic chick. Doctoral Thesis, University of Sussex.

Stephenson, R. M. and Andrew, R. J. (1981). Amnesia due to beta-antagonists in a passive avoidance task in the chick. *Pharmacology Biochemistry and Behaviour*, **15**, 597–604.

Stephenson, R. M. and Andrew, R. J. (1991). The effects of 5-HT receptor blockade on memory processing in the chick (in preparation).

Szabadi, E. C., Bradshaw, C. M. and Bevan, P. (1978). Recent advances in the pharmocology of adrenoceptors. *Proceedings of the 7th International Congress Pharmacology*. Elsevier Biomedical Press, Amsterdam.

Waterhouse, B. D. and Woodward, D. J. (1980). Interaction of norepinephrine with cerebrocortical activity evoked by stimulation of somatosensory afferent pathways in the rat. *Experimental Neurology*, **67**, 11–34.

Wikberg, J. E. S. (1979). The pharmacological classification of adrenergic alpha$_1$ and alpha$_2$ receptors and their mechanisms of action. *Acta Physiologica Scandinavica*, Supplementum **468**, 5–99.

Zaagsma, J. and Meems, L. (1976). Influence of protein binding on specific and nonspecific properties of beta adrenergic blocking agents. In *Adrenergic blocking agents* (ed. P. R. Saxena and R. P. Forsyth), pp. 321–3. Elsevier, Amsterdam.

17

Hormones and the timing of phases of memory formation

M. E. Gibbs, K. T. Ng, and S. Crowe

Day-old chicks normally peck readily at a small red glass bead. After pecking such a bead, which has been made unpleasant tasting by methylanthranilate (passive avoidance task: Chapters 1, 13), chicks avoid red beads but continue to peck a similar blue one. The retention timecourse following such training shows transient retention deficits or 'dips' which occur at 15 and 55 minutes after training. These dips delimit short-term, intermediate and long-term memory. The duration of the intermediate memory stage can be increased when certain hormones are given after training (Gibbs and Ng 1984 a,b). The hormones known to have this effect are those that are released in stressful experiences, such as adrenocorticotrophin (ACTH 1–24), corticosterone (CS) and arginine vasopressin (AVP), as well as testosterone. Intermediate memory consists of two phases, A and B, and a range of hormones have their effects on either phase. This chapter will concentrate on the effects of vasopressin. Retention time-courses will be presented which result when vasopressin is given to chicks which have their long-term memory formation blocked by cycloheximide, or their intermediate memory blocked by ouabain. Finally, the effect of training with a weak stimulus is investigated with respect to the presence of phase B and subsequent long-term memory formation.

In our original reports of the work (Gibbs and Ng 1977) retention was measured as percentage of chicks which avoided the red bead or the blue bead, and both sets of data were presented. Here we will present the percentage of chicks in groups of about 20 which avoid the red bead but continue to peck at the blue bead; in other words, chicks which fail to peck at the blue bead on test are removed from the final analysis. A 'discrimination ratio' is also reported in some cases; this is calculated as the number of pecks at the red bead over the total number of pecks at both the red and the blue bead, for all chicks pecking the blue bead on test. In all the experiments discussed in this paper, the chicks were pretrained to peck at both red and blue beads dipped in water (details: Gibbs and Ng 1977; Chapter 13).

Figure 17.1 gives the normal time course of memory formation. The data for this particular graph were collected over four separate experiments, which were carried out blind with different experimenters pretraining, training or testing the chicks, and with none of them knowing the interval between training and test until the completion of the data collection. Where more than one data point is shown for any time interval it means that there was a duplication of that time interval.

Two main dips or troughs in retention are clearly seen 15 and 55 minutes after training. One of the groups tested 15 minutes after training had a relatively high retention level; however, this was an abnormal group in which about half the chicks avoided the blue bead. These two dips or troughs in the retention function coincide with the end of short-term and intermediate memory, respectively, as defined by the drug intervention studies reviewed earlier (Ng and Gibbs: Chapter 13).

The intermediate stage of memory can be further divided into two parts, phase A and phase B, on the basis of susceptibility to disruption by the metabolic inhibitor 2,4-dinitrophenol (DNP). Intermediate memory, which lasts between 15 and 55 minutes after training under normal conditions (40 minutes duration), can be disrupted by the intracranial injection of DNP at any time up to 25 minutes after training. However, if the injection is given 30 minutes or more after training then DNP has no effect (Gibbs and Ng 1984c). Therefore, phase A can be abolished by DNP and lasts about 10 minutes, approximately from 15 to 25 minutes; phase B is not affected by DNP and lasts from 30 to 55 minutes after training (25 minutes). It is the second half of the intermediate memory stage. Other evidence for the existence of two phases in intermediate memory is presented in Chapter 13.

EFFECT OF HORMONES ON INTERMEDIATE MEMORY

Over the last few years we have been investigating the effects of several hormones on different stages in memory formation (Gibbs and Ng 1984b; Gibbs *et al.* 1986a, Gibbs *et al.* 1986b). Apart from testosterone, the hormones we have used are all released during stressful experiences; however, ACTH gives acute release of testosterone in mammals and so is not necessarily an exception (Gibbs *et al.* 1986b; Chapter 18). The results of administration of these hormones are shown schematically in Fig. 17.2. All the hormones except ACTH 4–10 extend the duration of intermediate memory, so that the second dip in the retention function occurs later than 55 minutes.

When vasopressin is administered immediately after training (within 6–10 seconds) the memory course alters (Fig. 17.3), such that short-term memory lasts for 10 minutes longer than normal with the first dip in

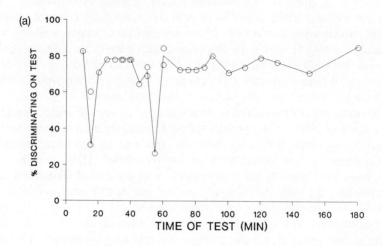

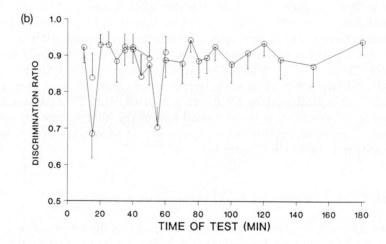

Fig. 17.1 Time-course of memory formation following training with an aversive red bead. Memory retention levels remain high (around 80 per cent discrimination) for all times of test except at 15 and 55 minutes after training. More than one datum point at any time of test represents a test of that interval in more than one of the four experiments. (a) Data are presented as per cent of chicks discriminating (1a), i.e. the per cent of chicks pecking the blue bead which avoided the red bead. In all 27 groups of chicks were used; after elimination of chicks avoiding the blue bead there were between 10 and 20 chicks per datum point (median 18). (b) With the data presented as discrimination ratio (text) a similar pattern is seen. Bars represent the standard error of the mean for each group of chicks.

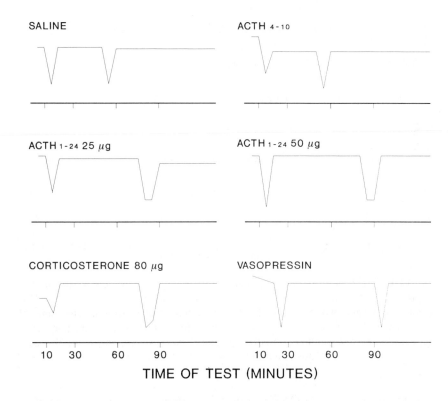

Fig. 17.2 Schematic representation of the results of the effects of hormones on the stages of memory formation inferred from the timing of the dips in retention. The hormones or saline were administered subcutaneously immediately after training and different groups of chicks tested at various intervals after training. Data taken from Gibbs and Ng (1984*a*, *b*, and unpublished data).

retention occurring 25 minutes after training. The second dip in retention is shifted from 55 minutes to 85–95 minutes after training, a prolongation of intermediate memory from 40 to 65 minutes. The dip in retention is now wider and shallower than in the normal situation, probably reflecting variability in the time of the dip across chickens or experiments.

In attempting to sort out how vasopressin affects intermediate memory, the first question we asked was whether the effect was on phase A or phase B. As DNP inhibits phase A and not phase B, the period over which the administration of DNP produces amnesia should give the timing of the two phases. Normally (in the absence of hormones) DNP can be injected up to 25 minutes after training to produce amnesia, but in the presence of

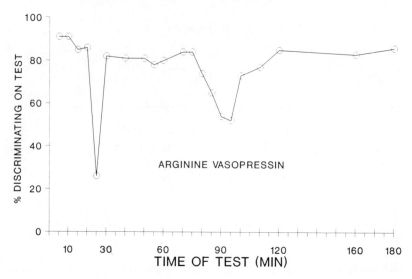

Fig. 17.3   Effect of arginine vasopressin on the timecourse of memory formation. Arginine vasopressin (0.1 ml of 0.2 i.u.) was given immediately after training. This graph represents two experiments; the data have been pooled. The time of appearance of the second dip was not the same in the two experiments and hence appears wider and shallower than it actually was. (Reanalysed from the data presented in Gibbs and Ng 1984*b*).

vasopressin (Fig. 17.4) DNP can be administered up to 65 minutes after training and still produce amnesia. In all these experiments the chicks were tested at 180 minutes after training. Phase A normally lasts 10 minutes (15–25 minutes) but in the presence of vasopressin it is extended to 40 minutes (25–65 minutes). Phase B is unaffected in duration, remaining at 25 minutes (30–55 minutes; 70–95 minutes).

CYCLOHEXIMIDE AND VASOPRESSIN

When CXM is given to chicks, no long-term memory is formed. The question asked was what happens when CXM is given to chicks which are treated with vasopressin? In these experiments (Fig.17.5*a*), intracranial CXM was given 5 minutes before training, and subcutaneous vasopressin (0.2 i.u.) was given immediately after the training trial. Vasopressin proved to prevent CXM from interfering with the formation of long-term memory. There was no evidence of amnesia, with good memory retention at 3 hours after training. It is possible that vasopressin acts by sustaining memory for times beyond the duration of action of CXM (Gibbs and Ng

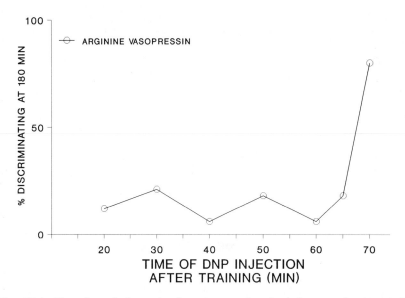

Fig. 17.4 Duration of phase A of memory under the influence of vasopressin. DNP, which inhibits phase A but not phase B, is effective in blocking memory when injected up to 65 minutes after training and vasopressin administration. In the absence of vasopressin, DNP will inhibit memory when given up to 25 minutes but not at 30 minutes after training. Chicks were tested 3 hours after training.

1984*a*). Short-term memory again lasted for 20 minutes, with the first dip occurring at 25 minutes.

However, high and stable evidence of retention during the intermediate memory stage lasted only until 65 minutes, that is until the end of phase A, as seen in Fig. 17.4. Between 65 and 90 minutes there appears to be a great deal of variability in retention levels. This may represent variability in the crossover from A to B or in the transition of B to long-term memory. In Fig. 17.5*a*, the part of the graph from about 60 to 100 minutes is derived from data from four separate experiments. The main feature during this period is a marked variability in the timing of the dip and the degree of retention levels from experiment to experiment.

In the presence of vasopressin alone, phase A (sensitivity to DNP) lasts for 65 minutes (Fig. 17.4). The same is probably true when both vasopressin and CXM are given (administration times the same as in Fig. 17.5). Preliminary experiments show that under these conditions DNP produces amnesia 10 minutes after injection when such injections occur 30, 40, or 50 minutes after training, but not when injections occur at 70 or 80 minutes. This suggests that when vasopressin is present from just after training, CXM which is given before training has little effect on the course

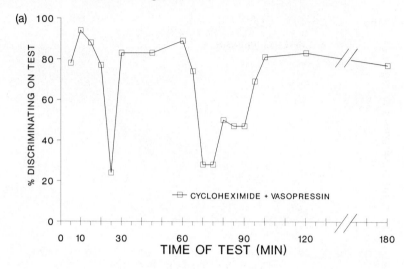

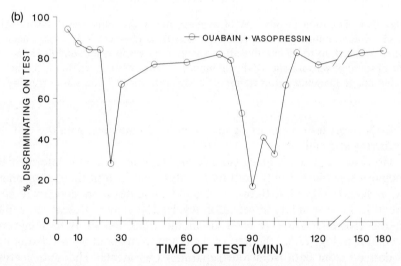

Fig. 17.5 (a) Memory loss due to cycloheximide is prevented by subcutaneous administration of vasopressin immediately after training. Cycloheximide was given intracranially 5 minutes before training. The extended second dip in retention levels seen between 70 and 90 minutes after training represents the means from four separate experiments. In these experiments the timing of the second dip was variable between, and even within experiments. The broadening of the trough may be viewed as resulting from variability in the timing of the transition from phase B to long-term memory. (b) Memory interruption by ouabain is prevented by the presence of vasopressin. Ouabain was administered intracranially 5 minutes before training and vasopressin given subcutaneously immediately after training. Chicks were tested at the times indicated after training.

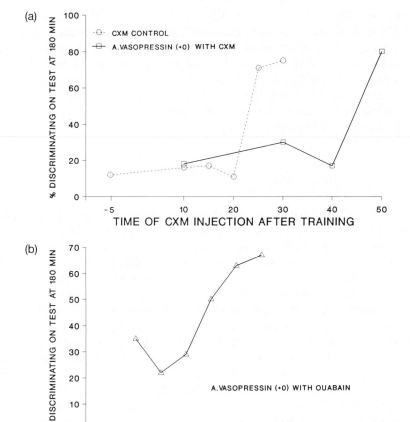

Fig. 17.6 (a) The ability of cycloheximide to interrupt memory formation is extended from 20 to 40 minutes when the chicks are treated with arginine vasopressin immediately after training. It is concluded that the formation of long-term memory has been delayed by vasopressin. (b) Similarly, the formation of intermediate memory can be delayed with the administration of vasopressin immediately after training. Normally ouabain does not inhibit memory formation if given 10 minutes after training, but, as seen in this graph, ouabain is still maximally effective when given to vasopressin-treated chicks 10 minutes after training.

of memory formation. The main change is a broadening (or increased variability) in the timing of the second dip.

Vasopressin (in a similar way to diphenylhydantoin (Gibbs and Ng 1984*a*) extended the sensitivity of long-term memory formation to cycloheximide (Fig. 17.6*a*). Vasopressin thus appears not to interfere directly with the action of CXM, but to shift the time at which there is sensitivity to CXM. It would seem that injected CXM has a relatively brief duration of action so that when given 5 minutes before training, it is no longer effective at the first point when sensitivity occurs in the presence of vasopressin. When CXM is injected at 10 minutes after training, its action evidently persists to a sensitive period. Sensitivity to inhibition by CXM in the presence of vasopressin ceases at 45–50 minutes, whereas in controls it disappears at 25 minutes.

OUABAIN AND VASOPRESSIN

When the intermediate memory inhibitor ouabain was injected 5 minutes prior to the training trial in the presence of vasopressin, the expectation was that there would be no intermediate memory (i.e. no memory present after the short-term memory stage). Unexpectedly, ouabain had little or no effect. Both dips were present at the timings expected in the presence of vasopressin alone (Fig. 17.5b). Clearly intermediate memory was intact.

As was the case with CXM, sensitivity of memory processes to inhibition by ouabain was extended in the presence of vasopressin (Fig. 17.6b). Normally, ouabain has no effect on memory when injected at 10 minutes after training; however, if vasopressin was given immediately after training, then ouabain was still maximally effective in producing amnesia even if administered at 10 minutes. It had no effect if given 20 minutes after training. A similar extension of sensitivity to ouabain to 15 minutes after training has been observed as a result of testosterone administration (Andrew 1980).

Ouabain appears to reduce the degree of extension of phase A by vasopressin. If chicks treated with ouabain and vasopressin are given DNP at times between 50 and 75 minutes after training (Fig. 17.7), phase A is present up to 55 minutes, and phase B begins at 60 minutes.

SUMMARY OF RESULTS WITH VASOPRESSIN

Vasopressin extends the duration of intermediate memory by extending phase A. The results with DNP suggest a very rapid transition from phase A to phase B. Long-term memory loss due to cycloheximide injected 5 minutes before training does not occur if vasopressin is given immediately after training, although there seems to be a period of marked instability in the memory retention function around the onset of phase B. In the presence of ouabain, which inhibits the formation of intermediate memory, there is again extension of intermediate memory, as well as no

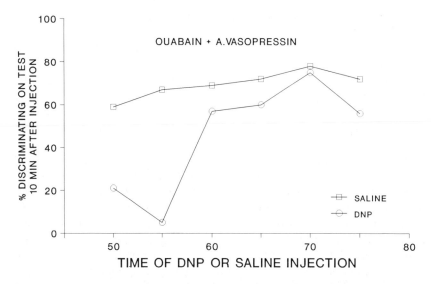

Fig. 17.7 Duration of phase A of intermediate memory in chicks treated with ouabain 5 minutes before, and with vasopressin immediately after training. DNP was effective in interrupting memory formation when given at 55 minutes after training but ineffective when given at 60 minutes, implying that phase B takes over the memory holding function at 60 minutes.

loss of long-term memory. Phase A is extended beyond its normal length and is followed by a phase B of normal length.

When a comparison is made between vasopressin and the other hormones, the results seem to fall into two classes. In the case of corticosterone and ACTH 1–24, both ouabain and cycloheximide effectively prevent the formation of long-term memory. Preliminary studies suggest the main difference between these two hormones and vasopressin is the lack of a rapid transition from phase A to phase B as shown by DNP administration; the transition here is much more gradual. The sensitivity to DNP does not persist until 65 minutes as occurs with vasopressin but falls away gradually from 30 minutes onwards. There is also the possibility that phase B may not be present or at least not expressed. When cycloheximide is given, memory loss occurs after 60 minutes and when ouabain is given DNP is ineffective between 60 and 75 minutes. A preliminary hypothesis from these results is that phase B is necessary for long-term memory formation.

LEARNING WITH A WEAK TRAINING STIMULUS

Another line of evidence for the necessity of phase B for long-term consolidation of memory comes from experiments using diluted methylanthranilate. It has been shown (Cherkin 1971; Gibbs 1983) that if the training bead is dipped in a weak solution of methylanthranilate rather than the 100 per cent anthranilate normally used in the chick passive avoidance experiments, there is no long-term memory, even though there is memory for some time after the training experience.

If chicks are trained using 20 per cent anthranilate dissolved in ethanol, then there is relatively good retention for 45 minutes after learning (Fig. 17.8*a*). There is the usual dip in retention at 15 minutes after training, but there is no long-term memory formation (Crowe *et al.* 1989 *a*, *b*). Intermediate memory lasts for 30 minutes (from 15 to 45 minutes). This is all phase A because if DNP is injected during this time, it is effective in inhibiting memory at all times of injection (0–50 minutes: see legend, Fig. 17.8). This implies that all the memory seen up to 45 minutes in Fig. 17.8 *a* is phase A. There is no phase B and no long-term memory. However, it is possible to get long-term memory formation by increasing the number of training trials. This can be done early after learning by introducing the training stimulus again at a time when a majority of the chicks will peck at it (i.e. during the first dip in retention levels 15 minutes after training). In the case of 20 per cent anthranilate in ethanol, a second trial is sufficient to consolidate the memory into long-term storage (Fig. 17.9*a*). There is a dip at 30 minutes, which presumably reflects the dip expected 15 minutes after the second presentation. There appear to be two further dips. The one at 45 minutes, if genuine, is unexpected. The second at 80 minutes is confirmed by a second time course (saline injection, Fig. 17.9*b*) and presumably represents the dip normally seen at 55 minutes (end of phase B). This 50 minute duration of intermediate memory (from 30 to 80 minutes) is longer than normal. DNP, in this experimental procedure (Fig. 17.9*b*), will interrupt intermediate memory if injected up to 55 minutes post-training, but has no effect if given 60 or 65 minutes after the original training period (note that injection was 10 minutes before test: legend). So with two training trials with 20 per cent anthranilate in ethanol there is a phase B and there is long-term memory formation.

In some preliminary studies with anthranilate diluted with water (1:400) (Crowe 1984), we obtained similar results (Fig. 17.10). With one presentation of weak anthranilate, there was no long-term memory, nor was there any long-term memory formation with two or three presentations of the training bead, 15 minutes apart. Even though intermediate memory was longer with three than with two presentations, repetition did not produce long-term memory until the fourth presentation. Using DNP as

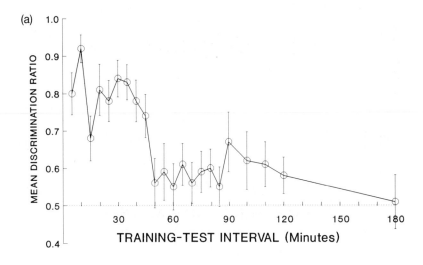

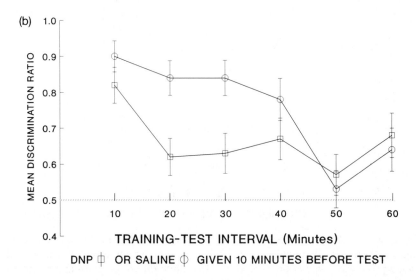

Fig. 17.8 (a) Retention function following training with 20 per cent anthranilate in ethanol. Short-term memory appears to be intact, with the first dip in retention occurring at 15 minutes. Intermediate memory survives until 45 minutes but then memory remains poor at all later testing times. (b) Duration of phase A of memory with 20 per cent anthranilate in ethanol. DNP is effective throughout the period for which memory survives (i.e. up to 40 minutes). Intracranial injections of DNP or saline were given 10 minutes prior to the retention test.

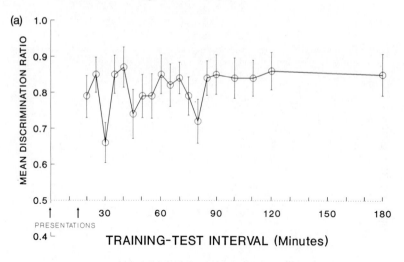

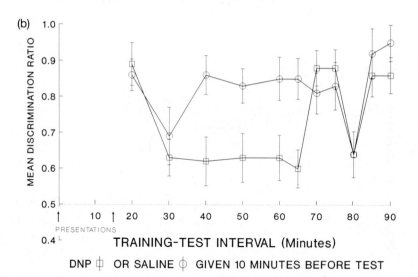

DNP $\boxdot$ OR SALINE ϕ GIVEN 10 MINUTES BEFORE TEST

Fig. 17.9 (a) Memory function following training with 20 per cent anthranilate in ethanol: there were two presentations of the stimulus 15 minutes apart. The second training trial was given at the time of the 15 minute dip in retention and retention levels were tested at the times shown after the original training. Note that there is now a dip at 30 minutes after the first presentation of the training stimulus, and another pronounced dip at 80 minutes. (b) Presence of both phase A and phase B of intermediate memory in the case of two presentations of the 20 per cent anthranilate training stimulus. DNP is effective in interrupting the memory when given between 30 and 55 minutes after training, but not effective when given at 60 or 70 minutes after training. The second dip, between intermediate and long-term memory, occurs at 80 minutes, as in saline controls.

the probe, we could show that there was no phase B until the experimental situation where there were four or more presentations. We have not been able to satisfactorily replicate these results with 1:400 anthranilate in water, but have shown subsequently that 10 per cent anthranilate in ethanol requires four presentations repeated every 15 minutes before long-term memory is formed.

Vasopressin given to chicks trained with one trial of 20 per cent anthranilate brings about long-term memory formation (Crowe *et al.* 1990). Intermediate memory is extended by 20 minutes in comparison to the hormone-free retention function. The second dip is postponed to 65 minutes after training. Phase B does occur, as DNP is ineffective given 35–50 minutes after training.

CONCLUSION

Obviously phase A can exist with no phase B or long-term memory occurring. So far there is no evidence that phase B can occur without leading to long-term memory. We are interested in what it is that triggers the formation of long-term memory and exactly when it occurs. We suspect that the trigger occurs very early on in memory formation, at the transition of phase A to B.

Arginine vasopressin will affect any of the processes we have postulated to be involved in the different memory stages. In the past we have used different inhibitory drugs to peel off the different stages of memory, but now we find that the different stages are amenable to manipulation by various physiological hormones and the data support our earlier pharmacological findings. It is interesting to speculate on the whole concept of the role of secondary messengers and hormones. It seems as if the biochemical cycles are applicable not only to the central nervous system but to a wide range of other tissues (e.g. kidney, muscle). Many of the agents that we have already used, and have found to modify the time-course of the different stages in memory formation, would on the basis of current knowledge be expected to modulate several cellular responses. For example, calcium, noradrenaline and cAMP can all be expected to be involved in the process of memory formation for both short-term and intermediate memory, and it is interesting to compare the actions of these agents with the results that one obtains by administering hormones. Hormones have memory effects which are of interest in their own right, but more importantly their actions may provide some insights into the basic cellular processes that are intimately involved in the storage of memory.

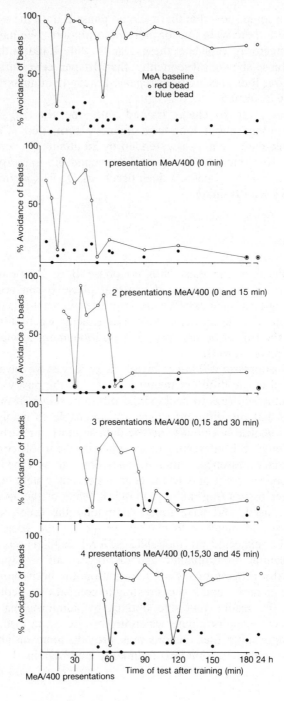

Fig. 17.10 Comparison of results from different numbers of presentations of 1/400 anthranilate. Although the duration of intermediate memory increases after two presentations of the training stimulus, it is not until four presentations of the bead (15 minutes apart) that there is formation of long-term memory.

REFERENCES

Andrew, R. J. (1980). Functional organization of phases of memory consolidation. *Advances in the Study of Behaviour*, **11**, 337–67.
Cherkin, A. (1971). Biphasic time course of performance after one-trial avoidance training in the chick. *Communications in Behavioural Biology*, **5**, 379–81.
Crowe, S. F. (1984). The effect of multiple presentation and hormonal modulation on weak memory traces: ability to produce long-term memory. Unpublished thesis, La Trobe University.
Crowe, S.F., Ng K. T., and Gibbs, M. E., (1989*a*). Memory formation processes in weakly reinforced learning. *Pharmacology Biochemistry and Behaviour*, **33**, 881–7.
Crowe, S. F., Ng, K. T. and Gibbs, M. E. (1989*b*). Effect of retraining trials on memory consolidation in weakly reinforced learning. *Pharmacology Biochemistry and Behaviour*, **33**, 889–94.
Crowe, S. F., Ng, K. T., and Gibbs, M. E. (1990). Consolidation of weakly reinforced learning experience by hormonal treatments. *Pharmacology Biochemistry and Behaviour*. (In press.)
Gibbs, M. E. (1983). Memory and behaviour: Birds and their memories. *Bird Behaviour*, **4**, 93–107.
Gibbs, M. E., deVaus, J. E., and Ng, K. T. (1986*a*). Effect of stress-related hormones on short-term memory. *Behavioural Brain Research*, **19**, 1–6.
Gibbs, M. E. and Ng, K. T. (1977). Psychobiology of memory. Towards a model of memory formation. *Biobehavioral Reviews*, **1**, 113–36.
Gibbs, M. E. and Ng, K. T. (1984*a*). Diphenylhydantoin extension of short-term and intermediate stages of memory. *Behavioural Brain Research*, **11**, 103–8.
Gibbs, M. E. and Ng, K. T. (1984*b*). Hormonal influence on the duration of short-term and intermediate stages of memory. *Behavioural Brain Research*, **11**, 109–16.
Gibbs, M. E. and Ng, K. T. (1984*c*). Dual action of cycloheximide. *Behavioural Brain Research*, **12**, 21–7.
Gibbs, M. E., Ng, K. T., and Andrew, R. J.(1986). Effect of testosterone on intermediate memory in day-old chicks. *Pharmacology, Biochemistry and Behavior*, **25**, 823–6.

18

Gonadal steroids and memory formation

P. G. Clifton

INTRODUCTION

In this chapter I have three aims. First, to review a number of studies which have examined the influence of gonadal steroids on the learning of the passive avoidance task so widely discussed in this book. Second, to examine the relationship between the effects of testosterone on this task and on a variety of other tasks and situations which have been studied in this species. Finally, I shall try to explore several issues which have not, as yet, received much experimental attention. Are these effect restricted to domestic fowl or, more generally, to birds, or may they also be observed in other vertebrates, especially mammals? Through what neural mechanisms are these effects produced and what neurotransmitter systems might be essential in mediating them?

THE ORIGINAL PHENOMENON

Our initial experiments uncovered a rather specific effect of testosterone on the bead task. We were using a slight variant of the standard procedure (Chapter 1) in which the birds, housed in pairs under white light, were initially pretrained on a sequence of two white, one red and one blue bead presentations. Each presentation lasted 10 seconds and was separated from the next by 5 minutes. After this the birds were left undisturbed for 2 hours. They were then given an aversive (methylanthranilate coated) presentation of a red bead similar to that used in pre-training. Finally, after a further 3 hours, the chicks were given test presentations of a red bead and, 5 minutes later, a blue bead. We recorded whether or not the birds pecked, the number of pecks and the number of behaviour patterns indicating overt avoidance. These included responses such as backing away from a bead and head shaking in its presence. The basic finding was that most birds given testosterone treatment 30 minutes before pre-training pecked the red bead at least once; birds treated only with vehicle, as expected, mostly did not peck at the test bead. Messent (1973) demonstrated opposition of training by pre-training with this experimental design

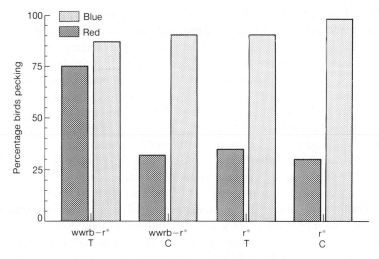

Fig. 18.1 The percentages of birds pecking either the red or blue test bead after aversive training on a red bead (r*), preceded by pre-training on two white, a red, and a blue bead (wwrb) and administration of either 12.5 mg testosterone oenanthate or vehicle, showing the basic enhancement effect of testosterone on pre-training. The raw data is taken from experiment 1 of Andrew *et al.* (1981), although in that paper mean pecking rates were presented. In all subsequent figures percentages are plotted and again, where necessary, the data has been reanalysed to present it in this form. Statistical analyses are given only where the data is presented for the first time (Figs 19.7 and 19.8).

several years earlier in an experiment which was itself a natural progression of Andrew's studies of attentional mechanisms in chicks (e.g. Andrew 1972). However, Messent gave the testosterone (as a long acting ester) two days or more before pre-training and training. The apparent rapidity with which testosterone was acting in our experiment was a surprise, since at that time the effects of steroids were almost always thought to involve an influence on genomic expression. This would inevitably be a much slower process than direct neural effects and therefore fitted well with the fact that steroids usually took many hours to produce any behavioural effect in the chick (Clifton and Andrew 1983).

These initial pilot studies said little about the underlying behavioural mechanisms. Were the testosterone-treated chicks unable to withold pecking to previously aversive bead? Had there been some gross effect on colour perception?

It soon became clear that underlying mechanism was not of this very general kind. Figure 18.1 shows the results of an experiment exactly like the one outlined above, except that two additional groups received testosterone or vehicle but *no* pre-training (experiment 1; Andrew *et al.*

1981). It is clear that only the group given both testosterone and pre-training pecked the red bead at higher than normal levels; there is no hint of similar effect in the testosterone-treated group given no pre-training. This is not the pattern that would be expected if these birds could not withold a pecking response to an object that had previously tasted unpleasant. Equally, it was clear that testosterone treatment was not simply producing a complete 'amnesia' for the red bead experience when it had been preceded by pre-training. This group of animals continued to show a reduced number of pecks at the red bead and some enhancement of overt avoidance behaviour, although the proportion of birds pecking the red bead was as high as that to the blue bead.

A second, and rather obvious test of the specificity of the effect was to ask whether the colour of the beads presented at pre-training influenced the opposition of training. In particular, did pre-training have to include a bead of the same appearance as that to be used in training? Our initial answer to this question was 'yes' (experiment 2; Andrew *et al*. 1981), but subsequently it became clear that this only held true when pre-training and training were separated by at least 30 minutes. Since the duration of the interval between pre-training and training also determines whether the phenomenon is seen at all, I will describe first the effects of varying that interval.

VARIED PRE-TRAINING–TRAINING INTERVALS

When the pre-training and aversive training experiences are separated by 2 hours then, in testosterone-treated birds, pre-training predominates in the sense that the birds are still prepared to peck the previously aversive bead. This suggests that recently experienced events are stored and become available to influence behaviour in a different way to more remote events. One approach to explaining such phenomena is to invoke a multiphase model of memory formation, and such a model had already been developed for the chick by Gibbs and Ng (1977; see Chapter 13). They suggested, initially on the basis of pharmacological interference with this task, that the memory for training passes through several stages. Each stage is serially dependent on the last and there may also be short transitional periods in which memory is relatively poor. Presumably, the memory of pre-training is supported in a similar way and so variation in the interval between pre-training and training might reveal something of the mechanisms underlying this testosterone-dependent phenomenon. Suppose, for example, that the effect was only seen when this interval exceeded 30–40 minutes. Since this would just allow the pre-training trace to establish in long-term memory, we could conclude that the effect

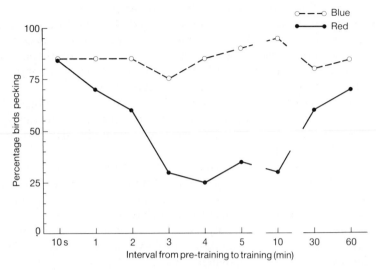

Fig. 18.2 Effects of varied pre-training–training intervals, showing the percentages of birds pecking either the red or blue test beads after training on a red bead and pre-training on a red bead. The interval between pre-training and training was varied as shown and the interval from training to test was held at 3 hours.

depended on interactions between a long-term trace (pre-training), and incoming information (training).

We carried out several experiments in which we systematically varied the pre-training—training interval. In the first we used exactly the same procedure as outlined earlier, with pre-training using small white (2), red and blue beads, training on a red bead and testing, 3 hours after training, on a red and a blue bead. In this experiment the interval between pre-training and training was varied between 10 minutes and 60 minutes. The timing here was between the red bead in pre-training and training. Since the blue pre-training bead followed 5 minutes after the red bead, the interval between the end of pre-training and training was only 5 minutes for the '10 minute' group. A large proportion of the testosterone-treated group pecked the red test bead when the interval was 30 minutes or more. At shorter intervals the proportion pecking did not differ from that seen in oil-treated birds. Inevitably in this experiment the timing of the pre-training–training was a little ambiguous, for pre-training itself lasted for 15 minutes. In addition, we could not examine the effect of very short intervals. The experiment was repeated using only a single red pre-training bead, allowing us to test intervals between 10 seconds and 60 minutes (Fig. 18.2). Again the birds were allowed 3 hours between training and testing. The results for the longer intervals duplicated those for the previous experiment; at intervals of 10 and 20 minutes the majority of birds, like similarly treated controls, failed to peck the red test bead, whereas at longer intervals they mostly pecked at this test bead (see also Chapter 19). There was little change in the numbers of birds pecking the blue bead at test. In fact, when the curves for the two experiments were superimposed they matched precisely, providing at least the timing in the first experiment was taken from the presentation of the red bead rather than from presentation of the first white or the final blue bead. The surprising result in this experiment was that at very short intervals, from 10 seconds to about 2 minutes, the testosterone-treated birds again tended to peck at the red test bead.

This result provided some puzzles. If there were two sets of intervals (less than 2 minutes and greater than 30 minutes) at which androgen-treated birds showed interference by pre-training with training, did this imply *two* different effects with the same behavioural outcome? If, on the other hand, these were two aspects of a single effect, could they be compatible with a serial model of memory formation for each of the two experiences? In fact, independent evidence already suggested subtle differences between the short and long interval effects. Messent (1973) had earlier described testosterone-dependent interference between pre-training and training with an interval of only 10 seconds; he also showed that the colour of the pre-training and training beads did not have to be the same. We already had preliminary evidence of colour specificity (i.e. the colour of the beads did have to be the same) when this interval was 2 hours. However, there were a large number of procedural differences between Messent's experiments and our own, in addition to the use of a very short interval. He had used internally illuminated glass spheres as stimuli and his chicks had been housed singly. We therefore directly compared the results from groups of birds given aversive red bead training preceded by either red or blue pre-training at intervals of both 10 seconds and 90 minutes. The result was clear (Fig. 18.3). At short intervals the pre-training bead need not be the same colour for interference to occur. At intermediate intervals no interference is expected, and at longer intervals interference is only seen when pre-training includes a bead of the same colour as the training bead. Subsequent experiments (e.g. Fig. 2 of Clifton *et al.* 1982) confirmed that the dependency of this short-term effect on the pre-training–training interval was very similar whether red or blue beads were used for pre-training; in both cases the effect disappeared when the interval exceeded 2–3 minutes, although there was a slight suggestion when pre-training with blue and training with red that the effect was already lost when the events were separated by 1 minute.

It now became possible to predict what might happen if the birds' memories for these two experiences were represented in a sequence of serially-dependent stores. In the case of short pre-training–training

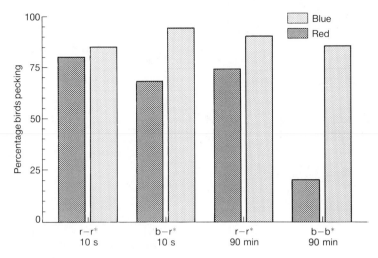

Fig. 18.3 Effect of colour specificity: A comparison of pre-training and training on either a bead of the same (red) or a different colour (blue) when the interval between the two experiences is either 10 seconds or 90 minutes.

intervals information relating to training might be held in the same short-term store which already holds the information concerning pre-training. Thus interference could result from interactions between these two representations in the same store. If this were the case then the results should quickly become apparent in the birds' behaviour. In the case of long pre-training-training intervals, the pre-training experience should already be represented in long-term memory before training occurred. Either interactions would have to occur between events represented in two different stores, or they would have to be postponed until both traces were in the same, long-term store.

VARIED TRAINING–TESTING INTERVALS

Since short- and long-term effects could be tentatively identified by the presence or absence of colour specificity in pre-training, it seemed sensible to examine the development of each effect separately after training. Messent (1973) had already suggested that the short-term effect developed almost immediately. In a replication of his experiment we used pre-training and training, both with a red bead, and separated by 10 seconds, with testosterone or vehicle given 30 minutes earlier. Different groups of birds were tested either 5 minutes or 3 hours after training. With both intervals the testosterone-treated birds tended to peck the red test bead and controls to avoid it (Fig. 18.4). This result contrasted strongly with

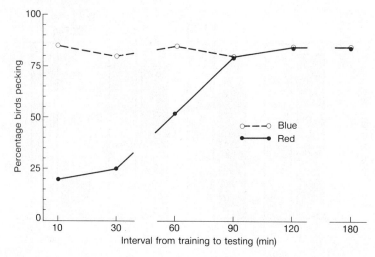

Fig. 18.4 The effect of increasing the interval between training and testing when pre-training was given 2 hours prior to training, showing the gradual appearance of a pre-training effect.

that obtained when pre-training and training were spaced by 2 hours. In this case separate groups of testosterone-treated birds were tested at between 10 minutes and 3 hours after training. The groups tested at shorter intervals (10 and 30 minutes) showed a low proportion pecking at the red test bead. Not until the interval was 90 minutes did the proportion of pecking increase to that typical of groups tested at the usual 3-hour interval. The timing of this gradual increase was very similar to that seen after birds were treated with the protein synthesis inhibitor cycloheximide (Gibbs and Ng 1977), which has been attributed to interference with the formation of 'long-term' memory.

Within a serial model of the Gibbs and Ng (1977) these two results can be fairly easily accommodated. If pre-training and training are separated by just a few seconds or minutes, interactions within the same short-term store could lead to some of the contradictory information provided by these two experiences failing to consolidate. In this case, for whatever reason, it is pre-training that predominates, in the sense that the birds remain prepared to peck at a red bead albeit with additional overt avoidance behaviour. When pre-training and training are separated by an intermediate interval, training predominates, perhaps because the processes that might lead to the consolidation of pre-training are in a vulnerable state and liable to change when contradictory information from training is presented. Finally, when pre-training and training are separated by a period which, in the Gibbs and Ng (1977) model, is sufficient to allow pre-training to begin consolidation into the long-term store, it becomes secure *in that store*. Thus training is unable to establish in the long-term store: however, this does not prevent it from remaining available from the previous stores that have a limited temporal span. This model has the advantage that it explains the timecourses of the effects we have observed without making many additional assumptions. The required additions to the model simply specify that when contradictory information is presented, then these contradictions will not be resolved until the information is represented in the same store, and that testosterone leads to more effective competition of pre-existing information within a store (either short- or long-term) with incoming information from either the environment or from an earlier store. Alternative explanations are considered below (p. 469).

VARIED INJECTION–TRAINING INTERVALS

In the introduction to this chapter, I suggested that a major surprise of our initial results was that the latency of this effect was rather short by comparison with facilitation by the same steroid of species-typical responses such as attack, copulation and vocal behaviour. In each of these cases the minimum latency is 2 days or more for a first administration of the hormone, although attack may show small changes within 7 hours in birds already primed with testosterone (Clifton and Andrew 1981).

We used the short-term effect, in which pre-training and training are completed within less than a minute, to determine the exact latency with which testosterone has its effects on this task. Separate groups of birds were tested 3 hours after training, having being injected between 60 and 10 minutes before training. The 10-minute interval produced little evidence for an effect (Fig. 18.5) but, providing that the interval was 20 minutes or greater, the effect was present. Taken with the prior evidence that, when pre-training and training are separated by only 10 seconds, enhanced pecking is observed at even very short training-test intervals, this result suggests that an upper estimate for the latency is between 10 and 20 minutes. Since testosterone was administered subcutaneously, this estimate includes the time required for appreciable levels to be found in the bloodstream (no more than 5 minutes; Andrew 1983) and for the steroid to be transported to the critical central structures and, if testosterone is not the active steroid, to be metabolized to the active form. An effect which, at the relevant neural site, was almost immediate would be perfectly compatible with these data.

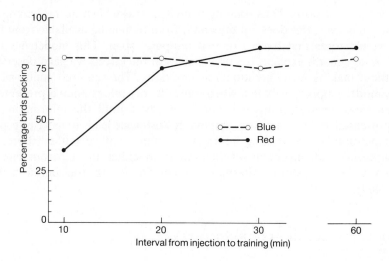

Fig. 18.5 The percentages of birds pecking the red and blue test beads when pre-training and training are separated by 2 minutes and are preceded, at an interval varying between 10 and 60 minutes, by testosterone administration, showing the short latency effect of testosterone.

STRUCTURE–ACTIVITY RELATIONSHIPS

In birds testosterone may be metabolized in one of three ways. Two pathways involve reduction to either 5-alpha-reduced compounds or 5-beta-reduced compounds (Massa *et al.* 1983). In both birds and mammals 5-alpha-reduced steroids, such as 5-alpha-dihydrotestosterone, are known to be behaviourally active. By contrast, despite one early contrary report (Balthazart and Hirshberg 1979), there is little evidence for behavioural effects of 5-beta-reduced metabolites. The high activity in this pathway in both young birds and long-term castrated individuals, who are refractory to the effects of testosterone, has suggested that its function may be as an 'inactivation shunt' (Hutchison and Steimer 1981). The third pathway of importance involves the aromatization of testosterone to oestradiol. Again oestradiol is known to be behaviourally effective in producing some effects of testosterone; aspects of sexual behaviour in mammals in one well-established example (Whalen and Luttge 1971). As a preliminary indication of structure-activity relationships, we carried out a dose–response study for testosterone, 5-alpha-dihydrotestosterone, 5-beta-dihydrotestosterone and 17-beta-oestradiol (Clifton *et al.* 1986). These steroids, injected as the propionates, were administered 30 minutes before pre-training on two white, one red, and one blue bead, in doses ranging from 10 ng to

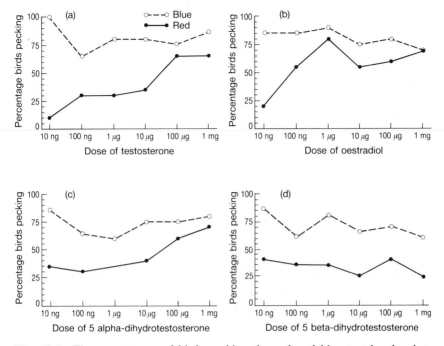

Fig. 18.6 The percentages of birds pecking the red and blue test beads when various steroids were injected 30 minutes before pre-training: (a) testosterone; (b) oestradiol; (c) 5-α-dihydrotestosterone; (d) 5-β-dihydrotestosterone. In each case propionates were used.

1 mg. Following the usual procedure the birds were trained on a methylanthranilate coated bead 2 hours after pre-training and tested on a red and then a blue bead after a further 3 hours (Fig. 18.6). 5-beta-dihydrotestosterone, in accordance with an 'inactivation-shunt' theory, was ineffective at any dose. 5-alpha-dihydrotestosterone became effective at a similar dose level (100 μg) to testosterone itself. However, the striking result was that oestradiol was effective at a dose of 100 ng (i.e. 100 times smaller than for the effective androgens). The result strongly suggested an oestrogenic effect.

This conclusion has been strengthened by the data from several previously unpublished experiments. MER-25 acts as a selective antagonist at oestrogen receptors (Södersten 1974), although in some situations it may also be a partial agonist (e.g. Roy and Wade 1976). In a first experiment with this compound we established that it could antagonize the effect of testosterone on our task. The birds were first injected with a dose of between 1 and 100 μg of MER-25. Thirty minutes later they were given 10 μg of testosterone in DMA. After another 30 minutes we began the

466   *P. G. Clifton*

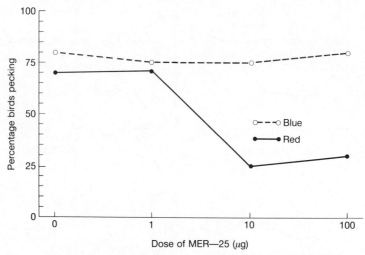

Fig. 18.7 Dose–response relationship: The percentages of birds pecking the red and blue test beads when testosterone administration was preceded by a varied dose of the anti-oestrogen MER-25. The numbers of birds pecking the red bead differ significantly with changes in the interval between injection and training $(\chi_3^2 = 16.68, p < 0.01)$.

regular sequence of pre-training (white, white, red, blue), training (aversive red) and testing (red, blue). Both 10 and 100 µg MER-25 antagonized the effect of testosterone, whereas 1 µg and the oil vehicle given alone were without effect (Fig. 18.7) and the resulting differences between groups were highly significant. A second experiment confirmed that this antagonism resulted from a specific effect rather than some combined effect of treatment with both compounds. In two groups of chicks either oil or 10 µg MER-25 was followed, after 30 minutes, by 10 µg of testosterone in DMA. In two further groups testosterone treatment *preceded* that with MER-25. As Fig. 18.8 demonstrates, MER-25 only antagonized the effect of testosterone if it was administered before the testosterone. Again, the differences between groups were highly significant. This pattern of results would be expected of a specific antagonism by MER-25, but would not be expected of a more general interaction between these two compounds.

Several other predictions can be made, although they have not been tested. For example, MER-25 should also interfere with the effects of oestradiol on this task; the effects of oestradiol should be stereoselective (the 17-alpha isomer should be much less active than the 17-beta isomer); inhibitors of the aromatization of testosterone to oestradiol such as ATD, which interfere with the facilitation of vocal behaviour by testosterone (Clifton and Andrew 1989), should also interfere with this effect of

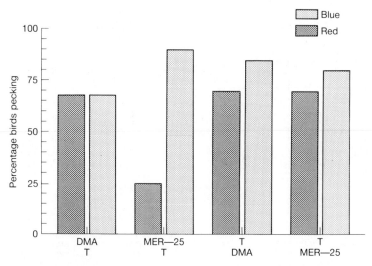

Fig. 18.8 Time-related effects of MER-25: The percentages of birds pecking the red and blue test beads when testosterone administration was preceded or followed by the administration of MER-25. The numbers of birds pecking the red bead differ significantly with treatment (χ^2_3 = 12.16. $p < 0.001$).

testosterone but should not interfere with the same behavioural effect when produced by oestradiol. The identification of an oestrogenic effect allows comparison with several other actions of steroids on avian behaviour. In particular, at least some of the effects of testosterone on attentional tasks are oestrogenic. For example, if male chicks are well trained to run down an alley for a food reward, they can be distracted either by changes in the object towards which they are running (the food dish), or in parts of the alley that are irrelevant to the current response (the side walls of the alley). Testosterone enhances distraction produced by the former manipulation but reduces distraction produced by the latter manipulation (Archer 1974). An appropriate dose of oestradiol dipropionate duplicates this effect (Clifton *et al.* 1988). This effect also occurs with short latency; the birds were administered the steroid 30 minutes before the test.

Since all of these oestrogenic effects have similar properties they may act through a single neural mechanism (see Chapter 19). However, not all effects that might potentially be interpreted in terms of attentional mechanisms act through oestrogenic mechanisms. Androgens retard the extinction of a conditioned taste aversion in both rats (Early and Leonard 1978) and chicks (Clifton and Andrew 1987) but, in both cases, this is an androgenic effect. Recent evidence from chicks indicates separate andro-genic and oestrogenic events during extinction of food-rewarded running

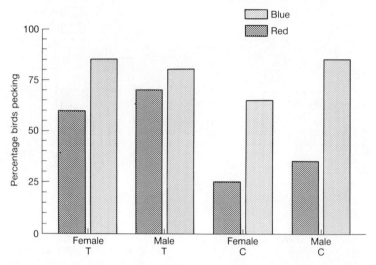

Fig. 18.9 Possible sex differences: The percentages of male or female birds pecking the red and blue test beads after administration of either testosterone or vehicle, showing similar responses of male and female chicks.

in an alley like the one described above. The former involves vigorous repetition of all responses that were previously successful (e.g. pecks at and approaches to the food dish) and the latter involves stabilization of attention on the food dish which, during extinction only, is covered with a transparent lid (Andrew and Klein, personal communication).

SEX DIFFERENCES

Many effects of gonadal steroids are sex dependent. Thus testosterone strongly facilitates attack in male chicks, of which pecking at objects larger than about 10 mm diameter is a prominent component. However the hormone has little effect on attack pecking in females, although enhanced attention to objects that would normally evoke such a response is clearly evident (Andrew 1966; Clifton *et al.* 1986). In this task male and female chicks respond very similarly to testosterone treatment. We demonstrated this using the familiar procedure of androgen treatment (12.5 mg testosterone oenanthate in 0.05 ml arachis oil) followed, after 30 minutes, by pre-training on two white, a red and a blue bead. Two hours later the birds were trained on a red bead and, after a further 3 hours, they were tested on first a red bead and then a blue bead. The results, seen in Fig. 18.9, show that the proportion of testosterone-treated and control birds pecking the red test bead were very different, but there is no evidence of any effect of sex on the proportion of birds pecking; data for mean pecking rates, presented by Clifton *et al.* (1986), showed a similar lack of effect. The dose of testosterone used in this experiment was well above threshold and it is important to note that there are small but consistent differences in threshold doses between male and female birds (Rainey 1983). However, it is not possible to say whether this represents a difference in the sensitivity of central structures to the steroids, or a result of peripheral sex differences.

A BEHAVIOURAL PERSPECTIVE

At this point it may be interesting to place our bead task in a wider context and to examine other behavioural models used to explain similar effects. For example, Best and Gemberling (1977) describe how, if rats are presented with a flavour 3.5 hours before it is used as a conditioned stimulus (CS) in flavour aversion training, the experience interferes with acquisition of the flavour-illness pairing. This interference, described as 'latent inhibition', is much reduced when the flavour is presented either 30 minutes or 1 week before the second exposure. Whitlow (1975) has described a similar effect in rabbits habituating to two tone presentations separated by a variable interval, although in this case the time scale was considerably abbreviated.

These results may be interpreted within the general framework of Wagner's (1981) Standard Operating Procedures (SOP) model. The model, which is essentially one of attentional mechanisms, proposes that when a stimulus is initially attended to, it is represented in an active (A1) state. This state, which ensures that the animal attends to the stimulus and can associate it with concurrent events (e.g. a bad taste in the mouth), is maintained by a rehearsal-like mechanism but decays fairly rapidly into a second A2 state. The stimulus will still be attended to, but will dominate attention to a lesser extent than in the A1 state; in particular it will not be capable of being associated with other events. The A2 state decays, rather more slowly, into an inactive (I) state. When either the same or a similar stimulus is presented on a second occasion then, providing the original representation is in the I state, it will be activated into either the A1 or the A2 state depending on its familiarity. However, representations in the A2 state cannot be moved into the A1 state. Thus the repeated presentation of a stimulus at an interval after which the first presentation has decayed to the A2 state interferes with learning based on that second presentation; Best and Gemberling's rats show reduced avoidance at test and Whitlow's rabbits show reduced habituation.

This model would also be able to account for our test data obtained 3 hours after varied pre-training intervals if we assume, first, that testosterone affects the processing of stimuli represented in the A1 state, and second, that because of the salience of beads and their great ability to evoke response, a representation of a bead in I will most likely be returned to A1 rather than A2 if the same bead is presented on a second occasion. At short intervals the representation of the red bead from pre-training would be in the A1 state when the red aversive bead was pecked. Testosterone could therefore influence, in favour of the pre-training representation, what remained in A1 and subsequently passed into A2 and then I; these birds would peck the red test bead. At intermediate intervals the representation of pre-training would be in the A2 state and so would not be returned to A1; as a result the representation of training would pass into the A1 state and would eventually pass into A2 and, finally, I. Testosterone would have no opportunity to influence processing and the animals would avoid the red test bead. Finally, with long pre-training–training intervals, the representation of pre-training would be in the I state at the time of training. It could then be retrieved to the A1 state with the same result as for short pre-training–training intervals. The model predicts, perhaps counterintuitively, that, in controls, either a less effective US at training or more effective pre-training should lead to *intermediate* pre-training–training intervals producing latent inhibition more readily than either short or long intervals. This would occur because, with intermediate intervals, the concurrent A2 representation of the red bead should block the association of the red test bead and its taste.

The formal operations underlying this account and that derived from the Gibbs and Ng model are obviously similar, even though they are couched in rather different language. However, there are two important results that might initially seem to favour an account in terms of stages of memory. Wagner's model would suggest that the results of short or long pre-training–training intervals should be identical, since in both cases the interactions occur while the stimuli are represented in the A1 state. Yet this is not the case, because the effects of long pre-training–training intervals only gradually become apparent, whereas those of short pre-training–training intervals are evident almost immediately. However, the model was not designed to explain time-courses of memory formation and, in any case, Wagner has suggested that the actual time-courses of the effects he discusses may vary widely from one situation to another. In addition, the long-term effect shows colour specificity whereas the short-term effect does not. One might suppose that the short-term representation would be the most accurate and hence colour specificity would, if there were any difference, be expected for the short-term rather than the long-term effect. Equally, it might be that, on retrieval from I, cues such as colour determine whether the activation is to A1 or A2. If a difference in colour between training and pre-training beads made it more likely that the pre-training I trace were activated to A2 rather than A1, then our result would be predicted. Thus much of our data can be accommodated within the general framework of this model. Clearly, it would be interesting to investigate the detailed time-courses of other situations that the Wagner model was designed to explain. The development of conditioned flavour aversions would be an obvious example for which there is already a large body of empirical data.

UNDERLYING MECHANISMS

The rapidity with which testosterone affects performance in this task clearly distinguishes it from actions of steroids which involve genomic interactions. However, there are a number of reports of gonadal steroids exerting rapid effects on neural activity. Kelly *et al.* (1977) showed that rapid inhibition by gonadal steroids of cell firing in the preoptic area was stereoselective; 17-β-oestradiol produced the effect whereas 17-α-oestradiol did not. They also failed to detect oestrogen-sensitive cells in several other sites (cortex, hippocampus, and thalamus). Orsini *et al.* (1985) reported that lateral hypothalamic/median forebrain bundle cells may show either non-specific steroid suppression of activity or selective increases in responding after microiontophoresis of testosterone. More recent papers have emphasized that extra-hypothalamic sites may also be responsive to steroids. In both the rat and guinea-pig hippocampus, cells can react with increased firing rates after a short period of exposure to low steroid concentrations. In this case hippocampal slices derived from male or female animals were responsive only to 'heterotypical' steroids (i.e. testosterone stimulated the female hippocampus and oestradiol the male hippocampus). No dose–response data were presented, so it is not possible to say whether this sex difference resulted from shifted thresholds or absolute insensitivity to certain steroids (Chiaia *et al.* 1983).

The underlying neurochemical basis of these effects is not clear, nor am I aware of studies in which hippocampal recordings have been made *in vivo* after peripheral administration of physiological doses of hormones. However, positive effects of this kind have been achieved in at least two other cases. Levesque and Di Paolo (1988) confirmed that an injection of 100 ng of 17-β-oestradiol produces increases in striatal dopamine metabolites, reflecting increased dopamine turnover, within 15 minutes. In addition, they demonstrated changes in the affinity states of striatal dopamine receptors. In addition, Becker and Cha (1989) have shown that amphetamine-stimulated release of dopamine varies over the oestrous cycle of female rats, suggesting modulation by natural variation in the levels of ovarian hormones; such actions should also be seen in the context of the greater likelihood of neuroleptic-induced motor disorders in women (Van Hartes-veltd and Joyce 1986). There is also increasing evidence for an involvement of ascending dopamine systems in attentional mechanisms (Robbins and Everitt 1987), so they must be prime candidates for further experimental study of the phenomena described here, given the similar profile of the attentional and memory effects outlined on p. 467.

Finally, Smith *et al.* (1987 *a,b*) have demonstrated effects of oestradiol and progesterone on the responsiveness of cerebellar Purkinje cells to excitatory and inhibitory amino acids. Typically, oestradiol enhanced the response of Purkinje cells to glutamate within 10–35 minutes of peripheral administration. 17-α-oestradiol had a smaller and transient effect but tamoxifen, and anti-oestrogen, was unable to inhibit the effect. Low steroid doses produced specific increases in responsiveness to glutamate, although higher doses also increased background firing rates. Progester-one, administered under similar conditions, enhanced responses to GABA; this effect does not involve protein synthesis, since it was not reversed by anisomycin. The latter action may be closely related to a barbiturate-like effect of progesterone derivatives at the GABA receptor (Harrison *et al.* 1987). Other steroids, including certain oestrogen metab-olites, act as antagonists at the same receptor site (Majewska 1987).

This restricted literature reveals rapid effects of gonadal steroids on both amino acid and catecholamine neurotransmitters through which the behavioural effects discussed earlier may act. Recent evidence indicates that such studies may not simply be of academic interest. Plasma levels of dehydroepiandrosterone (DHEA), an important precursor of both andro-gens and oestrogens, are reduced in aged individuals and in those with Alzheimer's disease (Sunderland *et al.* 1989). Flood *et al.* (1988) have shown that i.c.v. or s.c. administration of DHEA can reverse the amnesia produced by cholinergic blockade (scopolamine) or protein synthesis inhibition (anisomycin). Testosterone, in the chick, also reverses the amnesia produced by protein synthesis inhibition (Gibbs, Andrew, and Clifton, unpublished). In mice DHEA also reverses the milder amnesia that results from normal ageing (Flood and Roberts 1988). If the effects described by Flood have a similar structure–activity relationship to that reported for our work, then further behavioural studies in chicks, in which temporal and drug parameters can be quickly and easily varied, would be strongly justified.

Acknowledgements

I would like to acknowledge support from the AFRC (UK), and the contribution of Richard Andrew to the ideas developed in this chapter.

REFERENCES

Andrew, R. J. (1966). Precocious adult behaviour in the young chick. *Animal Behaviour*, **14**, 485–500.

Andrew, R. J. (1972). Recognition processes and behaviour, with special reference to the effects of testosterone on persistence. *Advances in the Study of Behavior*, **44**, 175–208.

Andrew, R. J. (1983). Specific short latency effects of oestradiol and testosterone on distractibility and memory formation in the young domestic chick. In *Hormones and behaviour in higher vertebrates*, (ed. J. Balthazart *et al.*), pp. 463–73. Springer-Verlag, Berlin.

Andrew, R. J., Clifton, P. G., and Gibbs, M. E. (1981). Enhancement of effectiveness of learning by testosterone in domestic chicks. *Journal of Comparative and Physiological Psychology*, **95**, 406–17.

Archer, J. (1974). The effects of testosterone on the distractibility of chicks by irrelevant and relevant novel stimuli. *Animal Behaviour*, **22**, 397–404.

Balthazart, J. and Hirschberg, D. (1979). Testosterone metabolism and sexual behaviour in the chick. *Hormones and Behavior*, **12**, 253–63.

Becker, J. B. and Cha, J. H. (1989). Estrous cycle-dependent variation in amphetamine-induced behaviours and striatal dopamine release assessed with microdialysis. *Behavioural Brain Research*, **35**, 117–25.

Best, M. R. and Gemberling, G. A. (1977). Role of short-term processes in the conditioned stimulus preexposure effect and the delay of reinforcement gradient in long-delay taste aversion learning. *Journal of Experimental Psychology: Animal Behavior Processes*, **3**, 253–63.

Chambers, K. C. (1987) Sexual dimorphism as an index of hormonal influences on conditioned food aversions. *Annals of the New York Academy of Sciences*, **443**, 110–25.

Chiaia, N, Foy, M., and Teyler, T. J. (1983). The hampster hippocampal slice: II. Neuroendocrine modulation. *Behavioral Neuroscience*, **97**, 839–43.

Clifton, P. G. and Andrew, R. J. (1981). A comparison of the effects of testosterone on aggressive responses by the domestic chick to the human hand and to a large sphere. *Animal Behaviour*, **29**, 610–20.

Clifton, P. G., and Andrew, R. J. (1987). Gonadal steroids and the extinction of conditioned taste aversions in young domestic fowl. *Physiology and Behavior*, **39**, 27–31.

Clifton, P. G. and Andrew, R. J. (1989). Contrasting effects of pre- and post-hatch exposure to gonadal steroids on the development of vocal, aggressive and sexual behaviour of young domestic chicks. *Hormones and Behavior*, **23**, 572–89.

Clifton, P. G., Andrew, R. J., and Gibbs, M. E. (1982). Limited period of action of testosterone on memory formation. *Journal of Comparative and Physiological Psychology*, **96**, 212–22.

Clifton, P. G. and Andrew, R. J. (1983). The role of stimulus size and colour in the elicitation of testosterone-facilitated aggressive and sexual responses in the domestic chick. *Animal Behaviour*, **31**, 878–86.

Clifton, P. G., Andrew, R. J., and Rainey, C. J. (1986). Effects of gonadal steroids on attack and memory processing in the domestic chick. *Physiology and Behavior*, 37, 701–7.

Clifton, P. G., Andrew, R. J., and Brighton, L. (1988). Gonadal steroids and attentional mechanisms in young domestic chicks. *Physiology and Behavior*, 43, 441–6.

Early, C. J. and Leonard, B. E. (1978). Androgenic involvement in conditioned taste aversion. *Hormones and Behavior*, 11, 1–11.

Flood, J. F. and Roberts, E. (1988). Dehydroepiandrosterone sulfate improves memory in aging mice. *Brain Research*, 448, 178–81.

Flood, J. F., Smith, G. E., and Roberts, E. (1988). Dehydroepiandrosterone and its sulfate enhance memory retention in mice. *Brain Research*, 447, 267–78.

Foy, M. R. and Teyler, T. J. (1983). 17-alpha-estradiol and 17-beta-estradiol in the hippocampus. *Brain Research Bulletin*, 10, 735–9.

Gibbs, M. E. and Ng, K. T. (1977). Psychobiology of memory: towards a model of memory formation. *Biobehavioral Reviews*, 1, 113–36.

Gibbs, M. E. and Ng, K. T. (1979). Behavioral stages in memory formation. *Neuroscience Letters*, 13, 279–83.

Harding, C. F., Sheridan, K., and Walters, M. J. (1983). Hormonal specificity and activation of sexual behavior in male zebra finches. *Hormones and Behavior*, 17, 111–32.

Harrison, N. L., Majewska, M. D., Harrington, J. W., and Barker, J. L. (1987). Structure-activity relationships for steroid interaction with the γ-aminobutyric acid-A receptor complex. *Journal of Pharmacology and Experimental Therapeutics*, 241, 346–53.

Hutchison, J. B. and Steimer, T. (1981). Brain 5-beta reductase: a correlate of behavioral sensitivity to androgen. *Science*, 213, 244–6.

Kelly, M. J., Moss, R. L., Dudley, C. A., and Fawcett, C. P. (1977). The specificity of the response of preoptic-septal area neurons to estrogen: 17-alpha-estradiol versus 17-beta-estradiol and the response of extrahypothalamic neurons. *Experimental Brain Research*, 30, 43–52.

Komisarak, B. and Beyer, C. (1972). Differential antagonism, by MER-25, of behavioral and morphological effects of estradiol benzoate in rats. *Hormones and Behavior*, 3, 63–70.

Levesque, D. and DiPaolo, T. (1988). Rapid conversion of high into low striatal D2-dopamine receptor agonist binding states after an acute physiological dose of 17-beta-estradiol. *Neuroscience Letters*, 88, 113–18.

Majewska, M. D. (1987). Antagonist-type interactions of glucocorticoids with the GABA-coupled chloride channel. *Brain Research*, 418, 377–82.

Massa, R., Bottoni, L., and Lucini, L. (1983). Brain testosterone metabolism and sexual behaviour in birds. In *Hormones and behaviour in higher vertebrates* (ed. J. Balthazart *et al.*), pp. 230–6. Springer-Verlag, Berlin.

Messent, P. R. (1973). Distractibility and persistence of chicks. D. Phil. Thesis, University of Sussex, UK.

Orsini, J. C., Barone, F. C., Armstrong, D. L., and Wayner, M. J. (1985). Direct effects of androgens on lateral hypothalamic neuronal activity in the male rat: I A microiontophoretic study. *Brain Research Bulletin*, 15, 193–297.

Rainey, C. (1983). Steroid specificity and memory in the chick. D. Phil. Thesis, University of Sussex, UK.

Robbins, T. W. and Everitt, B. J. (1987). Psychopharmacological studies of arousal and attention. In *Cognitive neurochemistry*, (ed. S. M. Stahl, S. D. Iverson and E. C. Goodman). Oxford University Press.

Roy, E. J. and Wade, G. N. (1976). Estrogenic effects of an antiestrogen, MER-25, on eating and body weight in rats. *Journal of Comparative and Physiological Psychology*, **90**, 156–66.

Sodersten, P. (1974). Effects of an estrogen antagonist MER-25, on mounting behaviour and lordosis behaviour in the female rat. *Hormones and Behavior*, **5**, 111–21.

Smith, S. S., Waterhouse, B. D., and Woodward, D. J. (1987*a*.) Sex steroid effects on extrahypothalamic CNS. I. Estrogen augments neuronal responsiveness to iontophoretically applies glutamate in the cerebellum. *Brain Research*, **422**, 40–51.

Smith, S. S., Waterhouse, B.D., and Woodward, D. J. (1987*b*.) Sex steroid effects on extrahypothalamic CNS. II. Progesterone, alone and in combination with estrogen, modulates cerebellar responses to amino acid neurotransmitters. *Brain Research*, **422**, 52–62.

Sunderland, T., Merril, C. R., Harrington, M. G., Lawlor, B. A., Molchan, S. E., Martinez, R., and Murphy, D. L. (1989). Reduced plasma dehydroepian-drosterone concentrations in Alzheimer's disease. *Lancet*, 570.

Van Hartesvelt, C. and Joyce, J. N. (1986). Effects of estrogen on the basal ganglia. *Neuroscience and Biobehavioral Reviews*, **10**, 1–14.

Wagner, A. R. (1981). SOP: A model of automatic memory processing in animal behavior. In *Information processing in animals: memory mechanisms* (ed. N. E. Spear and R. R. Miller), pp. 5–47. Lawrence Erlbaum, Hillsdale, NJ.

Whalen, R. E. and Luttge, W. G. (1971). Testosterone, androstenedione and dihydrotestosterone: effects on mating behavior of male rats. *Hormones and Behavior*, **2**, 117–25.

Whitlow, J. W. (1975). Short-term memory in habituation and dishabituation. *Journal of Experimental Psychology: Animal Behavior Processes*, **1**, 189–206.

19

Cyclicity in memory formation

R. J. Andrew

Much of the argument in this chapter depends on evidence that the trace(s) held in right and left hemisphere contain differing accounts of the same experience, and that events during memory formation give the opportunity for comparison and reconciliation of these two accounts. The first section therefore considers the probable nature of the differences between right and left hemisphere traces in chicks using both eyes and in monocular chicks. I then present evidence that brief episodes of unusually good retrieval (retrieval events) recur cyclically, following learning in the chick, and that these cycles have different periods in the right and left hemispheres. There is clearly a close causal connection between retrieval cycles and phases of memory: the first retrieval events coincide in time (Fig. 19.1) with the transitions between the main phases of memory formation, which are described in Chapter 13. The third section discusses how the two sets of phenomena may be related. I next examine in more detail the nature of the processes which appear to occur at those retrieval events, which are of most importance in memory formation. The implications of postponement of features of memory formation by hormones (Chapter 17) are then considered and the chapter concludes with more general issues.

DIFFERENCES BETWEEN TRACES IN THE TWO HEMISPHERES

A major assumption of this chapter is that, following learning, the two hemispheres contain different versions of the experience. As a result, interaction between the hemispheres can bring about sharply timed change in the information available to the hemisphere which controls response at test. Hemispheric specialization in the chick is considered in Chapter 21. Briefly, the right hemisphere tends to store a detailed description of the experience as a unique event set in a specific spatial context. The left hemisphere tends to relate selected properties of the stimulus to consequences of response, and as a result, is better able to categorize stimuli, and to decide on the appropriate response.

Much of the evidence which follows derives from experiments in which

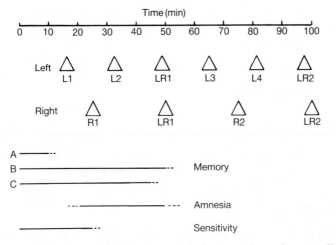

Fig. 19.1 Cyclicity in retrieval. The model shows points of unusually good retrieval which repeat cyclically in right and left hemispheres following learning (timed at 0 minutes). The right hemisphere cycle has a period of about 25 minutes, and the left hemisphere cycle one of about 16 minutes. These are estimates based on the timings of R1, L1, and L2 (text). They result in a slight progressive shift in phase relations such that at LR2 the two cycles are less completely in phase than at LR1. It is, of course, impossible to tell on present evidence whether such a shift is really to be expected. There is evidence (McKenzie, unpublished) that the cycles continue beyond 100 minutes, at least under some conditions. A number of other procedures show sudden change to occur at or very close to these retrieval events; uncertainty in the timing of those illustrated here is shown by the dotted portion of the lines. After ouabain (A) memory disappears a little before L1 (Chapter 13); after anisomycin (B) it persists up to LR1 (Chapter 13). Training with diluted aversant (Chapter 17) produces inhibition of pecking up to just before LR1 (C). After hypoxia, there is temporary amnesia (Chapter 14) starting just after L1, and finishing at LR1. Sensitivity to a number of amnestic agents disappears sharply between R1 and L2 (Chapters 13, 16, 17).

only one eye is in use. Here the differences between the information held in the two hemispheres are likely to be more profound. Indeed, it is usually assumed that in birds the memory trace forms only in the hemisphere contralateral to the eye which is used in monocular viewing. This is probably often true when the lateral visual field is used to fixate the stimulus. Goodale and Graves (1980) review a large literature, and show that interocular transfer* fails when there is lateral viewing, whether vision is restricted to one eye by covering the other, or by the head

---

* In tests of interocular transfer, animals are trained with one eye in use and then tested with the other in use. Transfer is held to be complete when such animals show as good retention as others which are tested with the same eye in use at training and testing (see also Chapter 3).

position of the bird. Here then the non-seeing hemisphere itself appears to hold little relevant information; it also has little or no access to the trace held by its partner. Predominant use of the lateral visual field during viewing may explain, for example, failure of chicks to show interocular transfer when trained to distinguish two simultaneously presented patterns whilst pecking for heat reward (Gaston 1979).

In contrast, Goodale and Graves (*loc cit.*) showed that frontal fixation allowed interocular transfer in pigeons. In chicks, good interocular transfer has long been known (Cherkin 1970) to occur in the aversive bead task (in which the bead is fixated frontally). The question is, does interocular transfer here depend upon access at test to a trace laid down in the hemisphere which was fed by the uncovered eye at training, or does a trace of some sort form at some point after training in both hemispheres?

It is worth remembering that, even with both eyes in use, it is common in birds for the left and right visual systems to work largely independently. When birds are using the standard resting position with diverged optical axes, or during independent scanning by the two eyes, even the frontal visual fields of the two eyes see different stimuli (Wallman and Pettigrew 1985); only after convergence is binocular viewing possible. It is therefore almost certain that for much of the time in normal vision each eye provides an input which is confined for initial analysis to the contralateral visual system; binocular units presumably either cease to function or disregard ipsilateral input. However, it is not clear what may happen during viewing with one frontal visual field, when one eye is covered. It is possible that binocular units in the ipsilateral visual system may make use of the input from the seeing eye (Pettigrew 1979; Denton 1981); it will be, after all, the only one which they receive.

The earliest stages of memory formation following bead training do seem to be predominantly carried out by the hemisphere fed by the uncovered eye (hereafter the 'contralateral' hemisphere). Bell and Gibbs (1977) administered amnestic agents 2 minutes after training to one or the other hemisphere, and showed that injection of the ipsilateral hemisphere at this time had no effect. Delayed loss of memory resulted from injection of the contralateral hemisphere, at times characteristic of the agent employed. Up to the time of loss, memory could be demonstrated through either eye; after the time of loss, amnesia was shown, again irrespective of eye. This strongly suggests that the hemisphere which is ipsilateral at training depends (at least at first) on access to the trace held in its partner to guide response. However, a subsequent study (Hodge *et al.* 1981) noted that such evidence does not exclude spontaneous duplication of the trace in the untrained hemisphere after the periods of early sensitivity to amnestic agents are over. Greif (1976) reached a similar conclusion, having found that large bilateral lesions on the hyperstriatum 2 or more hours after learning cause amnesia, but similar unilateral lesions, whether of the trained or untrained hemisphere, are without effect.

It is likely, in fact, that some version of the experience is stored in the ipsilateral hemisphere following learning. Gaston (1980) argued that monocular exposure to a green sweet solution, followed by the induction of illness, sets up quite different traces in the two hemispheres. Tests using the same eye as at training showed aversion to the appearance of the solution (i.e. green colour) but not to its taste. In contrast, tests with the other eye showed aversion to the taste of the solution, but not to its appearance. The hemisphere which could not see at training (or could not see well: above) of course had as good access to taste information as its partner.

It is possible that any trace in the ipsilateral hemisphere also contains from the start at least some visual information. As has already been noted, it potentially receives direct visual input from the frontal visual field of the uncovered eye through the ipsilateral projections which allow binocular input to visual units in birds (Chapters 3, 20). The effectiveness of such a direct input (if indeed it occurs) is likely to be reduced further by overall depression of visual function in the ipsilateral hemisphere, deprived as it is of all direct input from its own eye. Nevertheless, some visual information may be available early in trace formation in the ipsilateral hemisphere. In addition, the ipsilateral hemisphere presumably feels the bead in the bill and tastes something bitter, if methylanthranilate is present. Traces are thus likely to be set up simultaneously in both hemispheres (although of very different character). Even in the monocular condition, then, memory formation timed from learning should proceed in both hemispheres, and allow interactions with the same timings as in normal memory formation with both eyes in use.

CYCLIC REPETITION OF EPISODES OF GOOD OR BAD RETRIEVAL

There is long standing evidence for cyclicity in ease of recall following learning in the rat. A single period of poor retrieval was described by Kamin (review, Brush 1971). Longer time courses (Holloway 1978) revealed cyclically recurring periods of poor retrieval with a cycle length of 12 hours (or possibly some smaller interval: the sampling interval was, in general, 6 hours). In the chick, brief periods of poor retrieval (Gibbs and Ng 1977; Chapter 17) and of good retrieval (Andrew and Brennan 1985) have both been described. The possibility that such periods might repeat cyclically in the chick was first raised by Andrew (1985). It will be shown here that, in the chick, episodes of good retrieval recur in the left hemisphere with a period of about 16 minutes, and in the right hemisphere with a period of about 25 minutes. As a result, good retrieval coincides in both hemispheres at about 50 minutes after learning (and at 100 and perhaps 150 minutes: Fig. 19.1).

The evidence for the existence of these cycles will be presented as follows:

1. A wide variety of procedures have shown that two transitions, which are of great importance in memory formation, occur at 25/30 and 50/55 minutes after training.
2. Closer study of the periods around 25 and 30 minutes revealed good retrieval associated with the right hemisphere at about 25 minutes, and with the left hemisphere at a time around 32 minutes.
3. A retrieval test, which is likely to be particularly sensitive to changes in right hemisphere performance, revealed a 25-minute cycle in left-eyed birds, running through at least three cycles, with the first retrieval event at 25 minutes.
4. A procedure involving unilateral hemispheric injection with the amnestic agent, sotalol, revealed brief episodes of sensitivity in the left hemisphere, which repeated cyclically with a period of a little over 16 minutes. The first clear episode of sensitivity was about 32 minutes, and so coincided with the episode of good retrieval through the left hemisphere, which is mentioned above.
5. A first episode in the left hemisphere at about 16 minutes was thus strongly suggested by the properties of the cycle, but not revealed with certainty by sotalol. Evidence from other tests is cited to show that such an episode indeed exists.

Transitions at 25/30 and 50/55 minutes

Delayed loss of memory following the administration of protein synthesis inhibitors (anisomycin, cycloheximide) very soon after learning occurs between 50 and 55 minutes (Chapter 13; Gibbs and Ng 1977, 1984); temporary amnesia ceases at about the same time (Chapter 14). The same transition is also followed by a brief worsening of retrieval at 55 minutes (Chapter 17).

The earlier transition was first revealed by a sudden loss of sensitivity between 25 and 30 minutes to the β-adrenergic antagonist sotalol (Stephenson and Andrew 1981). Changes at exactly this time were subsequently demonstrated by two other procedures: reappearance of ability of a first experience with a clean red bead to compete with subsequent training with an ill-tasting bead (Clifton *et al.* 1982: Chapter 18) and loss of sensitivity to a quite different amnestic agent: dinitrophenol (Gibbs and Ng 1984; Chapters 13, 17). The periodic relationship between the timing of onset of these two transitions (25 and 50 minutes) provided the first hint of possible cycles in retrieval.

Retrieval events at the 25/30 transition

Two such events, one at 25 and one at 30–32 minutes were first demonstrated in binocular birds. They were then shown by tests with monocular
birds (involving both simple recall and experiments in which sotalol was
give unilaterally) to be associated with an event in the right hemisphere at
25 minutes, and the left hemisphere at about 32 minutes (Andrew and
Brennan 1985).

Cyclicity in right hemisphere

Direct evidence for cyclic repetition of the right hemisphere retrieval
events has been provided by a test which was originally designed to study
differences in the way which left and right-eyed birds analyse stimuli.
Briefly, in standard habituation tests, beads are offered for pecking in
pairs of presentations each 15 seconds in duration, with an interval of 5
seconds; pairs of presentations are separated by 120 minutes. Pecking
shows a predictable and relatively steep habituation. The degree of
dishabituation due to specific changes in the properties of the bead
indicates what sort of change is judged to be significant. Left-eyed birds
(right hemisphere) show much more interest in changes in appearance and
position than do right-eyed birds: indeed, right-eyed birds (left hemisphere) make use of only the most general features of the bead as they
first saw it, when assessing later presentations (Andrew 1983a; Chapter
21). Such birds treat beads illuminated internally with red or violet light,
and unlit beads as fully equivalent, for example, The very precise character
of the information retained and used by left-eyed birds, in contrast,
suggested that this test should be unusually sensitive to changes in the
ability of the right hemisphere to recall.

Systematic variation of the interval between pairs of presentations
revealed maximal habituation (i.e. best recall) not only at 25 minutes, when
it would be predicted from the results which have already been presented,
but also at 49 and 75 minutes (Fig. 19.2). The times of tests were chosen
before cyclicity was suspected, so that it is difficult to tell whether cyclicity
continues after 75 minutes; by 115 minutes habituation seems to remain very
marked in left-eyed birds, independently of timing of test.

Cyclicity in left hemisphere

Andrew and Brennan (1985) injected either right or left hemispheres with
the amnestic agent sotalol, in birds using right or left eye in a 2 by 2
design; memory was disturbed only when injection coincided with a
retrieval event in the injected hemisphere (25 minutes, right; 32.5 minutes,
left hemisphere). Unexpectedly, even this was true only if the injected

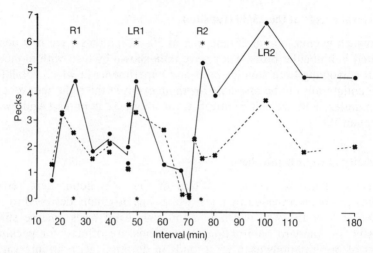

Fig. 19.2 Memory shown by habituation of pecking. The mean difference in number of pecks evoked at the first, and a subsequent presentation of a violet-lit bead, is shown for chicks using either the right or the left eye (RE, LE); the other eye was covered by a temporary paper patch. The larger the measure, the greater was the habituation, and so (presumably) the better the memory of the first presentation. The time between presentations varied from 16 to 180 minutes; every point is for a separate group of chicks (usually 18–20). Note the coincidence of the three peaks with the predicted timings of good retrieval through the right hemisphere (R1, LR1, R2, LR2: as in Fig. 19.1). A fourth peak could be present at 100 minutes, preceded by a trough: the spacing of points leaves this open. Beyond 100 minutes (110 minutes here; 120 minutes in Chapter 21) LE birds show marked habituation and RE birds only moderate habituation irrespective of time of test. (Statistical analysis and methods: see Appendix.)

hemisphere was ipsilateral to the eye in use. Since the contralateral hemisphere is almost certain to contain a trace describing training (which is evidently resistant to direct action of sotalol), it was argued that amnesia was here being produced by disruption of interaction between the hemispheres. Andrew and Brennan (*loc. cit.*) suggested that this most probably involved disturbance of information transfer from the injected hemisphere, during the retrieval event, so that the hemisphere containing the main trace received and incorporated degraded information. This hypothesis will be developed further, and used later to explain a number of other experimentally-induced amnesias.

Memory disturbance was shown in the original study by either the appearance of pecking of aversive (red) bead, or by marked depression of pecking at the neutral (blue) bead, presumably due to generalization. Interestingly for present purposes, the latter index also showed a sudden appearance of sensitivity at 65 minutes in the original study.

A replication of this study with a fuller time course has recently (McKenzie, personal communication) revealed cyclically repeating points of sensitivity, which coincided with the postulated left hemisphere retrieval events from L2 to LR2 (Fig. 19.3). The series of events should begin at about 16 minutes, but the presence of a first event at this time was not very clear in this time-course. Note that action at 65 minutes (L3: Fig. 19.3) replicates an earlier finding (above).

The first left hemisphere event

Here I present, firstly, evidence from binocular birds for good retrieval between 15 and 20 minutes, which corresponds, in the same experiments, with a similar period coinciding with the 32 minute episode (L2). Secondly, I describe an experiment which shows that both these periods of good retrieval are associated with the left hemisphere.

The first body of evidence comes from competition tasks (Andrew *et al.* 1981; Chapter 18). In such tests a chick is first presented with a clean bead and then, after a variable interval, with a bead of identical appearance but coated with an unpleasantly tasting substance, methylanthranilate. The two presentations thus provide contradictory information about one property of the bead: taste. Tasks of this sort have also been used in the rat (review, Andrew 1985). The interval between the two presentations determines whether the information derived from the first, or the second presentation determines behaviour at subsequent recall tests. The effectiveness of the first experience in such competition rises sharply between 25 and 30 minutes (Clifton *et al.* 1982), exactly at the time when the left hemisphere retrieval episode L2 occurs. It thus seemed possible that competition tests might reveal a corresponding earlier episode. Note that good retrieval of the pretraining trace seemed likely *a priori* to increase competition with training.

In the original study (Clifton *et al. loc. cit.*; Chapter 18) competition was considered to require the action of testosterone on memory formation following the first experience. However, re-analysis of time-courses from all available experiments covering the first 30–35 minutes following the first experience (Rainey 1982) shows that competition is also present in normal uninjected chicks. The time courses are shown in Fig. 19.4. The experiments were carried out before there was any thought of cyclicity in retrieval and the spacing of the intervals is, as a result, not optimal. Nevertheless, competition resulting in unusually high rates of pecking at test is clear between 15 and 21 minutes and at 30 and 32 minutes, but is absent at 10 and 25 minutes. Other features of the timecourses are considered later.

A return to the data for the time course for testosterone-treated birds, which is presented in Clifton *et al.* (1982), confirms that opposition occurs

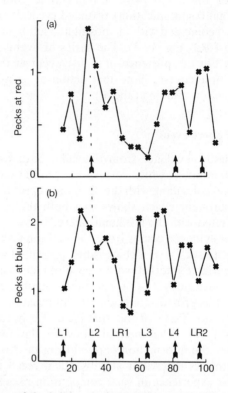

Fig. 19.3 Injection of the left hemisphere with sotalol. Chicks with the right eye covered by a temporary paper patch were trained with a red bead coated with ill-tasting methylanthranilate. At test, a clean red bead, and then after about 5 minutes, a clean blue bead was presented. The experiments were carried out with Ray McKenzie. The left hemisphere (i.e. that receiving no direct visual input at training or test) was injected at various intervals following training with the β-antagonist sotalol. Disturbances of memory formation are revealed by peaks of pecking at the red aversive bead or by depression of pecking at the blue bead; disturbance was already known to occur with this procedure following injection at about 32 minutes (Andrew and Brennan 1985). At every left hemisphere retrieval event (L1 to LR2: symbols as in Fig. 19.1) such disturbance occurs, but nowhere else. (Statistical analysis and methods: see Appendix.)

at the time of L1 and L2. In the original analysis, it was assumed that rates of pecking at the neutral blue bead could be used as a baseline against which to normalize changes in rate of pecking at the red training bead; as a result, opposition was detected only up to 2 minutes after pre-training and from 30 minutes onwards. However, it is clearly also present at 15 and 20 minutes; here it results in elevation of pecking rates at both types

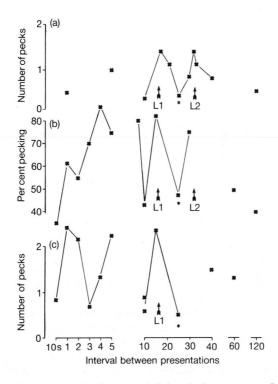

Fig. 19.4 Competition and the first two left-hemisphere events. In competition tests (see text) a clean red bead is presented, followed after a varying interval by training with a red bead coated with ill-tasting methylanthranilate. Pecking at test, which is shown here, is low when training is effective, but high when competition with training due to the first presentation is effective. The three time-courses shown here, which are taken from experiments carried out by Chris Rainey, show that competition is present at about the time of the (postulated) first left-hemisphere retrieval event (L1: Fig. 19.1), but is absent at 10 minutes and 25 minutes (R1). In (a) the timecourse includes L2, which is also marked by a peak. Competition also develops as the interval is lengthened from very short periods (10 seconds, 1 minute). At 3 minutes it may disappear briefly (c: special experimental conditions); unusual processes at 3 minutes are suggested by other evidence (see text). Statistical analysis and methods are given in the Appendix.

of bead (Fig. 19.5), rather than elevation of pecking at the red bead alone, coupled with some depression of pecks at the blue bead. Note that as a result, the period of competition which begins at 30 minutes closely resembles that which immediately follows learning.

The pecking scores of the control birds did not show competition in these experiments. However, another measure, avoidance, did; the timing

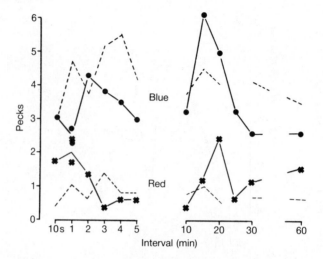

Fig. 19.5 Effects of testosterone on competition. The figure shows rates of pecking at the aversive (RED) and the neutral (BLUE) bead in a competition experiment (see text; e.g. Fig. 19.4). Data are re-analysed from Clifton *et al.* (1982). Chicks received 10 μl of testosterone (continuous lines) or vehicle alone (dashed lines) 30 minutes before pre-training; testosterone given before or in a restricted period after pre-training with a red bead is known to enhance competition (see text). Clifton *et al.* (1982), using a measure based on the difference between red and blue scores, showed competition to be present at 10 seconds and 1 minute, but then to disappear, reappearing at 30 minutes. When red and blue scores are examined separately, the 15–20 minute period can be seen to be marked by elevation of both blue and red scores. Once again, then, there is evidence of effects occurring at about the time of L1.

It is not clear why competition is not shown here by the pecking scores of controls. However, a second measure, avoidance of the bead at test, did reveal competition in the period 15–20 minutes (see Appendix, where statistical treatments are also given).

of the peak of competition at 15–20 minutes appeared to be identical in controls and birds receiving testosterone (legend, Fig. 19.5).

A final series of experiments used monocular chicks to show that both peaks of competition were associated with left hemisphere retrieval events. Andrew and Brennan (1985) developed a procedure to explore the period immediately after training, which avoided the use of an ill-tasting substance, the after-affects of which obscure changes during the first minute or so after training. A red illuminated bead was presented continuously over 60 seconds; by the end of this period, pecking was replaced by avoidance (turning away). At test the level of avoidance was used as a measure of goodness of recall. Andrew and Brennan (1985) presented data only for the period including R1 and L2, which were the events of

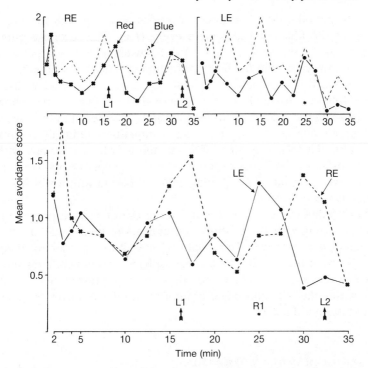

Fig. 19.6 Memory shown by avoidance of a red-lit bead. The bead was presented persistently for 60 seconds to a chick with both eyes uncovered. Initial pecking was replaced at the end of the 60 seconds by repeated turning away and avoidance of fixation. The mean number of such acts at test (AVOIDANCE) is shown here for birds using either right or left eye (RE, LE); the other eye was temporarily covered by a paper patch. The main curve shows response to a red bead at test in LE and RE; response to the red bead, and to a subsequently presented blue bead, are compared in the upper panels. The portion of the time-course between 22.5 and 35 minutes has already been published (Andrew and Brennan 1985).

RE birds show peaks in response, indicating good retrieval at times centring on about 16 minutes and 32 minutes, coinciding with the retrieval events at L1 and L2; LE birds show a single peak at 25 minutes (R1). The peak at 3 minutes in RE birds is not predicted by the model; however, there is other evidence (see text) for change at 3 minutes. At all peaks except L1, red and blue scores coincide and vary together both during the peak and in the troughs on either side of it. L1 is unusual in that a blue peak precedes the red; a similar independent variation of response to the two beads at this time can be seen in Fig. 19.5. Statistical treatments and methods are given in the Appendix.

interest in that publication. A more complete time-course (Fig. 19.6) from 2 minutes after the end of training to 35 minutes, shows firstly the points of good retrieval at R2 and L2, which have already been described, and secondly, two earlier left hemisphere retrieval events. One, which occurs over the period 15–17.5 minutes, coincides precisely with the predicted timing of the first left hemisphere event (L1). The second occurs at 3 minutes. It differs from the other left hemisphere retrieval events in its extreme brevity, and in the fact that its timing is not precisely what would be expected if it were part of the main cycle. Its significance is discussed later. However, it should be noted here that the time-courses shown in Fig. 19.4 suggest special conditions at, and just after minute 3, when (at least under one condition of testing) competition suddenly disappears. Note also that the elevation of competition, which develops within a minute or so of the initial experience in these experiments, corresponds well in overall duration and timing with the period within which hypoxia is effective (see below).

There is thus evidence for a complete series of left hemisphere retrieval events, starting with L1. Competition appears to be associated only with left hemisphere retrieval. This would agree well with predominant control of response in this test by the left hemisphere; this possibility is returned to below. Competition would then depend upon prevention of establishment within the left hemisphere of information derived from training with the ill-tasting red bead.

PHASES OF MEMORY FORMATION

In the multiphase model of memory formation in the chick (Gibbs and Ng 1977; Chapters 13 and 17) the timings of the transitions between the main phases coincide with those of the retrieval events occurring in the same period of time. Why is this so? I consider first processes occurring at LR1, when left and right hemisphere retrieval events coincide. I argue that, because of this, it is at LR1 that differences between the information held in the two hemispheres are chiefly resolved. At earlier events, when only one version is retrieved, the processing which follows (which may include interaction between the hemispheres) will be based initially and predominantly on that version, and so will take a different course.

Three of the most important phenomena, from which multiphase models have been deduced, indicate major reorganization at about 50 minutes of the information content of the trace which is used to control behaviour at test. These are:

1. *'Amnesia' following training with dilute aversant.* Training with dilute aversant (Chapters 1, 15, 17) is followed by inhibition of pecking at the aversive bead which, under appropriate conditions, disappears suddenly when pecking reappears at 50 minutes (Chapter 17). This has been

interpreted as forgetting, due to failure to form LTM. However, it is unlikely that genuine and complete amnesia is involved. Habituation tests (above: e.g. Fig. 19.2) using beads with no taste at all indicate that memory of specific properties can last for at least 120 minutes. The hypothesis of interaction between the hemispheres at LR1 offers an alternative explanation. Let us assume (cf. p. 476 and Chapter 21) that the right hemisphere holds at this time a detailed description of the presentation of the bead, but that association with taste is not very clear. Remember that behavioural signs that bad taste has been detected often develop only several seconds after pecking. The left hemisphere holds a more selected description of the bead, but clearly associates this with the after-effects of pecking. After dilute aversant, however, the left hemisphere information about taste either less definitely proscribes pecking, or is less clearly associated with pecking (or both). As a result, reconciliation of the two versions at LR1 results in further reduction in the effectiveness of the inhibition of pecking. It is important for the argument which follows [2, 3] that a further assumption is made (which has already been discussed), namely that it is predominantly the left hemisphere which determines what response should be made at test, and test therefore chiefly reveals change in the information held in the left hemisphere (Andrew 1985).

2. *Temporary amnesia.* As Allweis shows in Chapter 14 (see also Allweis *et al.* 1984) the induction of temporary amnesia by hypoxia (with a return of inhibition of pecking at LR1) strongly suggests parallel routes of memory formation, which allow a trace to survive in one route, even when the route immediately accessible to retrieval has been disrupted. The hypothesis which I am advancing here would make processes of memory formation in the two hemispheres the two parallel routes which are required to explain temporary amnesia. It will be assumed that hypoxia acts asymmetrically to disrupt the trace in the left hemisphere. Evidence for asymmetric action of amnestic agents is considered in 3. Since response to the bead at test is predominantly due to the left hemisphere, this results in amnesia. The character of the disturbance, however, is such that at LR1 information held by the right hemisphere is used to restore an effective trace in the left hemisphere.

3. *Delayed loss.* A number of very different amnestic agents, acting at different times, both close to and well after learning, cause delayed loss of memory at the time of LR1.

To explain this, I assume that such agents are also asymmetric in their action. Andrew and Brennan (1985) and Patterson *et al.* (1986; Chapter 15) have provided evidence that when amnestic agents are given to right or left hemisphere, injection may be effective in only one; which it is may depend on time of injection. Asymmetry of action could result from:

(1) asymmetry in sensitivity at the cellular level;
(2) asymmetry in the extent and/or timing of the processes and structures affected by the agents;
(3) asymmetry in the effects on the trace of a given degree of disturbance at the cellular level: a trace which records a limited number of key features might remain usable after disturbance which would make a detailed record useless, for example.

When delayed loss occurs at LR1, I assume that it was the information held in the right hemisphere which was affected by the amnestic procedure. The degradation of the right hemisphere material is assumed to be such that attempts at reconciliation at LR1 disturb the information held by the left hemisphere to a point at which it is no longer adequate to cause inhibition of pecking at test.

A second set of phenomena, the sharply timed endings of sensitivity to different groups of amnestic agents, also may coincide with early retrieval events (Fig. 19.1). At least three different routes of action of amnestic agents can now be seen to be possible; two of them (b and c) would tend to cause sensitivity to end at about the time of a particular retrieval event:

(a) Amnestic agents may act on the cellular basis of the trace during consolidation. Different steps in consolidation will be sensitive to different agents (Chapters 10, 13–16). Some steps may be sharply timed; however, there is no obvious reason why these should coincide with retrieval events.

(b) When the information held in memory is changed as a result of retrieval events, consolidation presumably begins again for at least a subset of the neurons responsible for storage; as a result, sensitivity to amnestic agents might also return briefly. This may be compared with the hypothesis suggested by Lewis (1979), who argued that the trace is set up rapidly following learning, and then enters a state ('inactive memory') in which it is invulnerable to amnestic agents. Sensitivity returns only with activation of the trace. Lewis considered as a cause of activation only reminiscence due to the perception of cues associated with training. In the chick it may be necessary to consider also activation due to endogenously timed processes.

(c) Amnestic agents may also affect the trace indirectly, by disturbing mechanisms for transfer or temporary storage of information at the time of a retrieval event, thus disturbing inputs to the trace. One possible consequence of such disturbance is the incorporation into the trace of degraded information.

I shall not attempt here to discuss which agents may act in which way. However, note that, whilst the arguments which I have so far presented do not necessarily challenge current ideas about the sequence of cellular events during consolidation in the chick, they do mean that the timings of transitions between phases need not relate to steps in a single progressive process of consolidation within a single neuronal population.

DIFFERENCES BETWEEN DIFFERENT RETRIEVAL EVENTS

It is likely that different steps in memory formation are associated with each of the early retrieval events. Only a brief and preliminary discussion is possible here.

Period immediately after the initial experience

Consolidation of records of the experience is presumably under way. However, information derived from the experience is also needed at once for two rather different purposes. Firstly, it is used to control attention. When, for example, a chick is searching for food, it uses information from a successful peck to find other similar items, and to direct search to similar sites (Andrew 1976; Klein and Andrew 1986; Rogers and Andrew 1989). Secondly, some record of the experience needs to be related to subsequent experiences which are judged to be relevant; after pecking a bead coated with methylanthranilate, these would include the development after a brief but variable delay, of a bad taste in the mouth.

It is not obvious at first sight why such use of information should come to a sharp and consistently timed end. Nevertheless, there is evidence that, in chicks which have been treated with testosterone, a limit to the duration of stabilization of such information is reached at around 2 minutes. This is evident in competition experiments (above); testosterone enhances competition due to pre-training over very short intervals up to intervals of about 2 minutes (Fig. 19.5; Chapter 18). It is interesting that a brief left hemisphere retrieval event appears to occur at 3 minutes (Fig. 19.6); evidently there is an important transition period during minutes 2 and 3, during which two (or more) changes occur.

One possible explanation for mechanisms which bring to an end the period in which temporarily stored information (derived from the original experiment) is used to select and assess stimuli, is as follows. The availability of such information allows the animal to assess the relevance of subsequent experiences to the original one. Additional information which ought to be related in memory to the original experience will, as a result, be gathered; this information will be termed here 'secondary material.' The processes leading up to and including the left hemisphere retrieval event at 3 minutes may provide the means by which (at least in the left hemisphere) appropriate secondary material is stored for future association with the original record.

L1 and hypoxia

Hypoxia is effective in a period 2.5–5 minutes after training; it is without effect at 0 and 9 minutes (Chapter 14). It thus acts at and just after the time of the 3 minute event; if the arguments set out in the preceding section are correct, then hypoxia may affect some aspect of the storage of secondary material for future association with a record of the original experience (probably held in the left hemisphere).

This in turn may explain the delay before temporary amnesia develops following hypoxia: this occurs around or perhaps a little after 15 minutes (i.e. close to L1). It has already been argued that delayed loss at LR1 may result from interaction between the left hemisphere record (which is here argued to be used to control response) and degraded right hemisphere material. A corresponding explanation for delayed loss after hypoxia might be interaction at L1 between the left hemisphere record of the original experience (here assumed not to be directly vulnerable to hypoxia) and secondary material, which was degraded at storage by hypoxia.

R1 and L2

The abrupt termination of sensitivity to a number of amnestic agents imediately after 25 minutes suggests that the record in the right hemisphere is vulnerable at R1.

There is evidence from competition experiments (above) that the material available for retrieval at L2 differs from that available at L1. There are two possible explanations: this may be due to change consequent on L1 (e.g. incorporation of secondary material) or to change associated with R1. It is impossible to tell from the evidence at present available whether one or the other (or both) are correct.

LR1

As has already been discussed, the coincidence at LR1 of retrieval events in both hemispheres may allow comparison and reconciliation of the records held in the two hemispheres. In normal memory formation, this may be important in that it would allow the left hemisphere to change its record as a result of access to a relatively detailed and unprocessed record in the right hemisphere.

Further learning

One possible additional function of retrieval events, which may hold both for the early events and for cycles continuing after LR1, is to bring about investigation of the place and the type of stimulus involved in the original experience. Further learning about important experiences is likely to be useful.

CHANGES IN TIMING DUE TO HORMONES

Gibbs (Chapter 17) shows that two features of memory formation are substantially postponed by treatment with hormones such as vasopressin. These are:

(1) the end of sensitivity to certain amnestic agents;
(2) brief periods of apparent amnesia ('dips in retention') which normally occur at 15 and 55 minutes.

Both types of features are closely associated with retrieval events in normal memory function, so their postponement requires discussion here. I confine myself to evidence from the effects of testosterone because its effects on attention are relatively well understood in the chick (below; Chapter 18), and these give some clues as to the way in which it affects memory formation. It should be noted that peptide hormones such as ACTH also affect both attention and memory formation (review, Andrew 1985).

The most obvious possible cause of systematic postponement of features of memory formation, once the existence of cyclic repetition of retrieval events is accepted, is a lengthening of the cycles themselves. However, there is evidence that this does not occur. Firstly, the timings of events associated with L1 and L2 are not appreciably changed (Fig. 19.5) by levels of testosterone which are fully effective in postponing the dip which normally occurs at 55 minutes by at least 30 minutes (Gibbs *et al*. 1986). At the same time, the character of the processes which occur at L1 and L2 is markedly changed by the hormone (facilitation of competition: above), so that the hormone is acting (and acting very effectively) in this period.

Secondly, when testosterone is injected at a series of times from 120 minutes before to 50 minutes after training (Gibbs *et al*. 1986), the relationship between the length of time for which testosterone is able to act on memory formation, and the degree of postponement of the 55 minute dip, is the reverse of what would be expected if testosterone postponed the dip by extending each of the stages of memory formation which precede the dip. Injection before learning, allowing the whole of memory formation up to the dip to be affected, produced only 5 minutes postponement, whereas the nearer to the normal time of the dip the injection came, the greater the postponement, up to a limit of 40 or 45 minutes. Andrew (1985) pointed out that the relationship between the length of time between injection and 55 minutes, and the degree of postponement, suggested that the crucial variable was the intensity of the central action of testosterone at the time of the dip (or just before it, at LR1).

It is thus necessary to consider whether postponement can be explained without postulating any change in the timing of the cycles of retrieval events. The fact that testosterone acts on processes associated with a number of retrieval events (L1 and L2: enhanced competition; LR1: just discussed), suggests a hypothesis. This is that retrieval events, and processes associated with them, provide the opportunity for events like dips in retention and sensitivity to certain amnestic agents. Postponement occurs when the opportunity provided by a retrieval event is missed because of effects of the hormone; a later retrieval event would then provide a second opportunity.

There is evidence that opportunities of the sort postulated do recur in association with each of a series of left hemisphere retrieval events. Recurring sensitivity to sotalol at each event from L2 to LR2 has already been discussed. In tests with monocular chicks (McKenzie, unpublished) dips in retention occurred at about 5 minutes after each of the series of left hemisphere retrieval events (LR1, L3, L4 and LR2), and not at any other time in this period.

In the case of the dip at 55 minutes there is some evidence as to the way in which postponement may be brought about. The argument is best set out in steps:

(a) It has already been noted that the postponement of the 55 minute dip appears to depend on action at about the time of LR1. The same may well be true of another effect of testosterone. When testosterone is given after pre-training, it facilitates competition with subsequent training (2 or more hours later) up to a time of injection somewhat after 30 minutes following pre-training (Clifton *et al.* 1982; Chapter 18); when latency of action is taken into account this brings the latest time at which onset of action is effective in enhancing competition to around 50 minutes (very approximately). Action of testosterone at LR1 thus seems reasonable.

(b) It has been argued that interaction between the hemispheres, allowing reconciliation of different versions of the original experience, is important at LR1. Testosterone might have its effects at LR1 by interfering with this process; resulting enhancement of competition would be explained, if such enhancement were to be caused by the exclusion of right hemisphere material from the final version of the trace in the left hemisphere.

(c) In competition between pre-training and training over short intervals, testosterone opposes the acceptance at training of information discrepant with that obtained at pre-training. It is likely that this is due to an effect, the stabilization of information held in temporary storage for use in the selection and assessment of stimuli, which underlies the effects of testosterone on attention (Chapters 18, 21). Clearly there is some resemblance between this sort of effect and interference with acceptance at LR1 of material from a different version of the trace held by the other hemisphere. Equally, there is a fundamental difference: in the first case, the source of the discrepant material is perceptual input, whereas in the second case, it is derived from material held in memory. An explanation of this sort must assume that similar mechanisms (or even the same, since both have to be assumed to be similarly affected by hormones) are used to search for, and assess both stimuli in the external world, and also centrally held information.

(d) It remains to consider why dips in retention should occur at all. On the hypothesis advanced by Gibbs and Ng (Chapters 13, 17), such dips mark a shift of retrieval from one store to another. This hypothesis fits well with the arguments advanced here: a dip would occur at the point following a retrieval event such as LR1, when information brought into use in temporary storage at the time of the retrieval event begins to be lost, and retrieval has to shift in consequence back to the main trace.

One interesting cause of such loss of temporarily held information appears to be the approach of another retrieval event. Even under the most effective hormonal regime, postponement of the 55 minute dip reaches a limit at LR2 (Gibbs *et al.* 1986; Andrew 1985). The same seems to be true of the 15 minute dip: postponement here reaches a limit at 25 minutes, the time of R1 (Chapter 17). It may be that the coincidence of the normal timing of the 15 minute dip with L1 itself also represents termination of temporary storage at the onset of the retrieval event.

CONCLUSION

Most of the previous three sections has been concerned with the ways in which retrieval cycles might explain the, by now, very detailed and complicated body of experimental evidence about phases of memory formation in the chick. I turn here to wider implications of the existence of such cycles. It is worth noting that these implications probably hold for mammals as well. The existence of cyclic changes in ease of retrieval in mouse and rat has already been noted; the close resemblance between the evidence for phases of memory in chick and rat (Chapter 14) also makes it likely that the basic features of the chick retrieval cycles will be found in mammals.

The chick cycles are surprisingly precisely timed. One reason for this is likely to be the need to ensure the correct sequence of changes in phase relations between cycles in the two hemispheres. Another possible reason stems from the fact that one experience follows another in a continuous sequence during working life; if processing the information derived from each experience cannot be completed during the experience itself, but must be continued at some later time, then some system of queuing is necessary. This would be ensured for experiences adjacent in time, if retrieval cycles for each experience were timed from the beginning of each experience. Interference between retrieval events would of course still occur for experiences separated by more than one cycle length. However, the problems which this might cause are probably reduced by the fact that waking periods, and so sequences of experiences, are limited in duration. It may not be a coincidence that in this chick waking and sleep alternate cyclically with an overall period of very roughly 30 minutes (Guyomarc'h 1975); as a result, continuous series of experiences are likely not greatly to exceed the duration of a single left hemisphere cycle.

Long timecourses (to be presented elsewhere) suggest that variation in duration of retrieval cycles may not exceed about 1 per cent in the chick. This is easily matched by the accuracy of free-running circadian rhythms in some vertebrates: thus in hamsters, a rhythm with a mean period of 24.12 hours had a standard error, in one particular population, of 0.04 hours (Elliott 1981). A connection between retrieval cycles and circadian rhythms has in fact been suggested for the rat: both are abolished by lesioning the suprachiasmatic nucleus (Stephen and Koracevic 1978). Tapp and Holloway (1981) argue for a role of the circadian rhythm in memory formation in the rat on the grounds that amnesia results if the phase of the rhythm is shifted by providing a light/dark transition immediately after learning.

Whatever their relationship with longer cycles, the retrieval cycles themselves seem likely to be directly driven by clocks with the same period as the cycle. Presumably, each experience takes its timing from the phase of the clock at which it occurs; the information deriving from the experience is then retrieved when that phase recurs.

A central issue raised by the existence of retrieval cycles is: why should there be processing of information (as distinct from consolidation of the neuronal basis of the initial record of the experience) once learning is over? One answer is that an experience has to be analysed in more than one way, and the results of each type of analysis need storing. It will often be necessary to store a relatively complete account of the experience. At the same time, there has to be an immediate interpretation on the basis of selected cues, so as to allow rapid and appropriate response. Further, it is not necessarily clear in advance when the experience will end: after-effects of response and changes in the stimulus itself may provide new and relevant information.

As a result, various versions of the experience and associated happenings are likely to need reconciliation. The evidence presented in this chapter relates almost entirely to the possibility that the differing specializations of the two hemispheres result in different versions of the experience being held in the right and left hemispheres, which then interact at times, and in ways determined by the retrieval cycles. However, it is also possible that something of the same sort of interaction occurs between different cerebral structures within a hemisphere.

Retrieval events may also provide a means for bringing about return to particularly interesting stimuli and situations for further investigation, guided now by information which has undergone processing. It may be that, in addition to continual direct response to external happenings, there is spontaneous provision of material from memory which also tends to initiate response, with sometimes one source and sometimes the other determining behaviour.

The brain structures involved in retrieval events are largely unknown. Stephenson (1981, Chapter 16) has shown in one case of drug action at the time of a retrieval event (sotalol at 25 minutes, R1), that injection is effective only far posterior to the anterior half of the brain. Most other amnestic agents appear to act anteriorly. Such anterior action was shown in the same study for a second drug (timolol, another beta-antagonist, but with markedly different effects on memory formation: Chapter 16), which had no effect posteriorly. Further, the structures which have been identified as showing learning-induced change (Chapters 8, 10, 11) or as sensitive to amnestic agents soon after learning (Chapter 15) also lie in the anterior half of the forebrain.

Structures in the posterior part of the forebrain fall into two major divisions: the posterior neostriatum lies central to the ventricle and the main part of the hippocampal formation lies peripheral to it. Both structures are likely to receive drugs as a result of posterior injection, and it is impossible at present to localize action any further. However, it is intriguing to consider the hippocampus as perhaps involved in finding information in memory, and in transferring it for incorporation into an altered version of an earlier record.

Acknowledgements

The work described here owes much to many collaborators, in particular John Archer, Anthony Brennan, Peter Clifton, David Feld, Marie Gibbs, Richard Klein, Ray McKenzie, Peter Messent, Kim Ng, Christopher Rainey, Lesley Rogers, and Robert Stephenson. It was supported at various times by the AFRC and SERC of the UK.

REFERENCES

Allweis, C, Gibbs, M. E. Ng, K., and T. Hodge, R. J. (1984). Effects of hypoxia on memory consolidation: implications for a multistage model of memory. *Behavioral Brain Research*, **11**, 117–12.

Andrew, R. J. (1976). Attentional processes and animal behaviour. In *Growing points in ethology* (ed. P. P. G. Bateson and R. A. Hinde), pp. 95–133. Cambridge University Press.

Andrew, R. J. (1983*a*). Lateralisation of emotional and cognitive function in higher vertebrates, with special reference to the domestic chick. In *Advances in vertebrate neuroethology* (ed. J. P. Ewert, R. R. Capranica, and D. J. Ingle), pp. 477–509. Plenum, New York.

Andrew, R. J. (1983*b*) Specific short-latency effects of oestradiol and testosterone on distractibility and memory formation in the young domestic chick. In *Hormones and behaviour in higher vertebrates* (ed. J. Balthazart, E. Pröve, and R. Gilles), pp. 463–73. Springer-Verlag, Berlin.

Andrew, R. J. (1985). The temporal structure of memory formation. *Perspectives in Ethology*, **6**, 219–59.

Andrew, R. J. and Brennan, A. (1985). Sharply timed and lateralised events at time of establishment of long term memory. *Physiology and Behaviour*, **34**, 547–56.

Bell, G. A. and Gibbs, M. E. (1977). Unilateral storage of monocular engram in day old chick. *Brain Research*, **245**, 263–70.

Brush, F. R. (1971). Retention of aversely-motivated behaviour. In *Aversive conditioning and learning* (ed. F. R. Bush), pp. 401–65. Academic Press, New York.

Cherkin, A. (1970). Eye-to-eye transfer of an early response modification in chick. *Nature*, **227**, 1153.

Clifton, P. G. Andrew, R. J., and Gibbs, M. E. (1982). Limited period of action of testosterone on memory formation in the chick. *Journal of Comparative and Physiological Psychology*, **96**, 212–22.

Denton, C. J. (1981). Topography of the hyperstriatal visual projection area in the young domestic chick. *Experimental Neurology*, **74**, 482–98.

Elliott, J. A. (1981). Circadian rhythms, entrainment and photoperiodism in the Syrian Hamster. In *Biological clocks in seasonal reproductive cycles* (ed. B. K. and D. E. Follett), pp. 203–17. Scientechnica, Bristol.

Gaston, K. E. (1979). Lack of interocular transfer of pattern discrimination learning in chicks. *Brain Research*, **171**, 339–43.

Gaston, K. E. (1980). Evidence for separate and concurrent avoidance learning in the two hemispheres of the normal chick brain. *Behavioral and Neural Biology*, **28**, 129–37.

Gibbs, M. E. and Ng K. T. (1977). Psychobiology of memory: towards a model of memory formation. *Biobehavioral Reviews*, **1**, 113–36.

Gibbs, M. E. and Ng, K. T. (1984). Dual action of cycloheximide on memory formation in day-old chicks. *Behavioral Brain Research*, **12**, 21–7.

Gibbs, M. E. Ng, K. T., and Andrew, R. J. (1986). Effect of testosterone on intermediate memory in day old chicks. *Pharmacology, Biochemistry and Behaviour*, **25**, 823–6.

Goodale, M. A. and Graves, J. A. (1980). The relationship between scanning patterns and monocular discrimination in the pigeon. *Physiology and Behavior*, **25**, 39–43.

Goodale, M. A. and Graves, J. A. (1982). Interocular transfer in the pigeon: retinal locus as a factor. In *Analysis of visual behaviour* (ed. D. J.. Ingle, M. A. Goodale, and R. Mansfield), pp. 197–209. MIT Press. Cambridge, Mass.

Greif, K. F. (1976). Bilateral memory for monocular one-trial passive avoidance in chicks. *Behavioral Biology*, **16**, 453–62.

Guyomarc'h, J. C. (1975). Les cycles d'activité d'une couvée naturelle de poussins et leur coordination. *Behaviour*, **53**, 31–75.

Hodge, R. J. Gibbs, M. E., and Ng, K. T. (1981). Engram duplication in the day old chick. *Behavioural and Neural Biology*, **31**, 283–98.

Holloway, F. A. (1978). State dependent retrieval based on time of day. In *Drug Discrimination and State Dependent Learning*, (ed. B. T. Ho, D. W. Richards, and D. L. Chute). Academic Press, New York.

Klein, R. M. and Andrew R. J. (1986). Distraction, decisions and persistence in runway tests, using the domestic chick. *Behaviour*, **99**, 139–56.

Lewis, D. J. 1979 Psychobiology of active and inactive memory. *Psychological Bulletin*, **86**, 1054–1083.

Patterson, T. A., Alvarado, M. O., Warner, I. T., Bennett, E. L., and Rosenzweig, M. R. (1986). Memory stages and brain asymmetry in chick learning. *Behavioral Neuroscience*, **100**, 850–9.

Pettigrew, J. D. (1979). Binocular visual processing in the owls telencephalon. *Proceedings of the Royal Society of London B*, **204**, 435–54.

Rainey, C. J. (1982). Steroid specificity and memory in the chick. D. Phil thesis. University of Sussex, UK.

Rogers, L. J. and Andrew, R. J. (1989). Frontal and lateral visual field use by chicks after treatment with testosterone. *Animal Behaviour*, **38**, 394–405.

Seybert, J. A., Wilson, M. A., and Archer, A. L. (1982). The Kamin effect as a function of time of training and associative-nonassociative processes. *Bulletin of the Psychonomic Society*, **19**, 227–30.

Stephan, F. K. and Koracevic, N. S. (1978). Multiple retention deficit in passive avoidance in rats is eliminated by suprachiasmatic lesions. *Behavioural Biology*, **22**, 456–62.

Stephenson, R. M. (1981). Memory processing in the domestic chick (*Gallus gallus*): a psychopharmacological investigation. D. Phil thesis, University of Sussex, UK.

Stephenson, R. M. and Andrew, R. J. (1981). Amnesia due to β-antagonists in a passive avoidance task in the chick. *Pharmacology and Biochemistry of Behaviour*, **15**, 597–604.

Tapp, W. N. and Holloway, F. A. (1981). Phase shifting circadian rhythm produces retrograde amnesia. *Science*, **211**, 1056–8.

Wallman, J. and Pettigrew, J. D. (1985). Conjugate and disjunctive saccades in two avian species with contrasting oculomotor strategies. *Journal of Neuroscience*, **5**, 1418–28.

APPENDIX

Figure 19.2.   Each presentation of the violet-lit bead (402 nm, half-peak width 30 nm) was for 15 s. Presentations were given in pairs, separated by 5 s; the measure shown is the difference between scores obtained at the first of each pair of presentations. There was overall heterogeneity over time ($F_{17,406} = 2.51$, $p = 0.005$), with no difference between the RE and LE curves ($F_{1,406} = 1.68$). At an interval of 120 minutes LE chicks are known to show markedly greater habituation than RE chicks (Andrew 1983a and Chapter 21); the same was true of similar intervals here (100–180 minutes: EYE, $F_{1,64} = 8.92$, $p = 0.004$). Over the period 16–80 minutes, there are 15 LE groups; the three peaks occur at the three times at which they were predicted ($p = 0.025$, Fisher exact).

Figure 19.3.   Birds were pre-trained by the presentation of a small white bead, a red bead, and a blue bead (all clean), before training. Eye patches were worn only at the time of presentations. Injection at 32.5 minutes was expected to disturb memory formation, whereas at 25 minutes it should be without effect (Andrew and Brennan, 1985): an ANOVA restricted to 25 and 30 minutes showed the same to be true here (red scores: TIME, $F_{1,28} = 8.29$, $p < 0.01$). In the blue scores there are five clear troughs, each of which coincides with a left-hemisphere retrieval event (L1, LR1, L3, L4). L2 is marked by a uniquely defined amnesic point in the red scores; note that with full amnesia, generalization of inhibition of pecking to the blue bead would not be expected. The trough at LR1 includes 55 minutes as well as 50 minutes; this is a second point of sensitivity and counts against the hypothesis. There are 19 times at which the seven observed points of sensitivity could have occurred ($p = 0.02$, Fisher exact).

Figure 19.4.   Each point represents a separate group of chicks (usually 16–20). All available experiments are given. The timecourses are best considered as a sequence, using earlier timecourses to predict the timing of change in later ones. A brief time-course (not shown), using the standard Sussex red bead (Chapter 1) gave rates of 1.49, 3.39, and 2.50 pecks, with intervals of 10, 15, and 20 minutes (INTERVAL, $F_{2,65} = 10.46$, $p < 0.001$). This allows prediction of little or no competition at 10 minutes, and maximal at 15 minutes, perhaps persisting to some extent to 20 minutes. Time-course (a) used red-lit beads (Kodak filter 92) (using the rounded tip of a test-tube-shaped glass vessel, of the same diameter as the standard bead). The comparisons suggested by the previous time-course were significant or suggestive (10 versus 17 minutes, $F_{1,29} = 4.23$, $p = 0.049$; 21 versus 25 minutes, $F_{1,25} = 3.92$, $p = 0.059$). The increase from 25 minutes to 32 minutes (R1 to L2) is significant ($F_{2,36} = 3.31$, $p = 0.048$). Time-course (b) used a standard red glass bead. The percentage (rather than the mean rate) of birds pecking at test is shown because quantitative data for two intervals (10 seconds and 30 minutes) were missing. There was overall heterogeneity across interval ($\chi^2_{13} = 58.02$, $p < 0.001$: two replications for 10 minutes). The predicted peaks and troughs were all present (10 versus 15 minutes, $F_{1,112} = 7.27$, $p = 0.008$; 15 versus 25 minutes, $F_{1,95} = 12.51$, $p < 0.001$; 25 versus 30 minutes, $\chi^2_1 = 4.22$, $p < 0.05$). Note that competition is absent as in (a), at 120 minutes, and also at very short intervals (10 seconds versus 15 minutes, $\chi^2_1 = 13.41$, $p < 0.001$). There appears to be marked competition at 4, 5, and 7 minutes (4 versus 10′ minutes, $F_{1,111} = 15.91$, $p < 0.001$). Time-course (c) also used red beads; at test, instead of the usual 10 seconds presentation, there were three presentations of 5 seconds separated by 5 second intervals. Total pecks are analysed here. There was heterogeneity across time ($F_{11,227} = 2.56$, $p = 0.004$). Once again, there was a peak at 15 minutes, flanked by troughs at 10 and 25 minutes (10 versus 15 minutes, $F_{2,57} = 3.42$, $p = 0.04$; 15 versus 25 minutes, $F_{1,38} = 5.51$, $p = 0.02$). The absence of competition at 10 seconds is confirmed (10 seconds versus 1 minute, $F_{1,37} = 4.56$, $p = 0.039$), as is its presence at 5 minutes (5 versus 10 minutes, $F_{2,57} = 5.22$, $p = 0.008$). However, in contrast to timecourse (c), competition disappears at 3 minutes; the difference is perhaps associated with the brevity of presentation.

Figure 19.5. The test occurred 180 minutes after training. The red bead was presented first; the intervals shown are for this presentation. The blue bead was presented about 5 minutes later. Each point represents a different group of chicks (typically, $n = 18$–20).

Overall rates of pecking varied significantly with interval ($F_{15,509} = 2.77$, $p < 0.001$), largely because of variation in the testosterone curve (HORMONE × INTERVAL, $F_{11,509} = 2.15$, $p = 0.016$). A major reason for this variation in overall rate is the peak in both red and blue rates at 15 and 20 minutes (restriction to 10, 15, 20 minutes: INTERVAL, $F_{2,112} = 5.95$, p = 0.004), which is present only in testosterone curves (HORMONE × INTERVAL, $F_{2,112} = 4.79$, $p = 0.01$). In other parts of the curves, red and blue scores varied inversely for testosterone groups but not for controls (INTERVAL × COLOUR, $F_{15,509} = 3.46$, $p < 0.001$; HORMONE × INTERVAL × COLOUR, $F_{11,509} = 3.57$, $p < 0.001$). This is due to two periods of marked competition in which elevated pecking at the red bead is accompanied by rather low pecking at the blue bead. The first occurs up to 1 minute, disappears sharply at 3 minutes, with 2 minutes intermediate; the second occurs at 30 and 60 minutes. Both transitions result in significant change (restriction to 10 seconds to 3 minutes, COLOUR × INTERVAL, $F_{6,215} = 3.03$, $p = 0.007$; HORMONE × COLOUR × INTERVAL, $F_{4,215} = 3.86$, $p = 0.005$; restriction to 25–30 minutes, COLOUR × INTERVAL, $F_{2,75} = 4.23$, $p = 0.014$). Testosterone thus enhances competition in all of the three periods in which it has been shown to occur in controls (Fig. 19.4): immediately after learning, at 15 and 20 minutes, and at 30 and 32.5 minutes.

It is not clear why competition is not shown here in control pecking scores. However, a second measure—avoidance of the bead at test—did reveal competition: in testosterone-treated birds avoidance was low when marked competition produced high pecking rates. Over the period involving intervals 10–20 minutes both testosterone and control groups varied almost identically (TIME, $F_{2,112} = 7.57, p < 0.001$; HORMONE $\times$ TIME, $F_{2,112} = 0.42$); both showed no competition at 10 minutes and marked competition at 15 and 20 minutes.

Figure 19.6. The red-lit bead (6 mm diameter; peak at 624 nm, half-peak width 15.4 nm) was presented for 10 seconds at test; times are for this presentation, starting from the beginning of training. Test with a blue-lit bead (486 nm) followed within 30 seconds. All available experiments (replications at 2, 3, 10, 25, and 32.5 minutes) are shown; the mean at 25 minutes is, as a result, slightly altered from that previously published. Scores for both red and blue (novel) beads are considered in the ANOVAs. The peaks result in overall heterogeneity over time (2–22.5 minutes, $F_{13,487} = 3.73$, $p < 0.001$; 22.5–35 minutes, $F_{7,254} = 4.79$, $p < 0.001$). The two previously undescribed peaks are both significant (2–7.5 minutes, $F_{6,249} = 2.64, p = 0.017$; 10–22.5 minutes, $F_{6,238} = 2.55$, $p = 0.021$); the remaining peaks are discussed by Andrew and Brennan (1985). At all times, RE and LE birds were matched in a fully counterbalanced manner; it is thus important that at each peak RE and LE scores for the red bead test differ significantly (3 minutes, $F_{1,71} = 15.00$, $p < 0.001$; 17.5 minutes, $F_{1,32} = 5.33, p = 0.028$; 25 minutes $F_{1,64} = 4.63$, $p = 0.035$; 32.5 minutes, $F_{1,61} = 17.78$, $p < 0.001$). The relationship between red and blue scores differs between RE and LE. In the block 2–22.5 minutes, the difference between these scores is larger in LE (EYE $\times$ COLOUR, $F_{1,487} = 8.59$, $p = 0.004$); this difference does not vary significantly with time. In the block 22.5–35 minutes, EYE $\times$ TIME $\times$ COLOUR is significant ($F_{7,254} = 3.02, p = 0.005$), because the difference between red and blue scores disappears at, and on either side, of R1 in LE birds, and of L2 in RE birds.

PART VI

Lateralization

Introduction

R. J. Andrew

Asymmetries of hemispheric function are of great importance to studies of learning, memory formation, and development of behaviour in the chick, as earlier chapters have made clear. This final section provides accounts of what is known of the development and nature of lateralization in the chick.

Rogers (Chapter 20) describes remarkable shifts in hemispheric sensitivity to insult, which indicate special states in the left hemisphere on day 8 and in the right hemisphere on days 10 and 11. Shifts in which hemisphere controls behaviour accompany these shifts in sensitivity. Corresponding changes occur in behaviour; an earlier transition comparable to that occurring between day 8 and day 10 may occur at day 4 (Chapter 6). The functions of these shifts in hemispheric control remain to be explored. They may not only determine the behaviour of chicks on particular days, but also what is likely to be learned on those days. It is also possible that they relate in some way to sudden and major maturational changes in structures of first one and then the other side of the CNS.

Sex differences in the pattern of the shifts are marked and are open to various interpretation (Chapters 20, 21). Another remarkable set of findings relate to induction of anatomical and functional asymmetries by asymmetric exposure to light during later fetal life. These not only provide a novel experimental approach, but also raise questions for studies of natural development: it is clearly important to know whether natural incubation produces variable degrees of asymmetric exposure and so phenotypic variation in some aspects of lateralization.

Hemispheric specialization includes specialization for modes of analysis of perceptual input (Chapter 21). In the chick, the right hemisphere appears to be specialized for analysis of experiences as unique detailed events, associated with a particular position in space. The left hemisphere is specialized rather to assign stimuli to one of a number of categories, taking into account selected important cues, and relating the experience to after-effects of any response to the stimulus performed by the chick. Relations between the hemispheres appear to range from simultaneous and complementary activity to strong control by one hemisphere (Chapter 21).

The possible ways in which hemispheric specialization might generate asymmetries in learning-induced change (for example) have been considered in general terms in earlier sections. However, it is worth noting that in the future it may be possible to use accumulating knowledge about hemispheric specialization to produce hypotheses about the functioning of brain structures which have asymmetric involvement in learning and memory formation. The special and protracted importance of the left IMHV in memory formation, for example, might indicate involvement of the IMHV in processes which are especially characteristic of the left hemisphere: these could include the selection of particular features of a stimulus, and relating them to after-effects separated in time from the initial experience.

20

Development of lateralization

L. J. Rogers

During early development the chicken undergoes a number of precisely timed changes in behaviour, and it would seem that these changes are at least partly due to shifts in dominance from one side of the brain to the other, in many instances from one forebrain hemisphere to the other. Behavioural functions lateralized to one hemisphere predominate at one age and those of the other hemisphere at another age. At yet another age in the developmental plan, both sides of the brain may be equally involved in controlling the behaviour even though, as in the case of imprinting (see Chapter 8), each may play a different role in that context.

These shifts of control from left-to-right-to-both sides of the brain are manifest as changes in the level or the type of responses which can be elicited from either the left or right eye of the chicken at different ages. Andrew and Brennan (1983) have shown that on day 5 post-hatching male chickens presented with a fearful stimulus, a violet bead, show significantly more fear responses when they are tested monocularly using their right eye as opposed to their left. At this age the fear responses of binocularly tested chicks are equivalent to those tested with the right eye, which suggests dominance of the right eye. On day 8 chicks tested using their left eye were found to give more fear responses than those using their right, and at this age the level of fear scored in the binocularly tested chicks was equivalent to that of those using the left eye, suggesting a shift to dominance of the left eye. On days 9 and 10 there are striking transitions in fear behaviour between the three groups. On day 9 these transitions are sharply defined and rather complex, but days 10 and 12 appear to show a clear result of low levels of fear in both of the monocularly tested groups (i.e. no lateralization) and very high levels of fear in the binocularly tested group. In other words, dominance no longer occurs and the hemispheres appear to be functionally coupled.

The shifts in laterality of function correlate with changes in cellular function which occur first on one side of the brain and then the other. It is possible to unmask lateralization of brain function in the chicken by injecting into one or the other hemisphere pharmacological agents which

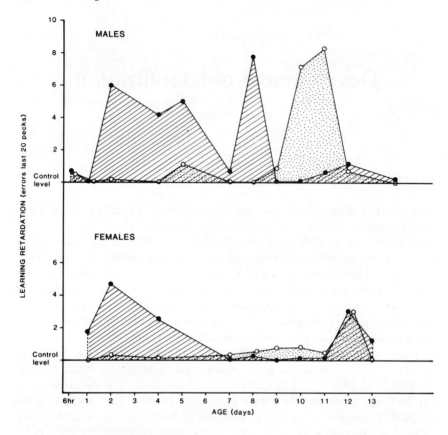

interfere with cellular processes essential to the subsequent functioning of the brain. For example, administration of cycloheximide to the left hemisphere of the 2-day-old male chicken permanently retards visual discrimination learning measured in a task requiring the chick to find grains of food scattered on a background of small pebbles which make the food difficult to see (Rogers and Anson 1979; for details of the task see Rogers *et al*. 1974). It also slows visual and auditory habituation learning. In contrast, treatment of the right hemisphere at this age has no effect on subsequent learning ability. If learning of the visual discrimination test is scored on day 14 post-hatching and the cycloheximide injection into the left or right hemisphere is given at various ages throughout the first week of life, changes in susceptibility to the drug are seen (Rogers and Ehrlich 1983; Rogers 1986; and see Fig. 20.1). From day 2 to 5 or 6 inclusive the left hemisphere is susceptible to the long-lasting effects of the drug (note that day 6 was not actually tested), on day 7 neither hemisphere is susceptible, on day 8 there is a sudden renewal of the susceptibility of the left hemisphere and this is followed on day 9 by, once again, neither

Fig. 20.1 Unilateral administration of cycloheximide to the left or right hemisphere of the chicken at various ages after hatching reveals separate development time-courses for each hemisphere. Each chick was injected once only at a given age with 20 μg of cycloheximide in 25 μl of 0.9 per cent saline. The contralateral hemisphere received 25 μl of saline. All were tested for visual discrimination learning on day 14 post-hatching. The task required search for grains of chick food scattered on a background of small pebbles (Rogers *et al.* 1974), and a total of 60 pecks were allowed. The number of pecks at pebbles (errors) were scored for each block of 20 pecks, and the number of errors in the last block of 20 pecks (pecks 41–60) was taken as an indication of learning ability and plotted in the figure relative to control levels. A higher error score indicates greater retardation of learning. For clarity the standard errors around these mean values have not been included in the figure: standard error never exceeded 2.0 and was mostly around 1.0. The controls received saline into both hemispheres, and they made a mean of only two errors in the last 20 pecks. This was taken as the baseline score. There were eight to ten chicks per point on the curves. The data for learning following cycloheximide treatment of the left hemisphere is presented as the hatched area, and that following treatment of the right hemisphere as the dotted area. In males, note that the cycloheximide disrupts development of the left hemisphere before it does so when given to the right hemisphere. This may indicate that the left hemisphere develops in advance of the right. In females treatment of the left hemisphere on day 2 leads to a significant slowing of learning relative to controls ($p < 0.05$), and also on day 4. On day 12 treatment of either the left or right hemispheres of females causes a slight but significant retardation of learning. The data for bilateral treatment of the hemispheres with cycloheximide have not been included. In males bilateral treatment retards learning if administered on any day after day 2 and before day 8 but not when given at any other age. In females, bilateral treatment has no effect on subsequent learning no matter at which age it is administered. Note that data reported previously (Rogers and Ehrlich 1983; Rogers 1986) have shown that cycloheximide treatment of the right hemisphere of males on day 2 causes some slight retardation in learning of this task, albeit significantly less than treatment of the left hemisphere. Treatment at this age has been repeated many times and, apart from the initial experiment reported previously, no effect of treating the right hemisphere has been found. The data reported for day 2 in this figure is the frequently repeated measure for that age. In addition, the data points at days 4, 5, 7, 8, 9, 10 and 11 days in males have been repeated twice and the placement of the lateralized peaks was found to be consistent across experiments (day 3 has not been tested).

hemisphere being affected. On days 10 and 11 the right hemisphere is susceptible while the left is not, and thereafter neither hemisphere responds to cycloheximide treatment.

By comparing the effects of bilateral treatment of the hemispheres with cycloheximide with those of unilateral treatment it is possible to deduce whether the hemispheres are working independently or whether their function is coupled. Bilateral treatment of both hemispheres with cycloheximide has been shown to retard visual discrimination learning when it is given after day 1 and prior to day 8 post-hatching (Rogers 1986). By day 8 bilateral treatment of the hemispheres has a slight tendency to retard visual discrimination learning but the effect is no longer significant (Rogers *et al.* 1974; Rogers 1986). On the other hand, unilateral treatment of the left hemisphere on day 8 causes a marked, highly significant retardation of learning (Fig. 20.1). Thus, on day 8 an imbalanced treatment state (with cycloheximide in one hemisphere and without it in the other) is more effective in causing retardation than the balanced, bilateral treatment. This differs from the effects of earlier treatment between days 2 and 5 inclusive (possibly including day 6 which has not been tested), at which stage retardation results equally from bilateral treatment and from unilateral treatment of the left hemisphere. Similarly, unilateral treatment on days 10 and 11, this time of the right hemisphere, causes retarded learning but bilateral treatment is completely without effect. The retarded learning resulting from unilateral treatment of the left hemisphere on day 8 and the right hemisphere on day 10 or 11 therefore appears to be qualitatively different from that resulting from treatment between days 2 to 5 or 6. From this data, it has been argued previously (Rogers 1986) that up to the end of the first week of life post-hatching, the hemispheres of the chick brain operate independently for this visual discrimination learning task at least, and that from day 8 on the hemispheres are coupled in such a way that an imbalance between them can be registered. For other forms of information processing interhemispheric communication, such as via the tectal or anterior commissures, may well be present prior to the end of the first week of life (and may possibly be involved in interocular transfer).

Consistent with this hypothesis of coupling from day 8 on, if the supraoptic decussation is sectioned on day 2 there is no effect on the asymmetry revealed by cycloheximide treatment on day 4 while that normally revealed by the same treatment on day 8 no longer occurs, and that normally revealed by treatment on day 10 is in the reverse direction (Rogers *et al.* 1986). This suggests that the left–right coupling which occurs from day 8 onwards may be via the supraoptic decussation.

Although these effects of sectioning the supraoptic decussation were manifest at the time of testing in the visual discrimination learning task (between days 13 and 15 in this case), the fact that the groups given unilateral treatment with cycloheximide on day 8 gave different results from those treated similarly on day 10 indicates that the effects of prior sectioning of the decussation depended on the age at which the cycloheximide treatment occurred rather than the time of testing on the visual task (cf. Andrew 1988). The difficulties of extrapolating backwards to generate a timecourse are, however, recognized. Also, although cycloheximide disturbs amino acid pools for only some 20–30 minutes, the interaction of this disturbance with neural activity may be more prolonged. Thus, it may not be possible to tie the precise timing of when coupling commences to day 8 rather than day 9, this latter age being the time of coupling suggested by Andrew and Brennan (1983).

There are also direct effects of sectioning the supraoptic decussation on learning performance in the task itself, as seen in chicks which have not received prior treatment with cycloheximide. Chicks with sectioned decussations and tested binocularly on the visual discrimination task show retarded learning, unlike unoperated controls (Rogers *et al.* 1986). Therefore, sectioning the decussation appears to generate conflict between the hemispheres, thus slowing the ability to learn this task.

Rogers and Ehrlich (1983) have presented evidence that the supraoptic decussation continues to undergo structural changes as it develops during the first week post-hatching. Although the precise end-point of this development could not be determined, it is tempting to suggest that its termination is marked by the two brief periods of unilateral susceptibility to cycloheximide, first of the left hemisphere on day 8 and secondly of the right on days 10 and 11, a sequence possibly related to the switching on of connections first from one side and then the other. These two very transient periods of unilateral susceptibility are separated by a period on day 9 when neither unilateral or bilateral treatment with cycloheximide has any subsequent effects of learning. This 'resistant', perhaps 'dormant', period remains intriguing but inexplicable.

The sharply timed cellular processes underscoring the effects of cycloheximide seemingly confirm the developmental timings of the transitions in eye dominance in the studies by Andrew and Brennan (1983, 1984), which single out day 9 as the important pivot point for a shift between a state of dominance of either the left or right hemispheres to subsequent non-dominance with coupling between the hemispheres. Other studies by R. J. Andrew's group have shown that days 8, 9, 10, and 11 are ages at which important changes in behaviour occur. For example, on day 8, free-ranging chickens have been found to show a sudden appearance of monocular fixation of their adult conspecifics and of the tester observing them (see Chapter 6), and they show a preference for using the right eye for this fixation (Workman 1987). The preferred eye used for fixation switches as rapidly as do the changes in hemispheric susceptibility to cycloheximide. Already by day 9 there is no significant preference for using one eye or the other, but by day 11 there is a significant preference to fixate the observer using the left eye (and right hemisphere). In other words, the timecourse for the shift in eye dominance for fixating the observer corresponds quite precisely with the results obtained with cycloheximide treatment. If we assume that, due to the complete decussation of the optic nerve fibres in the bird, dominance of the left eye means use of the right hemisphere and vice versa, then at a given age the controlling hemisphere is the one sensitive to cycloheximide (left hemisphere on day 8, right on days 10 and 11).

Day 8 is singled out as an exceptional day for eye use in searching for food using topographical cues. Andrew (1988) has reported the results of a task in which chicks were trained to search for food in one corner of an open field using relatively distant cues marked on the wall of the arena in that corner and closer cues marked on two bottles in the tray next to the food. The chicks were tested either when the walls were rotated 180° to the tray or when the bottles were moved to a new site. They were tested monocularly in ages ranging from day 7 to 14. At all ages, except day 8, those using their left eye showed advantage in finding the food by using the topographical cues on the walls of the cage, while the right eye was used for distinguishing food from other targets. On day 8 the right eye system assumed a transient dominance for control of searching and it used only the nearby cues on the bottles. Apart from day 8, chicks of all ages tested using the right eye searched at random.

A similar right-eye dominance on day 8, followed by the pivot point of no dominance on day 9 and then left-eye dominance from day 10 on has been shown for pecking at visual stimuli presented simultaneously in the peripheral visual fields of both eyes (M. Dharmaretnam, personal communication). Prior to day 8 there was no eye dominance for this task.

Considered together, these sharp changes in behaviour which occur in male chicks at the end of the first week of life seem to show rather good correspondence to age-dependent changes in susceptibility of the hemispheres to cycloheximide. The sharp peak in susceptibility of the left hemisphere to the drug on day 8 coincides with an equally sharp and transient change to dominance of the right eye for fixating the observer, directing the pecking response and guiding food searching behaviour. If, at this point, we assume that these visual behaviours are guided primarily by the hemisphere contralateral to each eye, and largely speaking this is so, visual inputs to the right eye would be processed almost exclusively by the left hemisphere. In correlation with this, certain biochemical events in the left hemisphere assume importance on day 8 and so are vulnerable to disruption by pharmacological agents. This biochemical and behavioural importance of the right eye–left hemisphere then declines as rapidly as it appeared, to be superceded on days 10 and 11 by dominance of the left eye for fixating the observer, driving the pecking response and searching for food. A correlated upsurge of biochemical events occurs in the right hemisphere on days 10 and 11, now making this hemisphere more vulnerable to pharmacological disruption.

Since the left and right hemispheres of the chicken subserve different behavioural functions, the right hemisphere for analysing the position of stimuli in space and the left for categorizing stimuli (see Chapter 21 for more detail on this), the shift in dominance from the left hemisphere on day 8 to right on days 10 and 11 may explain certain changes in overt behaviour which occur at this time. Indeed, on day 10 there is a sudden increase in the amount of time which chickens spend out of view of their brood hen (reported in Andrew 1988). Andrew suggests that this is due to an increase in exploration driven by the left hemisphere which is interested in distant, topographical stimuli.

LATERALIZATION OF CELLULAR PROCESSES

It is of interest to discover what biochemical processes are disrupted by the cycloheximide treatment. Cycloheximide inhibits ribosomal protein synthesis, but a series of experiments have shown that this is not the direct mechanism by which it disrupts the lateralized developmental events occurring in the chicken forebrain (Hambley and Rogers 1979; Rogers and Hambley 1982). Rather, by inhibiting protein synthesis in the young brain it causes an accumulation of amino acids, glutamate and aspartate in particular, in brain pools. Glutamate and aspartate are putative neurotransmitters which excite neurons by acting on receptors located on the cell membranes. Injected on their own on day 2, glutamate and aspartate have been shown to mimic the action of cycloheximide in causing permanent retardation of learning (Hambley and Rogers 1979; Howard *et al.* 1980). One may hypothesize that they do so by exciting neurons at random during a sensitive period when precisely patterned neural activity is required, and the sensitive period for this activity occurs first in the left hemisphere and then in the right.

Different receptor numbers for these neurotransmitters in the left hemisphere may, at least in part, explain this hemisphere's greater susceptibility to glutamate and aspartate in early life. McCabe and Horn (1988) have recently shown that imprinting of chickens triggers a large increase in the number of N-methyl-D-aspartate receptors (receptors for glutamate and aspartate) in the medial part of the hyperstriatum ventrale (IMHV) in the left hemisphere, as measured some 22–38 hours after hatching. The elevation in receptor number was assessed only in the IMHV of each hemisphere, as that is the region known to be involved in imprinting (see Chapter 8), but no measurements were made in other regions of the forebrain. Nevertheless, the presence of more receptors for glutamate in the left hemisphere would mean that there is an increased opportunity for a given dose of glutamate to excite cells, which may well explain the sensitivity of the left hemisphere, and not the right, to glutamate and cycloheximide in chicks of this age.

It should be noted here that cycloheximide and glutamate no longer have an effect in retarding learning when they are administered after day 12; yet, males older than this show asymmetry when tested monocularly (see later). The early developmental events, which can be disrupted by glutamate and cycloheximide treatment, may therefore be precursors to long-term or permanent lateralization of information processing for behavioural control.

SEX DIFFERENCES IN LATERALIZATION

So far, the time-course for males only has been discussed. Females treated with cycloheximide or glutamate in the left hemisphere on day 2, like males, show subsequent retarded learning of the visual discrimination task and those treated in the right hemisphere do not (see Fig. 20.1). This effect is still just evident on day 4; however, by day 7 and from then on neither hemisphere of the female is susceptible apart from a slight, but significant, increase in susceptibility of the left and right hemispheres on day 12. Thus, in females, development of the right hemisphere is never severely disrupted by cycloheximide treatment, and moreover bilateral treatment of the forebrain hemispheres in females has no effect on learning the visual discrimination task, no matter at what age the treatment occurs. The peak in susceptibility to cycloheximide which occurs on day 2 in females is therefore like the peak which occurs on day 8 in males and, in the same way as argued for males, the lack of effect of bilateral treatment at this age may be said to indicate that hemispheric coupling may occur as early as day 2 in females. This has not yet been tested. Nor has the behaviour of females been tested on the same large battery of tests as already described for males, but there is at least some evidence that behaviours which peak on day 10, such as time spent in exploration out of sight of the hen, occur less strongly in females than in males (Andrew 1988). Also, in some tasks which have revealed lateralization by testing the chicks monocularly, females have been found to show less marked lateralization. For example, in the task testing fear responses to the violet bead, Andrew and Brennan (1984) found no lateralization between the eyes in females tested at several ages between days 2 and 10. Both of the eyes in the females followed the same pattern of responding as did the males using the right eye.

Lateralization of learning the visual discrimination task requiring the chick to discriminate food from pebbles can be revealed by monocular testing on this task. Mench and Andrew (1986) tested three-day-old chicks on this task and found that male chicks learned faster when using the right eye than when using the left, which is consistent with the right eye—left hemisphere being more concerned with categorizing stimuli and recognizing them against a background of distracting stimuli. In this study by Mench and Andrew (1986) females of the same age also showed laterality, with the right eye learning faster than the left. Male chicks aged 14–16 days show the same laterality in this task as do younger ones, whereas females aged 14–16 days show no left-right eye difference, both eyes learning as well as the right eye of the male (Zappia and Rogers 1987). By day 23–24 males no longer have lateralization on this task (see later, and Fig. 20.5).

Another test has similarly shown that older females (2 weeks old) show no asymmetry whereas males have asymmetry. Vallortigara *et al.* (1988) investigated learning to discriminate between two identical boxes on the basis of their position. While males learnt the task faster when the negative box was placed to the right of the positive box, females showed no left or right advantage.

Although the data are, as yet, scanty, one might tentatively suggest that very young females have lateralization of visual learning, but older females have no lateralization of this brain function, both of their eyes performing as the right eye of the male. Alternatively, monocular testing may reveal lateralization at one level of organization, and cycloheximide or glutamate treatment of the hemispheres may reveal it at another, higher order level of organization. If so, there may be lateralization in both sexes at a higher level of information processing but there may be a sex difference in the organization of visual pathways which provide input to this level. The sex difference is perhaps a matter of age and development of visual pathways from eye to forebrain, the eyes of the females achieving equal access to lateralized cognitive functions earlier than in the male (see later).

Thus far, only visual functions and their lateralization have been discussed. Another category of behaviour, aggressive and sexual, is also lateralized in the chicken brain. It occurs equally in both sexes and persists into adulthood. Howard *et al.* (1980) have found that chicks treated in the left hemisphere with glutamate or cycloheximide subsequently showed elevation of copulation and attack behaviour, just as if they had received a dose of testosterone. Treatment of the right hemisphere does not elevate the levels of these behaviours. Males and females show this effect equally well (Bullock and Rogers 1986). Also, the effect may not be confined to a sensitive period, as treatment of the left hemisphere is still effective on day 11.

There is an important distinction between the mode of action of cycloheximide or glutamate treatment of the left hemisphere which leads to elevated attack and copulation and that which retards visual discrimination learning. The latter effect only occurs if the chicken observes specific visual patterns for at least 3 hours after the drug treatment, these being intersecting lines or spots (Rogers and Drennen 1978; Sdraulig *et al.* 1980). The chickens can be protected from either drug's effect by being held in white buckets, or buckets with non-intersecting lines on the wall, for 3 hours after treatment. No such protection is afforded from the effect of these drugs on attack and copulation (Rogers and Hambley 1982). This implies that the effect on visual learning does indeed involve an interaction between glutamate and active neurons in the visual system (first in the left forebrain hemisphere and then in the right), whereas the effect on attack and copulation involves a completely different neural system. Visual mechanisms do not appear to be involved in the effect of cycloheximide on subsequent attack and copulation. The two effects may also interface with completely different levels of neural processing, the retarded learning effect occurring at the level of information input, and the attack and copulation at the level of decision making or in output pathways to the centres in the hypothalamus which control these behaviours.

Functional lateralities between the eyes are also present for attack and copulation. Monocular testing of young, male chicks treated with testosterone leads to the expected elevation in copulation scores when the chicks are tested using the left eye, but no increase above control levels is seen when the testosterone-treated chicks are tested using the right eye (Rogers *et al.* 1985). Neural systems fed by the left eye activate attack and copulation, whereas those fed by the right eye suppress it. This suggests that the left hemisphere inhibits attack and copulation and the right hemisphere activates them. Hence, one route by which testosterone may act to facilitate copulation and attack may be to decrease the likelihood of control by the left hemisphere.

It is interesting to compare the above with the effects of testosterone treatment on monocular performance on the visual discrimination task. In the visual discrimination learning task testosterone treatment of males has different effects on the learning performance of each eye system (Zappia and Rogers 1987). It prevents the learning which normally occurs in monocular males using the right eye, and has a lesser but significant effect of improving learning of those using the left eye. Male chicks which have been treated with testosterone oenanthate therefore learn the visual discrimination task when using their left eye but not when using the right. This is effectively the reverse of that seen in controls, although testosterone-treated chicks using the left eye do not learn as well as controls using their right eye. That is, for performance on this task testosterone has a greater effect on the right eye–left hemisphere than on the left eye-right hemisphere. Incidentally, similar testosterone treatment of young females does not generate in them any lateralization for visual discrimination learning (Zappia and Rogers 1987), indicating that testosterone does not act in a simple, unitary sense in this context.

Lateralization for the control of agonistic behaviour has also been found in adult fowls (copulation was not scored). Hens accustomed to living in battery cages had monocular polypeepers, which occlude the frontal field of vision used for binocular vision, applied to either the left or right eye and they were then released into a large cage in groups of 14 birds (Rogers and Workman, in preparation). There were two control groups, one without polypeepers and the other with binocular polypeepers. Agonistic encounters and avoidance behaviours were scored and found to be significantly reduced in those chicks wearing binocular polypeepers and those with the monocular polypeepers on the left eye (Fig. 20.2). The groups without polypeepers and those with the monocular polypeepers on

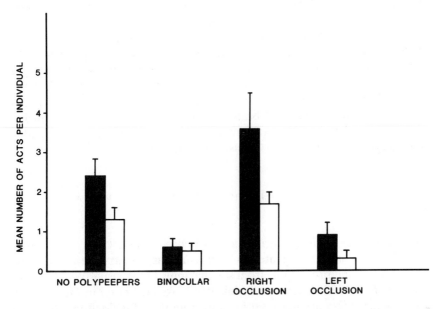

Fig. 20.2 Adult hens have been scored for agonistic encounters (*black bars*) and avoidance behaviour (*open bars*) in the following four groups of 14 hens each: wearing no polypeepers, wearing binocular polypeepers which occlude the frontal vision of each eye, occlusion of the frontal field of the right eye with a monocular polypeeper and occlusion of the frontal field of the left eye with a monocular polypeeper. Agonistic encounters involved sparring, pecking the other hen and rearing up in threat posture. Avoidance behaviour was scored as running away after an encounter with another hen. The mean number of acts and standard errors have been plotted. This data was collected by Workman and Rogers (in preparation).

the right eye displayed high levels of agonistic and avoidance behaviours. Thus, even in adult females attack behaviour is elicited by stimuli perceived with the left eye, just as occurs in young testosterone-treated chicks. Adult males have not yet been tested, but, if any sex difference occurs in this form of lateralization, it is not a case of presence in males and absence in females (as for visual discrimination learning in the second week of life), but rather it may be a matter of relative degree or ease in eliciting the behaviour from the left eye.

Phillips and Youngren (1986) have shown that placement of kainic acid-induced lesions in the archistriatal region of the forebrain in chicks aged 5 days post-hatching reveals asymmetry for fear behaviour tested some 12 days later. Lesions of the right archistriatum reduce the amount of distress calling in an unfamiliar environment to a significantly greater extent than do lesions of the left hemisphere. There were no sex differences in their results.

Laterality would appear to occur at many different levels of brain organization in the chicken, just as it has been shown to be present in the rat both at the hemispheric level, where it is mediated via the corpus callosum (Denenberg *et al.* 1980, 1986; Berrebi *et al.* 1988), and at the hypothalamic level (Nordeen and Yahr 1982). It is worth mentioning that the archistriatum of the avian brain is connected with the habenular nuclei, and in 2-day-old males the habenular nucleus on the right side is significantly larger than on the left (Gurusinghe and Ehrlich 1985).

STRUCTURAL ASYMMETRY IN THE THALAMOFUGAL VISUAL PROJECTIONS

The differences in visual learning ability between the left and right eyes of males may be in part generated by a structural asymmetry in the organization of the visual projections from the thalamus to the visual Wulst (Boxer and Stanford 1985; Rogers and Sink 1987). As illustrated in Fig. 20.3, in young males there are more projections from the left side of the thalamus (which receives its input from the right eye) to the right visual Wulst, or hyperstriatum, than there are from the right side of the thalamus (which receives its input from the left eye) to the left hyperstriatum. These projections cross from one side of the brain to the other in the supraoptic decussation (SOD), which has already been shown by lesioning experiments to play a role in lateralization in males (see earlier). Both sides of the thalamus send a large number of projections to their respective ipsilateral hyperstriata. The presence of asymmetry in the contralateral projections was first reported by Boxer and Stanford (1985) using the horseradish peroxidase technique to trace the projections from thalamus to hyperstriatum. They used 8-day-old chicks.

Rogers and Sink (1987) have confirmed the presence and direction of this asymmetry in male chicks aged 2–6 days and 12–16 days. Fluorescent dyes were used to label the neurons projecting to the hyperstriata in the left and right sides of the forebrain. In our first experiments True Blue was injected into either the left or right hyperstriatum, but more recently we have confirmed the earlier finding using a double-labelling technique, True Blue being injected into the hyperstriatum on one side of the forebrain, and fluorogold into the other. The order of injection was randomized. These markers are taken up by those neurons which project to the site of injection and are transported retrogradely to the neuronal cell bodies where they accumulate. Thus, after sectioning the brain it is possible to count the number of cell bodies labelled with either True Blue or fluorogold at the thalamic level, and so obtain quantitative measures of

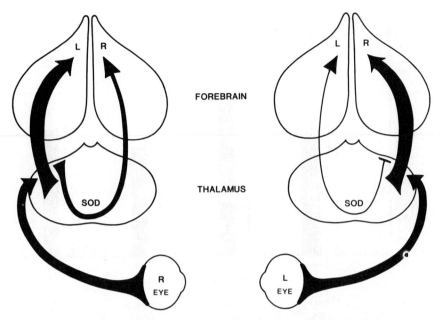

Fig. 20.3   This represents the asymmetrical organization of visual pathways in the thalamofugal system for males. The figure on the left illustrates those pathways fed by the right eye and arising from the left side of the dorsolateral thalamus. There is a large ipsilateral projection to the left hyperstriatum in the forebrain and a somewhat smaller projection (approximately 40 per cent of the number of ipsilateral projections) to the right hyperstriatum. The latter crosses from the left to right side of the brain via the supraoptic decussation (SOD). The figure on the right illustrates the organization of visual projections fed by the left eye and arising from the right side of the thalamus. The ipsilateral projection to the right hyperstriatum is equivalent to that on the other side, but the contralateral projection to the left hyperstriatum is much smaller than its counterpart on the other side (only 15 per cent of the number of ipsilateral projections).

the thalamofugal projections to the visual regions of the hyperstriata. As it is necessary to allow some 4 days survival of the chicks after injection so that the dyes can accumulate in the cell bodies, the time-windows sampled ranged from days 2–6, 12–16, and so on. Cell bodies in the thalamus are labelled both ipsilaterally and contralaterally to each injection site, the ipsilateral ones being more numerous. By calculating the ratio of the number of contralateral cells to ipsilateral cells for each dye separately it is possible to control for variations in the amount of dye injected (C/I ratios in Fig. 20.4; see Adret and Rogers 1989). The C/I ratio in male chicks was significantly higher for injections placed in the right hyperstriatum than for those in the left hyperstriatum, meaning that the left side of the thalamus has a larger number of projections to the right hyperstriatum

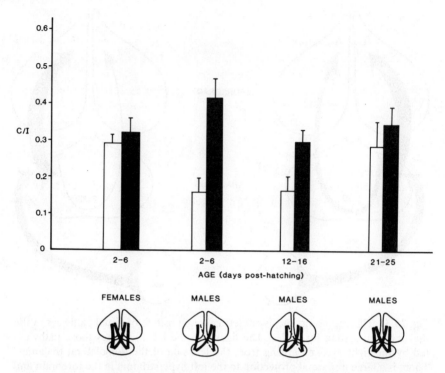

Fig. 20.4 The ratio of the number of contralateral cell bodies to ipsilateral cell bodies labelled relative to each injection site in the left or right hyperstriatum has been plotted for one age-group of female chicks and three age-groups of males. The group of females was injected on day 2 post-hatching and killed on day 6 and this was matched by a group of males of the same age. The other groups of males were injected on day 12 and killed on day 16 or injected on day 21 and killed on day 25. The *open bars* give the mean *C/I* ratios (plus standard errors) for injections into the left hyperstriatum, and the *black bars* for injections into the right hyperstriatum. True Blue and fluorogold were injected into opposite sides of the hyperstriatal region of the forebrain, the order being randomized. Note that there is no asymmetry in the female group ($n = 10$), but significant asymmetry occurs in males of the day 2–6 and 12–16 groups ($p = 0.004$, $n = 9$ and $p < 0.02$, $n = 11$ respectively). There is, however, no asymmetry in the day 21–25 age group of males ($n = 8$). The diagrams underneath illustrate the organization of the thalamofugal projections to the hyperstriata. All the data has been collected for white leghorn crossed with black australorp chickens.

than does the right side of the thalamus to the left hyperstriatum. As each side of the thalamus receives projections from its contralateral eye only, these results demonstrate that the right eye of chicks aged up to 16 days connects to the visual hyperstriata on both sides of the forebrain, whereas the left eye connects to the right hyperstriatum but has a relatively underdeveloped projection to the left hyperstriatum.

If we assume that the thalamofugal system is in some way involved in the visual processing required for learning to discriminate grain from a background of small pebbles, and there is some support for this (see earlier), this organization of the thalamofugal projections in males may perhaps explain the better learning performance of chicks using the right eye. Instead of it being a question of the right eye being connected to the left hemisphere and the left eye to the right hemisphere, with the circuits for learning this task being located in the left hemisphere (as suggested earlier), the right eye may have superior learning ability because it connects to the hyperstriata in both hemispheres, whereas the left eye is limited to the right hemisphere. This situation would not be inconsistent with location of the learning circuits in the left hemisphere only, but, alternatively, better learning may occur when both hemispheres can receive the visual input. There are crossed efferent projections from the hyperstriata to the thalamus via the supraoptic decussation, which may be involved if the latter is the case.

Two additional pieces of evidence are worth considering, given the suggestion that the thalamofugal system may be involved in determining the left-right differences in visual discrimination learning, although it is recognized that the thalamofugal system is unlikely to have an exclusive role in visual tasks of this sort. First, in males aged 21–25 days there is no longer any asymmetry in the organization of the thalamofugal projections to the hyperstriata (Fig. 20.4). The contralateral projections from the right side of the thalamus to the left hyperstriatum have developed by this age. Therefore, by this age both eyes of the male are equally well connected to the hyperstriata on either side of the forebrain, and from this it was predicted that the visual learning should occur equally well with either eye in males of this age. This is indeed the case (Fig. 20.5). Males aged 23–24 days were tested monocularly on the task requiring search for grains on a background of pebbles, and both eyes learned the task well.

Second, female chicks examined on day 6 after injection on day 2 have no asymmetry in these visual projections from thalamus to hyperstriata (Fig. 20.4, and for the same result in a feral strain of chicks, see Adret and Rogers 1989). Both sides of the thalamus have as many contralateral projections to the hyperstriata as does the left side of the thalamus (right eye) in the male. This lack of asymmetry in females is consistent with our earlier finding that females in their second week of life learn the pebble floor task equally well with either eye and at a rate equivalent to young males using the right eye (Zappia and Rogers 1987). It is not, however, consistent with the study by Mench and Andrew (1986) which reported that 3-day-old females show lateralization on this task. As left-right differences have been demonstrated in 2-week-old females tested on

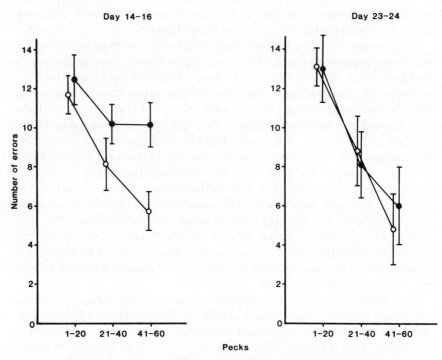

Fig. 20.5   Male chicks have been tested monocularly on the visual discrimination task (as in Fig. 20.1). The number of errors (pecks at pebbles) for each block of 20 pecks is plotted as mean scores ± standard errors for groups of 8–10 chicks. The *open circles* represent those tested using their right eye, and the *black dots* those using their left eye. Two age groups have been tested; day 14–16 and day 23–24. A fall in the curve indicates learning. Note that chicks using their left eye on day 14–16 show no significant learning, while those using their right eye learn. No lateralization occurs in the older chicks.

topographical tests (see Chapter 21), it is clear that the thalamofugal projections cannot be considered to have an exclusive role in determining functional lateralization. Nevertheless, the organization of these projections may contribute to at least some of the sex differences in laterality of function in young chicks.

Although young male chicks show only transient asymmetry in the thalamofugal projections to the hyperstriata and transient lateralization for visual discrimination learning ability, this does not imply that all of their forms of lateralization are transient. The transient asymmetry in thalamofugal projections of males may generate a different degree of hemispheric specialization than that present in females, or a different pattern of such specialization, which persists into adulthood. Crossed projections are necessary for driving binocular units which are used for depth perception by stereopsis, shown in owls to be a property of the visual hyperstriatum (Pettigrew 1979). In the young male chickens tested binocularly the right hemisphere receives such inputs simultaneously from the left and right eyes, while the left hemisphere does so to a much more limited extent. Thus, the right hemisphere may be more responsible for making judgements of depth. This may persist as its specialized property beyond the first weeks of life into adulthood and explain the greater use of the right hemisphere in, say, topographic learning (Andrew 1988).

ROLE OF SUPRAOPTIC DECUSSATION AND TECTAL COMMISSURE IN LATERALIZATION

The contralateral projections which travel from one side of the thalamus to the hyperstriatum on the other opposite side of the forebrain cross the mid-line of the brain in the supraoptic decussation, and, as mentioned earlier, sectioning the supraoptic decussation affects lateralization occurring on and after day 8 of life. Yet, given the presence of asymmetry in the thalamofugal projections in male chicks injected on day 2 and sacrificed on day 6, one might question why sectioning the supraoptic decussation had no effect on the asymmetry present on day 4 (see earlier). A recent experiment may provide more information about this.

The metabolic activity of neurons in the hyperstriata was measured in male chicks of various ages using the radioactive 2-deoxyglucose (2-DG) technique. The 2-DG accumulates in metabolically active neurons. The chicks were injected with 2-DG and housed in groups with a wide variety of visual stimuli for 30 minutes prior to sacrifice. Very low levels of activity were found in the hyperstriata of chicks aged 2 days post-hatching, but in chicks aged 13, 17 or 23 days there was strong labelling of the hyperstriata with 2-DG, and preliminary data for day 7 suggest quite good labelling at that age (Rogers and Bell 1989). Maier and Scheich (1987) have reported a similar absence of labelling of the hyperstriata with 2-DG in guinea fowl chicks aged 1 and 4 days, even in animals re-exposed to their imprinting stimulus, but strong labelling in those aged 7 days. The lack of an effect of sectioning the supraoptic decussation on asymmetry in 4-day-old chicks may therefore result because the thalamofugal system is relatively inactive at this age.

In a recent study (Bell and Rogers, in preparation) we have been able to demonstrate high levels of metabolic activity in the hyperstriatum dorsale (HD) in 2-day-old chicks placed in the optomotor apparatus after injection of 2-DG. As the HD is the sub-region of the hyperstriatum which receives the thalamofugal projections, it would appear that this specific form of visual input drives the thalamofugal system. Interestingly, these same chicks showed very low levels of metabolic activity in the hyperstriatum accessorium, a region which receives input from the HD and is very active in older chicks (Rogers and Bell 1989).

Thus it would appear that in the first week post-hatching the thalamofugal system is relatively inactive, or perhaps selectively active for certain forms of visual stimulation or in certain tasks. Rogers and Bell (1989) have suggested that the two visual systems of the chick become fully functional at different rates, and that the ectostriatal (or tectofugal) visual system subserves the majority of early visual behaviour. If so, then superior learning performance by the right eye on day 3 (Mench and Andrew 1986) may depend solely on use of the tectofugal visual system and on the learning circuits being located in the left hemisphere. It would perhaps be timely to investigate whether lateralization occurs in the tectofugal system of the newly hatched chicken, either at a structural or a functional level. It should also be noted that in their first week of life chicks learn the visual discrimination task much more slowly than older chicks even when tested binocularly, which may possibly relate to use of only the one visual system.

Incidentally, it is between days 0 and 4 post-hatching that the hyperstriatum accessorium undergoes its greatest degree of increase in the density of spine synapses and in the synapse/neuron ratio (Bradley 1985). This is somewhat puzzling, as one might expect these changes to be occurring in response to early visual input and, if so, one would expect them to be accompanied by elevated metabolic activity of neurons in the hyperstriatum. Focused activity of the hyperstriatum accessorium for particular sorts of learning may, however, explain this, and past experience may also play a role. Brown and Horn (1978, 1979), for example, have shown that exposing 1-and 2-day-old chicks to a flashing light for 3 hours increases the number of unit responses which can be electrophysiologically recorded from the hyperstriatum accessorium, compared to dark-reared controls. By contrast, these researchers found that the unit reponses recorded from the HD were not influenced by visual experience. Visual experience increases the volume of the dendritic spines in the hyperstriatum accessorium, but does not alter the synaptic apposition length, the volume of the boutons or the mean number of synapses per micrograph (Bradley and Horn 1979). Although it is tempting to suggest that the low level of 2-DG labelling in the hyperstriatum of the young chicks in our experiment was due to prior lack of visual experience, they had all received exposure to the normal range of stimuli present in the laboratory and were housed in groups from hatching until day 2 and after the injection of 2-DG. Further studies are needed to clarify this.

Nevertheless, there appear to be a series of timed events which comprise phases of development in the chicken. In males, asymmetry in the thalamofugal projections occurs at a structural level up to somewhere between day 16 and 25 post-hatching, but for the first week this asymmetry is either not used or used very rarely in specific situations. In the second and third weeks, the thalamofugal system has become fully functional and its input to the forebrain is asymmetrical. By the end of the third week this input has become symmetrical, and functional lateralization occurring from this time on cannot stem from lateralized inputs from thalamus to forebrain. The first 2 weeks of post-hatching development are also singled out as a period of synaptogenesis, to be followed by synaptic maturation (see J. Rostas Chapter 7).

Incidentally, we have very recently found that there is a high level of metabolic activity in the hyperstriata in embryos at day 19 of incubation (Rogers and Bell, in preparation). The brief period of low levels of 2-DG labelling which occurs post-hatching may therefore represent an active shutting down or focussing of neural activity in the hyperstriatum accessorium during this phase of development.

Apart from the supraoptic decussation, other neural pathways which connect the left and right sides of the avian brain are the tectal commissure, the posterior commissure and the anterior commissure. The former, at least, appears to have a part in maintaining functional asymmetry, as demonstrated in the pigeon (Güntürkün and Bohringer 1987). Like young male chicks, adult pigeons learn to discriminate grain from pebbles better when using the right eye (Güntürkün and Kesch 1987), and similarly they show superior performance in an operant task of pattern discrimination when they use the right eye (Güntürkün 1985). Sectioning the tectal commissure (along with the nearby posterior commissure) reverses the direction of this lateralization (Güntürkün and Bohringer 1987). These data would seemingly locate the lateralization of visual learning in the tectofugal system, possibly at the level of the tectum itself. The hyperstriatum does, however, have efferent projections to the tecta (via the tractus septomesencephalicus; Bagnoli *et al.* 1980), and so there is a possibility for involvement of the thalamofugal system. Given the reciprocal connections between tectum and forebrain, the forebrain may be the source of lateralization which is finally established at tectal level. Although the pigeon has been the species on which most studies investigating the organization of the thalamofugal visual system have been conducted, no attempt has yet been made to investigate whether this species has asymmetry of organization in these projections and there has been no investigation of their development.

FACTORS AFFECTING THE DEVELOPMENT OF LATERALIZATION

The direction of lateralization in the chicken brain is determined by light exposure of the embryo prior to hatching. For the last several days prior to hatching the embryo is oriented in the egg in such a way that its left eye is occluded by the body and the right eye remains exposed to receive light input entering via the shell and membranes (Rogers 1986). This posture of the body occurs at the stage at which the central visual connections in the forebrain are becoming electrophysiologically functional and when light stimulation can evoke motor responses in the embryo (Freeman and Vince 1974). The eye itself opens and closes during this period; yet, even when closed it is covered by transparent eye-lids which allow light to pass through.

Chickens hatched from eggs incubated in darkness during the last 3 days of incubation no longer show functional lateralization at the group (or population) level. When glutamate is injected unilaterally into the hemispheres on day 2 post-hatching, there is no longer a difference in attack and copulation scores between those injected in the left and those in the right hemispheres (Rogers 1982; Zappia and Rogers 1983). The scores for each group appear to be bimodally distributed, although this could only be tested for significance with larger numbers of chicks; half of the individuals had low scores and the other half high scores. In other words, it would seem that each individual chick hatched from an egg incubated in darkness retains lateralization of brain function, but half of the chicks so incubated have the lateralization in one direction and half in the other. Light exposure therefore appears to synchronize or align the direction of laterlization so that all individuals are lateralized in the same direction. As little as 2 hours of light exposure (varying in intensity from 100 to 500 lux) on day 19 of incubation is sufficient to align the direction of lateralization in the group (Rogers 1982). The brevity of light exposure which has an effect on lateralization is reminiscent of the equally brief exposure to a visual stimulus which, as found by Bradley and Horn (1979), produced morphometric changes in the hyperstriatum accessorium of 1-and 2-day-old chicks (see earlier). Light exposure of the right eye may enhance the development of visual projections from that eye, increase blood flow to the contralateral hemisphere (Bondy and Morelos 1971) and thereby stimulate a number of developmental processes in that hemisphere. In so doing it may establish or trigger the development of the left hemisphere in advance of the right, as already demonstrated with unilateral treatment of the hemispheres with cycloheximide (see earlier) and so lay the basis for all, or a wide range, of lateralities in function.

By withdrawing the embryo's head from the egg on day 19/20 of incubation, it has now been possible to reverse the direction of functional lateralization in the forebrain (Figs. 20.6 and 20.7; Rogers 1990). This result clearly establishes the role of light in determining the direction of lateralization in the chicken brain.

The embryos' heads were withdrawn from their eggs on day 19/20 and patches were applied to the right or left eyes. The latter situation mimicked the natural condition and was used as a control. Those with occlusion of

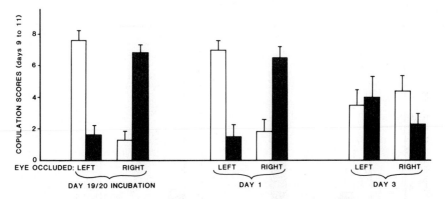

Fig. 20.6 Reversal of lateralization for control of copulation by occlusion of the right eye. Monocular eye patches were applied to either the left or right eyes for 24 hours on day 19/20 of incubation, day 1 post-hatching or day 3 post-hatching. The lateralization for copulation was revealed by injecting glutamate into the left hemisphere (*open bars*) or right hemisphere (*black bars*) on day 2 post-hatching for the first two groups and day 4 post-hatching for the third group. Copulation was scored from day 6 to 11 inclusive, and the figure represents data averaged across days 9–11. Means and standard errors are plotted (n = 8–10 per group). Controls received occlusion of the left eye (mimicking the normal situation) and test animals received occlusion of the right eye. Note the reversal of lateralization by occlusion of the right eye on day 19/20 of incubation and on day 1 post-hatching.

the left eye were found to have the same lateralization for attack, copulation, and visual learning discrimination as seen in chicks which hatched from unmanipulated eggs exposed to light before hatching. This laterality was revealed by unilateral treatment of the hemispheres with glutamate on day 2 post-hatching: those injected in the left hemisphere showed elevated attack and copulation scores (Fig. 20.6: note that the scores for copulation only are given, as attack scores were similar) and retarded learning (Fig. 20.7). In contrast, the embryos which had had occlusion of the right eye and light exposure of the left eye showed elevation of attack and copulation and retarded visual discrimination learning following glutamate treatment of their right hemispheres, while treatment of the left had no effect. The direction of lateralization was reversed at the group level; that is their laterality was aligned in the opposite direction to that of controls.

The sensitive period for this effect extends to day 1 post-hatching. The eggs were incubated in darkness and the chicks kept undisturbed in the dark incubator for the first 24 hours, at which time eye patches were applied in darkness to either one of the eyes. They were then exposed to light for 24 hours with the eye patches in place, after which time the patches were removed and rearing proceeded as normal. Unilateral

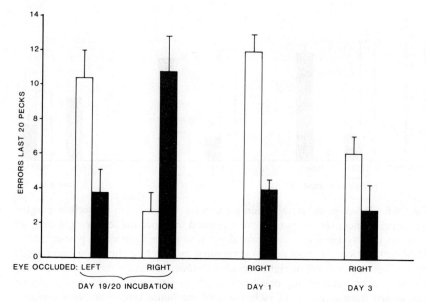

Fig. 20.7   Reversal of lateralization for visual discrimination learning. The mean number of errors, and standard errors, are plotted for the last 20 pecks (as in Fig. 20.1). The eyes were occluded as described in Fig. 20.6. Note the reversal of lateralization by occlusion of the right eye on day 19/20 of incubation, but not by the same procedure on day 1 or 3 post-hatching.

treatment of the hemispheres with glutamate on day 2, 5 minutes after removal of the patches, revealed the normal direction of lateralization for attack and copulation in those chicks which had had occlusion of the left eye and reversed lateralization in those which had had occlusion of the right eye (Fig. 20.6). Occlusion of the right eye at this age, however, fails to reverse the direction of lateralization for visual discrimination learning (Fig. 20.7). Thus, the sensitive period for plasticity in the neural pathways used for visual discrimination learning is shorter than that for attack and copulation performance.

Extending the period of incubation and rearing in darkness to day 3 post-hatching causes some problems in later behavioural testing for attack and copulation. In this case the unilateral treatment with glutamate was given on day 4, 5 minutes after removal of eye patches, which had been applied on day 3. In normal, light-exposed chicks treated with glutamate at this age, treatment of the left hemisphere, but not the right, retards learning and elevates attack and copulation, but in the dark-reared chicks which had received occlusion of the left eye there were no differences between the attack and copulation scores for the groups injected on the left and right sides. For those which had received occlusion of the right eye there was also no significant difference in copulation scores between those injected in the left versus the right hemisphere (Fig. 20.6). Given the effect of dark-rearing on the performance of the controls, it is not possible to draw any conclusions from these data for attack and copulation. However, dark-rearing had less effect on performance in the visual discrimination learning task, and chicks which had received occlusion of the right eye on day 3 showed the normal lateralization of retarded learning after unilateral treatment with glutamate (Fig. 20.7), confirming that the sensitive period for reversal of lateralization for visual discrimination learning ends before day 1 post-hatching.

As mentioned already, as little as 2 hours of light exposure of embryos on day 19 of incubation is sufficient to align the direction of functional lateralization in the population, while 1 hour of light exposure is ineffective (Rogers 1982). It was considered of interest to know how stably this direction of lateralization is held by the brain once it has been established. To test this, embryos were exposed to 1,2, or 6 hours of light on day 19 of incubation prior to having their heads withdrawn from the egg, and eye-patches applied to the right eye for 24 hours, while the left eye was exposed to light. The aim of this procedure was to attempt to reverse the direction of lateralization (Rogers, 1990). Reversal of lateralization occurred in those embryos exposed to light for 1 hour before the occlusion of the right eye, and this is expected as 1 hour of light is insufficient to establish the direction of lateralization. Reversal of lateralization also occurred in those exposed to light for 2 hours before occlusion of the right eye, but not in those exposed to light for 6 hours. Thus, while 2 hours of light exposure on day 19 of incubation is sufficient to determine the direction of lateralization, more than 2 hours (but less than 6 hours) is necessary to 'fix' this direction so that it can no longer be reversed by light exposure of the left eye. In other words, neural plasticity remains for a short period of time after asymmetrical light input has established the direction of lateralization. Thereafter, the direction appears to be stabilized, and separate time-courses of development proceed in each hemisphere.

Recent studies in our laboratory have shown that light exposure of the male embryo on day 19 or 20 of incubation establishes the direction of asymmetry in the visual projections from either side of the thalamus to the hyperstriatum (Rogers and Sink 1987). As described above for the studies investigating reversal of functional lateralization, the heads of embryos were withdrawn from the egg on day 19/20 of incubation and eye patches were applied to either the left (mimicking the normal situation) or right eye. The patches remained in place for 24 hours while the embryos received light exposure via the unoccluded eye, after which time the patches were removed and rearing continued as usual in the light. On day 2 post-hatching, fluorescent dyes were injected into the hyperstriatum on each side of the forebrain, and 4 days later the number cells labelled in the thalamus were counted. Fig. 20.8 presents the data for calculations of the ratio of the number of cell bodies labelled on the side contralateral to the injection site to those labelled on the ipsilateral side (*C/I* ratio).

The control group, which consisted of chicks which had received occlusion of the left eye, had the normal direction of asymmetry in the visual projections. The *C/I* ratios were higher following injections in the right hyperstriatum than following injections in the left, meaning that the left side of the thalamus had a much larger number of projections to its contralateral hyperstriatum than the right side of the thalamus to its contralateral hyperstriatum. Those chicks which had received occlusion of the right eye were found to have the asymmetry of their projections from thalamus to hyperstriatum in the reverse direction. It is therefore lateralized light stimulation of the eyes which establishes the direction of the structural asymmetry in these visual projections from thalamus to forebrain in males.

The direction of the asymmetry in these visual projections correlates with the direction of functional asymmetry, such that the eye which learns the visual discrimination task is the one which projects to the side of the thalamus with the largest number of connections to its contralateral hyperstriatum. This eye is therefore well connected to both hyperstriata, whereas the eye which does not learn this task is well connected to one hyperstriatum but only poorly to the other.

For an eye to be well connected to both hyperstriata it must receive light input before or just after hatching. The following experiment shows that each eye operates independently in its response to light stimulation in this way. An additional group of embryos was incubated in darkness until hatching had occurred, and then the chicks were exposed to light. Each eye therefore received light exposure simultaneously. As before, the fluorescent dyes were injected on day 2 post-hatching. There was no asymmetry in the visual projections from thalamus to hyperstriata in these birds (Fig. 20.8). Both sides of the thalamus had large numbers of connections to their respective contralateral hyperstriata. Light exposure of both eyes simultaneously stimulated the growth of these visual projections from the thalamus equally on both sides of the brain.

The absence of asymmetry in the visual projections in this latter group correlates with the earlier finding by Zappia and Rogers (1983) of an absence of functional lateralization for attack and copulation at the group level in chicks hatched from eggs similarly incubated in darkness and exposed to light only after hatching. The chicks in this study would have had no asymmetry in the organization of their thalamofugal projections. Even though the organization of the thalamofugal visual projections may have no direct association with lateralization of attack and copulation behaviours, asymmetry of light input to the eyes of the embryo clearly influences both the functional lateralization of the forebrain and the asymmetrical organization of the visual projections.

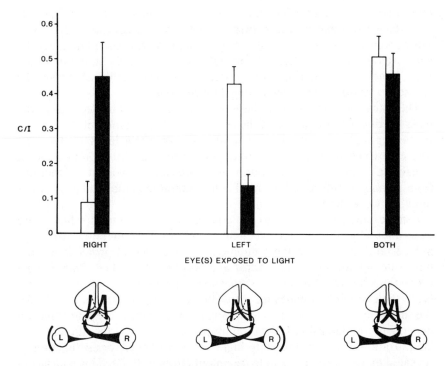

Fig. 20.8 The effect of lateralized light input to the eyes on the organization of the thalamofugal visual pathways in males. *C/I* ratios have been plotted as in Fig. 20.4, the *open bars* being the ratios for injections in the left hyperstriatum and the *black bars* for those in the right hyperstriatum. The dyes were injected on day 2 post-hatching. The wording under each column represents the eye occluded for 24 hours. Note that the unoccluded eye was exposed to light. Occlusion of the left eye on day 19/20 of incubation, which mimics the normal situation, leads to the same asymmetry as reported for unmanipulated male chicks (as in Fig. 20.4). Occlusion of the right eye at this age reverses the direction of asymmetry (middle columns of data). Simultaneous light input to both eyes, on day 1 post-hatching after incubating in darkness, removes the asymmetry; the contralateral thalamofugal projections have developed equally on both sides.

Another interesting aspect of the effect of light in stimulating the growth of the thalamofugal projections is that once the contralateral projections from one side of the thalamus have developed, as a result of asymmetrical light input to the eyes, the contralateral pathway from the other side of the thalamus is inhibited from growing until some 2–3 weeks after hatching (see Fig. 20.4). This is so despite the fact that following the 24 hours of monocular exposure to light, as in the experiment reported in Fig. 20.8, the chicks were kept in the light and had both eyes open. Development of one set of contralateral projections in response to light input inhibits, for more than 2 weeks after hatching, the growth of its counterpart from the eye which had been occluded prior to hatching. In contrast, when both sets of contralateral projections are stimulated to grow simultaneously, by allowing both eyes to receive their first exposure to light simultaneously, there is no such inhibition and, apparently, no competition between the two sets of contralateral thalamofugal projections.

The transient asymmetry in these thalamofugal visual projections of the male is a direct consequence of the asymmetrical orientation of the embryo in the egg and the consequent lateralization of visual input to the eyes. The eye which receives light input, in a sense, 'wins' its complement of thalamofugal projections to both hemispheres and prevents the other eye from gaining its full complement of contralateral thalamofugal projections until 2–3 weeks later.

Female chickens appear to be equivalent to the males which were experimentally able to receive light simultaneously in both eyes (and indeed females do have large numbers of contralateral projections from both sides of the thalamus: Adret and Rogers 1989). The thalamofugal projections of the female may develop independently of light input. Nevertheless, while females may possibly lack responsiveness to light for the development of their thalamofugal projections, they are indeed dependent on lateralized light input for determining the direction of lateralization at other, probably higher, levels of their brain function as revealed by unilateral glutamate treatment (Rogers 1982). This conclusion is reached as, in all of the experiments demonstrating lateralization of function by occlusion of the embryo's right eye coupled with exposure of the left to light, the effects were the same for males and females. Of course, it is also possible that the lateralized light input received by the embryo influences development of the tectofugal visual system and that it does so in both females and males.

REFERENCES

Adret, P. and Rogers, L. J. (1989). Sex difference in the visual projections of young chicks: a quantitative study of the thalamofugal pathways. *Brain Research*, **478**, 59–73.
Andrew, R. J. (1988). The development of visual lateralization in the domestic chick. *Behavioural Brain Research*, **29**, 201–9.
Andrew, R. J. and Brennan, A. (1983). The lateralization of fear behaviour in the male domestic chick: a development study. *Animal Behaviour*, **31**, 1166–76.
Andrew, R. J. and Brennan, A. (1984). Sex differences in lateralization in the domestic chick. *Neuropsychologia*, **22**, 503–9.
Bagnoli, P., Grassi, S., and Magni, F. (1980). A direct connection between visual wulst and tectum opticum in the pigeon (*Columba livia*) demonstrated by horseradish peroxidase. *Archives of Italian Biology*, **118**, 72–88.

Berrebi, A. S., Fitch, R. H., Ralphe, D. L. Denenberg, J. O., Friedrich, V. L., and Denenberg, V. H. (1988). Corpus callosum: region-specific effects of sex, early experience and age. *Brain Research*, **438**, 216–24.

Bondy, S. C. and Morelos, B. J. (1971). Stimulus deprivation and cerebral blood flow. *Experimental Neurology*, **31**, 200–6.

Boxer, M. I. and Stanford, D. (1985). Projections to the posterior visual hyperstriatal region of the chick: an HRP study. *Experimental Brain Research*, **57**, 494–8.

Bradley, P. (1985). A light and electron microscopic study of the development of two regions of the chick forebrain. *Developmental Brain Research*, **20**, 83–8.

Bradley, P. and Horn, G. (1979). Neuronal plasticity in the chick brain: morphological effects of visual experience on neurones in the hyperstriatum accessorium. *Brain Research*, **162**, 148–52.

Brown, M. W. and Horn, G. (1978). Effects of visual experience on unit responses in hyperstriatum of chick brain. *Journal of Physiology (Canada)*, **278**, 48P.

Brown, M. W. and Horn, G. (1979). Neuronal plasticity in the chick brain: electrophysiological effects of visual experience on hyperstriatal neurones. *Brain Research*, **162**, 142–7.

Bullock, S. P. and Rogers, L. J. (1986). Glutamate induced asymmetry in the sexual and aggressive behaviour of young chickens. *Pharmacology, Biochemistry and Behaviour*, **24**, 549–54.

Denenberg, V. H., Hofmann, M., Garbanati, J. H., Sherman, C. F., Rosen, G. D., and Yutzey, D. A. (1980). Handling in infancy, taste aversion and brain laterality in rats. *Brain Research*, **200**, 123–33.

Denenberg, V. H., Gall, J. S., Berrebi, A., and Yutzey, D. A. (1986). Callosal mediation of cortical inhibition in the lateralized rat brain. *Brain Research*, **397**, 327–32.

Freeman, B. M. and Vince, M. A. (1974). *Development of the avian embryo*. Chapman and Hall, London.

Güntürkün, O. (1985). Lateralization of visually controlled behaviour in pigeons. *Physiology and Behaviour*, **34**, 575–7.

Güntürkün, O. and Bohringer, P. G. (1987). Lateralization reversal after intertectal commissurotomy in the pigeon. *Brain Research*, **408**, 1–5.

Güntürkün, O. and Kesch, S. (1988). Visual lateralization during feeding in pigeons. *Behavioural Neuroscience*, **101**, 433–5.

Gurusinghe, C. J. and Ehrlich, D. (1985). Sex-dependent structural asymmetry of the medial habenular nucleus of the chicken brain. *Cell Tissue Research*, **240**, 149–52.

Hambley, J. W. and Rogers, L. J. (1982). Retarded learning induced by intracerebral administration of amino acids in the neonatal chick. *Neuroscience*, **4**, 677–84.

Howard, K. J., Rogers, L. J., and Boura, A. L. A. (1980). Functional lateralization of the chick forebrain by use of intracranial glutamate. *Brain Research*, **188**, 369–83.

Maier, V. and Scheich, H. (1987). Acoustic imprinting in guinea fowl chicks: age dependence of 2-deoxyglucose uptake in relevant forebrain areas. *Developmental Brain Research*, **31**, 15–27.

McCabe, B. J. and Horn, G. (1988). Learning and memory: regional changes in

N-methyl-D-aspartate receptors in the chick brain after imprinting. *Proceedings of the National Academy of Science, USA*, **85**, 2849–53.

Mench, J. A. and Andrew, R. J. (1986). Lateralization of a food search task in the domestic chick. *Behavioural and Neural Biology*, **46**, 107–14.

Nordeen, E. J. and Yahr, P. (1982). Hemispheric asymmetries in the behavioural and hormonal effects of sexually differentiating mammalian brain. *Science*, **218**, 319–94.

Pettigrew, J. D. (1979). Binocular visual processing in the owl's telencephalon. *Proceedings of the Royal Society of London B*, **204**, 435–54.

Phillips, R. E. and Youngren, O. M. (1986). Unilateral kainic acid lesions reveal dominance of right archistriatum in avian fear behaviour. *Brain Research*, **377**, 216–20.

Rogers, L. J. (1982). Light experience and asymmetry of brain function in chickens. *Nature*, **297**, 223–5.

Rogers, L. J. (1986). Lateralization of learning in chicks. *Advances in the Study of Behaviour*, **16**, 147–89.

Rogers, L. J. (1990). Light input and the reversal of functional lateralization in the chicken brain. *Behavioural Brain Research*, **38**, 211–21.

Rogers, L. J. and Anson, J. M. (1979). Lateralization of function in the chicken forebrain. *Pharmacology, Biochemistry and Behaviour*, **10**, 679–86.

Rogers, L. J. and Bell, G. A. (1989). Different rates of functional development in the two visual systems of the chicken revealed by [^{14}C] 2-deoxyglucose. *Developmental Brain Research*, **49**, 161–72.

Rogers, L. J. and Drennen, H. D. (1978). Cycloheximide interacts with visual input to produce permanent slowing of visual learning in chickens. *Brain Research*, **158**, 479–82.

Rogers, L. J. and Ehrlich, D. (1983). Asymmetry in the chicken forebrain during development and possible involvement of the supraoptic decussation. *Neuroscience Letters*, **37**, 123–7.

Rogers, L. J. and Hambley, J. W. (1982). Specific and non-specific effects of neuro-excitatory amino acids on learning and other behaviours in the chicken. *Behavioural Brain Research*, **4**, 1–18.

Rogers, L. J. and Sink, H. S. (1987). Transient asymmetry in the projections of the rostral thalamus to the visual hyperstriatum of the chicken, and reversal of its direction by light exposure. *Experimental Brain Research*, **70**, 378–98.

Rogers, L. J. Drennen, H. D., and Mark, R. F. (1974). Inhibition of memory formation in the imprinting period: irreversible action of cycloheximide in young chickens. *Brain Research*, **79**, 213–33.

Rogers, L. J. Zappia, J. V., and Bullock, S. P. (1985). Testosterone and eye-brain asymmetry for copulation in chickens. *Experimentia*, **41**, 1447–9.

Rogers, L. J., Robinson, T., and Ehrlich, D. (1986). Role of the supraoptic decussation in the development of asymmetry of brain function in the chicken. *Developmental Brain Research*, **28**, 33–9.

Sdraulig, R., Rogers, L. J., and Boura, A. L. A. (1980). Glutamate and specific perceptual input interact to cause retarded learning in chicks. *Physiology and Behaviour*, **24**, 493–500.

Vallortigara, G., Zanforlin, M., and Cailotto, N. (1988). Right-left asymmetry in position learning of male chicks. *Behavioural Brain Research*, **27**, 189–91.

Workman, L. (1987). Lateralization of brain function and behavioural ontogeny in the chick under natural conditions. D.Phil. thesis, University of Sussex.

Zappia, J. V. and Rogers, L. J. (1983). Light experience during development affects asymmetry of forebrain function in chickens. *Developmental Brain Research*, **11**, 93–106.

Zappia, J. V. and Rogers, L. J. (1987). Sex differences and reversal of brain asymmetry by testosterone in chickens. *Behavioural Brain Research*, **23**, 261–7.

21

The nature of behavioural lateralization in the chick

R. J. Andrew

Evidence from the chick suggests lateralization for two major modes of analysis of a stimulus or experience, which must be carried out simultaneously by any animal capable of complex behaviour (Andrew 1988). The system fed by the left eye predominantly analyses and records detailed and specific properties of stimuli, including their spatial relations; such analysis is necessary if the novelty of a stimulus is to be estimated, and if the organization of the environment is to be learnt. The system that is fed by the right eye is chiefly concerned to select cues which allow stimuli to be assigned to categories which accommodate a range of differing exemplars; such analysis allows rapid and effective choice of the response appropriate to a stimulus (even if that stimulus is in various respects novel).

A second aim of this chapter is to present evidence which suggests that the right and left visual systems can interact in the chick in a variety of ways when assessing and responding to a stimulus. Such interaction is basic to the functioning of lateralized systems. It has proved difficult to pin down in human studies: Allen (1983) considers a variety of theoretically possible types of interaction, all of which have recently been postulated. It is important to establish what sort of interaction actually occurs, since deductions about the nature of hemispheric specialization depend upon the sort of interaction which is believed to occur.

There is increasing evidence for marked asymmetry in the processes of memory formation in the chick (Chapters 8–11, 19). It is likely that this is intimately related to hemispheric specialization of the sort discussed in this chapter. How this might be is discussed briefly in a final section.

HEMISPHERIC SPECIALIZATION IN THE CHICK

This is a convenient point to define a number of terms. Chicks with one eye covered are referred to as right- or left-eyed (RE, LE). The visual structures (including ones concerned with high-level analysis) which lie contralateral to the viewing eye are 'right and left VS'; this excludes commissural projections to the other side of the brain. 'Right- or left-eye systems' (RES, LES) are terms used of the functional system that analyses what is seen by an eye. It is likely that the differences between LE and RE chicks, which are described here, are largely due to differences between the right and left VS. However, evidence of varying involvement of ipsilateral structures under certain circumstances will be presented here; in view of this, it is convenient to have a term which does not imply exclusively contralateral processing. 'RES' and 'LES' are nevertheless used here only where there is good reason to believe that control is predominantly by the contralateral VS; in male chicks, at least, this appears usually to be the case.

Differences between RES and LES have now been demonstrated in the chick using two very different classes of stimuli. These are beads which are small and nearby and evoke pecking, and larger spheres which are presented at a distance and are treated as social companions. Any differences between RES and LES which are revealed by tests with both types of stimuli are unlikely to be associated with particular stimulus properties or motivational states. In both cases, the procedures which were used depended upon response to various degrees of transformation of a familiar stimulus. As a result, the chick (or the eye system) is left to decide what degree of change is important; this is more likely to reveal preferred strategies of analysis than would discrimination driven by powerful reinforcement. It turns out that transformations which evoke response are mostly so great as to be readily discriminable from the original stimulus. This is further evidence that differences between RES and LES do not depend (at least in the main) on differences in lower level visual mechanisms.

Bead experiments

In the first type of experiment (Andrew 1983*b*), beads which could be illuminated internally with coloured light were presented in two pairs of 15s presentations (AB,CD), separated by intervals as follows: A-5s-B-120 minutes-C-5s-D. Standard habituation curves for a violet bead are shown in Fig. 21.1 for 2-day-old chicks; their main features have been repeatedly replicated. In males, the pattern in the CD sector was standard: at C the RE curve was high and the LE curve was low, followed by convergence at D, due to a steep fall in the RE curve and a shallow one in the LE curve.

In females, both sectors showed a pattern different from that present in males, with RE and LE curves identical at the first presentation of each pair (A and C), but then diverging because of a very steep fall in the LE curve.

Habituation is clear in the standard curves. The extent to which different beads are treated as similar was studied by using a range of stimuli in the

538   R. J. Andrew

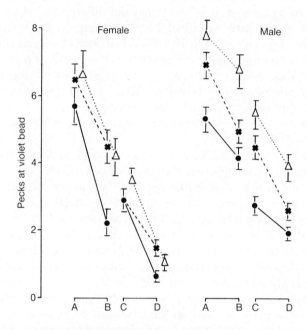

Fig. 21.1 Pecks at a violet bead: habituation curves. A violet-lit bead was presented for a first pair of presentations (each of 15s), separated by a 5 second interval (AB) and then, after 120 minutes, for a second similar pair (CD). The curves are based on all available experiments (females: 3; males: 6); two female and four male experiments included binocular groups. The ANOVAs reported here always compare corresponding populations (e.g. females with males tested in the same period of time). Each condition in each experiment (LE = left-eyed; RE = right-eyed; BIN = binocular) involved 20 chicks, in almost all cases. *Monocular curves.* In females, the LE curve was lower than the RE ($F_{1,81} = 10.09, p < 0.01$) and diverged from it within each pair of presentations (EYE x TEST: $F_{3,242} = 5.36$. $p < 0.01$). In males, the LE curve was also lower than the RE ($F_{1,155} = 15.76$, $p < 0.001$), but it converged with the RE curve within each pair of presentations (CD, EYE x TEST: $F_{1,155} = 4.48, p = 0.036$). Male curves were higher than ($F_{1,171} = 11.13, p < 0.001$), and differed in shape from female curves (SEX x TEST: $F_{3,512} = 5.03, p < 0.01$). Both differences were largely due to LE curves, which were higher in males ($F_{1,85} = 9.60, p < 0.01$), and fell less steeply within AB and CD sectors but more steeply between pairs of presentations (SEX x TEST: $F_{1,85} = 15.64$, $p < 0.001$). *Binocular curves.* In females, the BIN curve was higher than LE ($F_{1,61} = 5.21, p = 0.026$) but identical with RE. In males, all three eye conditions differed in level ($F_{2,173} = 18.53, p < 0.001$); both RE and LE curves were lower than BIN ($F_{1,116} = 8.06, p = 0.005; F_{1,116} = 37.41, p < 0.001$). Female BIN curves were lower ($F_{1,61} = 17.02, p < 0.001$), and fell more steeply than male (SEX x TEST: $F_{3,183} = 5.15, p = 0.002$). LE = continuous lines; RE = dashed lines; BIN = dotted lines.

first pair of presentations in place of the violet bead. These were a red-lit bead (R), a non-illuminated bead (N) and the bare tip (T) of the rod on which the beads were presented: they represented progressively larger transformations of the violet bead (V). The degree of transfer of habituation to the violet bead at the second pair of presentations (here termed A'B') was then estimated by comparison with the standard curves. The two sexes showed similar changes in pattern as the size of the transformation increased, but shifted so that each male pattern matched a female pattern produced by a smaller transformation (Fig. 21.2).

LE and RE birds differ in similar (but not identical) ways in both sexes. RE males treat violet, red and non-illuminated beads as more or less equivalent. It is very unlikely that this is due to inability to discriminate; indeed, following training with an ill-tasting red bead, it is RE males which draw a sharp distinction, inhibiting pecks at red beads, but pecking freely at blue ones, whereas LE males generalize inhibition of pecking to blue beads (Andrew and Brennan 1985). RE females do not treat the three classes of bead as so fully equivalent but the biggest change is still between the curves for the non-illuminated bead and the rod tip (Fig. 21.2).

In both sexes, LE birds respond to smaller changes than do RE birds. This is true not only for changes in the intrinsic properties of the beads but also in their spatial relations: LE birds show dishabituation following a change in the position from which the violet bead approaches, whereas RE chicks are quite unaffected (Andrew 1983b; below). All of these differences between the behaviour of LE and RE birds are argued here to reflect differing specialization of LES and RES.

There is also a sex difference in the behaviour of LE birds. LE females are more strongly affected by any given transformation than LE males: in Fig. 21.2, LE curves in females following prior experience of V, R, or N can be seen to correspond to LE curves for males after experience of R, N, or T, respectively. This, and the marked sex differences in the standard habituation curves for the violet bead, will be discussed further, when differences in the pattern of interaction between the right and left VS are being considered.

Imprinting objects

Comparable specialization of RES and LES is suggested by experiments in which chicks chose between an object (a table tennis ball) like that with which they lived ('familiar' stimulus), and some transformation of it (Vallortigaro and Andrew 1990). Both were usually red with a white bar on one face. At test (day 3), the two balls were presented, one at each end of a runway, in the centre of which the chick was placed.

LE males chose to associate with the familiar test object, when transformation was from a horizontal to a vertical bar or from an oblique bar (45°

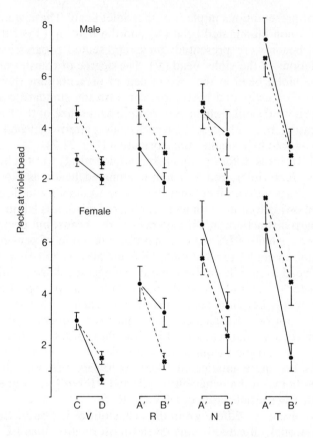

to the horizontal) to an oblique bar tilted the other way. However, transformation from horizontal to oblique resulted in choice of the unfamiliar test object (Fig. 21.3). RE males, in contrast, chose at random under all three conditions (although they spent just as much time close to one or other ball). Only when a marked overall transformation was used (balls changed by the removal of the horizontal bar) did RE males choose. They then, like LE males, chose the familiar object. Binocular groups behaved throughout like LE groups.

When the horizontal bar was extended to form an equatorial belt right around the ball in the home cage, transformation to a vertical meridian also resulted in RE males choosing the familiar object. The change as seen by the chick during test differed little from what was seen at choice between horizontal and vertical bars. It is thus unlikely that inability to distinguish horizontal and vertical bars explains the failure of RE males to choose between them.

When females (Fig. 21.3) chose between horizontal and vertical, or horizontal and oblique bars, RE as well as LE and binocular groups chose

Fig. 21.2 Transfer of habituation. The curves show rates of pecking at a violet-lit bead (V) over a pair of 15 second presentations (refer to Fig. 21.1). In each case the chicks had already seen a similar bead (V) or some transformation of it (R = red-lit; N = not lit; T = rod tip without bead) in a pair of presentations 120 minutes earlier. The curves for chicks which had previously seen a violet bead have already been presented (Fig. 21.1). *Males.* Prior experience of R produced a pattern at first presentation of V (A'B') almost identical with that standardly obtained at the second pair of presentations of V (CD). After N (two experiments) a quite different pattern was obtained: RE and LE coincided at A' but diverged at B' (EYE x TEST, $F_{1,63} = 7.88$, $p < 0.01$). Comparison with all of the standard V habituation curves showed the LE curve here to be higher than CD curves (A' and C: $F_{7,109} = 2.14$, $p < 0.05$; B' and D: $F_{7,116} = 4.46$, $p < 0.001$). After T (two experiments), RE and LE curves coincided. The high rates of response suggested that experience of T had no effect, but comparison with standard AB curves showed that A' was suggestively higher, and B' suggestively lower than the corresponding A and B values (in both cases, $p = 0.067$, Mann Whitney). *Females.* After R (two experiments), uniquely for females, the LE curve sloped less steeply than the RE curve (EYE x TEST: $F_{1,62} = 9.29$, $p = 0.003$). This resulted in significantly higher values at B' than after experience of V ($F_{4,71} = 11.08$, $p < 0.001$). The RE curve, in contrast, was similar to that following V experience. After N, both RE and LE were similar. Their overall level showed little sign of transfer of habituation; however, unlike the standard curves with no prior experience (Fig. 21.1), the LE curve was a little above the RE curve, which fell as steeply as the LE. After T, females showed exactly the same pattern as with no prior experience (RE higher than LE: $F_{1,30} = 5.69$, $p = 0.024$; LE falls more steeply: EYE x TEST, $F_{1,30} = 9.75$, $p = 0.004$). *Male/female.* Note the resemblance between prior R in females and prior N in males, and between prior N in females and prior T in males. LE = continuous lines; RE = dashed lines.

the familiar test object. However, as in the bead tests, lateralization can be demonstrated in females under appropriate conditions (Vallortigaro and Andrew 1990). When females chose between a familiar chick, with which they had been living up to the time of test, and a stranger (of apparently identical appearance), LE and binocular females chose the familiar chick but RE females chose at random. In the same task LE and binocular males chose the stranger and RE males chose at random. Since this is the pattern of choice also shown by males to the smallest rotation of the bar (horizontal to oblique), it suggests that LE males begin to choose the unfamiliar when transformations are judged to be relatively small or minor. It remains to be seen whether sufficiently small transformations would result in a similar choice of unfamiliar object by LE females; this would provide a complete parallel with the bead data.

Once again the differences between LE and RE males suggest that LES is interested in small changes, which tend to be ignored by RES. The fact that RE males do respond to change in an equatorial belt which is visible in the home cage as an invariant property of the ball from whatever angle

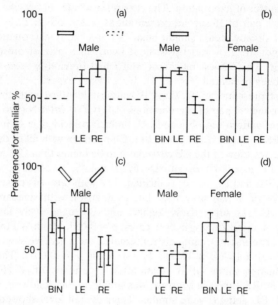

Fig. 21.3 The mean percentage of chicks choosing the familiar stimulus (rather than a transformation of it) is shown; SEM are shown as bars. In all cases, the familiar stimulus was a red table tennis ball bearing a white bar on one face. Transformations involved rotation or removal of the bar. BIN = binocular birds; LE = left-eyed birds; RE = right-eyed birds. (a) Choice between a familiar ball with a horizontal bar and one without a bar. Both LE ($t_{(15)} = 2.40, p < 0.05$) and RE males ($t_{(15)} = 3.60, p < 0.01$) tended to choose the familiar stimulus. (b) Choice between a familiar ball with a horizontal bar and a ball with a vertical bar. Males: BIN ($t_{(30)} = 2.17, p < 0.05$) and LE birds ($t_{(30)} = 8.50, p < 0.001$) tended to choose the familar stimulus. RE birds chose at random. Females: BIN, LE and RE birds all chose the familar stimulus ($t_{(31)} = 4.63, p < 0.001$). (c) Choice between a familiar ball with an oblique bar tilted either to the right (left hand of each pair of histograms) or to the left, and a ball with a bar tilted the other way. BIN ($t_{(29)} = 3.11, p = 0.004$) and LE males ($t_{(29)} = 3.36, p = 0.002$) tended to choose the familiar stimulus, whilst RE males chose at random. (d) Choice between a familiar ball with a horizontal bar and a ball with an oblique bar. Males: LE birds chose the transformed ball ($t_{(39)} = 3.00, p < 0.01$), RE birds chose at random. Females: BIN, LE and RE birds all chose the familiar ball ($t_{(31)} = 4.23, p < 0.001$).

it is viewed, suggests that RES may record invariant features accurately and respond to their transformation.

Topographical cues

Chicks were trained to find food buried under sawdust at a particular spot within a large tray; the spot could be located by cues within the tray as well as by using topographical features of the environment (Rashid and Andrew 1989). At test, no food was present and the tray was rotated through 180°, so that the use of near and far cues could be distinguished. RE males searched assiduously but almost at random in such a test, whereas LE males concentrated search in the two areas indicated by near and by far cues. Females showed much the same differences between RE and LE groups as did males (Rashid 1988); in both sexes these differences were present for at least the first two weeks of life.

It is thus likely that LES interest in spatial relations of individual objects extends to interest in, and knowledge of the layout of the environment.

Pebble floor test

In this test (Chapters 1 and 20), chicks are presented with familiar food grains scattered amongst pebbles (encountered in the test for the first time), which roughly matched the food in size and hue. Food and pebbles are usually at first pecked in roughly equal proportions, but with experience, as the test proceeds, pecks at pebbles become rarer and rarer. The decline in pecks at pebbles is much faster on day 3 of life in RE birds of both sexes than in the counterpart LE groups (Mench and Andrew 1986). This decline clearly requires the chick to learn to discriminate between pebbles and food (Chapter 1), but some caution is needed in interpreting the differences between LE and RE chicks. Many pecks at pebbles are likely to reflect interest in them as novel objects; others are no doubt mistaken attempts to seize a food grain. The interest of LE birds in smaller changes in the properties of beads than those which interest RE birds, suggests that exploratory pecks at pebbles are likely to be commoner in LE birds; this may explain much of the difference between RE and LE in rates of decline of pebble pecks.

It will also be remembered that LE males chose much more clearly between the imprinting object and transformations of it; evidently the differences between RES and LES cannot readily be explained as due to a lesser ability of either to carry out 'visual discrimination'.

HEMISPHERIC SPECIALIZATION: GENERAL ISSUES

Much of what has just been described is reminiscent of features of human lateralization. I turn at this point to a brief comparison of human and chick data, in order to show that the chick may be a good model system in which to study basic properties of lateralization, which are probably common to both birds and mammals.

Human lateralization has been reviewed many times (e.g. Bradshaw and Nettleton 1983) and many attempts have been made to summarize its basic features (e.g. Witelson 1985). Here I will treat these features as falling under three main headings, and argue that all three are paralleled sufficiently closely in the chick as to suggest that they are likely to be widely present in higher vertebrates.

Motor behaviour

Special involvement of the human left hemisphere in motor command is associated with asymmetry of function in the nigrostriatal system (Tucker and Williamson 1984). In humans, the links between handedness and cognitive lateralization are clearly close and presumably explain the overwhelming preponderance of right-handedness (Porac and Coren 1981). The separate nature of the lateralization of motor control is much clearer in rats, where nigrostriatal asymmetry varies in direction between individuals largely independently of (for example) functional asymmetries in frontal cortex (Ross and Glick 1981).

Involvement of the left hemisphere in motor control in pigeons is suggested by the fact that section of the left forebrain bundle (the main outflow from the forebrain) markedly reduces rates of key pecking without affecting discrimination; right section has no effect (Güntürkün and Hoferichter 1985). Chicks use predominantly the right foot to detach a small sticky object from the bill (Rogers and Workman, unpublished).

Emotional behaviour

Fear, horror and disgust tend to be associated with human right hemisphere function (Flor-Henry 1979; Heller and Levy 1981) and happiness and laughter with left hemisphere function (Ahern and Schwartz 9185). Expression of emotion is more intense on the left side of the face, presumably because of right hemisphere control (Sackeim *et al.* 1978). There appear to be no human data which bear on the possible lateralization of the control of sexual and aggressive behaviour. In rats, ablation of the right neocortex tends to depress mouse killing, whereas ablation of the left neocortex elevates such behaviour (Denenberg 1984). Left hemisphere opposition to, and right hemisphere involvement with certain species-specific behaviour (classed in humans as associated with intense emotion) seems likely.

In the chick, facilitation of copulation and attack during right hemisphere control is suggested by the effects both of unilateral hemisphere insult and of covering one eye (Chapter 20). Association of LE viewing with intense distress calling has been reported (Andrew *et al.* 1982), but requires investigation over a wider range of ages.

Cognitive processes and attention

In normal right-handed humans, the right hemisphere has the advantage in the analysis of spatial relations and topography (De Renzi 1982), and in the recognition of complex and relatively unfamiliar stimuli (Bradshaw and Nettleton 1983). More generally, the right hemisphere is better at tasks involving the analysis of complex information which cannot readily be fitted into an existing 'descriptive system' (Goldberg and Costa 1981). Attention is global rather than focussed when the right hemisphere is in charge; memory is likely to be of an organized scene rather than of the presence of particular single items (Zaidel 1987).

In the chick the LES (right hemisphere) is especially concerned with spatial relations, including relation to distant topographical features. Its interest in a wide range of properties of a stimulus also suggests global attention.

The properties of the human left hemisphere are dominated by its verbal abilities. However, it is generally accepted that naming can be largely excluded in studies involving 'nonsense' complex visual stimuli. As such stimuli become more familiar, left hemisphere advantage in their recognition becomes more likely, presumably because effective routines have been elaborated for this purpose (Goldberg and Costa 1981). The left hemisphere tends to group visual stimuli by the functions which they might serve, rather than their general appearance (Warrington 1982). There is also special involvement of the left hemisphere in the emission of appropriate practised response to each in turn of a series of stimuli (Witelson 1985).

In the chick it appears that the RES (left hemisphere) is concerned to select cues which allow stimuli to be assigned to categories, despite variation between stimuli in a variety of other properties.

The resemblances between human and chick hemispheric specialization are thus extensive. The simple behavioural repertoire of the chick makes it easier to see what the basic function of such specialization might be. Any higher vertebrate must carry out two different types of analysis simultaneously when assessing a new stimulus. It must use detailed records of previous comparable experiences to decide the novelty of the stimulus, and it must elaborate a detailed record of the stimulus for future use. In the chick the LES is likely to be chiefly responsible for such analysis.

At the same time the chick must use appropriate cues, based on past experience, to try to assign the stimulus to a category, and so to decide what response (if any) should be given. This must be done despite variation in many other properties, including position; it should take into account possible after-effects of response. The RES has been argued here to be chiefly responsible for such analysis.

R. J. Andrew

HEMISPHERIC INTERACTION

A number of issues raised by studies of memory formation and the development of learning abilities in the chick will require a proper understanding of hemispheric interaction for their resolution. I review briefly here what is at present known of such interaction.

A wide variety of patterns of interaction between the human cerebral hemispheres has been postulated. Allen (1983) considers the following: the hemispheres might collaborate, each taking responsibility for different processes or types of analysis; both might process similarly, and in parallel; both might be involved, but with one largely determining response and the other carrying out only subsidiary tasks; one might be entirely responsible for analysis and response, with the other completely suppressed.

There is evidence that several, and perhaps all of these patterns of interaction occur in the chick. Three are fairly well established by current evidence: (1) both VS view the stimulus and analyse it differently; as a result, both affect response; (2) one VS is dominant; its analysis of its own direct visual input determines response; (3) one VS is dominant but receives little or no direct visual input (at least from the stimulus which is the object of attention). Here the dominant VS constrains analysis by its subordinate partner, which must be responsible, however, for at least the first stages of perceptual analysis.

Much of the evidence for the existence of these different patterns of interaction comes from comparison of the behaviour of male and female chicks. Females are more likely in any given situation to show control by one VS alone.

Strategies 1 and 2 both occur in the experiments which measured habituation and dishabituation of pecking at beads. When the curves for binocular and monocular groups are compared in the standard habituation tests with violet beads (Fig. 21.1), there is a clear sex difference: in females, the curves for RE and binocular groups coincide, whereas in males, the curve for the binocular group is substantially higher than that of either of the monocular groups. Appropriate prior experience (e.g. with the non-illuminated bead: data not shown here) leaves scores for all three groups similar (and initially high). It is thus unlikely that the higher scores of binocular males reflect absence of interference with pecking by the eye patch; the same conclusion follows from the absence of binocular elevation in females. Instead, the most likely explanation is that when the violet bead is not preceded by any comparable experience, both RES and LES are involved in analysis, and both simultaneously order response in males (strategy 1). In females, RES largely or entirely dominates response to the violet bead when both eyes are in use (strategy 2).

Strategy 2 is apparently also shown in response to changes in the social companion (above). When males choose between the imprinting object and its transformations, the LES appears to be responsible for behaviour when both eyes are in use. The same is true of females, at least during choice between familiar and strange chicks. This, together with the evidence just cited from bead tests, implies that either ES may take charge according to the nature of the task.

The first evidence for strategy 3 comes from the standard habituation curves for the violet bead (Fig. 21.1). In females, the scores of LE and RE groups coincide at the first presentation of each pair (Fig. 21.1); however, the subsequent marked divergence shows that there are differences in the way in which the two types of female assess the violet bead. The most likely explanation of the masking of such differences at the first presentation is that the same VS controls response at that time, whichever eye is in use.

It is likely that the left VS is the controlling one in this particular case: there are several lines of evidence which indicate that both LE and RE females behave like RE males at the first presentation of the violet bead. This is clear for the course of development of fear response in such tests (Andrew and Brennan 1983): following day 2 (when all groups of chicks show similar low levels), there are marked changes over days, in which RE and LE females exactly parallel RE males. LE males follow a quite different course.

In two different dishabituation procedures, the divergence of the curves for the RE and LE females comes about because LE females begin to behave like LE males, and quite differently from RE birds of either sex. Firstly, when the position of entry of the bead is varied between first and second pairs of presentations, neither LE nor RE females are affected at first presentation, just as is true of RE males (Andrew 1983*b*). However, at the second presentation of the pair, LE (but not RE) females show slight but significant dishabituation due to position change (Andrew, unpublished).

Secondly, following first experience of a red bead, LE females show the same continuing interest at the second experience (which involves the violet bead), as is usual in LE males (cf. R-V for LE females and N-V for LE males in Fig. 21.2).

VIEWING AND HEMISPHERIC INTERACTION

Measurements of head position whilst chicks view valent stimuli (such as a hen), for the first time, have recently provided direct evidence for strategy 3 in birds able to use both eyes quite freely (Dharmaretnam and Andrew, unpublished). In order to present this evidence it is, necessary briefly to consider developmental changes in hemisphere dominance in the chick. There is a substantial body of evidence which indicates special states of activity in the left hemisphere on day 8 and in the right hemisphere on days 10 and 11. There is also marked and unusual bias towards control of response by the left VS on day 8 and the right VS on days 10 and 11. The whole topic is reviewed in Chapters 6 and 20.

Stimuli of interest to a chick, which are presented at a little distance, are predominantly viewed with the lateral visual field of one or other eye. It was expected that there would be predominant use of the RE on day 8 and of the LE on days 10 and 11, and this was what was found for chicks viewing a human being (Workman and Andrew 1989). It is also true of both male and female chicks when looking at a hen (Dharmaretnam, personal communication; Chapter 6): the RE is used almost exclusively on day 8 and the LE on day 11 (which appears to be the peak point of bias to the LES). However, unexpectedly, females show a precisely reversed pattern of change with age when presented with a simple novel stimulus (a small flashing light).

The evidence of control of response by a non-seeing VS in monocular tests (above) suggests that in 'reversed viewing' the normally dominant VS continues to control both which eye is used in viewing (here that ipsilateral to the dominant VS), and the sort of analysis which is carried out. The initial stages of perceptual analysis presumably remain the responsibility of the subordinate viewing VS: since the lateral visual field is used there is unlikely to be any involvement of ipsilateral visual projections. Reversed viewing is thus the most clear-cut example of strategy 3. It would seem to require transfer of information (at perhaps a relatively high level of analysis) which is fast and effective, despite the fact that lateral visual fields are in use.

At least two functions seem possible for reversed viewing. Firstly, the subordinate VS may be left to keep an eye (literally) on the novel stimulus, whilst the dominant VS explores its environs for other change. A second possibility is that the subordinate VS is constrained to view the stimulus, so that the dominant VS can discover what its partner knows about a stimulus, which it has itself judged to be quite novel.

Stabilization of attention and hemispheric interaction

In chicks testosterone opposes shifts of attention (Chapter 18). The effect appears to depend on the stabilization of information held in temporary storage for use in the selection and assessment of stimuli (Chapter 19). Sex differences in the way in which this effect is expressed in behaviour provide further evidence of a greater tendency in females for one VS to take control of the action of both itself and its partner.

Such sex differences were first discovered (Andrew 1972) in a food search test, in which two familiar types of food (which differed strikingly in colour) were scattered over a test floor. Each chick began search with a run of choice of one of the two types. Untreated males commonly shifted after varying periods to equally consistent selection of the other type. Stabilization of attention postponed and prevented this shift. A second effect was that search within particular clumps of food was made more persistent, often continuing until local exhaustion of preferred food resulted in a peck at a grain of the second type; consistent selection of the original type then resumed in a new clump (Andrew and Rogers 1972).

Positions where food has been found are remembered by testosterone-treated males, which return to such positions during search, unlike controls (Rogers and Andrew 1989). These two different effects of testosterone may well be mediated by separate stabilization of attention associated with each of the two VS. This might be expected to result in the case of the right VS (LES) in more persistent use of cues of position, and in the case of the left VS (RES) in more persistent choice of a particular category of food.

Females (Andrew 1972), in contrast, consistently chose only one type of food throughout the test; this held over a wide range of doses of testosterone, as well as for controls. They showed no hint of any increased persistence of search in particular areas, even though females do show increased stabilization of attention due to testosterone under appropriate circumstances (below). The absence of any effect here is consistent with the evidence already discussed for relatively complete control of food search in females by the left VS: as a result search would be sustained on a particular type of food with or without testosterone; position would be less important.

The most revealing results are those from tests in which chicks, which have been trained to traverse a runway to reach a food dish, are presented with change either in the object of attention (the dish) or features irrelevant to the task (runway walls). In both sexes, testosterone enhances response to change in the object of attention (Klein and Andrew 1986; Andrew and Klein, unpublished). The food dish itself is only an intermediate target; prolongation of examination of change in its appearance, rather than shifting attention at once to the food within it, is likely to result from stabilization in use of the information which specifies the dish as target of attention.

In contrast, response to change in features irrelevant to the task is affected by testosterone in males but not in females. In males, stabilization of attention by testosterone has two effects. Firstly, the chick is better able to resume progress to the dish after brief examination of the stimulus; secondly, after a second or third such trial, the novel stimulus becomes established as a second point of attention, without loss of the first, so that the chick alternates between food dish and novel stimulus (Klein and

Andrew 1986). Controls are more distracted by the novel stimulus. They may come to ignore it, but not to alternate its examination with that of the food dish. Again, the changes produced by testosterone would be well explained by stabilization of attention in both VS; the right VS (LES) is the more likely to be interested in novelty and the left VS (RES) may well be more concerned with carrying out a practised task, such as traversing the runway to the food dish. Females show little distraction by the novel stimulus, and no effect of testosterone on such distraction as occurs (Andrew and Klein, unpublished). Here too, female behaviour would be explained by predominance of left VS control, so that there is little decrease in distractibility left for testosterone to produce.

Clinching evidence that both sexes show stabilization of attention by testosterone when faced with changes in the point of attention is provided by competition tests (see Chapters 18 and 19 for description). Both sexes show hormonally enhanced competition when a second experience with a red bead provides information which is discrepant with an immediately previous first experience (Andrew 1983a).

GENERAL DISCUSSION

A proper account of the ways in which hemisphere specialization and interaction may affect learning and memory formation is a matter for the future. However, a number of points are already clear.

Masking

In female chicks monocular tests do not necessarily reveal the special properties of the VS which is contralateral to the uncovered eye. Fortunately, strategy 3 (control of responses by the ipsilateral VS) has so far proved to be used very little by males (except under special conditions not discussed here). However, monocular tests clearly require cautious interpretation in female chicks. Masking may well explain the evanescence of some right-left differences in females (Chapter 20): when learning is measured in pebble floor tests, RE and LE birds differ on day 3 in the same way whether they are male or female (Mench and Andrew 1986). These differences disappear in females, but not males, by days 14–16 (Zappia and Rogers 1987). It is unlikely that this is caused by a difference between the sexes in the general timecourse of development of lateralization, since this appears to be identical in the two sexes up to at least day 12 (Chapter 6).

The findings in the older females would be well explained by masking due to control by the left VS in LE, as well as RE birds. This may occur in older, but not young females because of a general decrease in interest in objects like pebbles with increasing age, due to the cumulative effects of selecting and eating food grains, and of pecking without success at a variety of other inedible features of the environment. Any reduction in interest in pebbles is likely to reduce involvement of the right VS in the test.

More complete control by the dominant hemisphere in females may also explain the absence of the sensitivity to unilateral intrahemispheric injection of cycloheximide, which is so marked in males on days 8, 10 and 11 (Chapter 20). In males, such sensitivity appears to be present only if the injected dominant hemisphere (which may be right or left according to age) is able to interact with an uninjected, and so presumably relatively normal partner. In females, injection of the dominant hemisphere may disturb the other, because of close control by the dominant hemisphere, to a point at which this condition is not satisfied.

Hemispheric interaction and memory formation

The evidence reviewed here suggests that hemispheric interaction is important at the time of an experience, and that it probably takes two forms. One is control by one hemisphere of the way in which the other processes information, and even what stimulus it examines. It is likely that transfer of information between hemispheres also occurs: it is difficult, for example, to see how reversed viewing could function without some transfer. At the same time, under appropriate conditions, the two hemispheres can function relatively independently, whilst assessing the same stimulus.

If, as is argued in Chapter 19, the processes which are initiated at retrieval events are to some extent similar to those which occur at the time of learning, then the hemispheric interactions which have just been discussed may give some hints as to the range of types of interaction which might occur at events during memory formation.

On the same hypothesis, hormonal effects on attention may have their counterpart during memory formation. It is therefore worth noting the evidence (above) which suggests that hormonal stabilization may affect attention independently in the two hemispheres, when they are functioning relatively separately.

Hemispheric specialization and memory formation

It has already been argued (Chapter 19) that hemispheric specialization is likely to bring about the initial elaboration of rather different accounts of an experience in the two hemispheres. This in turn provides a reason why opportunities for further processing may be needed during memory formation, when the two accounts can be reconciled and interrelated. It was argued that such reconciliation was associated in particular with the first point (LR1), at which retrieval events occur simultaneously in left and right hemisphere.

The evidence presented here and in Chapter 19 suggests that, initially, the right hemisphere is likely to hold a relatively detailed and complete account of the experience, including the spatial context in which the stimulus appeared. The corresponding account in the left hemisphere is likely to stress conspicuous or valent cues, and to relate them to consequences of response to the stimulus. This last would require more protracted processing immediately following the experience, which would have to take into account sequences of events in time.

All of this argument applies to memory formation following learning in which both hemispheres to some extent function independently. It remains to be seen what may happen when both eyes are in use, but one VS strongly constrains analysis by its partner. This might be expected to be likely in females (which have been very little used in the standard aversive bead task). Two outcomes of learning under such conditions seem possible. The subordinate system might learn little or nothing, or it might record the product of analysis by the dominant system. In either case, it seems almost certain that memory formation would take a somewhat different course from that so far studied.

Equally interesting for future research are possible differences in the overall content of what is finally learned, under these two strategies of hemispheric functioning.

Learning-related asymmetries

An impressive range of asymmetries in the distribution of learning-induced change and in the effects of unilateral injection of amnestic drugs or of unilateral lesions are described in Chapters 8–11. It seems likely that such asymmetries relate in some way to the hemispheric specialization, and patterns of hemispheric interaction which have been described in this chapter. Two effects are worth considering now; others will no doubt be discovered in the future.

Firstly, if the task is such as to be largely the responsibility of one hemisphere, learning-induced change and sensitivity may be confined in part or entirely to one hemisphere.

Secondly, when both hemispheres are involved in learning, the differences between them in predominant type of analysis may result in different structures being active in each during learning and memory formation. If true, this would suggest (for example) that the IMHV, which normally shows learning-induced change chiefly in the left hemisphere, might be particularly important in processing which involved the selection of particular cues, and their association with subsequent reinforcement and other consequences of responses to the stimulus.

Acknowledgements

The studies on which this chapter has been based owe much to collaboration with Anthony Brennan, Meena Dharmaretnam, David Feld, Ray McKenzie, Joy Mench, Norma Rashid, Lesley Rogers, and Lance Workman. Support was provided by the SERC and AFRC of the UK.

REFERENCES

Ahern, G. L. and Schwartz, G. E. (1985). Differential lateralization for positive and negative emotion in the human brain: EEG spectral analysis. *Neuropsychologia*, **23**, 745–55.

Allen, M. (1983). Models of hemispheric specialization. *Psychological Bulletin*, **93**, 73–104.

Andrew, R. J. (1972). Changes in search behaviour in male and female chicks, following different doses of testosterone. *Animal Behaviour*, **20**, 741–50.

Andrew, R. J. (1983a). Specific short-latency effects of oestradiol and testosterone on distractibility and memory formation in the young domestic chick. In *Hormones and behaviour in higher vertebrates* (ed. J. Balthazart, E. Pröve, and R. Gilles), pp. 463–73. Springer-Verlag, Berlin.

Andrew, R. J. (1983b). Lateralization of emotional and cognitive function in higher vertebrates, with special reference to the domestic chick. In *Advances in vertebrate neuroethology* (ed. J. P. Ewert, R. R. Capranica, and D. J. Ingle), pp. 477–510. Plenum, New York.

Andrew, R. J. (1988). The development of visual lateralization in the domestic chick. *Behavioural Brain Research*, **29**, 201–9.

Andrew, R. J. and Brennan. A. (1983). The lateralization of fear behaviour in the male domestic chick: a developmental study. *Animal Behaviour*, **31**, 1166–76.

Andrew, R. J. and Brennan, A. (1985). Sharply timed and lateralized events at time of establishment of long-term memory. *Physiology and Behaviour*, **34**, 547–56.

Andrew, R. J. and Rogers, L. J. (1972). Testosterone, search behaviour and persistence. *Nature*, **237**, 343–6.

Andrew, R. J. Mench J., and Rainey, C. J. (1982). Right-left asymmetry of response to visual stimuli in the domestic chick. In *Analysis of visual behavior* (ed. D. J. Ingle, M. A. Goodale, and R. J. W. Mansfield), pp. 197–209. MIT Press, Cambridge, Mass.

Bell, G. A. and Gibbs, M. E. (1977). Unilateral storage of monocular engrams in day-old chicks. *Brain Research*, **124**, 263–70.

Bradshaw, J. L. and Nettleton, N. C. (1983). *Human cerebral asymmetry*. Prentice-Hall, New York.

Denenberg, V. H. (1984). Effects of right hemisphere lesions in rats. In *The right hemisphere: neurology and neuropsychology* (ed. A. Ardila and F. Ostrosky-Solis), pp. 241–62. Gordon and Breach, New York.

De Renzi, E. (1982). Disorders of space, exploration and cognition. John Wiley, New York.

Flor-Henry, P. (1979). Laterality, shifts of cerebral dominance, sinistrality and psychosis. In *Hemisphere asymmetries of function in psychopathology* (ed.) P. Flor-Henry, pp. 3–19. Elsevier, Amsterdam.

Goldberg, E. and Costa, L. D. (1981). Hemisphere differences in the acquisition and use of descriptive systems. *Brain and Language*, **14**, 144–73.

Güntürkün, O. and Hoferichter, H-H. (1985). Neglect after section of a left telencephalotectal tract in pigeons. *Behavioural Brain Research*, **18**, 1–9.

Heller, W. and Levy, J. (1981). Perception and expression of emotion in right-handers and left-handers. *Neuropsychologia*, **19**, 263–72.

Klein, R. M. and Andrew, R. J. (1986). Distraction, decision and persistence in runway tests using the domestic chick. *Behaviour*, **99**, 139–56.

Mench, J. A. and Andrew, R. J. (1986). Lateralization of a food search task in the domestic chick. *Behavioral and Neural Biology*, **46**, 107–14.

Porac, C. and Coren, S. (1981). *Lateral preferences and human behavior*. Springer-Verlag, Heidelberg.

Rashid, N. Y. (1988). Lateralization of topographical learning and other abilities in the chick. D. Phil Thesis, University of Sussex, Brighton, UK.

Rashid, N.Y. and Andrew, R. J. (1989). Right hemisphere advantage for topographical orientation in the domestic chick. *Neuropsychologia*, **7**, 937–48.

Rogers, L. J. and Andrew, R. J. (1989). Frontal and lateral visual field use by chicks after treatment with testosterone. *Animal Behaviour*, **38**, 394–405.

Ross, D. A. and Glick, S. D. (1981). Lateralized effects of bilateral frontal cortex lesions in rats. *Brain Research*, **210**, 379–87.

Sackeim, H. A., Gur, R. C., and Saucy, M. C. (1978). Emotions are expressed more intensely on the left side of the face. *Science*, **202**, 434–6.

Thompson, W. R. and Wright, J. S. (1979). 'Persistence' in rats: effects of testosterone. *Physiological Psychology*, **7**, 291–4.

Tucker, D. M. and Williamson, P. A. (1984). Asymmetric neural control systems in human self-regulation. *Psychological Review*, **91**, 185–215.

Vallortigaro, G. and Andrew, R. J. (1990). Lateralization of response by chicks to change in a model partner. *Animal Behaviour*. (In press.)

Warrington, E. K. (1982). Neuropsychological studies of object recognition. *Philosophical Transactions of the Royal Society of London B*, **298**, 15–53.

Witelson, S. F. (1985). On hemispheric specialization and cerebral plasticity from birth. In *Hemispheric function and collaboration in the child* (ed. C. T. Best), pp. 33–85.

Workman, L. and Andrew, R. J. (1987). Asymmetries of eye use in birds. *Animal Behaviour*, **34**, 1582–4.

Zaidel, D. W. (1987). Hemispheric asymmetry in memory for pictorial semantics in normal subjects. *Neuropsychologia*, **25**, 487–95.

Zappia, J. V. and Rogers. L. J. (1987). Sex differences and reversal of brain asymmetry by testosterone in chickens. *Behavioural Brain Research*, **23**, 261–7.

Author Index

Subject Index

acetylcholine, *see* cholinergic systems
accumbens, nu. 67, 68, 321
ACTH 86, 350, 440–1
actin 189
active avoidance 370–2
activity cycles 144–5, 162, 496
adenosine 373–5
adenylate cyclase 435
adrenergic antagonists, *see* alpha-adrenergic
    antagonist; *also see* beta-adrenergic
    antagonists
ageing 472
aggression 18
Aix sponsa 149
alpha-adrenergic antagonists 420–1
alpha-amino-isobutyrate 358, 384, 397
5-alpha-dihydrotestosterone 464–5, 467–8
amino-acids, non-essential 354, 358
amnesia, delayed 347, 350, 423–5, 430,
    450–3, 477–8, 489, 492
amnesia, temporary (DPHTA) 347, 350,
    423–5, 430, 450–3, 477–8, 489, 492
amnesic syndrome 217, 248
amnestic agents, *see* alpha-amino-
    isobutyrate; amino-acids, non-essential;
    anisomycin; anti-thy-1-antibodies;
    ascites; benzodiazepines; beta-
    adrenergic antagonists; 2-deoxy-
    galactose; 2,6-diaminopurine;
    diethyldithiocarbamate; dinitrophenol;
    electro shock; emetine; ethacrynic acid;
    fucose; glutamate; halothane; 5-HT
    antagonists; hypoxia; information
    transfer; lanthanum chloride; lithium
    chloride; mellitin; phase of circadian
    rhythm; potassium chloride;
    propanolol; puromycin; saline,
    intracerebral; scopolamine; sotalol;
    timolol; trifluoperazine
amphetamine 358, 471
amygdala 63, 67–8, 78, 80, 246
anaesthesia 6, 296, 372
anisomycin 292, 333, 354, 361, 370, 384,
    396–8, 401–2, 411, 429, 472, 477, 480
ANOVAs, interpretation of interactions
    126
ansa lenticularis 72
anseriform birds, *see* duck
anti-thy-1 antibodies 354, 357
aphasia 270

Aplysia 193, 279–80, 288, 323
arachidonic acid 288
archistriatum 67, 72–3, 77–81, 83
archistriatum pars caudalis 67, 78
    pars intermedialis 62, 78, 245
    medial 67, 78
    posterior 245–6
    nu. robustus 323
    rostral 78
    ventrale 308
arginine vasopressin, *see* vasopressin,
    arginine
ascites 354
aspartate 513
association learning, *see* learning,
    association
asymmetry, cerebral, *see* visual system,
    asymmetries of thalamofugal
asymmetry, fetal position 525–6
asymmetry, functional, *see* lateralization;
    see also learning-induced change,
    asymmetry in
atenolol 420–1
atlas of chicken brain 7, 48, 66
ATP 358, 390–1
attack 468, 515–7, 526–30, 544
attention and search 491, 549
attention, stabilization of 11, 36, 350, 467,
    472, 491, 495, 549–51
auditory system 78–9, 81, 83, 97, 238
autoshaping 10
autoradiography 42–3
aversion 17
aversion, conditioned 10, 291, 467, 479
aversive bead task, *see* passive avoidance
    task
avoidance, memory of 487–8

B-50 284
basal ganglia 62–3, 67–9, 71, 321; *also see*
    parolfactorius, lobus *and*
    palaeostriatum augmentatum
basalis, nu. 62, 67, 72, 78–81
benzodiazepines 36
beta-adrenergic antagonists 349, 362,
    420–32; *also see* nadolol; propanol;
    sotalol; timolol
beta-adrenergic systems 419–36